MRCP Part 2

450 BOFs

This book is due for return on or before the last date shown below

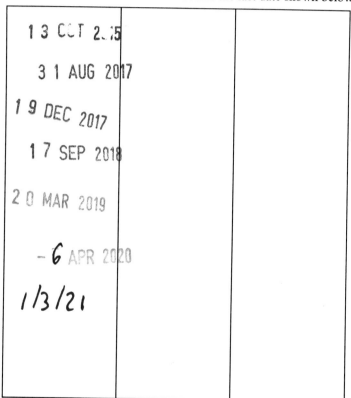

1 3 OCT 2015		
3 1 AUG 2017		
1 9 DEC 2017		
1 7 SEP 2018		
2 0 MAR 2019		
– 6 APR 2020		
1/3/21		

SWNHS

C204678

D0230810

MRCP Part 2

450 BOFs

Carolyn Allen MBChB MRCP
Consultant Physician, Rotorua Hospital, Rotorua, New Zealand

Suzanne Forbes BSc MBChB MRCP
Specialist Registrar in Nephrology, Royal London Hospital, UK

David Hunt MBBS BSc PhD MRCP
Clinical Teaching Fellow, Newham University Hospital, UK

Heather Lewis MBChB MRCP
Specialist Registrar in Gastroenterology, Newham University Hospital, UK

Ravi Menon MBBS MRCP MD
Honorary Clinical Lecturer, Newham University Hospital, UK

Luke Moore MBChB MRCP(Lond.) FRCPath MSc MPH DTM&H
Lecturer, Division of Infectious Diseases & Immunology,
Imperial College, London, UK

Edited by
Aruna Dias BSc MBBS MRCP
Consultant Gastroenterologist,
Newham University Hospital, UK

Eric Beck MBBS FRCP FRCPG FRCPE
Former Chairman of MRCP(UK) Part 2 Board
and former Member of the MRCP (UK) Part 1 Board
University College London, UK

JP
medical
publishers

London • Philadelphia • Panama City • New Delhi

© 2013 JP Medical Ltd.
Published by JP Medical Ltd
83 Victoria Street, London SW1H 0HW, UK
Tel: +44 (0)20 3170 8910   Fax: +44 (0)20 3008 6180
Email: info@jpmedpub.com   Web: www.jpmedpub.com

The rights of Carolyn Allen, Suzanne Forbes, David Hunt, Heather Lewis, Ravi Menon, Luke Moore, Aruna Dias and Eric Beck to be identified as authors of this work have been asserted by them in accordance with the Copyright, Designs and Patents Act 1988.

All brand names and product names used in this book are trade names, service marks, trademarks or registered trademarks of their respective owners. The publisher is not associated with any product or vendor mentioned in this book.

Medical knowledge and practice change constantly. This book is designed to provide accurate, authoritative information about the subject matter in question. However, readers are advised to check the most current information available on procedures included and check information from the manufacturer of each product to be administered, to verify the recommended dose, formula, method and duration of administration, adverse effects and contraindications. It is the responsibility of the practitioner to take all appropriate safety precautions. Neither the publisher nor the authors assume any liability for any injury and/or damage to persons or property arising from or related to use of material in this book.

This book is sold on the understanding that the publisher is not engaged in providing professional medical services. If such advice or services are required, the services of a competent medical professional should be sought.

Every effort has been made where necessary to contact holders of copyright to obtain permission to reproduce copyright material. If any have been inadvertently overlooked, the publisher will be pleased to make the necessary arrangements at the first opportunity.

ISBN: 978-1-907816-45-1

British Library Cataloguing in Publication Data
A catalogue record for this book is available from the British Library

Library of Congress Cataloging in Publication Data
A catalog record for this book is available from the Library of Congress

JP Medical Ltd is a subsidiary of Jaypee Brothers Medical Publishers (P) Ltd, New Delhi, India

Publisher: Richard Furn
Development Editor: Thomas Fletcher
Design: Designers Collective Ltd

Indexed, copy-edited, typeset, printed and bound in India.

Preface

'Assessment drives learning' is a crucial mantra; it emphasises the broad educational value of the best of five (BOF) MCQs in this book. Its value is further enhanced by the inclusion of explanatory answers, making this a valuable source of continuing medical education and continuing professional development. However, the prime readership will, of course, be candidates preparing for the written Part 2 MRCP examination.

In this book you will find authentic questions, comprehensively covering the curriculum, devised by 'battle-hardened', recently successful examinees who are now teachers. The chapters reflect the specialties covered by the MRCP Part 2 exam. The number of questions per specialty is directly proportional to the weight each specialty area will carry in the exam. Each chapter covers a broad range of topics within the specialty, and questions range in difficulty between relatively easy and very difficult, as in the exam itself. For each answer, there is a section explaining why that answer is the most appropriate and also why the other options are not correct.

The emphasis of the Part 2 examination is in testing the application of basic medical science knowledge to more clinical situations. By passing the Part 1 examination, you have already demonstrated your command of this knowledge. This book gives you an opportunity to practise applying it. Apart from practice, there are no special techniques or tricks to be learned to pass the exam because the examiners take considerable care to use plain English and avoid including ambiguities or clues when setting questions. Nevertheless, always remember the general exhortation for all written examinations: 'read the question carefully before answering!'

The final ingredient required for success is what we all wish you – 'Good Luck'.

Eric Beck
January 2013

Contents

Contents

Exam revision advice

Format

The MRCP(UK) exam consists of three elements. Part 1 is a written exam, whereas Part 2 is split into a written exam and a clinical exam (PACES). Part 2 can be attempted only by candidates who have passed Part 1 within the previous 7 years. The Part 2 written exam and PACES can be attempted in either order.

The MRCP(UK) Part 2 written exam has a three-paper format. Each paper lasts 3 hours and consists of 90 multiple choice questions. The examination lasts 2 days, with two of the papers taken on the first day and the remaining paper on the second day. As in the Part 1 exam, questions take a best of five (BOF) approach, where the most appropriate answer must be selected from a choice of five possibilities, with questions covering the full range of medical specialties. However, one major difference between the two exams is that a proportion of Part 2 questions will be illustrated with a medical image (e.g. ECG, radiograph, CT, MRI, blood film, photograph of a clinical finding), interpretation of which is key to correctly answering the question. The composition of the papers is demonstrated in **Table 1**.

There is no specific syllabus for the MRCP(UK) Part 2 examination, but the Royal Colleges recommend that candidates refer to the Specialty Training Curriculum for General Internal Medicine, prepared by the Joint Royal Colleges of Physicians Training Board.

Table 1 Composition of the MRCP Part 2 exam	
Specialty	**Number of questions per 100***
Cardiology	10
Dermatology	5
Endocrinology and metabolic medicine	10
Gastroenterology	10
Haematology, immunology	5
Infectious diseases and genitourinary medicine	10
Neurology, ophthalmology, psychiatry	10
Oncology and palliative medicine	5
Renal medicine	10
Respiratory medicine	10
Rheumatology	5
Therapeutics and toxicology	10
Total	**100**

*Figures should be taken as an indication of the likely number of questions – the actual number may vary by up to 2%. A proportion of the questions will be on adolescent medicine and medicine for elderly people.

The MRCP(UK) Part 2 exam is now marked using a process called equating. Using the equating system means that rather than being given a percentage overall score, candidates will instead be given an 'overall scaled score'. This score is a number between 0 and 999, which is calculated from the number of questions a candidate has answered correctly (out of the maximum possible) and takes into account the relative difficulty of the exam. Since no two exams contain the same questions, it is inevitable that some papers may be slightly harder (or easier) than others, and equating is a statistical process that addresses this. At present, the equated score required to pass MRCP(UK) Part 2 is 425.

Candidates are strongly advised to visit the MRCP(UK) website for further details of the exam.

How to prepare for MRCP (UK) Part 2

Here are some general tips to help prepare for the exam:
- Start early – it is advisable to start revision at least 3 months before the exam date.
- Approach revision specialty by specialty.
- Cover all topics, particularly focusing on the topics from which a greater number of questions will be drawn.
- Remember to think laterally when revising – for example, a question on vasculitis could appear in the renal, rheumatology, respiratory, neurology or dermatology sections.
- Tackle the questions as you would in the exam, by reading the rubric carefully and thinking of what the correct answer might be before reading the A–E options. Next, select which of the options best fits the answer that you were thinking of.
- There are no 'trick' questions, but there are definitely questions that are not as straightforward as they may initially appear. Read the question *very carefully*. In this book only the *minimum* relevant information necessary to get the correct answer is provided. In the actual exam the questions may be longer but the information given may not necessarily be useful.
- Use the information in the answer to confirm and expand upon what you already know, or to help understand and remember why a certain answer is more appropriate than others.
- As a large part of the exam is on the practical application of knowledge, you will be expected to know the current guidelines of the various medical societies, which can be found on their websites. Review these before the exam.

Medical Society websites

Association of British Neurologists – http://www.theabn.org
British Association of Dermatologists – http://www.bad.org.uk
British Cardiovascular Society – http://www.bcs.com
British Infection Association – http://www.britishinfection.org
British Society of Gastroenterology – http://www.bsg.org.uk
British Society for Haematology – http://www.b-s-h.org.uk
British Society for Rheumatology – http://www.rheumatology.org.uk
British Thoracic Society – http://www.brit-thoracic.org.uk

European Federation of Neurological Societies – http://www.efns.org

National Institute for Health and Clinical Excellence (NICE) – http://www.nice.org.uk

Renal Association – http://www.renal.org

Society for Endocrinology – http://www.endocrinology.org

Acknowledgements

We are deeply indebted to the many people who provided helpful suggestions through all stages of preparing this book. We would especially like to thank the following individuals:

Dr Peter Byrne, Consultant Psychiatrist, Dr Iyas Assalman, Specialist Registrar in Psychiatry, Newham University Hospital and Dr Jelena Jankovic, Consultant Psychiatrist, at Dudley and Walsall Mental Health Partnership NHS Trust for reviewing the psychiatry questions.

Dr Chulanie De Silva, Consultant Rheumatologist at Norfolk and Norwich University Hospital, for reviewing the rheumatology questions.

Dr Olivia Kreze, Consultant Haematologist, and Kathir Mahadevan, Section Leader of the Haematology Laboratory at Newham University Hospital, for supplying the blood films and reviewing the haematology questions.

Dr Mark Blunden, Consultant Nephrologist, and Michael Sheaff, Professor of Pathology, at the Royal London Hospital for providing the renal biopsy images and reviewing the renal questions.

Dr Catherine Harwood, Consultant Dermatologist at the Royal London Hospital, and Dr Ferina Ismail, Consultant Dermatologist at the Royal Free Hospital, for providing the dermatology images and reviewing the dermatology questions.

Dr Sean O'Sullivan, Consultant Neurologist at Cork University Hospital, Ireland, and Dr Benjamin Turner, Consultant Neurologist at the Royal London Hospital, for reviewing the neurology questions.

Dr Shamira Perera, Consultant Ophthalmologist at the Singapore National Eye Centre, Singapore, Dr Sam Khandhadia, Clinical Research Fellow at University Hospitals Southampton, and Anila Nair at the Newham Diabetic Retinal Screening Service for providing the ophthalmology images and reviewing the ophthalmology questions.

Dr Francesca Ng, Speciality Registrar in Radiology at Northwick Park Hospital, Dr Hussein Kamel, Consultant Radiologist at Newham University Hospital, Enhui Yong at Barts and the London Medical School, and Dr Ava Jackson and Dr Hafiz Syed, Consultant Stroke Physicians at Newham University Hospital, for providing the radiological imaging.

We are very grateful to Dr Aruna Dias, Consultant Gastroenterologist and Physician, Newham University Hospital, for his constant help and tireless support throughout all stages of writing and editing this book. We would also like to thank Dr Eric Beck for giving his time to provide helpful editorial input. We are very appreciative of the dedication and commitment that Hannah Applin, Richard Furn and Thomas Fletcher from JP Medical have shown to us at all times.

CA, SF, DH, HL, RM, LM

Dedication

To our families.

Plate 1

Figure 2.1

Figure 2.2

Figure 2.3

Figure 2.5

Figure 2.4

Plate 2

Figure 2.6

Figure 2.7

Figure 2.8

Figure 2.9

Figure 2.10

Figure 2.11

Plate 3

Figure 4.1

Figure 4.2

Figure 4.4

Figure 4.7

Figure 5.1

Figure 5.3

Plate 4

Figure 5.4

Figure 5.5

Figure 5.6

Figure 5.7

Figure 5.8

Figure 5.9

Plate 5

Figure 6.3

Figure 7.2

Figure 7.4

Figure 7.6

Figure 7.8

Figure 7.10

Plate 6

Figure 7.12

Figure 7.13

Figure 7.15

Figure 7.17

Figure 7.19

Figure 7.21

Plate 7

Figure 9.1

Figure 9.2

Figure 9.4

Figure 9.6

Figure 9.7

Figure 9.8

Plate 8

Figure 12.1

Chapter 1

Cardiology

Questions

1. A 28-year-old man presented with a history of acute-onset chest pain lasting 30 minutes. Pain was central and was described as stabbing and of 6/10 severity but had since gone down to a dull ache. He worked as a swimming instructor and had no symptoms prior to this. He had no significant past medical history. His father had had a myocardial infarction aged 52 years and his mother had suffered from angina since the age of 56 years.

   On examination, his body mass index was 29 kg/m², pulse 98 beats per minute, blood pressure 130/90 mmHg and respiratory rate 34 breaths per minute. Heart sounds were normal and rest of the physical examination was non-contributory.

   Investigations:

haemoglobin 12.9 g/dL (13.0–18.0)	creatinine 88 µmol/L (60–110)
white cell count 8 × 10⁹/L (4–11)	albumin 38 g/L (37–49)
neutrophil 6 × 10⁹/L (1.5–7.0)	alanine transaminase 32 U/L (5–35)
sodium 139 mmol/L (135–145)	alkaline phosphatase 67 U/L (45–105)
potassium 4.4 mmol/L (3.5–5.0)	bilirubin 4 mmol/L (1–22)

   Chest X-ray: normal

   Electrocardiogram: (see **Figure 1.1**)

   What is the most appropriate next step in management?

   A   Aspirin, clopidogrel, low-molecular-weight heparin, intravenous morphine, high-flow oxygen and transfer for primary percutaneous coronary intervention
   B   Aspirin, sublingual nitrates, bisoprolol, statin and ramipril, and put on the list for coronary angiogram for the next day
   C   Therapeutic dose of low-molecular-weight heparin and order a CT pulmonary angiogram
   D   No acute treatment needed but monitor vital signs, repeat ECG and wait 12 hours for troponin results
   E   Echocardiogram to look for the presence of pericardial effusion

2. A 59-year-old man was admitted to hospital with acute-onset chest pain which had lasted more than an hour. He was pale, sweaty and clammy.

   On examination, his pulse rate was 100 beats per minute and regular, blood pressure 86/50 mmHg and respiratory rate 24 breaths per minute. Jugular venous pressure was +10 cm. On auscultation, a third heart sound was heard in the left 4th intercostal area close to the sternum. Chest auscultation revealed vesicular breath sounds only.

   The ECG tracing is shown in **Figure 1.2** [the precordial leads (V1–V6) are right sided].

   What is the most appropriate next step in management?

   A   Dopamine infusion
   B   Intravenous glyceryl trinitrate infusion

C   Intravenous 0.9% saline
D   Levosimendan infusion
E   Noradrenaline infusion

Figure 1.1

Figure 1.2

3. A 47-year-old man was admitted with peripheral oedema, cough, hoarseness of voice and shortness of breath. He had a history of hypertension and was on bendrofluazide 2.5 mg once daily. The only other past history of note was a treated sexually transmitted infection 25 years ago.

   On examination, his pulse was 96 beats per minute and regular, blood pressure 160/40 mmHg and respiratory rate 26 breaths per minute. There was a long, high-pitched, decrescendo diastolic murmur in the left 3rd intercostal space, close to the sternum, which was equally well heard in the right 3rd intercostal space.

   Investigations:

   > Chest X-ray:
   > cardiomegaly
   > pulmonary venous congestion

   What is the most appropriate test to confirm the diagnosis?

   A   Antiacetylcholine esterase antibodies
   B   High-resolution CT of the chest followed by biopsy
   C   IgG antibodies against *Borrelia burgdorferi*
   D   Rapid plasma reagin test
   E   Video-assisted thoracoscopic biopsy

4. A 33-year-old man of Turkish origin was seen in the emergency department with a history of fever, malaise and shortness of breath for the last 15 days. He had no significant past history of note. He had travelled to Turkey several times over the last few years. He did not have any pets or any other contact with animals.

   On examination, his temperature was 39.1°C, pulse 110 beats per minute and regular, blood pressure 110/40 mmHg and respiratory rate 22 breaths per minute. Auscultation revealed a systolic murmur at the apex radiating to the left axilla.

   Investigations:

   > haemoglobin 11.2 g/dL (13.0–18.0)   lymphocytes 4 × 10⁹/L (1.5–4.0)
   > white cell count 9 × 10⁹/L (4–11)   sodium 139 mmol/L (135–145)
   > platelets 248 × 10⁹/L (150–400)   potassium 4.5 mmol/L (3.5–5.0)
   > neutrophils 4 × 10⁹/L (1.5–7.0)   creatinine 98 µmol/L (60–110)
   >
   > Urine dipstick: protein 1+, white blood cells 1+, red blood cells 1+
   >
   > Echocardiogram:
   > moderate mitral regurgitation
   > vegetation (2 mm × 2 mm) on the anterior mitral valve leaflet
   > billowing of anterior mitral valve leaflet
   >
   > Blood cultures (three samples): negative after 5 days

   He was started on benzylpenicillin and gentamicin with no clinical improvement. What is the most appropriate next diagnostic test?

   A   Bartonella antibodies
   B   Brucella antibodies
   C   Fungal cultures
   D   Surgical biopsy and culture of the vegetation
   E   Transoesophageal echocardiogram to look for root abscess

5. A 38-year-old man was admitted to hospital with a 3-week history of leg swelling, decreased appetite, increased abdominal girth, tiredness and shortness of breath. He had no significant past medical or family history. He had no recent contact with pets and his only travel history of note was to South Africa, 3 years ago.

On examination, his pulse was 108 beats per minute and regular, blood pressure 110/60 mmHg and respiratory rate 24 breaths per minute. His venous pressure was elevated at +12 cm with sharp x and y descents. There was a sustained inspiratory rise in mean jugular venous pressure (Kussmaul's sign). Cardiac auscultation was normal and abdominal examination revealed shifting dullness and slight hepatosplenomegaly.

Investigations:

haemoglobin 12.0 g/dL (13.0–18.0)

white cell count 8×10^9/L (4–11)

neutrophils 4×10^9/L (1.5–7.0)

lymphocytes 4×10^9/L (1.5–4.0)

platelets 234×10^9/L (150–400)

sodium 137 mmol/L (135–145)

potassium 4.2 mmol/L (3.5–5.0)

creatinine 97 µmol/L (60–110)

brain natriuretic peptide 110 ng/L (<100)

Abdominal ultrasound:

mild hepatosplenomegaly and ascites

liver echogenicity was mildly increased

Electrocardiogram:

normal left ventricular function and size with ejection fraction of 65% (>55)

pulmonary artery systolic pressure 30 mmHg (15–30)

interventricular septum shift to left on inspiration tissue

Doppler echocardiography showed normal early relaxation velocity

Cardiac catheterisation:

equalised right and left ventricular diastolic pressures at 50 mmHg

there was a 'dip and plateau' (square root) pattern of the ventricular pressures

right atrial pressure 18 mmHg (0–8)

What is the most likely diagnosis?

A   Arrhythmogenic right ventricular cardiomyopathy
B   Cardiac amyloidosis
C   Constrictive pericarditis
D   Haemochromatosis
E   Restrictive cardiomyopathy

6. A 46-year-old woman was referred to the cardiology clinic with a history of shortness of breath on exertion for the last 6 months. The only significant past history was a febrile illness in childhood with joint pains. She was originally from Pakistan but had recently emigrated to the UK.

On examination, her pulse rate was 88 beats per minute, irregularly irregular, blood pressure 110/68 mmHg and respiratory rate 16 breaths per minute. She had a 2/6 mid-diastolic murmur at the apex and mild pitting pedal oedema.

Investigations:

Echocardiography:

enlarged left atrium (3.2 cm × 4.0 cm)

mitral valve stenosis with transvalvar gradient 15 mmHg (normal) and valve area of 1.3 cm^2 (4–6) with commissural fusion and only minimal calcification

trace mitral regurgitation

pulmonary artery systolic pressure (PASP) 50 mmHg (15–30)

What is the most appropriate next step in the management?

A   Echocardiographic surveillance with surgery if PASP rises to >60 mmHg
B   Mitral valve repair
C   Mitral valve replacement
D   Percutaneous balloon mitral valvotomy
E   Surgical mitral valvotomy

7.   A 63-year-old man was referred to the cardiology clinic after an annual health evaluation at work showed T-wave inversion in the lateral leads of his ECG. His past medical history included type 2 diabetes, hypertension and asthma. He was on metformin, gliclazide, ramipril and salbutamol inhaler.
      On examination, his pulse was 82 beats per minute and regular, blood pressure 110/70 mmHg and respiratory rate 14 breaths per minute. The rest of the physical examination was normal apart from a left carotid bruit.
      Blood tests were normal apart from a serum creatinine level of 130 µmol/L (60–110).
      Exercise tolerance test using a modified Bruce protocol showed a 1-mm ST depression in the anterior leads, which recovered after 2 minutes.

Investigations:

Coronary angiography:
85% stenosis in the proximal left anterior descending (LAD) artery
90% stenosis in the right coronary artery (RCA)
60% stenosis of the left main stem (LMS)
65% stenosis of the left circumflex artery (LCx)
ejection fraction 50% (>55)

What is the most appropriate next step in management?

A   Coronary artery bypass graft (CABG) surgery
B   Maximise medical therapy by adding a statin and starting insulin
C   Maximise medical therapy by adding high-dose statin and nicorandil
D   Percutaneous coronary intervention with stents to the RCA and LAD
E   Percutaneous coronary intervention with stents to the RCA, LAD and LCx

8.   A 72-year-old woman was admitted with shortness of breath on exertion for the last week. She had also had palpitations during this period. She had hypertension, for which she was on ramipril 5 mg once daily. On examination, her pulse rate was 140 beats per minute and irregular, blood pressure 130/70 mmHg, respiratory rate 24 breaths per minute and temperature 37.3°C. Pulse oximetry showed oxygen saturation on air of 96%. Heart sounds were normal and chest was clear to auscultation.

Investigations:

sodium 141 mmol/L (135–145)	haemoglobin 12 g/dL (11.5–16.5)
potassium 4.5 mmol/L (3.5–5.0)	white cell count 8 × 10⁹/L (4–11)
urea 9 mmol/L (2.5–7.5)	platelets 135 × 10⁹/L (150–400)
creatinine 90 µmol/L (45–90)	

Chest X-ray: normal

Electrocardiogram: see **Figure 1.3**

What is the most appropriate next step in management?

A   Commence digoxin intravenous loading and enoxaparin therapeutic dose
B   Direct current synchronised cardioversion with enoxaparin 1 mg/kg immediately before
C   Oral digoxin loading and enoxaparin therapeutic dose
D   Oral metoprolol and enoxaparin therapeutic dose
E   Verapamil 5 mg intravenously and enoxaparin therapeutic dose

Figure 1.3

9.   A 45-year-old man was admitted to the emergency department with a history of palpitations which started 4 hours ago. He reported no chest pain, shortness of breath or dizziness. On examination, his pulse was 160 beats per minute and irregular, blood pressure 80/60 mmHg, respiratory rate 28 breaths per minute and oxygen saturation on air was 90%.

Admission ECG showed wide QRS complex atrial fibrillation at 170 beats per minute. He had a synchronised DC shock and postcardioversion pulse rate was 80 beats per minute and blood pressure 110/70 mmHg.

Postcardioversion ECG is shown (see **Figure 1.4**).

Figure 1.4

What is the most appropriate management?

A   Digoxin, start at 62.5 µg and titrate up
B   Intravenous adenosine after vagal manoeuvres
C   Metoprolol 25 mg three times daily and titrate up
D   No medical therapy
E   Verapamil 40 mg three times daily and titrate up

10. A 36-year-old man was seen in the emergency department with chest pain. This was his second presentation with chest pain in the last 6 months. He was diagnosed as having musculoskeletal pain during the last admission. He described the chest pain as central, crushing and radiating to the jaw. He had no significant past history of note and was not on any medication. He mentioned that he used cocaine occasionally and in fact had used it a few hours ago. On examination, his temperature was 37.5°C, pulse 110 beats per minute and regular, blood pressure 170/100 mmHg and respiratory rate 18 breaths per minute. His pupils were dilated. Heart sounds were normal. ECG showed a 2-mm ST depression in the anterolateral leads.

Which one of the following should not be given to this patient?

A   Angiotensin-converting enzyme inhibitors
B   Aspirin
C   Benzodiazepines
D   Beta blockers
E   Nitroglycerin (sublingual)

11. A 35-year-old man was seen in the cardiology clinic after an episode of syncope. It lasted less than a minute and he was not confused afterwards. He had no history of palpitations or other significant past medical history. His paternal uncle had died suddenly at the age of 39 years and his grandfather at the age of 36 years. ECG showed left ventricular (LV) hypertrophy.

Investigations:

Transthoracic echocardiogram:
LV free wall thickness of 0.8 cm and septal thickness of 2.2 cm (both 0.6–0.9)
LV outflow tract gradient of 20 mmHg (0)
LV ejection fraction – 68% (>55)
mild mitral regurgitation
systolic anterior motion of anterior mitral leaflet noted
mild tricuspid regurgitation with pulmonary artery systolic pressure of 30 mmHg (15–30)

Holter monitor showed two episodes of non-sustained ventricular tachycardia lasting <10 seconds each. Exercise testing showed normal blood pressure and heart rate response. Exercise tolerance was good. No arrhythmia noted during exercise testing.

What is the next most appropriate step in management?

A   Alcohol septal ablation
B   Dual chamber pacemaker implantation to improve left ventricular outflow tract (LVOT) gradient
C   Implantable cardioverter defibrillator (ICD)
D   Initiate beta-blocker therapy
E   Septal myomectomy

12. A 59-year-old man presented with shortness of breath. He had breathlessness on minimal exertion but no chest pain; there was some swelling of his feet. Past history included ischaemic heart disease with two previous myocardial infarctions and a three-vessel coronary artery bypass graft (CABG). He also had a history of hypertension and hyperlipidaemia.

He had been under the care of the heart failure clinic for 8 months and was on ramipril 5 mg once daily, bisoprolol 7.5 mg once daily, simvastatin 40 mg once daily, aspirin 75 mg once daily, spironolactone 12.5 mg once daily and furosemide 40 mg twice daily.

On examination, his temperature was 37.2°C, pulse rate 56 beats per minute and regular, blood pressure 104/50 mmHg and respiratory rate 18 breaths per minute. He had pitting pedal and ankle oedema. Jugular venous pressure was +9 cm, the apex was displaced laterally but the hearts sounds were normal. ECG showed sinus rhythm with a PR interval of 180 ms, intraventricular conduction block with QRS duration of 160 ms and poor R-wave progression in the anterior chest leads.

Stress echocardiogram revealed an akinetic segment in the anterior wall of the left ventricle (LV), dilated LV with an ejection fraction of 30% (>55) and mild mitral regurgitation. There was no evidence of reversible ischaemia.

What is the most appropriate therapeutic option?

A Amiodarone
B Biventricular pacemaker–defibrillator
C Coronary angiogram with percutaneous coronary intervention to any blocked vessels detected
D Dual-chamber pacemaker
E Implantable cardioverter defibrillator

13. A 39-year-old woman was admitted with upper abdominal pain and a small amount of haematemesis. She was known to have a cardiac murmur. She was treated with proton pump inhibitors and was scheduled to have an upper gastrointestinal endoscopy. She had been under cardiology follow-up for the cardiac murmur and had had an echocardiogram 2 months ago. She was asymptomatic from the cardiac point of view.

Investigations:

Echocardiogram:
mitral valve prolapse with moderate mitral regurgitation
LV end diastolic diameter 42 mm (39–53)
LV ejection fraction 65% (>55)
pulmonary artery systolic pressure 32 mmHg (15–30)
other valves normal

Electrocardiogram: sinus rhythm and no abnormalities

What is the most appropriate course of action?

A Chlorhexidine mouthwash for infective endocarditis prophylaxis prior to endoscopy
B Intravenous amoxicillin 2 g (30–60 minutes) prior to endoscopy
C No infective endocarditis prophylaxis required
D Oral amoxicillin 2 g (30–60 minutes) prior to endoscopy
E Postpone endoscopy until a stress echocardiogram can be arranged

14. A 56-year-old man was seen in the clinic after being diagnosed with hypertension and was put on amlodipine 5 mg once daily. There was no other significant past history. He smoked five cigarettes per day and had a small glass of wine most days. On examination, his pulse was 88 beats per minute, blood pressure 156/88 mmHg and respiratory rate 14 breaths per minute. Heart sounds were normal and chest was clear. On abdominal examination, a pulsatile mass was felt in the upper abdomen.

Ultrasound of the abdomen showed a 4.2 cm diameter suprarenal abdominal aortic aneurysm. Watchful waiting was initiated and an ultrasound 6 months later showed a 5.3-cm aneurysm.

What is the next most appropriate step in management?

A   Aggressive medical management with blood pressure target of <125/75 mmHg and statin therapy, monitor every 6 months and repair if aneurysm size >6 cm

B   Endovascular repair of the aneurysm

C   Open surgical repair of the aneurysm

D   Repeat ultrasound or CT in 3 months' time and advise repair if aneurysm diameter exceeds 5.5 cm

E   Repeat ultrasound or CT in 6 months' time and advise repair if aneurysm diameter exceeds 5.5 cm

15. A 71-year-old man was referred to the emergency department with a history of central chest pain at rest. It lasted 15 minutes and had resolved by the time he reached the emergency department. He had had chest pain on and off for the last week. Episodes lasted 15–20 minutes and were often relieved by sublingual glyceryl trinitrate spray. He had a history of medically treated angina for the last 8 years. His other past medical history included hypertension and hypercholesterolaemia. He was on atenolol 50 mg once daily, ramipril 2.5 mg once daily, simvastatin 40 mg once daily and aspirin 75 mg once daily.

     On examination, his pulse was 68 beats per minute, blood pressure 106/66 mmHg and respiratory rate 22 breaths per minute. He was immediately started on enoxaparin and clopidogrel 300 mg followed by 75 mg once daily. The rest of the medications were continued.

Investigations:

Blood tests showed:	troponin 10.9 µg/L (<0.04)
creatinine 98 µmol (60–110)	

Electrocardiogram: (see **Figure 1.5**)

Figure 1.5

What is the most appropriate next step in management?

A   Add glycoprotein IIb/IIIa inhibitor

B   Immediate left heart catheterisation

C   Maximise medical therapy by adding nicorandil and substituting simvastatin with atorvastatin 80 mg once daily

D   Plan left heart catheterisation within the next 96 hours

E   Thrombolyse with alteplase immediately

16. A 17-year-old boy was referred to the emergency department after suffering from palpitations and shortness of breath at a party. He had no past history of note apart from asthma for which he was on salbutamol and budesonide inhalers. He had one previous admission to an intensive therapy unit because of acute severe asthma. He admitted to taking an unknown substance that his friends gave him during the party. There was no previous history of illicit drug use.

    On examination, his pulse was 200 beats per minute and regular, blood pressure 104/54 mmHg, respiratory rate 24 breaths per minute and oxygen saturation 96% on air.

    ECG (see **Figure 1.6**):

Figure 1.6

What is the next most appropriate step in management?

    A   Adenosine 6 mg intravenous bolus followed by saline bolus
    B   Amiodarone 150 mg intravenously over 10 minutes
    C   DC cardioversion with 100 J energy
    D   Metoprolol 5 mg intravenously over 1 minute
    E   Verapamil 2.5 mg intravenously over 2.5 minutes

17. A 60-year-old man was seen at a screening visit for a community-based research trial on diet and lifestyle modification to prevent diabetes. He had no significant past medical history and was not on any medications. He was found to have an irregular heart beat and a subsequent ECG showed atrial fibrillation at a rate of 110 beats per minute.

    Blood tests, including urea and electrolytes, full blood count, thyroid and liver function tests, were normal.

    His general practitioner started him on bisoprolol 2.5 mg once daily and referred him for an echocardiogram which showed normal atrial dimensions and good left ventricular function. Considering that he was asymptomatic and by patient preference, rate control was accepted as the management strategy.

What is the next most appropriate step in management?

A   Low-molecular-weight heparin followed by warfarin to a target international normalised ratio of 2–3

B   Low-molecular-weight heparin for 4 weeks followed by aspirin 325 mg once daily

C   Oral aspirin 75 mg once daily

D   Oral aspirin 75 mg once daily and dipyridamole 200 mg twice daily

E   Start on warfarin and maintain the international normalised ratio at 2–3

18. An 86-year-old man was brought to the emergency department following an episode of chest pain. It is 8/10 in severity. He also had an episode of brief loss of consciousness a few weeks ago. On closer questioning he mentioned that he had been finding it increasingly difficult to do activities such as shopping and gardening. He had shortness of breath when walking more than 10–15 metres. His other past medical history included osteoarthritis of the hips, for which he had a right hip replacement 10 years ago. He used one stick and was unable to cook or shop for himself.

     On examination, his pulse was 86 beats per minute, blood pressure 110/85 mmHg, and respiratory rate 18 breaths per minute. He had a weak pulse, heaving apex and an ejection systolic murmur loudest at the aortic area and radiating to the carotids.

Investigations:

> Electrocardiogram: sinus rhythm and left ventricular (LV) hypertrophy
>
> ---
>
> Echocardiogram:
> mild LV dilatation with LV hypertrophy
> LV ejection fraction 50% (>55)
> calcified aortic valve with valve area of 0.8 cm² (3–4)
> transvalvar gradient 55 mmHg (0)
> mitral valve normal E/A (early to late ratio) 0.9 (0.98–2.78)
> pulmonary valve normal
> mild tricuspid regurgitation
> pulmonary artery systolic pressure 32 mmHg (15–30)

What is the most appropriate next step in management?

A   Arrange social and palliative care

B   Balloon aortic valvotomy

C   Medical management including high-dose statins

D   Open aortic valve replacement

E   Transcatheter aortic valve implantation

19. A 45-year-old woman was referred to the clinic with a history of shortness of breath for the past 6 months. She had progressive exertional breathlessness and now could walk only a few hundred metres. She also had one episode of loss of consciousness. She had noticed swelling of her ankles for the last 3 weeks. Her only past medical history was of hay fever in childhood. She was a non-smoker and only drank 3–4 units of alcohol a week. She was not on any medication. Her general practitioner had started her on salbutamol and beclomethasone inhaler with no improvement.

     On examination, her pulse was 88 beats per minute, blood pressure 140/86 mmHg, respiratory rate 20 breaths per minute and oxygen saturation 94% on room air.

Investigations:

Full blood count, urea and electrolytes, liver function test: normal
Autoantibody screen: negative
Chest X-ray: clear lung fields, normal cardiac size

Lung function tests:
forced expiratory volume in 1 second 2.9 L (120% predicted)
forced vital capacity 3.5 L (130% predicted)
total lung capacity 5.8 L (120% predicted)
carbon monoxide diffusion in the lung 92%

Echocardiogram:
left ventricle size normal
LV (left ventricular) ejection fraction 64% (>55)
normal aortic and pulmonary valves
right ventricle dilated, mild tricuspid regurgitation
pulmonary artery systolic pressure – 60 mmHg

CT of the chest: normal
Ventilation–perfusion ($\dot{V}/\dot{Q}$) scan: low probability for thromboembolic disease

What is the most appropriate next investigation?

A   Bronchoalveolar lavage
B   Cardiac catheterisation
C   CT-guided lung biopsy
D   CT pulmonary angiography
E   Sweat chloride testing

20. A 28-year-old woman was admitted with shortness of breath on minimal exertion and pedal oedema. She had a caesarean section 2 months ago following a failure of induction with oxytocin at term. During the pregnancy she had gestational hypertension but no evidence of pre-eclampsia. Her previous two deliveries were normal. She was a non-smoker and did not drink any alcohol.

   On examination, her pulse was 94 beats per minute and regular, blood pressure 100/50 mmHg, respiratory rate 20 breaths per minute and temperature 36.7°C. Jugular venous pressure was elevated at 12 cm, first and second heart sounds were normal, and there was a left ventricular third heart sound as well as a long systolic murmur at the apex.

Investigations:

sodium 139 mmol/L (135–145)	creatinine 96 μmol/L (45–90)
potassium 4.3 mmol/L (3.5–5.0)	troponin I 0.9 μg/L (<0.04)
urea 9 mmol/L (2.5–7.5)	

NTpBNP (N-terminal pro-brain natriuretic peptide) 1860 pg/mL (<300)
Thyroid function test: normal
Serology for cytomegalovirus, Coxsackievirus and HIV: negative
Antinuclear antibody: negative

Chest X-ray:
cardiomegaly with upper lobe venous dilatation
small bilateral pleural effusions

Contd...

Contd...

> Electrocardiogram: sinus tachycardia, left axis deviation, P mitrale and tall R waves in V4–V6
>
> Echocardiogram:
> dilated left ventricle with end-diastolic diameter 6.2 cm
> LV ejection fraction 35%
> mild mitral and tricuspid regurgitation
> dilated left atrium
> pulmonary artery systolic pressure 35 mmHg (15–30)

What is the most likely diagnosis?

A   Cor pulmonale due to pulmonary thromboembolism
B   Hypertensive heart failure
C   Idiopathic dilated cardiomyopathy unmasked by pregnancy
D   Myocardial infarction related to coronary vasculitis
E   Peripartum cardiomyopathy

21. A 56-year-old man presented to the emergency department with sudden severe pain in the central chest and back that occurred while he was playing tennis. He had a past history of hypertension for which he was on amlodipine 5 mg once daily. He was an ex-smoker. The pain was 7/10 in severity and associated with mild sweating and nausea.

    On general examination, he was 188 cm tall and weighed 82 kg. Heart rate was 98 beats per minute and regular, blood pressure 190/98 mmHg, respiratory rate 20 breaths per minute and oxygen saturation on air 96%. Heart sounds were normal but there was a short early diastolic murmur at the 3rd left intercostal space.

Investigations:

> Electrocardiogram: sinus tachycardia and chest X-ray was normal

What would be the most appropriate next investigation?

A   Cardiac troponin
B   CT angiography
C   D-dimer
D   Transthoracic echocardiogram (TTE)
E   Ventilation–perfusion ($\dot{V}/\dot{Q}$) scan

22. A 57-year-old woman was admitted with a history of progressive shortness of breath. She did not have any chest pain. She had a past history of hypertension (for which she was on ramipril 10 mg once daily and amlodipine 2.5 mg once daily), hypercholesterolaemia (on simvastatin) and had had a breast carcinoma, which was resected 10 years ago.

    On examination, her pulse was 98 beats per minute and regular, blood pressure 106/58 mmHg, respiratory rate 24 breaths per minute and oxygen saturation on air 95%. Jugular venous pressure was elevated with an inspiratory increase in pressure. Heart sounds were normal. Chest was clear to auscultation. Abdominal examination showed an enlarged tender liver and moderate ascites. There was pitting oedema up to mid-shin level. There was an inspiratory decrease in blood pressure of 15 mmHg.

Investigations:

> Chest X-ray: enlarged cardiac silhouette with normal lung
>
> Echocardiogram:
> pericardial effusion with 1.4 cm fluid between pericardium and right ventricle
> right atrial collapse during diastole
> right ventricular collapse in early diastole
> LV ejection fraction 62% (>55)

What is the next most appropriate step in the management?

A   Abdominal ultrasound
B   Cardiac MRI
C   CT of the chest, abdomen and pelvis
D   Diagnostic pericardiocentesis
E   Therapeutic pericardiocentesis

23. A 27-year-old woman was seen in the clinic with a history of progressive shortness of breath for the past 3 weeks. She was 16 weeks' pregnant and was awaiting an antenatal clinic appointment. She had no significant past medical history. However, her mother mentioned that she had a heart murmur at birth but she had been subsequently lost to follow-up.

  On examination, her pulse was 98 beats per minute, blood pressure 106/58 mmHg, respiratory rate 18 breaths per minute and oxygen saturation on air 95%. The first heart sound was soft and there was wide fixed split of the second with accentuation of P2. There was a parasternal heave. There was a 2/6 ejection systolic murmur at the second left intercostal space and a 2/6 pansystolic murmur at the apex.

Investigations:

> Electrocardiogram: first-degree heart block and left axis deviation

What is the most likely diagnosis?

A   Ostium primum atrial septal defect
B   Ostium secundum atrial septal defect
C   Patent foramen ovale
D   Trilogy of Fallot
E   Ventricular septal defect

24. A 54-year-old man was admitted to the coronary care unit with central chest heaviness and shortness of breath of 2 hours' duration. ECG showed ST elevation in V3–V6 and I and aVL, and he subsequently underwent primary percutaneous coronary intervention with stenting to the left circumflex artery.

  He was discharged from the hospital on the fourth day after admission on aspirin, clopidogrel, ramipril, atorvastatin and bisoprolol. There was no significant past medical history.

  Two weeks later he came to the emergency department with recurrent chest pain, malaise, tiredness and diffuse joint aches. He described the chest pain as sharp, over the precordium and left chest, and radiating to the left shoulder.

Investigations:

haemoglobin 13.8 g/dL (13.0–18.0)	sodium 141 mmol/L (135–145)
white cell count 16×10^9/L (4–11)	potassium 3.9 mmol/L (3.5–5.0)
platelets 375×10^9/L (150–400)	urea 8 mmol/L (2.5–7.5)
erythrocyte sedimentation rate 80 mm/1st h (0–20)	creatinine 102 µmol/L (60–110)
	troponin I 0.45 µg/L (<0.04)
C-reactive protein 145 mg/L (<10)	bilirubin 5 mmol/L (1–22)
neutrophils 12×10^9/L (1.5–7.0)	albumin 40 g/L (37–49)
lymphocytes 3×10^9/L (1.5–4.0)	alanine aminotransferase 45 U/L (5–35)
monocytes 1×10^9/L (0–0.8)	alkaline phosphatase 68 U/L (45–105)

Electrocardiogram: concave upwards ST elevation in leads I, II, aVL, aVF and V2–V6

Chest X-ray: normal cardiac contour and a small left pleural effusion

Pleural tap:

white cell count 20 x 10^9/L (<1)   protein 43 g/L (30)

lactate dehydrogenase (LDH) 150 U/L = [plasma LDH 120 U/L (10–250)]
(normal pleural fluid to serum ratio 0.6)
no malignant cells or culture
Gram and acid-fast bacillus stain and cultures: negative

Echocardiogram:
dilated left ventricle with end-diastolic diameter 5.7 cm
LV ejection fraction – 35% (>55)
mild mitral and tricuspid regurgitation
dilated left atrium
pulmonary artery systolic pressure 35 mmHg (15–30)

On examination, his temperature was 38.9°C, pulse 70 beats per minute, blood pressure 110/60 mmHg and respiratory rate 18 breaths per minute. There was mild pitting pedal oedema. Jugular venous pressure was not elevated and cardiac auscultation revealed normal heart sounds and a scratchy sound, best heard in the left lower sternal edge on leaning forward. There was reduced air entry in the left lower lobe with dullness to percussion.

What is the most appropriate next step in management?

A   Aspirin 300 mg four times daily
B   Blood cultures and start ceftriaxone and gentamicin intravenously
C   Pleural biopsy
D   Urgent coronary angiogram
E   Viral serology for Coxsackievirus, cytomegalovirus, HIV and Epstein–Barr virus

25. A 24-year-old man was seen in the clinic with gradual shortness of breath on exertion. He was from Burkina Faso originally and had been in the UK for the last 2 years. He had had these symptoms for the past few years, but now his exercise tolerance was reduced to 400 metres on the flat; he could manage only one flight of stairs.

His past history was of recurrent respiratory illnesses and two bouts of malaria. His mother who had accompanied him said that he used to have episodes of shortness of breath with blue lips in childhood which was relieved by squatting down.

On examination, his temperature was 37.5°C, pulse 98 beats per minute, blood pressure 104/65 mmHg, respiratory rate 18 breaths per minute and oxygen saturation 92% on room air. He had finger clubbing and central and peripheral cyanosis. The apex beat was undisplaced but there was a parasternal heave. There was a normal first heart sound, a single second sound, best heard in the right 2nd intercostal space and an ejection systolic murmur in the left second intercostal space.

ECG (see **Figure 1.7**):

Figure 1.7

What is most likely diagnosis?

A   Atrial septal defect with reversal of shunt
B   Eisenmenger's disease
C   Fallot's tetralogy
D   Noonan's syndrome
E   Patent ductus arteriosus with reversal of shunt

26. A 48-year-old man was seen in the emergency department with shortness of breath for the last few days. He was an ex-smoker and had been diagnosed with chronic obstructive pulmonary disease previously. He was on salbutamol, ipratropium, fluticasone and tiotropium inhalers. There was no other past history of note.

On examination, his temperature was 37.4°C, pulse 152 beats per minute, blood pressure 110/60 mmHg, respiratory rate 30 breaths per minute and oxygen saturation 90% on air. Chest auscultation revealed bilateral polyphonic wheeze, but no crepitations and equal air entry.

He was given hydrocortisone 100 mg intravenously, salbutamol and ipratropium nebulisers, and started on oxygen 4 L/min.

ECG (see **Figure 1.8**):

Figure 1.8

What is the most appropriate next step in management?

A   Adenosine 6 mg rapid intravenously
B   DC cardioversion
C   Digoxin 500 µg intravenously
D   Flecainide 300 mg orally
E   Verapamil 5 mg intravenously

27. A 56-year-old man was admitted with congestive cardiac failure. On the third day after admission he collapsed in the ward. The initial rhythm was asystole. Cardiopulmonary resuscitation (CPR) was initiated with chest compression and the airway was secured.

What is the most appropriate next step in management?

A   DC cardioversion monophasic 360 J × 1
B   Intravenous adrenaline 10 mL of 1 in 10 000 solution (1 mg/10 mL)
C   Intravenous adrenaline 10 mL of 1 in 1000 solution (1 mg/mL)
D   Intravenous atropine 3 mg single dose
E   Intravenous calcium gluconate 10 mL

28. A 68-year old woman was admitted with a history of chest pain of 2 hours' duration, which woke her up from sleep. Her ECG showed ST elevation in the lateral leads as well as T inversion. She had been referred 2 months earlier to a rapid access chest pain clinic and had been discharged after having a normal exercise tolerance test. On closer questioning she had had episodes of chest pain lasting up to 15–20 minutes for the last year. She could not recall any specific triggering factors. Her only other past medical history was of osteoarthritis affecting her knees, hips and fingers. She was on diclofenac and a paracetamol–codeine combination for pain relief.

     Troponin I was positive at 1.8 µg/L (<0.04). She was started on aspirin, clopidogrel, bisoprolol, ramipril and simvastatin.

She underwent a left heart catheterisation on the day of admission, which showed only minor <50% blockages in the coronary arteries. Left ventricular size and function were within normal limits. Clopidogrel was discontinued. Serial ECGs showed resolution of the previous ST depression.

What is the most appropriate next step in management?

A   Optimise the dose of non-steroidal anti-inflammatories and opiates for pain relief
B   Repeat coronary angiogram and do flow studies across the area of blockage
C   Stop all medications and follow up as an outpatient
D   Stop beta-blockers and start diltiazem and nitrates
E   Titrate beta-blockers and add nitrates if episodes of chest pain persist

29. A 57-year-old man was referred by the general practitioner for shortness of breath on exertion. There was no chest discomfort or coughing. He had a past history of type 2 diabetes and hypertension. He had been on holiday in Spain 2 months ago where he had some chest discomfort and shortness of breath for 2 days, which he attributed to the heat and humidity. After coming back, he had progressive shortness of breath which took him to the general practitioner.

On examination, his temperature was 37.2°C, pulse 100 beats per minute, blood pressure 100/60 mmHg and oxygen saturation 94% on room air. Jugular venous pressure was +12 cm, his apex was difficult to locate, and he had a left-sided third heart sound (S3). There were some basal crackles in his lungs.

ECG (see **Figure 1.9**):

Figure 1.9

What is the most likely cause of his symptoms?

A   Acute anterior ST segment elevation myocardial infarction with left ventricular failure (LVF)
B   Brugada's syndrome
C   Left main stem artery stenosis with recurrent angina and LVF
D   Previous anterior myocardial infarction with left ventricular aneurysm and LVF
E   Previous anterior myocardial infarction with LVF and papillary muscle dysfunction

30. A 79-year-old man was admitted with two episodes of syncope. Over the last 3 months, he had had episodes of dizziness and had lost consciousness twice. There were no seizures and he was

not disoriented after regaining consciousness. He was on amlodipine for hypertension and simvastatin for high cholesterol. There was no other relevant past medical history.

ECG (see **Figure 1.10**):

Figure 1.10

What is the most likely diagnosis?

A   First-degree heart block
B   Sinus bradycardia with sinus pause
C   Complete heart block
D   Trifascicular block
E   2:1 second-degree heart block

31. A 78-year-old woman was admitted with weakness in her right arm and difficulty in speaking which started the day before. On admission, her temperature was 37.3°C, pulse 92 beats per minute, blood pressure 160/100 mmHg and oxygen saturation 96% on air. Her chest was clear, heart sounds were normal and there was right hemiparesis.

She later had a short run of non-sustained ventricular tachycardia (NSVT) on the monitor. A subsequent CT of the head confirmed a left middle cerebral artery infarct. She was started on antiplatelet agents.

ECG (see **Figure 1.11**):

What is the next most appropriate management?

A   Start amiodarone and evaluate for implantable cardioverter defibrillator (ICD) implantation, once acute phase resolves
B   Start beta-blockers; monitor cardiac markers and serial ECGs
C   Arrange for percutaneous coronary intervention in the next 2–3 days
D   Arrange urgent echocardiogram
E   Consider thrombolysis or primary percutaneous intervention urgently

Figure 1.11

32. A 28-year-old man was admitted with acute-onset shortness of breath and chest pain. He had a non-productive cough. He had just flown back to London from a trip to Shanghai. His immunisations were up to date and he reported no night sweats or myalgia. He had no significant past history of illnesses apart from childhood asthma and was not on any medication. He did not smoke.

     On examination, his temperature was 37.6°C, pulse 110 beats per minute, blood pressure 100/50 mmHg, respiratory rate 20 breaths per minute and oxygen saturation 91% on air. He had a pleural rub and some crackles in the left lower zone; a third heart sound was heard in the left lower sternal edge.

     ECG (see **Figure 1.12**):

Figure 1.12

What is the most appropriate diagnostic investigation?

A   CT angiogram for aortic dissection
B   CT pulmonary angiogram
C   D-dimer assay
D   Echocardiogram
E   Peak flow assessment

33. A 46-year-old man was admitted with history of abdominal pain, diarrhoea and dizzy spells. CT of the abdomen had revealed a mass in the head of the pancreas 2.3 × 1.2 cm in size. There was no lymph node enlargement or other lesions on the CT. He was awaiting the results of a gut hormone panel and was being investigated for a neuroendocrine tumour, and a CT-guided biopsy of the mass was planned. He did not have any significant past medical history and was not on any medications.

    The next morning, he collapsed with sudden onset of severe right-sided chest pain. His pulse was 140 beats per minute, blood pressure 70/40 mmHg, respiratory rate 34 breaths per minute and oxygen saturation 87% on air. ECG showed sinus tachycardia and a partial right bundle-branch block (RBBB) pattern.

    Despite being resuscitated with intravenous fluids, oxygen, heparin and inotropes, after 10 minutes the blood pressure was still 60 mmHg systolic and oxygen saturation 88% on 15 L O_2/min.

What is the most appropriate next step in management?

A   Coronary angiography and stenting
B   CT pulmonary angiogram
C   Emergency echocardiogram
D   Start clopidogrel and abciximab
E   Start intravenous alteplase

34. A 26-year-old man was admitted with shortness of breath on walking 200 metres. He had progressive shortness of breath over the past year. He was a heavy smoker but had cut down in the last year. He had no significant past history apart from being told that he had a heart murmur as a child. He was taking no medication.

    On examination, there was no central cyanosis but he had clubbing of his toes and a systolic murmur at the left upper sternal edge radiating to the left infraclavicular region.

What is the most likely cause?

A   Patent ductus arteriosus with reversal of shunt
B   Rupture of sinus of Valsalva into the right ventricle
C   Tetralogy of Fallot
D   Total anomalous pulmonary venous return
E   Ventricular septal defect with reversal of shunt

35. A 54-year-old woman was seen in the clinic with a history of fever, night sweats and malaise. She also had shortness of breath on brisk walking and climbing stairs. She had no significant past history of illnesses, no recent travel history and no relevant family history. She was not on any medications apart from paracetamol taken on an as required basis.

    On examination, her temperature was 38.9°C, pulse 88 beats per minute, blood pressure 110/60 mmHg and oxygen saturation 94% on room air. Her chest was clear but there was a mid-diastolic murmur with an added sound which was variable on position.

Investigations:

Electrocardiogram: sinus rhythm and P mitrale

Echocardiogram:
mass attached to the atrial septum and prolapsing into the left
ventricle with a transmitral valve mean gradient of 14 mmHg (0)

What is the most likely diagnosis?

A   Left atrial myxoma
B   Leiomyosarcoma of the interatrial septum
C   Mitral regurgitation with infective endocarditis
D   Mitral stenosis with infective endocarditis
E   Mitral valve prolapse with infective endocarditis

36. A 35-year-old man was admitted with a 6-month history of shortness of breath on exertion. There was no history of chest pain, ankle swelling or syncope. He gave a history of occasional palpitations at rest, but there was no history of dizziness or light-headedness. There was no relevant family or past medical history.

On examination, his pulse rate was 78 beats per minute, blood pressure 140/90 mmHg, respiratory rate 16 breaths per minute and temperature 37.3°C. Brisk carotid pulses were noted and he had a triple apical impulse. On auscultation, he had a short systolic murmur medial to the apex radiating towards the base of the heart and a prominent fourth heart sound. Murmur increased on standing and diminished on squatting. Handgrip also diminished the murmur whereas Valsalva's manoeuvre increased it.

What is the most likely diagnosis?

A   Bicuspid aortic valve with aortic stenosis
B   Dilated cardiomyopathy with left bundle-branch block
C   Hypertrophic cardiomyopathy
D   Left atrial myxoma
E   Mitral valve prolapse and mitral regurgitation

37. A 59-year-old man was admitted with a 2-day history of chest pain and shortness of breath. He had a past history of type 2 diabetes controlled with metformin and pioglitazone. He was also on ramipril for hypertension.

He was admitted and started on aspirin, clopidogrel, fondaparinux and subcutaneous twice daily mixed insulin. He had a coronary angiogram and insertion of two stents to the posterior descending artery and left circumflex artery.

On the third day of admission, his shortness of breath was more severe with a pulse rate of 98 beats per minute and blood pressure 110/70 mmHg. On examination, jugular venous pressure was elevated at 10 cm and auscultation revealed a gallop rhythm and a grade 3 systolic murmur, heard best at the apex and radiating to the base. There was no radiation to the axilla. There were crackles at both lung bases.

What is the most likely diagnosis?

A   Dressler's syndrome
B   Left ventricular free wall rupture
C   Mitral regurgitation due to anterolateral papillary muscle rupture
D   Mitral regurgitation due to posteromedial chordal rupture
E   Ventricular septal rupture

38. A 68-year-old man was referred because of recurrent episodes of syncope. Each lasted less than 2 minutes and was not associated with confusion, palpitations or aura. Two episodes occurred in the morning while he was dressing to go out to work and another occurred when he turned his head sharply while at work. He had no significant past medical history and was not on any medication.

Physical examination was unremarkable. Carotid sinus massage produced a 6 s asystole and 40 mmHg drop in systolic pressure. Despite altering his clothing and appropriate advice, he had another episode of syncope while driving.

What is the most appropriate next step in management?

A   Dual chamber permanent pacemaker insertion
B   Implantable cardioverter defibrillator insertion

    C   Start doxazosin
    D   Start fludrocortisone
    E   Start midodrine

39. A 26-year-old man of Romanian origin was admitted with history of shortness of breath. He had had fever with rigors and chills intermittently for the last week. For the past day he had had weakness and pain in the left arm. He did not have any significant past medical history and denied any recreational drug use.

    On examination, his temperature was 39.4°C, pulse 112 beats per minute, blood pressure 92/50 mmHg, respiratory rate 24 breaths per minute and oxygen saturation 94% on air. Jugular venous pressure was elevated +6 cm and there was an early diastolic murmur best heard in the 3rd left intercostal space in expiration. Auscultation of the lungs revealed bi-basal crackles. There was some weakness in the left hand.

Investigations:

haemoglobin 10.2 g/dL (13.0–18.0)	lymphocytes 3 × 10⁹/L (1.5–4.0)
mean corpuscular volume 84 fL (80–96)	sodium 138 mmol/L (135–145)
white cell count 26 × 10⁹/L (4–11)	potassium 5.0 mmol/L (3.5–5.0)
platelets 349 × 10⁹/L (150–400)	urea 8 mmol/L (2.5–7.5)
neutrophils 23 × 10⁹/L (1.5–7.0)	creatinine 114 μmol/L (60–110)

Urinalysis: protein 2+, blood 2+, leukocytes +, nitrites negative

Electrocardiogram: sinus tachycardia

Transoesophageal echocardiogram:
normal left ventricular size with hyperdynamic systolic function
left ventricular (LV) ejection fraction 60% (>55)
aortic valve bicuspid with three masses on the leaflets as well as leaflet disruption
largest mass 7 mm in size
moderate aortic regurgitation with high LV end-diastolic pressure
fluid present around the aortic annulus

Ultrasound: infarct of left kidney

What is the most appropriate next step in management?

    A   Immediate aortic valve surgery under antibiotic cover
    B   Start antibiotics and monitor clinical condition
    C   Start antibiotics and plan aortic valve replacement after 48 hours of antibiotics
    D   Start antibiotics, unfractionated heparin and monitor
    E   Start antibiotics, warfarin and monitor

40. A 50-year-old woman was admitted with a history of shortness of breath, swelling of her ankles, poor appetite, bruising and constipation. She could walk only 200 metres on the flat. She had noticed that she had bruises on her chest and around her eyes, but there was no history of any trauma. She did not have any significant past medical history and denied any recreational drug use.

    On examination, her temperature was 36.9°C, pulse 92 beats per minute, blood pressure 112/50 mmHg, respiratory rate 18 breaths per minute and oxygen saturation 94% on air. There was no pallor, cyanosis or jaundice.

    Ecchymotic patches were present around the eyes and on the trunk. Macroglossia was present with teeth marks around the edges of the tongue. Jugular venous pressure was elevated +6 cm and there was a left ventricular third heart sound (S3). Chest auscultation revealed bi-basal crackles.

Investigations:

haemoglobin 10.2 g/dL (11.5–16.5)	lymphocytes 3 × 10⁹/L (1.5–4.0)

haemoglobin 10.2 g/dL (11.5–16.5)   lymphocytes 3×10^9/L (1.5–4.0)
mean corpuscular volume 82 fL (80–96)   sodium 138 mmol/L (135–145)
white cell count 9×10^9/L (4–11)   potassium 5.1 mmol/L (3.5–5.0)
platelets 210×10^9/L (150–400)   urea 8.1 mmol/L (2.5–7.5)
neutrophils 6×10^9/L (1.5–7.0)   creatinine 134 µmol/L (45–90)

Urinalysis: protein 2+

Electrocardiogram: sinus rhythm, low-voltage complexes

Echocardiogram:
left atrium enlarged at 5.2 cm
LV (Left ventricular) mild enlargement
LV ejection fraction 40% (>55)
moderate LV hypertrophy with LV septal thickness of 2.0 cm (0.6–0.9)
posterior wall thickness of 1.7 cm (0.6–0.9)
LV diastolic dysfunction present
myocardium had a 'ground-glass' appearance

What is the most appropriate diagnostic investigation?

A   Abdominal fat pad aspiration
B   Left heart catheterisation
C   Serum angiotensin-converting enzyme level
D   Serum ferritin level
E   Urine metanephrines

41. A 50-year-old man was referred with chest pain. The pain was episodic with no particular
     relationship to exertion or food and was not relieved with antacids. The pain was central and
     occasionally constricting. He had a past history of hypertension and hyperlipidaemia, and was
     on amlodipine and simvastatin. There was no family history of premature heart disease. He
     was an ex-smoker. He worked as a company director and did not take much exercise. Alcohol
     consumption was moderate at 21 units/week.
         On examination, his temperature was 36.9°C, pulse 82 beats per minute, blood pressure
     152/90 mmHg, respiratory rate 18 breaths per minute and oxygen saturation 96% on air. Physical
     examination was otherwise unremarkable.

Electrocardiogram: sinus rhythm with no abnormalities

What is the most appropriate diagnostic investigation?

A   CT calcium score
B   CT coronary angiography
C   Exercise ECG using a modified Bruce protocol
D   Left heart catheterisation
E   Myocardial perfusion scan

42. A 51-year-old man was admitted with sudden-onset, central and constricting chest pain. There
     were no other symptoms. He had been admitted 3 weeks previously with similar symptoms. The
     ECG had shown ST elevation in the anterior leads and he had a paclitaxel-eluting stent inserted
     into the mid-LAD (left anterior descending) artery following primary percutaneous coronary
     intervention (PCI). He was discharged on aspirin, clopidogrel, omeprazole, irbesartan, bisoprolol
     and atorvastatin.

Investigations:

Electrocardiogram: 2-mm ST elevation in V1–V4

What is the most likely diagnosis?

A   Coronary artery aneurysm
B   Coronary artery dissection at the site of stent insertion
C   Dislodging of the stent
D   In-stent restenosis
E   In-stent thrombosis

43. A 22-year-old man was referred to the clinic after an episode of syncope. He was a university student and was also on the college basketball team. The syncopal episode occurred while he was playing and was preceded by palpitations. There were no preceding convulsions, aura or confusion. He had no previous medical illnesses and no family history of syncope.

On examination, his pulse was 62 beats per minute, blood pressure 110/70 mmHg, respiratory rate 14 breaths per minute and oxygen saturation 98% on air. Jugular venous pressure was not elevated but his apex showed a double impulse and there was a mid-systolic murmur.

Investigations:

Electrocardiogram: sinus rhythm with left ventricular hypertrophy and strain pattern

Echocardiogram:
left ventricular (LV) hypertrophy with LV septum 18 mm
posterior wall 14 mm thickness
LV outflow tract peak gradient at rest of 30 mmHg
LV ejection fraction 70% (55–65)
no systolic anterior motion of the mitral valve leaflets
mild LV diastolic dysfunction

24-hour Holter:
one episode of NSVT (non-sustained VT) lasting 8 seconds (rate 180/min) and not associated with symptoms

What is the most appropriate management?

A   Alcohol septal ablation
B   Amiodarone
C   Beta-blockers
D   Implantable cardioverter defibrillator (ICD) insertion
E   Surgical myomectomy

Answers

1. D No acute treatment needed but monitor vital signs, repeat ECG and wait 12 hours for troponin results

The ECG trace is suggestive of early repolarisation syndrome. There is a J wave present (elevation of the QRS complex – ST segment junction) in at least two leads (V4, V5 and V6 here) and concave upward elevation of the ST segment. Inferolateral leads are most commonly involved. If the right precordial leads (V1–V3) are involved, Brugada's syndrome and arrhythmogenic right ventricular cardiomyopathy (ARVC) must be ruled out.

Early repolarisation has been long considered a benign variant and is easily obliterated by exercise. However, recent attention has been focused on its possible relationship with sudden cardiac death.

Answers A and B are essentially treatment of ST elevation myocardial infarction and unstable angina, and is not appropriate in this instance.

Although the ECG pattern is suggestive of early repolarisation, it does not preclude underlying cardiac disease especially if there is a family history of premature ischaemic heart disease, and hence monitoring and checking a 12-hour troponin is appropriate.

The history and ECG pattern are not suggestive of pulmonary embolism or pericarditis and hence answers C and E are incorrect. The most common ECG abnormality in pulmonary embolism is tachycardia with occasionally incomplete or complete right bundle-branch block and other signs of right ventricular strain. Widespread concave upward elevation of the ST segment is observed in pericarditis, but J point elevation is not a characteristic pattern.

Haissaguerre M, et al. Sudden cardiac arrest associated with early repolarization. N Engl J Med 2008; 358:2016–2023.

2. C Intravenous 0.9% saline

The ECG shows inferior ST elevation myocardial infarction (MI) with right ventricular involvement. Those with inferior MI often tend to have right ventricular involvement as well. The best lead to assess right ventricular involvement is right-sided V4. To detect right ventricular myocardial infarction (RVMI), an ECG with right precordial leads should be done at admission for those presenting with inferior myocardial infarction.

Right ventricular involvement classically results in a triad of low blood pressure, elevated jugular venous pressure and absence of signs of pulmonary oedema (i.e. clear lung fields on auscultation). Right ventricular third heart sound is often heard.

RVMI leads to poor contractility of the right ventricle, leading to increased right atrial pressure, elevated jugular venous pressure and venous congestion, resulting in peripheral oedema. Also flow into the pulmonary artery is reduced resulting in reduced left ventricular preload and hence low systolic blood pressure.

Volume expansion with 0.9% saline is the first step in order to increase the left ventricular preload and systolic pressure. Once adequate volume expansion has been achieved (e.g. with one litre of normal saline) and if haemodynamic instability persists then dobutamine infusion or dobutamine with noradrenaline infusion may be tried. Levosimendan (a calcium sensitiser) is an additional therapy that may be beneficial in cardiogenic shock.

Dopamine use results in increased mortality in cardiogenic shock.

Glyceryl trinitrate would further reduce the left ventricular preload and is contraindicated in this situation.

Buerke M, et al. Pathophysiology, diagnosis, and treatment of infarction-related cardiogenic shock. Herz 2011; 36(2):73–83.

3. D Rapid plasma reagin test

The clinical features are suggestive of severe aortic regurgitation because of widening of the aortic root (aortic root aneurysm). Given the previous history of sexually transmitted infection, tertiary syphilis with cardiovascular manifestations must be considered. In advanced cases, aortic root aneurysm leads to severe volume overload of the left ventricle with gross left ventricular hypertrophy and dilatation (cor bovinum or bovine heart). Cough and hoarseness of voice may be due to compression of the bronchus and the left recurrent laryngeal nerve by the enlarged aortic root.

The standard serological test for syphilis consists of the rapid plasma reagin test or the VDRL (Veneral Disease Reference Laboratory) test (98% sensitive in tertiary syphilis) followed by a confirmatory test such as the FTA-Abs (fluorescent treponemal antibody – absorption) test.

Antiacetylcholine esterase antibodies are positive in myasthenia gravis (which may be associated with thymoma causing mediastinal widening). In this case symptoms are not suggestive of myasthenia.

Borrelia burgdorferi causes Lyme disease which may lead to a myocarditis or cardiac conduction blocks, but not aortic root widening.

Video-assisted thorascoscopic surgery biopsy and CT-guided biopsy are not indicated in cases of aortic root widening.

4. B Brucella antibodies

The clinical and echocardiographic features point to infective endocarditis. The lack of neutrophilia and relative lymphocytosis, in the presence of fever, points towards unusual organisms. There is no history to suggest an immunocompromised status. This, combined with the travel history, leads to the possibility of brucella endocarditis. Endocarditis is a rare feature in brucellosis; however, travel in the endemic area and typical presentation of culture-negative endocarditis should raise the suspicion. Brucellosis can be acquired by ingestion of unpasteurised milk.

Bartonella causes trench fever and cat scratch disease. The patient has no history suggestive of contact with cats. Although fungal cultures should be asked for in culture-negative endocarditis, there is no specific history here that would raise the suspicion of fungal endocarditis.

Although aortic root abscess is a possibility when the clinical condition does not improve after appropriate antibiotics, the situation here is of culture-negative endocarditis with relative lymphocytosis. Transoesophageal echocardiogram (TOE) is helpful especially in cases where transthoracic echocardiogram (TTE) is negative.

Treatment is usually with a combination of doxycycline, rifampicin and clotrimazole for up to 3 months. Often surgical treatment is required as well. Treatment is monitored by looking at the antibody titres. *Brucella melitensis* results in more severe infection compared with *Brucella abortus*.

5. C Constrictive pericarditis

The clinical picture is suggestive of right heart failure. Rapid *x* and *y* descents and elevated jugular venous pressure on inspiration (Kussmaul's sign) suggest either restrictive cardiomyopathy or constrictive pericarditis (cardiac tamponade would lead to distended neck veins with absent *y* descent and paradoxical pulse). The interventricular septal shift on inspiration again suggests a constrictive physiology rather than restrictive. The normal tissue Doppler (early relaxation myocardial velocity) suggests that myocardial relaxation was normal and hence right ventricular cardiomyopathy was less likely.

Cardiac catheterisation in constrictive pericarditis classically shows:
1. Elevated right atrial pressure
2. Relative equalisation of left and right ventricular diastolic pressures which are usually elevated
3. Kussmaul's pattern (elevation of right atrial and ventricular pressures on inspiration)
4. Elevated right ventricular systolic pressure

5. Exaggerated *x* and *y* descents in the right atrial pressure pattern
6. Dip and plateau pattern (square root sign) of the right or left ventricular pressures

Brain natriuretic peptide values, which are near normal, also support constrictive over restrictive physiology.

Correlation of these signs with the clinical symptoms and signs is essential. In many cases pericardial thickening is not evident on echocardiography. This is better seen with a high-resolution CT (HRCT) of the chest or MRI. However, the pericardium may not be thickened in constrictive pericarditis and thickened pericardium by itself does not prove constrictive physiology. Calcification of the pericardium is usually seen with tuberculosis.

Given the travel history, tuberculous constrictive pericarditis is a possibility here. However, many cases of pericarditis are idiopathic (thought to be due to past viral infections, e.g. with Coxsackievirus, adeno- or hepatitis viruses).

Cardiac amyloidosis results in a restrictive pattern of heart failure.

6. D Percutaneous balloon mitral valvotomy

The history and echocardiographic findings are suggestive of rheumatic mitral stenosis. Rheumatic mitral valve involvement is associated with leaflet thickening, calcification, chordal fusion and fusion of the commissures. Normal mitral valve area is 4–5 cm^2; however, symptoms of mitral stenosis start developing when the valve area drops below 1.5 cm^2. Symptoms can develop with exercise even when the valve area is between 1.5 and 2.5 cm^2.

Mitral stenosis results in left atrial dilatation and pulmonary hypertension. Severity of mitral stenosis is graded based on the valve area, pressure gradient across the valve and pulmonary systolic pressure (see **Table 1.1**).

Table 1.1 Assessment of severity of mitral stenosis

Severity	Valve area (cm^2)	Mean transvalvar gradient (mmHg)	Pulmonary artery systolic pressure (mmHg)
Mild	>1.5	<5	<30
Moderate	1–1.5	5–10	30–50
Severe	<1	>10	>50

Treatment depends on symptoms and severity of the valve stenosis. It also depends on the presence of associated valvar lesions such as mitral regurgitation or aortic lesions. Atrial fibrillation is common due to left atrial dilatation and would need anticoagulation and rate control. Patients with asymptomatic mild mitral stenosis should be monitored yearly in clinic and have an ECG and chest X-ray done. Echocardiography should be repeated if disease progression is suspected. No specific intervention or treatment is required.

In asymptomatic patients with moderate mitral stenosis, exercise evaluation should be performed and if it shows low capacity they should be offered percutaneous balloon valvotomy (PBV), if suitable, or surgical options. If it shows normal capacity, but has any of the high-risk features, PBV or surgical options must still be considered.

Patients with symptoms and severe mitral stenosis, and those with significant pulmonary hypertension (>50 mmHg systolic) should be offered PBS. However, people with significant mitral regurgitation, severe calcification of the leaflets or significant sub-valvar thickening and calcification are not suitable for balloon valvotomy, and are best treated with open valvotomy or mitral valve replacement.

Chandrashekhar Y, Westaby S, Narula J. Mitral stenosis. Lancet 2009; 374:1271–1283.

7. A Coronary artery bypass graft (CABG) surgery

This patient has diabetes and multi-vessel coronary artery disease. In such a setting, the outcomes with CABG are better. This is especially true with left internal mammary artery grafts to left anterior descending artery. His other indications for CABG as opposed to percutaneous coronary intervention (PCI) are three-vessel disease, left main stem involvement and mildly depressed left ventricular systolic function.

An additional point is the presence of a left carotid bruit, which needs to be resolved prior to surgery. Carotid Doppler should be followed by a decision to treat/not treat based on symptoms and degree of stenosis.

PCI is being increasingly used to treat patients with multi-vessel disease as well as in patients with left main stem disease, especially those who are not fit for surgery. There are no clear contra-indications for surgery in this patient and hence the best option here is CABG.

Maximising medical therapy by adding a statin and antianginal therapy is a logical decision in this patient. However, answer B is not correct as there are no clear grounds to switch to insulin with the information given in the question. Switching to insulin is a decision dependent on the overall glycaemic control and success with the current regimen. There is insufficient information here to make the decision.

Intensive glucose lowering with insulin–dextrose infusion did bring down mortality in acute ST elevation myocardial infarction (STEMI) in the DIGAMI 1 trial. However, subsequent trials have failed to yield the same benefit. Current guidelines only give it as a class II recommendation due to insufficient evidence. In this case, the patient does not have acute STEMI and hence the guidelines do not apply.

Answer C is also not the preferred one here as the angiographic picture is best treated by CABG.

Kushner, FG et al. 2009 Focused Updates: ACC/AHA Guidelines for the Management of Patients With ST-Elevation Myocardial Infarction (updating the 2004 Guideline and 2007 Focused Update) and ACC/AHA/SCAI Guidelines on Percutaneous Coronary Intervention (updating the 2005 Guideline and 2007 Focused Update): a report of the American College of Cardiology Foundation/American Heart Association Task Force on Practice Guidelines. Circulation 2009; 120:2271.

8. D Oral metoprolol and enoxaparin therapeutic dose

The ECG shows atrial fibrillation at a rate of 130 beats per minute. There are also some T-wave changes in the lateral leads.

The patient is haemodynamically stable and from the history it is likely that she developed the atrial fibrillation in the last week. Hence, there is no indication for DC cardioversion at present. Chemical or DC cardioversion should be attempted only after an adequate period of anticoagulation to prevent thromboembolism, since it is >48 hours after onset. If facilities for transoesophageal echocardiography (TOE) are available at short notice, then TOE can be used to look for the presence of left atrial thrombus and if absent, cardioversion can be carried out under heparin cover.

In this clinical scenario (haemodynamically stable atrial fibrillation 48 hours after onset), rhythm control and anticoagulation are preferred.

She does not have any contraindications for beta-blocker therapy from the history and examination, and she is clinically stable, hence beta-blockers would be the drugs of choice. Enoxaparin followed by warfarin is also indicated in a 72-year-old woman with history of hypertension and no other contraindication for anticoagulation.

Verapamil and diltiazem are the other first-line agents in cases where beta-blockers are contra-indicated. However, she is clinically stable, so there is no clear indication for intravenous verapamil.

Digoxin is no longer recommended as the first-line agent in atrial fibrillation.

Camm AJ, et al. Guidelines for the management of atrial fibrillation. Eur Heart J 2010; 31:2369–2429.

9. D No medical therapy

The ECG shows Wolff–Parkinson–White syndrome. Characteristics of Wolff–Parkinson–White syndrome in an ECG are:

1. Short PR interval <120 ms
2. Wide QRS complex >120 ms with slurred (slowed) initial deflection of the QRS complex (delta wave)
3. ST-T changes

These features, when associated with an episode of tachycardia, are called Wolff–Parkinson–White syndrome.

Wolff–Parkinson–White (WPW) syndrome is due to the presence of an abnormal conduction pathway between the atria and ventricles (bundle of Kent or accessory pathway). Apart from the atrioventricular (AV) node and the His–Purkinje fibres, the atria and ventricles are electrically isolated from each other. The bundle of Kent offers another pathway via the ventricular musculature for the electrical impulses to reach the ventricles from the atria. Impulses passing through this accessory pathway (AP) produce a wider, 'fusion' QRS complex as the ventricular muscle is activated first, as represented by the initial delta wave, followed by activation of the His–Purkinje system occurring via the normal conduction pathway. On the other hand, this accessory pathway bypasses the normal AV nodal delay, thus resulting in the shorter PR interval (pre-excitation). Concealed WPW syndrome occurs when the AP conducts retrogradely only from ventricles to atria and hence normal sinus beats show a narrow QRS complex with normal PR interval.

Typically the AP has more rapid conduction but a longer refractory period compared with the AV node. The most common arrhythmia in WPW syndrome is narrow complex AV re-entry tachycardia. The second most common is atrial fibrillation (AF), which occurs in about half of people with WPW syndrome. In individuals who have rapid conduction from the atria to the ventricles via the AP, the AP can conduct without the associated AV nodal delay resulting in rapid ventricular rates. This can result in shock and can lead to ventricular fibrillation (VF). QRS complexes are often wide in this instance and can change from beat to beat, especially if there are fusion beats from the conduction through the AV node as well.

In cases of AF with WPW syndrome and complexes showing pre-excitation, drugs that inhibit the AV node such as digoxin and verapamil are contraindicated. Hence digoxin, beta-blockers (apart from sotalol) and non-dihydropyridine calcium channel blockers such as verapamil and diltiazem should be only cautiously used in WPW syndrome with pre-excitation AF as they may increase the conduction through the AP. Digoxin and verapamil given intravenously tend to shorten the refractory interval of the AP, resulting in faster ventricular rates and may increase the risk of AF. When there is no haemodynamic compromise, procainamide, amiodarone or ibutilide can be used. If the patient is haemodynamically unstable, DC cardioversion should be used. There are, however, some reports stating that amiodarone could induce VF in pre-excitation AF.

In tachyarrhythmias without the pre-excitation, AV nodal slowing can be used. For long-term therapy, the best option is electrophysiological evaluation and ablation of the AP. For narrow complex tachycardias, beta-blockers and calcium channel blockers can be used. In this patient who presented with wide complex AF with haemodynamic compromise and ECG after cardioversion, showing the classic features of WPW syndrome, the best treatment would be catheter ablation which has over 90% success rate, regardless of age. If medical therapy is preferred for whatever reason, especially where ablation has failed or arrhythmias have recurred, class Ia, Ic or III drugs such as quinidine, flecainide, amiodarone and propafenone are preferred as they increase the refractoriness and slow the conduction rate of the AP.

European Heart Rhythm Association; European Association for Cardio-Thoracic Surgery. Guidelines for the management of atrial fibrillation: the Task Force for the Management of Atrial Fibrillation of the European Society of Cardiology (ESC). Europace 2010; 12(10):1360–1420.

Fengler BT, Brady WJ, Plautz CU. Atrial fibrillation in the Wolff–Parkinson–White syndrome: ECG recognition and treatment in the ED. Am J Emerg Med 2007; 25(5):576–583.

Thanavaro JL, Thanavaro S. Clinical presentation and treatment of atrial fibrillation in Wolff–Parkinson–White syndrome. Heart Lung 2010; 39(2):131–136.

10. D Beta-blockers

Cocaine blocks the re-uptake of noradrenaline and dopamine at the presynaptic adrenergic terminals, causing an accumulation of catecholamines at the postsynaptic terminal and is hence a powerful sympathomimetic. Cocaine can induce coronary ischaemia via arterial spasm as well as by increasing myocardial oxygen demand (increased heart rate and contraction because of adrenergic stimulation). Cocaine is also known to increase platelet adhesion and enhance thrombosis.

Coronary spasm is due to vasoconstriction via α-adrenergic stimulation as well as by increasing endothelin-1, which is a powerful vasoconstrictor. Aspirin would therefore be indicated since cocaine has effects on platelet adhesion. Benzodiazepines are also indicated especially in acute cocaine intoxication.

Angiotensin-converting enzyme inhibitors are also not contraindicated as they do not have much effect on the sympathetic system. Nitroglycerin is a vasodilator and is useful in reducing the high blood pressure induced by cocaine and also in relieving vasospasm.

Beta-blockers, on the other hand, can cause unopposed α-adrenergic stimulation and hence can enhance vasospasm and increase blood pressure. Hence, they are to be used with caution in acute cocaine intoxication.

Cord J, et al Management of cocaine-associated chest pain and myocardial infarction: a scientific statement from the American Heart Association Acute Cardiac Care Committee of the Council on Clinical Cardiology. Circulation 2008; 117:1897–1907.

11. C Implantable cardioverter defibrillator

The echocardiographic findings suggest hypertrophic cardiomyopathy.

Although there is systolic anterior motion of the anterior mitral valve leaflet, the mitral regurgitation is mild. The left ventricular outflow tract (LVOT) gradient is 20 mmHg and this, along with the absence of other symptoms, suggests that he does not need septal ablation or myomectomy. Although dual chamber pacing would improve the outflow tract obstruction, in isolation it is not indicated here. Sudden cardiac death is a very real threat in the case of hypertrophic cardiomyopathy and risk stratification is important.

The risk of sudden cardiac death is higher if:
- There is family history of sudden cardiac death related to hypertrophic cardiomyopathy
- One or more unexplained recent syncopal episodes
- Significant LV hypertrophy with wall thickness >30 mmHg
- Non-sustained ventricular tachycardia (NSVT) on ambulatory ECG monitoring
- Attenuated or hypotensive blood pressure response to exercise.

In those aged 18–50 years, the presence of one or more of these risk factors would merit consideration for an implantable cardioverter defibrillator (ICD) implantation. In those aged 65 years or more, a stronger risk factor profile needs to be present prior to ICD implantation.

There are other secondary risk factors to be considered as well, such as: LVOT gradient >30 mmHg, LV apical aneurysm, certain genetic mutations such as double sarcomere mutations and *LAMP2*, extensive delayed enhancement in cardiac MRI and end-stage phase with widespread scarring.

In this case, this young man has a strong family history of sudden cardiac death and episodes of NSVT in Holter monitoring, as well as a recent episode of unexplained syncope. Even in the absence of significant abnormalities in exercise testing, he would be a strong candidate for ICD implantation.

Marron BJ. Contemporary insights and strategies for risk stratification and prevention of sudden death in hypertrophic cardiomyopathy. Circulation 2010; 121:445–456.

12. B Biventricular pacemaker–defibrillator

This person has New York Heart Association (NYHA) class 4 symptoms. He is already under the care of the heart failure clinic and is on optimised medical therapy. His ECG shows a widened QRS complex, his echocardiogram shows an ejection fraction less than 35% and there is no reversible ischaemia.

Under these circumstances he has a significant risk of death due to arrhythmia. However, a single chamber ICD would not do anything for his symptoms.

A biventricular pacemaker–defibrillator, on the other hand, would allow for resynchronisation of right and left ventricles [cardiac resynchronisation therapy – (CRT)] and might result in an improvement of the symptoms.

Class 1 indication for cardiac resynchronisation therapy include: NYHA class 3–4 symptoms, LV dilatation, LV ejection fraction <35%, sinus rhythm and QRS duration ≥120 ms.

Guidelines for cardiac pacing and cardiac resynchronization therapy. Eur Heart J 2007; 28:2256–2295.

13. C No infective endocarditis prophylaxis required

There have been changes in the recent guidelines for infective endocarditis (IE) prophylaxis since it has been recognised that there is no firm evidence to suggest that routine IE prophylaxis is of any benefit. Some harm may be present due to the potential for anaphylaxis.

The National Institute of Health and Clinical Excellence and the European Society of Cardiology recommend that infective endocarditis prophylaxis be given only to those at the highest risk of IE and only for the most infection-prone procedures. Currently only people with prosthetic heart valves, previous IE and certain congenital heart diseases are recommended to have IE prophylaxis.

Most dental procedures, upper and lower gastrointestinal endoscopy, bronchoscopy, and obstetric and urological procedures need not be accompanied by IE prophylaxis. Thus mitral prolapse with or without mitral regurgitation alone does not necessitate prophylaxis and endoscopy alone is not one of the high-risk procedures. Stress echocardiography may provide helpful information including pulmonary artery systolic pressure, but is not required in this situation.

Guidelines on the prevention, diagnosis, and treatment of infective endocarditis. Eur Heart J 2009; 30:2369–2413.

14. C Open surgical repair of the aneurysm

The important question here is the rate of growth. In general, the larger the aneurysm diameter, the higher the risk of rupture. For size 4.0–5.4 cm the risk of rupture is between 0.5 and 5%.

Symptomatic aneurysms warrant repair. In asymptomatic aneurysms, ultrasound/CT monitoring is advised. The interval depends on size. If it is less than 4 cm, monitoring every 2–3 years is advised. The frequency is increased to 6 monthly when size exceeds 4 cm and if it exceeds 5 cm 3 monthly.

The American College of Cardiology (ACC) criteria suggest that aneurysm repair should be contemplated when the diameter exceeds 5.5 cm. However, the rate of expansion is also important. In this case, the aneurysm grew by 1.1 cm over a period of 6 months. If the rate of growth exceeds 0.5 cm every 6 months, then repair has to be considered.

Medical therapy would consist of good blood pressure control though the target of 125/75 mmHg has not been suggested. Beta-blockers have been tried with equivocal results. Statin therapy improves overall mortality but not aneurysm expansion. Smoking increases the rate of expansion.

Endovascular repair is being evaluated. Currently it is suggested for people who are poor surgical candidates. This person has no other major risk factors and would not fall into that category.

Hirsch A T, et al. ACC/AHA Guidelines for the Management of Patients with Peripheral Arterial Disease (lower extremity, renal, mesenteric, and abdominal aortic): a collaborative report from the American Associations for Vascular Surgery/Society for Vascular Surgery, Society for Cardiovascular Angiography and Interventions, Society for Vascular Medicine and Biology, Society of Interventional Radiology, and the ACC/AHA Task Force on Practice Guidelines (writing committee to develop guidelines for the management of patients with peripheral arterial disease)–summary of recommendations. J Vasc Interv Radiol 2006; 17:1383–1397.

15. D Plan left heart catheterisation within the next 96 hours

This patient presented with symptoms suggestive of unstable angina and has had a positive troponin. Hence he has a non-ST elevation myocardial infarction (NSTEMI). ECG shows ST–T changes suggestive of NSTEMI/unstable angina (UA).

The initial management of UA/NSTEMI is as suggested: continue aspirin, if already on it; if not load with 300 mg aspirin and continue at 75 mg once daily. The second antiplatelet agent of choice is usually a thienopyridine such as clopidogrel or prasugrel. The next step depends on the patient's risk status. To assess risk, either a TIMI or GRACE score is used. Initial conservative strategy is recommended for those at low risk of an event in 6 months. For those at medium or high risk, an early intervention strategy is recommended. In this case – given his age, past history, ECG changes and elevation of cardiac enzymes – he falls into the high-risk category. Hence early intervention strategy, i.e. left heart catheterisation within 96 hours, would be preferred. If he continues to have pain or if the pain recurs along with ECG changes immediate left heart catheterisation (LHC) can be considered.

The patient is already on dual antiplatelet therapy. The indication for addition of a third agent such as GP IIb/IIIa (glycoprotein IIb/IIIa) inhibitor should be made only if he gets recurrent chest pain on the dual therapy (prior to left heart catheterisation). Since there are no features suggestive of ST elevation in the ECG, there is no indication for thrombolysis.

Wright RS, et al. 2011 ACCF/AHA Focused Update of the Guidelines for the Management of Patients with Unstable Angina/Non–ST-Elevation Myocardial Infarction. J Am Coll Cardiol 2011; 57(19):1920–1959.
National Institute for Health and Clinical Excellence. Guideline CG94 Unstable angina and NSTEMI. London: NICE, 2010.

16. E Verapamil 2.5 mg intravenous over 2.5 minutes

His ECG is suggestive of narrow complex tachycardia at a rate of 210 beats per minute. Closer analysis suggests that it is probably AV re-entry tachycardia (AVRT) as evidenced by retrograde P waves visible in some leads with PR interval <70 ms.

Clinically there is no evidence of haemodynamic compromise, hence vagal manoeuvres should be tried first. However, that has not been given as an option in this question. In the absence of haemodynamic compromise, DC cardioversion is not immediately indicated.

Given that the patient has asthma, with a previous intensive therapy unit admission with severe asthma, adenosine is relatively contraindicated. Although the literature suggests that asthma is a relative contraindication and adenosine has been successfully used in people with asthma, the probability of a severe episode of asthma, in this instance, is high. This applies to metoprolol as well.

Digoxin is not beneficial in AVRT or AVNRT.

Due to its side-effect profile and slow onset of action, amiodarone is not preferred in this instance.

Verapamil has a longer duration of action and is well tolerated in asthma. In recent studies, verapamil 2.5–5.0 mg given at a rate of 1 mg/min intravenously has shown good results.

Blomstrom-Lundqvist C, et al. ACC/AHA/ESC guidelines for the management of patients with supraventricular arrhythmias: executive summary; a report of the American College of Cardiology/American Heart Association Task Force on Practice Guidelines and the European Society of Cardiology Committee for Practice Guidelines (Writing Committee to Develop Guidelines for the Management of Patients With Supraventricular Arrhythmias). Circulation 2003; 108:1871–1909.

17. C Oral aspirin at a dose of 75 mg once daily

The risk factors for thromboembolism in atrial fibrillation (AF) are shown in **Table 1.2**.

Table 1.2 Risk factors for thromboembolism in AF	
Major risk factors	**Relevant non-major risk factors**
Previous stroke	Cardiac failure
Transient ischaemic attack or systemic embolism	Hypertension
Vascular disease (previous myocardial infarction, peripheral vascular disease or atherothrombotic disease)	Diabetes
Age ≥75	Age 65–74

Any major risk factor or two non-major risk factors are sufficient grounds to start anticoagulation. If only one non-major risk factor is present then a clinical decision has to be made to start oral anticoagulation or aspirin. If no risk factors are present then one can opt for no therapy or oral aspirin alone.

The current ESC (European Society of Cardiology) guidelines use CHADS$_2$ to evaluate the need for anticoagulation.

C – Cardiac failure (moderate or higher)
H – Hypertension
A – Age >75
D – Diabetes
S$_2$ – Stroke or transient ischaemic attack (TIA) (2 points).

Score ≥2 suggests the need for anticoagulation. Recently the CHA$_2$DS$_2$–Vasc scoring system has been used where age 65–74 years gets one point and >75 years gets two points. The Vasc refers to vascular events such as previous myocardial infarction, peripheral vascular disease or atherothrombotic disease.

CHADS$_2$ ≥2 → oral anticoagulation
consider other risk factors (age >75 – 2 points, age 65–74 – 1 point, female sex 1 point, vascular disease 1 point each)

CHADS$_2$ <2

if other risk factors ≥2 then start on oral anticoagulation
if one other risk factor then consider oral anticoagulation or aspirin
if no other risk factors then consider no therapy or aspirin

If by either of these methods the patient does not qualify for anticoagulation, then you can decide on clinical grounds to start aspirin (75–325 mg once daily) or not to start anticoagulation.

In this case, his only risk factor is prediabetes and hence we have two options: either aspirin or no therapy. Since the latter is not an option, D is the correct answer.

Camm AJ, et al. Guidelines for the management of atrial fibrillation. Eur Heart J 2010; 31:2369–2429.

18. D Open aortic valve replacement

This 86 year old has severe aortic valve stenosis as evidenced by a valve area <1 cm^2 and a transvalvar gradient of >50 mmHg. The gradient is probably more than this since there is left ventricular (LV) dilatation and reduction in LV ejection fraction.

In this circumstance, the best option is aortic valve replacement. Balloon aortic valvotomy has a high complication rate and recurrence is common. Also the survival advantage is not greater than no intervention at all.

A sufficient evidence base is not yet present for percutaneous aortic valve replacement [or transcather aortic valve implantation (TAVI)] and it is currently recommended only for those who are a very poor surgical risk. A recent study found that the 1-year mortality rate for patients who are a poor surgical risk is similar for open and percutaneous valve replacements; however, the rate of neurological complications is much higher in the percutaneous group.

Table 1.3 Assessment of severity of aortic stenosis			
Severity	**Valve area (cm^2)**	**Mean transvalvar gradient (mmHg)**	**Peak jet velocity (m/s)**
Mild	>1.5	<25	<3
Moderate	1.0–1.5	25–40	3.0–4.0
Severe	<1.0	>40	>4.0

Based on: Bonow RO, et al. 2008 Focused update incorporated into the ACC/AHA 2006 guidelines for the management of patients with valvular heart disease. Circulation 2008; 118(15):e523–e661.

This patient was independent prior to hospital admission and had no significant past medical history apart from osteoarthritis. His surgical risk would primarily be from his age and slightly diminished LV function, so he would not fall into the very-high-risk group (EUROSCORE – 7 with a perioperative mortality rate of around 7–8%).

Medical management of aortic stenosis is limited because it is primarily a mechanical issue. Statins have no convincing evidence to suggest regression, or indeed reduction, in progression of the stenosis.

Smith CR, et al. Transcatheter versus surgical aortic-valve replacement in high-risk patients. N Engl J Med 2011; 364:2187–2198.

19. B Cardiac catheterisation

The blood tests and echocardiogram, along with the negative CT and $\dot{V}/\dot{Q}$ scan suggest a diagnosis of idiopathic pulmonary arterial hypertension (IPAH), previously called primary pulmonary hypertension.

Presentation with progressive exertional breathlessness, syncope and haemoptysis is commonly seen in IPAH. Physical examination might show a loud P2 (pulmonary second heart sound). Eventually pulmonary and tricuspid regurgitant murmurs may be heard. Similarly, elevated jugular venous pressure, enlarged liver and ascites with peripheral oedema may be seen as a consequence of right heart failure in later stages.

IPAH is more common among women. Other causes of pulmonary hypertension, such as congenital or acquired cardiac lesions, chronic obstructive lung disease, other lung pathology, pulmonary thromboembolic disease, vasculitides, should be screened for and excluded.

Other rare aetiologies include HIV, anorexic drugs such as fenfluramine and dexfenfluramine and recreational drugs such as metamphetamine and cocaine. Haemoglobinopathies such as sickle cell disease, homozygous β-thalassaemia and hereditary spherocytosis have been associated with pulmonary hypertension as well.

The gold standard for diagnosis of IPAH is right heart catheterisation (RHC). Echocardiography is a good screening test, but confirmation requires right heart catheterisation. RHC allows for measurement of oxygen saturation in the veins and in the chambers of the heart, and allows for an accurate measurement of right atrial, ventricular and pulmonary artery pressures. It also allows for the measurement of pulmonary capillary wedge pressures, pulmonary vascular resistance and, importantly for treatment, response to acute vasodilators. The definition of IPAH includes a mean pulmonary artery pressure >25 mmHg, pulmonary artery wedge pressure ≤15 mmHg and pulmonary vascular resistance >3 Wood units.

McLaughlin VV, et al. ACCF/AHA 2009 expert consensus document on pulmonary hypertension: a report of the American College of Cardiology Foundation Task Force on Expert Consensus Documents and the American Heart Association: developed in collaboration with the American College of Chest Physicians, American Thoracic Society, Inc., and the Pulmonary Hypertension Association. Circulation 2009; 119:2250–2252.

20. E Peripartum cardiomyopathy

Peripartum cardiomyopathy usually presents between the last trimester of pregnancy and 5 months after delivery. The most common time of diagnosis is between the last month of pregnancy and the first 2 months postpartum. Left ventricular dilatation is common and the LV ejection fraction is usually less than 45%.

The cause is unknown but genetic, immunological, viral and pregnancy-related haemodynamic factors have all been postulated. Factors that predispose to this condition include: multi-parity, family history, smoking, diabetes, hypertension, ethnicity, malnutrition, pre-eclampsia, advanced maternal age and teenage pregnancy. During diagnosis alcohol, thyroid disease, phaeochromocytoma, cocaine, valvular heart disease and pulmonary thromboembolism all need to be excluded.

In this instance, she had gestational hypertension, not pre-existing severe hypertension, and hence hypertensive heart failure is unlikely. Idiopathic dilated cardiomyopathy is usually unmasked in the first two trimesters rather than in the postpartum period.

There is no history suggestive of myocardial infarction and the ECG does not show evidence of myocardial infarction. The echocardiogram did not show any hypo- or akinetic regions.

Although pulmonary embolism-related heart failure remains a possibility, the echocardiogram does not show right heart dilatation or hypertrophy.

Spontaneous recovery is common in peripartum cardiomyopathy and up to 50% of women recover without sequelae. The recurrance rate in subsequent pregnancies is 30–50% and hence, in women who have not recovered the ventricular function, subsequent pregnancies must be discouraged. Even when the ejection fraction has normalised, counselling should be advised because of the incidence of recurrence.

Sliwa K, et al. Current state of knowledge on aetiology, diagnosis, management, and therapy of peripartum cardiomyopathy: a position statement from the Heart Failure Association of the European Society of Cardiology Working Group on peripartum cardiomyopathy. Eur J Heart Fail 2010; 12:767–778.

21. B CT angiography

The clinical picture of sudden severe central chest pain during activity in a middle-aged ex-smoker with a history of hypertension is suggestive of thoracic aortic dissection.

The ECG may show only non-specific ST–T changes. Chest X-rays may be normal or show mediastinal widening, small pleural effusion, abnormal aortic contour or the displacement of calcium in the aortic arch. Although pulmonary embolism is the other differential diagnosis, the history of sudden sharp chest pain with back pain, normal oxygen saturation and significant hypertension on admission, points much more towards aortic dissection. He has no predisposing conditions for pulmonary embolism.

The investigation of choice would be a CT angiogram. A transthoracic echocardiogram (TTE) does not have sufficient sensitivity; a transoesophageal echocardiogram (TOE) offers better sensitivity, but is not an option in this question. Cardiac troponin would be elevated in aortic dissection, pulmonary embolism and myocardial infarction. D-dimer would be elevated in both dissection and embolism and would be helpful only to rule out both conditions when pre-test probability is low.

A $\dot{V}/\dot{Q}$ scan is not useful in aortic dissection.

22. E Therapeutic pericardiocentesis

The clinical features suggest cardiac tamponade – especially the inspiratory drop of 15 mmHg pressure (paradoxical pulse).

The echocardiographic picture of right atrial and ventricular collapse supports the diagnosis of cardiac tamponade.

Given that the patient is symptomatic and that the clinical picture points towards tamponade, therapeutic pericardiocentesis is the urgent intervention of choice.

The other investigations would delineate the aetiology of pericardial effusion, especially as this is likely to be a malignant effusion related to the previous breast cancer. However, the immediate intervention here would be to aspirate the effusion.

23. A Ostium primum atrial septal defect

The physical examination features such as the fixed wide split of the second sound are suggestive of an atrial septal defect (ASD). There are several types of ASD. The most common is the ostium secundum ASD in which there is a failure of closure of the embryonic ostium secundum. The ejection systolic murmur at the pulmonary area is due to increased flow across the valve in ASD. This situation is exacerbated by pregnancy. In adults, features of pulmonary hypertension often include a loud P2 (pulmonary component of second heart sound) and a parasternal heave. This is due to the increased blood flow through the pulmonary circulation.

This woman has also has a pansystolic murmur at the apex. This is suggestive of mitral regurgitation. In ostium primum ASD, there is an atrioventricular valve cleft which has, in this case, resulted in an additional finding of mitral regurgitation. Often in these cases there is also a tricuspid valve incompetency.

Trilogy of Fallot consists of pulmonary valve stenosis, right ventricular hypertrophy and atrial septal defect [tetralogy of Fallot has ventricular septal defect (VSD) with over-riding aorta instead of the ASD]. Here again, the apical pansystolic murmur would not be present. Patent foramen ovale is usually clinically difficult to detect and VSD would give rise to a pansystolic murmur at the left sternal edge but not at the apex. Sometimes these VSDs affect the musculature and have multiple holes so as to resemble a Swiss cheese and these are difficult to close.

Given the constellation of clinical findings, the diagnostic possibility strongly favours ostium primum ASD.

24. A Aspirin 300 mg four times daily

This patient has developed low-grade fever, malaise, tiredness, chest pain and arthralgia, a few weeks after admission for acute myocardial infarction and percutaneous insertion of a coronary stent.

Physical examination reveals a pericardial rub and left pleural effusion. Investigations show a pericarditic ECG (ST elevation in non-classic distribution), an acute inflammatory picture (raised leukocytosis with leftward shift, raised C-reactive protein and erythrocyte sedimentation rate), signs of cardiac injury (raised troponin) and an exudative pleural fluid.

There is no definite evidence of infection or cardiac failure.

This picture, developing a few weeks after an acute myocardial infarction and percutaneous coronary intervention, is suggestive of postpericardial injury syndrome (PPIS) or Dressler's syndrome. Anti-heart antibodies may be seen in high titre. Following injury to the heart, autoantigens are exposed which subsequently leads to the formation of autoantibodies and an immunological reaction.

In the era before thrombolysis and primary percutaneous coronary intervention, this was much more common. However, whether due to reduced extent of myocardial damage resulting from early intervention or due to the multiple drugs such as angiotensin-converting enzyme inhibitors, antiplatelet agents and statins, all of which have anti-inflammatory actions, this syndrome is much less common in the modern era.

Treatment is mainly by anti-inflammatory agents such as non-steroidal anti-inflammatories and corticosteroids. However, both may increase the risk of myocardial rupture. European guidelines suggest ibuprofen whereas the American ones suggest aspirin.

Maisch B, et al. Guidelines on the diagnosis and management of pericardial diseases executive summary: the task force on the diagnosis and management of pericardial diseases of the European Society of Cardiology. Eur Heart J 2004; 25:587–610.
Antman EM, et al. Focused update of the ACC/AHA 2004 guidelines for the management of patients with ST-elevation myocardial infarction: a report of the ACC/American Heart Association Task Force on Practice Guidelines: developed in collaboration with the Canadian Cardiovascular Society endorsed by the AAFP: 2007. Writing Group to Review New Evidence and Update the ACC/AHA 2004 guidelines for the management of patients with ST-elevation myocardial infarction, writing on behalf of the 2004 Writing Committee. Circulation 2007; 117:296–329.

25. C Fallot's tetralogy

This patient has all the four components of Fallot's tetralogy:
1. Large VSD (ventricular septal defect)
2. Overriding aorta, i.e. aorta overrides the VSD and straddles both left and right ventricular outflow tracts
3. RV outflow tract (RVOT) obstruction/pulmonary valve stenosis
4. Right ventricular hypertrophy.

Since there is VSD with pulmonary stenosis and overriding aorta, the blood ejected from the RV also goes into the aorta, giving rise to a cyanotic congenital heart disease. The severity depends on the degree of RVOT obstruction. This determines the degree to which deoxygenated blood enters the systemic circulation.

Squatting increases systemic vascular resistance and hence forces the blood away from the systemic circulation towards the pulmonary circulation, relieving the dyspnoeic spells. Due to reduced blood flow through the RVOT, the pulmonary component of the second heart sound is usually soft or inaudible, leaving a single loud A2.

The ejection systolic murmur is due to turbulent blood flow in the RVOT. Often there is an ejection sound due to either stenotic pulmonary valve or overriding aorta, but not in this particular patient.

ECG usually shows right ventricular hypertrophy, with no p pulmonale and often a rightward QRS axis, as in this instance.

Perloff JK, Child JS. Congenital heart disease in adults, 2nd edn. Philadelphia, PA: Saunders, 1998.

26. E Verapamil 5 mg intravenous

This patient with chronic obstructive pulmonary disease has an atrial flutter with a ventricular rate of 150 beats per minute on the ECG. The atrial rate is 300 beats per minute with 2:1 block due to the high atrial rate. The usual dictum is to rule out an atrial flutter when the ventricular rate is 150 beats per minute.

Management of atrial flutter is very similar to that of atrial fibrillation (AF) and studies have shown that it increases the risk of thromboembolism, but less so compared with AF. Atrial flutters also have a tendency to convert to AF, reflected by the common usage flutter–fibrillation.

Management strategy depends on time of onset (</> than 48 hours), risk of thromboembolism (as decided by the CHADS$_2$ score) and haemodynamic instability. Haemodynamic instability would suggest the need for DC cardioversion immediately followed by anticoagulation.

Adenosine is ineffective as with AF. An atrial flutter of new onset (<48 hours) can be cardioverted either chemically or electrically. DC cardioversion is mostly done when the patient is unstable cardiovascularly and requires less energy than AF. Chemical cardioversion can be achieved using amiodarone, flecainide (pill-in-pocket approach for recurrent atrial flutters), ibutilide, dronedarone, etc.

However, in this instance we do not know the time of onset of atrial flutter, hence rhythm control is not appropriate prior to anticoagulation for 3–4 weeks. The alternative would be a transoesophageal echocardiogram to rule out atrial thrombus.

The appropriate treatment here would be ventricular rate control. The drug of choice would be a beta-blocker such as esmolol or metoprolol. However, this person has widespread wheeze and hence beta-blockers might not be appropriate. Hence verapamil, which is a calcium channel blocker with negative chronotropic properties, would be the drug of choice. Digoxin could be used but is not a first-line drug, in this instance.

Once good rate control has been achieved and anticoagulation started, he could then have an elective DC cardioversion. An echocardiogram would also be indicated prior to the DC cardioversion. Blood tests to rule out reversible causes such as thyrotoxicosis and electrolyte abnormalities must also be carried out. Radiofrequency ablation of atrial flutter is increasingly becoming the treatment of choice for patients with symptomatic atrial flutter without a clearly identifiable transient, reversible cause.

Stiell IG, Macle L; CCS Atrial Fibrillation Guidelines Committee. Canadian Cardiovascular Society atrial fibrillation guidelines 2010: management of recent-onset atrial fibrillation and flutter in the emergency department. Can J Cardiol 2011; 27(1):38–46.

27. B Intravenous adrenaline 10 mL of 1 in 10 000 solution (1 mg/10 mL)

This question hinges on the management of asystole in a cardiac arrest situation. According to the Resuscitation Council guidelines, the management of asystole is to maintain proper cardiopulmonary resuscitation (CPR) and to give intravenous adrenaline every 4 minutes (3–5 minutes). Atropine is no longer recommended for asystole and pulseless electrical activity (PEA); 1 mg of (intravenous) adrenaline is used, most commonly as 10 mL of 1 in 10 000 solution (1 mg/10 mL).

Though there is good cause to suspect hyperkalaemia in this instance, given that the patient is on both ramipril and spironolactone, the immediate priority is intravenous adrenaline. DC cardioversion is not recommended for asystole.

Resuscitation Council (UK). Guidelines for Adult Advanced Life Support. London: Resuscitation Council, 2010.

28. D Stop beta-blockers and start diltiazem and nitrates

This woman most likely has variant angina or Prinzmetal's angina. This is primarily due to coronary vasospasm, which non-steroidal anti-inflammatories can often worsen by blocking cyclo-oxygenase. Characteristically, the attacks often occur at rest and bear no relationship to exertion or food intake. Often the attacks occur at night.

Classically, chest pain is accompanied by ST elevation and minimal coronary artery disease on angiography. The ECG changes and symptoms are not in proportion to the angiography findings. Certain ethnic groups such as the Japanese have a higher incidence of variant angina.

Diagnosis depends on a typical history with ECG findings. In some cases, the diagnosis is made on changes in Holter recordings. Provocative agents such as acetylcholine or ergonovine during coronary angiography are also used to make the diagnosis.

Beta blockers, especially unselective ones, may worsen the vasospasm. However, people with significant concurrent atherosclerotic lesions may benefit from the negative chronotropic and inotropic actions. In general, beta-blockers are better avoided in variant angina.

The main drugs used for treatment are calcium channel blockers, such as diltiazem, and long-acting nitrates. In patients who have significant life-threatening arrhythmic episodes with vasospastic episodes, an implantable cardioverter defibrillator may be of benefit.

JCS Joint Working Group. Guidelines for diagnosis and treatment of patients with vasospastic angina (coronary spastic angina) (JCS 2008): digest version. Circ J 2010; 74(8):1745–1762.

29. D Previous anterior myocardial infarction with left ventricular aneurysm and LVF

The ECG shows ST elevation in anteroseptal leads with QS complexes suggestive of a previous myocardial infarction. His symptoms began 2 months ago and lasted 2 days initially. This was followed by progressive shortness of breath. The physical examination findings suggest left ventricular failure and diffuse apex. Persistence of ST elevation in the presence of Q waves and for several weeks after the onset of symptoms suggests a left ventricular aneurysm.

The onset of symptoms several weeks ago does not suggest acute anterior ST segment elevation myocardial infarction. Brugada's syndrome presents with episodes of syncope or presyncope and palpitations. It can also result in sudden cardiac death. ECG findings include ST elevation in V1 and V2 as well as partial right bundle-branch block pattern. Left main stem stenosis with recurrent angina would present with recurrent episodes of chest pain or its equivalent.

Papillary muscle dysfunction should not present with persistent ST elevation. Investigations in this instance should include an echocardiogram and coronary angiogram. Treatment would depend on the findings of the investigations but would include secondary prevention in the form of statins, angiotensin-converting enzyme inhibitors, beta-blockers and aspirin.

Left ventricular aneurysm (LVA) is an area of abnormal left ventricular shape with systolic paradoxical bulge, i.e. systolic dyskinesia. The usual cause is myocardial infarction. Other rare causes include hypertrophic cardiomyopathy, sarcoidosis and unknown (idiopathic). Differentials include LV pseudoaneurysm (which is often a contained rupture), which has a more serious prognosis and is more likely to rupture. Post-myocardial infarction, both aneurysm and pseudoaneurysm, is likely to develop. Complications of LVA include thromboembolism, refractory angina, congestive cardiac failure, arrhythmias and, rarely, rupture. Treatment depends on the size of the aneurysm, thromboembolic potential and likelihood of rupture. Anticoagulation with warfarin and treatment of heart failure are generally accepted; surgical treatment with left ventricular repair would depend on the factors outlined.

Makkuni P, Kotler MN, Figueredo VM. Diverticular and aneurysmal structures of the left ventricle in adults: report of a case within the context of a literature review. Tex Heart Inst J 2010; 37(6):699–705.

30. E 2:1 second-degree heart block

The ECG clearly shows one P wave with a normally conducted QRS complex and the second P wave which is not conducted. The heart rate is around 20 beats per minute. This is a 2:1

second-degree heart block; however, the distinction between Mobitz type I block and Mobitz type II block cannot be made from the ECG when a 2:1 block is present. In this situation, every other beat is not conducted and there is no opportunity to observe for possible PR prolongation that is characteristic of a Mobitz type I AV block. A long rhythm strip should be obtained or a previous ECG examined to try to find evidence of PR prolongation with non-conducted beats in a pattern other than 2:1.

Given the age, absence of any contributing factors and slowness of the heart rate, this is more likely to be Mobitz type II than type I.

Treatment depends on identifying and correcting reversible causes of slowed conduction such as myocardial ischaemia, increased vagal tone and drugs that depress conduction. There is a high likelihood of progression to complete heart block and hence a permanent pacemaker is indicated. However, in this case, the patient is symptomatic and heart rate is very low, hence there is justification for inserting a temporary pacemaker to tide the patient over until a permanent system can be put in.

Epstein AE, et al. ACC/AHA/HRS 2008 Guidelines for Device-Based Therapy of Cardiac Rhythm Abnormalities: a report of the American College of Cardiology/American Heart Association Task Force on Practice Guidelines (Writing Committee to Revise the ACC/AHA/NASPE 2002 Guideline Update for Implantation of Cardiac Pacemakers and Antiarrhythmia Devices): developed in collaboration with the American Association for Thoracic Surgery and Society of Thoracic Surgeons. Circulation 2008; 117:e350.

31. B Start on beta-blockers; monitor cardiac markers and serial ECGs

This woman has presented with a stroke affecting the right middle cerebral artery (MCA) territory. ECG changes are well known to be associated with central nervous system (CNS) events such as subarachnoid haemorrhage, thromboembolic stroke, subdural haemorrhage or intracerebral haemorrhage.

The common ECG abnormalities associated with these conditions include alterations in the repolarisation patterns such as ST–T segment changes, deeply inverted symmetrical T waves or peaked T waves and QT interval prolongation. These appear soon after the event or can evolve over several days. Cardiac arrhythmias such as ectopic ventricular beats, ventricular tachycardia and bradycardia can also be seen. Pathogenesis is commonly attributed to an adrenergic surge because of CNS trauma. Involvement of the insular cortex is shown to cause a surge of noradrenaline resulting in ECG changes, arrhythmias and occasionally death.

Symmetrical T-wave inversions can be seen in the ECG shown. This pattern is commonly associated with coronary artery stenosis, but in the setting of an acute stroke this pattern can be seen without any coronary disease. An echocardiogram in these patients can show regional wall motion abnormalities and in many instances a rise in serum cardiac markers can follow.

In many cases, these changes revert, the ECG normalises and long-term echocardiographic changes are not seen. Since the risk factors of acute ischaemic stroke and myocardial ischaemia are similar, myocardial perfusion imaging may be indicated in some individuals during the recovery period. However, at present there is no routine indication for proceeding to a coronary angiogram directly in this setting. Cardioprotection in this setting may be achieved by beta-blockers and angiotensin-converting enzyme inhibitors/angiotensin receptor blockers.

Since the patient was seen beyond the window for thrombolysis for the acute stroke, the management would be to initiate antiplatelet agents. Since she also had a short run of non-sustained ventricular tachycardia, adding a beta-blocker would be appropriate to control the adrenergic surge. She should be monitored in an intensive care/high dependency care setting. Serial ECG and cardiac markers would also be appropriate so that a decision on further evaluation of the coronary artery status can be made if the abnormalities persist.

Jauch EC, et al. Acute Stroke Management. Medscape: Neurology http://emedicine.medscape.com/article/1159752-overview (last accessed May 2012).
Sharma JC, et al. Cardio-protection in acute stroke. Int J Stroke 2007; 2(4):288–290.

32. B CT pulmonary angiogram

The electrocardiogram shows sinus tachycardia, S1Q3T3 pattern (deep S waves in I, Q waves in III and T-wave inversion in III) and partial right bundle-branch block. This combined with a history of recent long-haul flight, chest pain and shortness of breath as well as the pleural rub, reduced saturations and right ventricular S3 suggests pulmonary embolism.

A D-dimer assay is not needed when the clinical suspicion of pulmonary embolism is very high. Among the options given, a CT pulmonary angiogram is the most appropriate investigation. The other option would be a ventilation–perfusion scan, which is not among the options given.

Torbicki A, et al. Guidelines on the diagnosis and management of acute pulmonary embolism: the Task Force for the Diagnosis and Management of Acute Pulmonary Embolism of the European Society of Cardiology (ESC). Eur Heart J 2008; 29(18):2276–315.

33. E Start intravenous alteplase

This patient has had a massive pulmonary embolism (PE) with haemodynamic compromise. Despite being on low-molecular-weight heparin, inotropes and fluids, he is heading for a pulseless electrical activity cardiac arrest. The strongest predictor of poor outcome in a pulmonary embolism is low systolic pressure. It also indicates massive pulmonary embolism. The tumour in his pancreas and the hospital stay were probably instrumental reasons for developing the PE.

The only interventions to be considered at this stage are (a) thrombolysis of the pulmonary embolus with intravenous alteplase/streptokinase/tenecteplase or (b) pulmonary artery catheterisation and either direct thrombolysis or embolectomy. At this level of haemodynamic compromise, arranging a surgical thrombectomy is unlikely to be practical.

Similarly, catheter-based interventions may also not be practical for this patient unless experienced operators are available immediately and a catheter lab is also ready to receive the patient and is located close by.

Several regimens are available for thrombolysis of massive PE – outcomes with streptokinase and alteplase are similar. A 2-hour bolus of alteplase at a dose of 100 mg is commonly considered. In imminent collapse, as in this patient, a 0.6 mg/kg bolus at a maximum dose of 50 mg over 15 minutes is another alternative.

If thrombolysis fails, catheter-based intervention should be considered.

Marshall PS, et al. Diagnosis and management of life-threatening pulmonary embolism. J Intensive Care Med 2011; 26:275–294.

34. A Patent ductus arteriosus with reversal of shunt

This patient has differential clubbing, i.e. clubbing of toes but not hands (there is likely to be differential cyanosis as well, but not mentioned in the case report). This along with the murmur suggests patent ductus arteriosus with a reversal of a shunt. The murmur is continuous (i.e. systole–diastole) prior to reversal, but often confined to the systole after reversal of the shunt.

The most common location of ductus arteriosus is just below the origin of the left subclavian artery. Hence when there is a right-to-left shunt, the pulmonary arterial blood from the ductus is directed distal to the left subclavian artery origin.

35. A Left atrial myxoma

Myxomas are predominantly seen in women and 90% are sporadic. They can present with systemic symptoms such as fever, weight loss, malaise, night sweats, cachexia, rash, arthralgia, clubbing, Raynaud's disease, anaemia, leukocytosis, elevated erythrocyte sedimentation ratio (ESR) and thrombocytosis.

The characteristic tumour 'plop' sound is often heard early to mid-systole and is often variable with position. Because of obstruction to the mitral valve, symptoms and signs akin to mitral stenosis are often seen.

In some cases myxomas can be familial and associated with other abnormalities, the most well-defined being Carney's syndrome (myxomas, endocrine syndromes such as primary nodular adrenal cortical disease with or without Cushing's syndrome, testicular tumours and lentigines), LAMB (lentigines, atrial myxoma and blue naevi) and NAME (naevi, atrial myxoma, myxoid neurofibroma and ephelides).

Mitral stenosis, being a low-pressure lesion, is not commonly associated with infective endocarditis. Mitral regurgitation usually produces a pansystolic murmur. Mitral valve prolapse also produces a mid-late systolic murmur.

Atrial myxomas can also become infected, although they can cause embolisms when uninfected.

Pinede L, et al. Clinical presentation of left atrial cardiac myxoma. A series of 112 consecutive cases. Medicine (Baltimore) 2001; 80(3):159–72.

36. C Hypertrophic cardiomyopathy

The clinical examination findings are suggestive of hypertrophic cardiomyopathy (HCM). A brisk carotid upstroke is often seen in HCM (spike and dome carotid pulse).

A fourth heart sound is often better felt than heard and is felt as an apical impulse in late diastole. A triple apical impulse is often found in HCM, especially in people with left ventricular (LV) outflow tract obstruction.

Two impulses are felt in systole: early systolic, because of LV contraction, and late systolic, because of the near empty left ventricle undergoing isometric contraction and the palpable S4 in late diastole. Flow through the LV outflow tract results in a harsh systolic crescendo-decrescendo murmur that starts after the first heart sounds and ends before the second. These are heard slightly medial to the apex.

Manoeuvres that decrease the afterload, increase contractility or decrease the preload increase the murmur. Hence standing after squatting or the Valsalva manoeuvre increases the murmur whereas squatting and isometric handgrip exercises decrease it. In contrast, in aortic stenosis the murmur decreases on standing and increases on squatting.

The bicuspid aortic valve produces an ejection click and the aortic stenosis an ejection systolic murmur in the aortic area. The click is diminished if the valve is calcified. Dilated cardiomyopathy can result in mitral and tricuspid regurgitant murmurs. Left atrial myxoma can result in the so-called 'tumour plop' sound, especially on changing posture. Mitral valve prolapse results in a mid-systolic click and a late systolic murmur.

37. D Mitral regurgitation due to posteromedial chordal rupture

The systolic murmur in a post-myocardial infarction setting, radiating from apex to the base and musical in character, is most likely to be due to a chordal rupture. The anterolateral papillary muscle usually has a dual blood supply from the left anterior descending and left circumflex, whereas the posteromedial artery usually only has a supply from the posterior descending artery. This means that the anterolateral papillary muscle is more resistant to ischaemic injury.

The rupture of posteromedial papillary muscle or chordal detachment produces a flail leaflet and mitral regurgitation, which has an eccentric jet directed towards the posterior left atrial wall. The flail leaflet may be responsible for the musical nature of the murmur.

If the rupture is acute on the echocardiogram, the left atrium may be of normal size and the patient may develop pulmonary oedema rapidly.

Sharma SK, et al. Clinical, angiographic and anatomic findings in acute severe ischemic mitral regurgitation. Am J Cardiol 1992; 70(3):277–280.

38. A Dual chamber permanent pacemaker insertion

This patient has signs and symptoms of carotid sinus hyperactivity (CSH). Positive carotid sinus massage is defined as asystole >3 seconds or a 50 mmHg, or greater, fall in systolic blood pressure during 5 second carotid sinus massage. Asystole indicates cardioinhibitory CSH whereas a drop in blood pressure indicates vasodepressor CSH, and some patients have a combination of both.

Clinically, the differential diagnoses are vasovagal syncope (usually in younger individuals), sick sinus syndrome (no precipitating event unlike carotid sinus involvement) and orthostatic hypotension (posture dependent, diagnosed by tilt-table test).

Patients with vasodepressor CSH are more likely to be female, have less syncope and have had cardiovascular disease and associated orthostatic hypotension.

Treatment of CSH consists of lifestyle advice, including avoiding tight collars, increasing fluid intake and avoiding sudden neck movements. Various medical therapies have been tried including drugs that increase heart rate such as antimuscarinic agents, fludrocortisone and midodrine, with variable degrees of success. However, most of these are in small numbers. For cardioinhibitory CSH which is resistant to lifestyle changes, pacing offers the best outcomes.

Epstein AE, et al. ACC/AHA/HRS 2008 Guidelines for Device-Based Therapy of Cardiac Rhythm Abnormalities: a report of the American College of Cardiology/American Heart Association Task Force on Practice Guidelines (Writing Committee to Revise the ACC/AHA/NASPE 2002 Guideline Update for Implantation of Cardiac Pacemakers and Antiarrhythmia Devices) developed in collaboration with the American Association for Thoracic Surgery and Society of Thoracic Surgeons. J Am Coll Cardiol 2008; 51(21):e1–62.
Healey J, et al. The management of patients with carotid sinus syndrome: is pacing the answer? Clin Auton Res 2004; 14(1):80–86.

39. A Immediate aortic valve surgery under antibiotic cover

The history and clinical picture are suggestive of acute infective endocarditis on a bicuspid aortic valve. The normal left ventricular (LV) size and moderate aortic regurgitation with high LV end-diastolic pressure suggest acute aortic regurgitation with pulmonary oedema.

Clinically, he is in acute pulmonary oedema. Acute aortic regurgitation (AR) with pulmonary oedema warrants urgent aortic valve surgery. Broad-spectrum antibiotics should be started prior to surgery; however, there is no need to wait for 48 hours before surgery.

Surgery is urgently indicated if there is evidence of pulmonary oedema, rapidly rising left ventricular end-diastolic pressure, emboli (in this instance stroke and renal infarcts), periannular extension or cardiogenic shock. The role of anticoagulation in this setting is controversial, especially in the first 2 weeks. The priority is surgery to replace the aortic valve.

Prendergast BD, Tornos P. Surgery for infective endocarditis: who and when? Circulation 2010; 121(9):1141–1152.

40. A Abdominal fat pad aspiration

This patient presents with ecchymoses, macroglossia and features of congestive cardiac failure. The ECG shows low-voltage complexes, but the echocardiogram shows features of hypertrophy. This and the characteristic 'ground glass' or granular sparkling appearance of the myocardium should raise suspicion of cardiac amyloidosis.

To establish the diagnosis of amyloidosis, a tissue biopsy is the most definitive option. Abdominal fat pad aspiration is the best option. Endomyocardial biopsy is the gold standard; however, this is not often the first-line test.

The most common cause of cardiac amyloidosis is amyloid light (AL) chain amyloidosis due to clonal proliferation of plasma cells with overproduction of light chain (or occasionally heavy chain) immunoglobulin. Occasionally, this can be due to mature B-cell lymphoma. In the AL type, the kidneys are the most commonly involved organ, followed by the heart, which is also the case here. Cardiac involvement commonly takes the form of restrictive cardiomyopathy.

Treatment involves eliminating the plasma cells responsible for the clonal proliferation. Melphalan and dexamethasone along with cyclophosphamide, thalidomide derivatives and bortezomib have been used. Autologous stem cell transplants have also been used.

The other forms of amyloidosis that can affect the heart include familial amyloidosis associated with transthyretin, senile amyloidosis and AA type amyloidosis, which is associated with chronic inflammatory diseases such as rheumatoid arthritis and Crohn's disease.

Kapoor P, et al. Cardiac amyloidosis: a practical approach to diagnosis and management. Am J Med 2011; 124(11):1006–1015.

41. E Myocardial perfusion scan

The answer is based on the new NICE guidance for stable angina. This man has atypical angina.

Typical angina is defined as constricting chest discomfort in the chest, neck, shoulders, arms or jaw, which is brought on by exertion and relieved by nitrates or rest within 5 minutes. Typical angina has all three of these features, whereas atypical angina may have two of these and pain with one or none is felt to be non-anginal.

In people with atypical angina, further evaluation depends on the individual likelihood of coronary artery disease (CAD). This man has a 45–60% likelihood of CAD.

For people with a 10–30% risk and with clinical features supportive of atypical angina, the investigation of choice is CT calcium scoring. For those with a 30–60% likelihood of CAD, the test of choice is functional non-invasive imaging such as a stress echocardiogram, myocardial perfusion scanning, first-pass contrast-enhanced magnetic resonance perfusion or MRI for stress-induced wall motion abnormalities. In those with a 60–90% likelihood of CAD, the test of choice is invasive coronary angiography.

National Institute for Health and Clinical Excellence. Chest Pain of Recent Onset: Assessment and diagnosis of recent onset chest pain or discomfort of suspected cardiac origin. London: NICE, 2010.

42. E In-stent thrombosis

This patient most likely has had another acute ST elevation myocardial infarction in the same vessel territory 3 weeks after a stent insertion. In-stent restenosis is more likely after a few months rather than a few weeks after percutaneous coronary intervention. Coronary artery dissection can produce an acute myocardial infarction in the periprocedure time-frame. It can also increase the risk of in-stent thrombosis at a later date, but is unlikely to cause a myocardial infarction of itself. Dislodgement of the stent is very rare and was more common previously with manual crimping of the stent. This usually happens during the procedure.

Aneurysms following stent insertion are extremely uncommon.

The most likely pathology is subacute stent thrombosis. Although the balance of evidence does not show any increase in adverse events with the combination of proton pump inhibitors and clopidogrel, omeprazole in particular is known to affect the bioavailability of clopidogrel. This is especially true in the case of slow metabolisers (impaired cytochrome P450 CYP2C19 action which helps convert clopidogrel to its active metabolite). This is likely to be a factor here.

The most common cause of in-stent thrombosis remains the interruption to the dual antiplatelet therapy. Other factors include: vessel size, location of the lesion, undersized stent, incomplete stent apposition, residual stenosis and dissection.

The majority of in-stent thrombosis occurs within 30 days of the procedure. The incidence is about 1%. Late stent thrombosis has an incidence of 0.2–0.6% per year after the initial 30 days and is more likely in drug-eluting stents (DESs) rather than bare metal stents (BMSs).

In-stent restenosis, on the other hand usually presents as angina rather than myocardial infarction and is less common in DESs compared with BMSs.

Levine GN, et al. 2011 ACCF/AHA/SCAI Guideline for Percutaneous Coronary Intervention: a report of the American College of Cardiology Foundation/American Heart Association Task Force on Practice Guidelines and the Society for Cardiovascular Angiography and Interventions. Circulation 2011; 124(23):e574–651.

43. D Implantable cardioverter defibrillator (ICD) insertion

From the history, clinical examination and echocardiographic findings, this student has hypertrophic cardiomyopathy (HCM). Left ventricular wall thickness of 15 mm or more should raise suspicion of HCM.

The management of HCM depends on:
1. Left ventricular outflow tract (LVOT) obstruction and symptoms
2. Risk of sudden cardiac death
3. Atrial fibrillation.

Apart from one episode of syncope, he is not symptomatic. His peak LVOT gradient is 30 mmHg at rest. Ideally, a gradient after exercise or pharmacological intervention such as amyl nitrate should be obtained. A gradient >50 mmHg suggests the need for intervention such as drugs, alcohol ablation or surgical myectomy.

Risk of sudden cardiac death (SCD) depends on:
1. Previous episodes of ventricular fibrillation (VF)/ventricular tachycardia (VT)
2. Previous episodes of syncope
3. Family history of SCD in more than one first-degree relative
4. Episodes of non-sustained ventricular tachycardia (NSVT) on ambulatory monitor
5. LV wall thickness >30 mm
6. Abnormal blood pressure response during exercise ECG
7. LVOT gradient >30 mmHg.

Recommendations for ICD placement suggest that it should be a decision tailored on an individual basis depending on patient involvement. ICD insertion is suggested for patients with HCM and previous history of cardiac arrest, VF or haemodynamically significant VT.

An ICD for patients with HCM is also recommended with: sudden death due to HCM in a first-degree relative, LV wall thickness >3 cm and episode of syncope. NSVT and abnormal blood pressure response to exercise may be indications in the presence of other factors.

This student has both a recent history of syncope and a Holter recording showing an episode of NSVT. Thus, the appropriate treatment would be an ICD insertion.

American College of Cardiology Foundation/American Heart Association Task Force on Practice et al. 2011 ACCF/AHA guideline for the diagnosis and treatment of hypertrophic cardiomyopathy: a report of the American College of Cardiology Foundation/American Heart Association Task Force on Practice Guidelines. J Thorac Cardiovasc Surg 2011; 142(6):e153–203.

Chapter 2

Dermatology

Questions

1. A 54-year-old woman presented with symptoms of muscle weakness and myalgia. She had also noticed some stiffness and pain in the small joints of her fingers. She had recently been diagnosed with hypercholesterolaemia and started simvastatin 3 weeks ago. She had no other past medical history of note and took no other medication.

   On examination, she had an erythematous rash on her upper eyelids, some mild tenderness of the muscles in her upper limbs and a violaceous erythema over the extensor surface of her fingers. The rest of her examination was unremarkable.

   Investigations:

haemoglobin 13.2 g/dL (13.0–18.0)	creatine kinase 564 U/L (35–170)
white cell count 5.4 × 10⁹/L (4–11)	C-reactive protein 45 mg/L (<10)
platelets 168 × 10⁹/L (150–400)	

   antinuclear antibody 1/160 (negative)
   anti-Jo-1 antibody positive (negative)

   What is the most likely diagnosis?

   A   Cutaneous T-cell lymphoma
   B   Dermatomyositis
   C   Systemic lupus erythematosus
   D   Systemic sclerosis
   E   Trichinosis

2. A 63-year-old man presented with a rash on his left leg which had been rapidly progressing over a few hours. He gave a history of cutting his foot on a nail the day before. He had a past medical history of type 2 diabetes. His current medication was metformin and aspirin.

   On examination, he was in severe pain. He had a temperature of 38.5°C, pulse 140 beats per minute and blood pressure 76/40 mmHg. There was erythema and swelling of his left calf extending up to his knee with blistering of the skin. Palpation of his calf displayed severe tenderness associated with crepitus.

   What is the most likely causative organism?

   A   Group A β-haemolytic streptococcus
   B   Group B streptococcus
   C   Coagulase-negative staphylococcus
   D   *Pseudomonas aeruginosa*
   E   *Staphylococcus aureus*

3. A 70-year-old woman presented with blistering on her arms and legs which was preceded by itching. She had a past medical history of ischaemic heart disease and was recently admitted to hospital with congestive cardiac failure. Her current medication included aspirin, simvastatin, ramipril and furosemide.

On examination, she appeared well. There were no oral or mucosal lesions. She had tense blisters on the flexor aspects of her elbows and knees.

What is the most likely diagnosis?

A   Bullous pemphigoid
B   Cicatricial pemphigoid
C   Dermatitis herpetiformis
D   Epidermolysis bullosa
E   Pemphigus vulgaris

4.   A 48-year-old businessman presented with a non-pruritic rash. He was otherwise well. He had no past medical history and took no regular medications. He had travelled to New York 2 weeks ago and Thailand 2 months ago.
     On examination, he had a diffuse erythematous rash over his torso and limbs extending to his palms. The lesions were not ulcerated and there was no exudate. Inspection of his oropharynx revealed broad, flat, whitish lesions on his mucosal surface. Otherwise examination was normal.

Investigations:

haemoglobin 14.5 g/dL (13.0–18.0)	C-reactive protein 31 mg/L (<5)
white cell count 9.8 × 10⁹/L (4–11)	erythrocyte sedimentation rate 89 mm/1st h (0–20)
platelets 389 × 10⁹/L (150–400)	

What is the most likely diagnosis?

A   Coxsackievirus
B   *Coxiella*
C   Dengue
D   Hand, foot and mouth disease
E   Syphilis

5.   A 24-year-old woman presented with a pruritic rash. She had no significant past medical history and took no regular or new medications. She first noticed a few lesions on her abdomen which spread over 3 days to cover her trunk, all of her limbs and her face (see **Figure 2.1**).

Figure 2.1 *See colour plate section.*

Which one of the following is not associated with the aetiology of this condition?

A   Atenolol
B   Lithium
C   Streptococcal throat infection
D   Viral infection
E   Vitamin D deficiency

6. A 63-year-old woman presented with a 48-hour history of pain in the palm of her right hand and a spreading rash. She was a keen gardener and also had many cats. She reported a fever and rigors over the last 24 hours. She had experienced some palpitations earlier that same day.

     On examination, her temperature was 37.2°C, pulse 63 beats per minute, blood pressure 124/78 mmHg, respiratory rate 18 breaths per minute and oxygen saturation 99% on air. There was a non-confluent rash that extended across her torso and left leg (see **Figure 2.2**).

Figure 2.2 *See colour plate section.*

Investigations:

haemoglobin 11.8 g/dL (11.5–16.5)	platelets 435 × 10⁹/L (150–400)
white cell count 12.9 × 10⁹/L (4–11)	C-reactive protein 286 mg/L (<5)
neutrophils 10.8 × 10⁹/L (1.5–7.0)	erythrocyte sedimentation rate 45 mm/1st h (0–30)

Electrocardiogram: PR interval 300 ms with premature ventricular ectopics

What is the most likely diagnosis?

A   Bullous pemphigoid
B   Cat scratch fever (bartonellosis)
C   Cellulitis
D   Cutaneous diphtheria
E   Wegener's granulomatosis

7.   A 19-year-old female student presented with a slowly creeping skin eruption on her foot that was intensely pruritic. It had been present for the last 7 days and had extended from the initial 1 cm at which she first noticed it to now being 4–5 cm long. She had no other past medical history and reported no recent travel.

On examination, she was apyrexial and systemic examination was normal. On the lateral plantar aspect of her left foot there was a 5-cm serpiginous tract with overlying excoriations but little surrounding erythema. The rest of her cutaneous examination showed no other lesions.

Investigations:

haemoglobin 12.8 g/dL (11.5–16.5)	platelets 178 × 10⁹/L (150–400)
white cell count 4.5 × 10⁹/L (4–11)	C-reactive protein 2 mg/L (<5)
neutrophils 2.9 × 10⁹/L (1.5–7.0)	creatine kinase 54 U/L (35–170)
eosinophils 0.7 × 10⁹/L (0.04–0.4)	

What is the most likely diagnosis?

A   Cutaneous larva migrans
B   Filariasis
C   *Loa loa* filariasis
D   Schistosomiasis
E   Strongyloidiasis

8.   A 53-year-old man presented for investigation of a lesion he had noticed on his right lower leg. He had received a renal transplant 15 years ago for IgA nephropathy. His regular medications included ciclosporin, azathioprine and low-dose prednisolone.

On examination, he was generally well. There was a lesion on his right leg (see **Figure 2.3**).

Figure 2.3 *See colour plate section.*

Which one of the following is not considered a risk factor for the development of this condition?

A   Age at transplantation
B   Azathioprine
C   Human papillomavirus
D   Keratotic skin lesions
E   Sirolimus

9.   A 55-year-old man with known hepatitis C presented with cough, pleuritic chest pain and breathlessness. He also complained of a rash over his lower legs.

On examination, his pulse was 89 beats per minute, blood pressure 110/75 mmHg, respiratory rate 24 breaths per minute and oxygen saturation 92% on air. Auscultation of his chest revealed fine inspiratory crackles in both lung fields. Abdominal examination was normal. Inspection of his legs revealed an erythematous rash (see **Figure 2.4**).

Figure 2.4 *See colour plate section.*

Investigations:

haemoglobin 10.2 g/dL (13.0–18.0)	creatinine 125 µmol/L (135–145)
white cell count 8.9 × 10⁹/L (4–11)	bilirubin 23 mmol/L (1–22)
platelets 78 × 10⁹/L (150–400)	albumin 28 g/L (37–49)
erythrocyte sedimentation rate 88 mm/1st h (0–20)	alanine transaminase 135 U/L (5–35)
	alkaline phosphatase 198 U/L (45–105)
urea 6.7 mmol/L (2.5–7.5)	

What is the most likely diagnosis?

A   Livedo reticularis
B   Livedoid vasculitis
C   Mixed cryoglobulinaemia
D   Polyarteritis nodosa
E   Systemic lupus erythematosus

10. A 24-year-old male healthcare worker presented with a painful lesion on the pulp of his thumb. This had arisen over the last 24 hours with no history of trauma. He had no past medical history and took no regular medication.

    On examination, he was otherwise well. There was a painful lesion on his thumb (see **Figure 2.5**).

Figure 2.5 *See colour plate section.*

What is the most likely diagnosis?

A   Behçet's disease
B   Chancroid
C   Disseminated gonococcal infection
D   Herpes simplex
E   Syphilis

11. A 54-year-old woman presented with blisters on the back of her hands, forearms and face. She had noticed that the skin of the backs of her hands had become very fragile. She had also developed increased facial hair. She had a past medical history of chronic hepatitis C virus. She was not taking any current medication and had no other medical problems.

     On examination, she had bullae and erosions on the backs of her hands, forearms and face associated with scarring and pigmentary change. There was increased facial hair particularly around the temple and malar regions. She had no oral or genital lesions. The rest of the examination was normal.

What is the most likely diagnosis?

A   Bullous pemphigoid
B   Cicatricial pemphigoid
C   Epidermolysis bullosa
D   Pemphigus vulgaris
E   Porphyria cutanea tarda

12. A 52-year-man presented with painful lesions on both legs. He first noticed it about 3 weeks ago. He had type 1 diabetes with diabetic nephropathy and was a long-standing renal replacement patient, currently undergoing haemodialysis three times a week via a left brachiocephalic fistula. He had a history of atrial fibrillation with embolic stroke and took warfarin. He often missed dialysis sessions and was non-compliant with his medications which included Calcichew, alfacalcidol, atorvastatin and novomix insulin. He has been otherwise well and had had no recent procedures or changes to his medications.

     On examination, he was systemically well. On both legs there were painful lesions (see **Figure 2.6**).

Investigations:

haemoglobin 9.8 g/dL (aim 11–12 in dialysis)	phosphate 1.95 mmol/L (1.13–1.78 in CKD stage 5)
platelets 169 × 10⁹ L (150–400)	
international normalised ratio 2.2	parathyroid hormone 153 pmol/L (16.5–33.0 in CKD stage 5)
corrected calcium 2.71 mmol/L [2.1–2.37 in chronic kidney disease (CKD) stage 5]	

Figure 2.6 *See colour plate section.*

What is the most likely diagnosis?

A   Calciphylaxis
B   Cholesterol emboli
C   Disseminated intravascular coagulopathy
D   Malignant melanoma
E   Vasculitis

13. A 25-year-old woman who is 14 weeks' pregnant presented with a diffuse, macular rash over her torso and face. It was non-blanching. She was otherwise well.

    On examination, she was apyrexial with normal chest examination. Abdominal examination revealed a palpable smooth mass arising from her pelvis. There was a fine macular rash covering her torso. There was no neck stiffness.

Investigations:

haemoglobin 10.1 g/dL (11.5–16.5)	neutrophils 4.9 × 10^9/L (1.5–7.0)
mean corpuscular volume 77 fL (80–96)	platelets 345 × 10^9/L (150–400)
white cell count 5.7 × 10^9/L (4–11)	C-reactive protein 13 mg/L (<5)

Urine dipstick: negative

Urine β-human chorionic gonadotrophin: positive

What is the next most appropriate management step?

A   Intravenous aciclovir
B   Intravenous ceftriaxone
C   Intravenous immunoglobulin
D   Send rubella and parvovirus serology
E   Send varicella-zoster serology

14. A 65-year-old woman was admitted with left-sided abdominal pain and vomiting that was diagnosed as acute diverticulitis. She had a history of chronic cryptogenic cirrhosis and known diverticular disease.

On admission, she was hypotensive and septic, and developed both an acute liver and acute kidney injury. She was treated empirically with tazocin and gentamicin. Ten days later, she had a mildly pruritic, erythematous, maculopapular rash on both lower limbs (see **Figure 2.7**).

Figure 2.7 *See colour plate section.*

Investigations:

IgA 1.0 g/L (0.8–3.0)	C3 1.9 g/L (0.65–1.9)
IgG 8.0 g/L (6–13)	C4 0.18 g/L (0.15–0.5)
IgM 1.6 g/L (0.4–2.5)	

Antineutrophil cytoplasmic antibody: negative
Urine dipstick: negative
Hepatitis B and C serology: negative

What is the most likely cause of the rash?

A   Cryoglobulinaemia
B   Granulomatosis with polyangiitis (GPA) (Wegener's granulomatosis)
C   Henoch–Schönlein syndrome
D   Tazocin
E   Toxic shock syndrome

15. A 74-year-old man was referred to the dermatology clinic. He was a retired landscape gardener. He had noticed several small, very rough spots (all less than 5 mm diameter) on his scalp, ears and forearms, some of which had recently enlarged and become more red and scaly.

What would you advise him regarding his diagnosis?

A   It is benign and does not require follow-up
B   It may progress to squamous cell carcinoma
C   It may progress to malignant melanoma
D   It will not respond to cryotherapy
E   It will require treatment with chemotherapy

16. A 69-year-old man presented unwell with a rash. This had progressed over the last 12 hours after he received his first erythropoietin injection the day before. He had a past medical history of diabetes mellitus and chronic kidney disease.

His temperature was 35.6°C, pulse 125 beats per minute, blood pressure 85/52 mmHg and oxygen saturation 99% on air. Systemic examination was normal. He had a generalised, erythematous skin rash (see **Figure 2.8**).

Figure 2.8 *See colour plate section.*

Investigations:

haemoglobin 8.9 g/dL (13.0–18.0)	C-reactive protein 13 mg/L (<5)
white cell count 16.9 × 10⁹/L (4–11)	urea 2.9 mmol/L (2.5–7.5)
platelets 568 × 10⁹/L (150–400)	creatinine 348 μmol/L (60–110)

What is the most appropriate next step in management?

A   Intravenous flucloxacillin
B   Intravenous fluids
C   Intravenous methylprednisolone
D   Oral methotrexate
E   Topical steroids

17. A 34-year-old South African woman presented for investigation of a mole on her neck which had recently become darker and seemed to bleed after minor trauma. She had an urgent biopsy which confirmed the diagnosis of malignant melanoma.

Which one of the following is most appropriate concerning the patient's prognosis?

A   Nodal status at diagnosis is the most important factor in prognosis
B   Non-ulcerated tumours have a worse prognosis than ulcerated ones of the same Breslow thickness
C   Stage I disease confers a 75% 5-year survival rate
D   Stage III disease confers a 10% 5-year survival rate
E   Tumours on the head and neck carry a better prognosis than on the limbs

18. A 19-year-old man presented with a 5-day history of malaise, fatigue, odynophagia and a low-grade fever. A course of amoxicillin from his general practitioner did not improve his symptoms.

His temperature was 38.1°C, blood pressure 124/72 mmHg, pulse 86 beats per minute and regular, and respiratory rate 16 breaths per minute. There was cervical lymphadenopathy, a tender palpable liver edge and a fine maculopapular rash over his trunk. Examination of his oropharynx revealed the following appearance which was painless (see **Figure 2.9**).

Figure 2.9 *See colour plate section.*

Investigations:

haemoglobin 13.1 g/dL (13.0–18.0)	bilirubin 7 mmol/L (1–22)
white cell count 10.6 × 10⁹/L (4–11)	alanine transaminase 56 U/L (5–35)
neutrophils 8.9 × 10⁹/L (1.5–7.0)	aspartate transaminase 76 U/L (1–31)
lymphocytes 0.2 × 10⁹/L (1.5–4.0)	alkaline phosphatase 156 U/L (45–105)
platelets 179 × 10⁹/L (150–400)	albumin 38 g/L (37–49)
Monospot: negative	
Paul Bunnell test: positive	

What is the most likely diagnosis?

A Behçet's disease
B Cytomegalovirus infection
C Epstein–Barr virus infection
D HIV seroconversion
E Systemic lupus erythematosus

19. A 63-year-old woman was referred with a 2-year history of an ulcerating lesion over her right leg. She had received multiple courses of antimicrobials with little effect. Except for some constipation, she had no other complaints and no past medical history.

     On examination, she was well and general examination was normal. There was an obvious rash over her right leg (see **Figure 2.10**).

Figure 2.10 *See colour plate section.*

Investigations:

haemoglobin 9.7 g/dL (11.5–16.5)	alanine aminotransferase 31 U/L (5–35)
white cell count 7.4 × 10⁹/L (4–11)	alkaline phosphatase 109 U/L (45–105)
platelets 587 × 10⁹/L (150–400)	total protein 95
urea 5.8 mmol/L (2.5–7.5)	albumin 31 g/L (37–49)
creatinine 189 μmol/L (60–110)	corrected calcium 2.9 mmol/L (2.2–2.6)
bilirubin 5 mmol/L (1–22)	

What is the most appropriate next step in management?

A   Colonoscopy
B   Oral co-amoxiclav for 2 weeks
C   Oral prednisolone
D   Protein electrophoresis and urinary Bence Jones protein
E   Skin biopsy

20. A 28-year-old woman presented with a 3-week history of a pruritic rash on her left shin that had not responded to over-the-counter topical emollients. She was otherwise well and on no regular medications. She reported that her boyfriend had a similar lesion on his calf.
     On examination, there was a roughly circular scaly lesion with a leading edge. It was approximately 5 cm in diameter with obvious excoriations. Otherwise examination was normal.

Investigations:

haemoglobin 12.9 g/dL (11.5–16.5)	platelets 389 × 10⁹/L (150–400)
white cell count 4.8 × 10⁹/L (4–11)	C-reactive protein <5 mg/L (<5)

Urea and electrolysis and liver function test: normal

What is the most likely diagnosis?

A   Cellulitis
B   Cutaneous larva migrans
C   Erysipelas
D   Larva currens
E   Tinea pedis

21. A 68-year-old female haemodialysis patient presented with an intensely itchy rash on her lower limbs. She first noticed a few small marks on the skin which had progressed over the last 2 weeks. She denied any other symptoms and had taken no new medications.
     Both lower limbs displayed multiple skin lesions (see **Figure 2.11**).

Figure 2.11 *See colour plate section.*

Which one of the following is not associated with the development of this condition?

A   Chronic kidney disease
B   Diabetes
C   Hepatocellular carcinoma
D   Hypothyroidism
E   Ischaemic heart disease

22. A 56-year-old woman presented with blistering lesions on her face, scalp and back. She also had painful ulcers of her buccal mucosa for the past 6 weeks which had not healed. She had no other past medical history of note and took no medication.

On examination, she had flaccid blisters and erosions on the areas mentioned as well as multiple oral ulcers. Nikolsky's sign was positive.

Direct immunofluorescence showed IgG deposits on the surface of keratinocytes

What is the most likely diagnosis?

A   Behçet's disease
B   Bullous pemphigoid
C   Dermatitis herpetiformis
D   Epidermolysis bullosa
E   Pemphigus vulgaris

Answers

1. B Dermatomyositis

Dermatomyositis is a disorder that consists of characteristic skin manifestations and an inflammatory myopathy. The peak age of onset is 50 years, and women are affected twice as commonly as men. The characteristic cutaneous manifestations are a heliotrope rash, which manifests as an oedematous erythema on the upper eyelids, and Gottron's papules – a red/violaceous scaly eruption on the extensor surface of the fingers. Other characteristic features include a photosensitive eruption, particularly over the malar region of the face, V of the neck and a violaceous erythema on the extensor surfaces, as well as periungual changes. Criteria for the diagnosis of dermatomyositis include the presence of the characteristic cutaneous findings in association with three or four of the following: proximal muscle weakness, elevated serum creatine kinase, myopathic changes on electromyography or pathological findings compatible with inflammatory myositis. Underlying malignancy should be considered in patients with dermatomyositis. A positive antinuclear antibody is common in patients with dermatomyositis; anti-Jo-1 antibodies are often positive in polymyositis. The rash classically seen in systemic lupus erythematosus is a butterfly rash across the bridge of the nose and cheeks. Systemic sclerosis causes sclerosis of the skin rather than the rash described here. Cutaneous T-cell lymphoma causes cutaneous lesions that are not photodistributed, as in this case. Trichinosis usually causes an urticarial rash.

Callen JP. Dermatomyositis. *Lancet* 2000; 355(9197):53–57.

2. A Group A β-haemolytic streptococcus

This patient has necrotising fasciitis with features of toxic shock syndrome and the most likely causative organism is a group A β-haemolytic streptococcus. Necrotising fasciitis without features of toxic shock syndrome is most commonly polymicrobial in nature. All of the above organisms can cause necrotising fasciitis, but group A β-haemolytic streptococci are the most likely organisms when there are features of toxic shock syndrome present.

Hasham A, Matteucci, Stanley PRW. Clinical review: Necrotising fasciitis. BMJ 2005; 530:830–833.

3. A Bullous pemphigoid

Bullous pemphigoid is an autoimmune subepidermal blistering disorder with autoantibodies directed against the basement membrane zone of the skin. It presents with tense blisters which can have a generalised pattern of distribution with a predilection towards the flexural areas of the skin. The bullae can appear on normal skin as well as on skin affected by urticaria. Mucous membranes are less commonly involved than in pemphigus. It is usually a disease of elderly people. Pathological findings demonstrate a subepidermal blister with a mixed dermal inflammatory infiltrate with prominent eosinophils. It may be precipitated by drugs such as furosemide.

Cicatricial pemphigoid is also a subepidermal bullous disease but predominantly affects the mucous membranes including the conjunctiva. Dermatitis herpetiformis classically causes a papular, vesicular rash, often on the extensor surfaces, and is associated with a gluten-sensitive enteropathy. Epidermolysis bullosa is a group of inherited bullous disorders characterised by blisters often following mechanical trauma. Pemphigus vulgaris is an autoimmune intraepithelial blistering disease that presents with flaccid blisters that commonly burst prior to presentation.

Wojnarowska, F et al. Guidelines for the management of bullous pemphigoid. Br J Dermatol 2002; 147:214–221.

4. E Syphilis

This man presents with the global macular rash typical of secondary syphilis that extends to include the palms. The timeframe fits with the inoculation occurring during his trip to Thailand, possibly acquired from a sex worker. *Treponema pallidum* is a spirochaete bacteria transmitted through sexual intercourse that has several recognised stages:

- Primary syphilis usually presents as a painless ulcer at the site of initial inoculation – the penis, anus or mouth of men and the vagina/cervix, anus or mouth of women. In over 50% of men and 70% of women presenting with secondary syphilis the initial chancre cannot be recalled.
- Secondary syphilis classically presents, as in this case, with a diffuse papular or maculopapular rash affecting all areas including the palms and soles. Rarely hepatitis can result, and ocular manifestations can necessitate an ophthalmic opinion.
- Latent syphilis then ensues – transmission is more likely in the 2 years after acquisition (early latent) compared with longer than 2 years (late latent).
- Tertiary syphilis can occur up to 15 years after acquisition and can result in aortitis, neuropsychiatric disease and gummata.

Diagnosis is through dark ground microscopy from the primary chancre or through serological tests. Treatment is with a prolonged (3 weeks) course of parenteral penicillin.

Hand, foot and mouth disease is one of the few other causes of a macular/maculopapular rash that includes the palms and soles. It is caused by Coxsackievirus A16 and although prevalent in children is rare in adults. The oral lesions in hand, foot and mouth are more petechial than the condyloma latum described in this syphilis case. *Coxiella burnetii* is the causative organisms of Q fever and causes pneumonia or endocarditis. A rash can appear but would not affect the palms and soles. Similarly dengue can cause a widespread rash but cannot be caught in New York and the timeframe for this patient's trip to Thailand is too distant.

Stoner BP. Current controversies in the management of adult syphilis. Clin Infect Dis 2007; 44(3):S130–146.

5. E Vitamin D deficiency

This patient has developed guttate psoriasis. Guttate psoriasis is one of the many types of psoriasis and typically affects younger patients under the age of 30 years. It presents as a widespread rash with multiple small (<1–1.5 cm), red, scaly, tear-drop-shaped lesions over the limbs and trunk. As well as a genetic susceptibility, there are several environmental factors that are associated with the aetiology of guttate psoriasis. The most common trigger is streptococcal throat infection and it is thought that up to 80% of patients presenting with guttate psoriasis have a history of a throat infection 2–3 weeks beforehand. Viral infections, such as chickenpox, rubella and roseola, may also trigger an outbreak in children.

Certain drugs are associated with psoriasis outbreaks in susceptible individuals, and these include beta-blockers, angiotensin-converting enzyme inhibitors, lithium and chloroquine.

Although vitamin D analogues are used in the treatment of psoriasis and low levels of vitamin D are associated with poorer response to treatment, vitamin D deficiency is not documented as a cause of psoriasis.

6. D Cutaneous diphtheria

This woman has a cutaneous infective process that is causing systemic upset, cardiac rhythm disturbance and a rash distant to the initial inoculation, all consistent with a diagnosis of cutaneous diphtheria. Diphtheria is caused by the bacteria *Corynebacterium diphtheria* and *Corynebacterium ulcerans* and presents with two distinct syndromes – respiratory diphtheria with pharyngeal erythema, bull neck and membrane formation; and cutaneous diphtheria with a local area of necrosis, diffuse and widespread toxin-mediated erythema. Sequelae from diphtheria are through both the local effects (including airway compromise from the membrane/pharyngeal swelling in respiratory diphtheria) and the binary toxin produced by these bacteria. Diphtheria toxin can cause a myocarditis with conduction defects in 20% of cases and a peripheral neuropathy in 10% of cases. Treatment of the initial bacterial infection is with penicillin although antimicrobials that inhibit toxin production such as clindamycin can be useful. In those with toxin-mediated effects diphtheria antitoxin can be given. A vaccine is available combined with tetanus and pertussis and is highly effective. In areas of the world where immunisation programmes have become less effective (including many of the former Soviet states) diphtheria is on the rise again.

Cellulitis is a diffuse inflammation of the skin and, although the arm appearance in the photo may be construed as cellulitis, this diagnosis does not explain the remote rash or the cardiac abnormalities. Bullous pemphigoid is a blistering dermatosis related to immune system disorders. Cat scratch fever is caused by *Bartonella* and can cause the systemic upset noted in this patient but is not typically associated with conduction defects or with rashes, instead usually causing an adenopathic presentation. Wegener's granulomatosis is a vasculitis that can cause renal and pulmonary complications but its cutaneous manifestation is typically that of purpura unlike the contiguous erythema depicted in this case.

de Benoist AC, et al. Imported cutaneous diphtheria, United Kingdom. Emerg Infect Dis 2004; 10(3):511–513.

7. A Cutaneous larva migrans

Cutaneous larva migrans (CLM) is caused by dermal penetration of hookworms – typically canine hookworms – which lack the mechanism to penetrate beyond the subcutaneous tissues and become trapped causing cutaneous irritation. Infection causes a red, intensely pruritic, serpiginous eruption. The tracks advance by a few millimetres each day but will appear only near the original site of inoculation – in this way CLM is easily differentiated from the larva currens of strongyloidiasis. Typically the sole of the foot or the buttock is affected – areas that come into contact with ground where the hookworm resides, having previously been deposited there in dog faeces. Scratching can cause local trauma and may predispose to a secondary bacterial infection.

The itching stops and the tracts will fade when the hookworms die which may take up to 2 months. Treatment with topical anthelmintics can expedite the death of the worms and thiabendazole is efficacious when used in this manner and induces fewer side effects than systemic albendazole therapy.

Brenner MA, Patel MB. Cutaneous larva migrans: the creeping eruption. Cutis 2003; 72(2):111–115.

8. E Sirolimus

This transplant recipient has presented with a squamous cell carcinoma (SCC) on his leg. In the general population it is the second most common form of non-melanoma skin cancer (NMSC) to basal cell carcinoma, although this ratio is reversed in transplant recipients. It is a malignant tumour of epithelial origin, and the clinical appearance is variable, but is typically described as a non-healing ulcer or growth with 'heaped-up' edges.

NMSCs are increased in organ recipients and all transplant recipients should be regularly followed up and educated about risk of sun exposure. It is estimated that up to 50% of all malignancies in transplant recipients are skin cancers. There is evidence that in this population the two major risk factors are amount of sunlight exposure and age at transplantation. Level and duration of immunosuppression are also clearly implicated, including calcineurin inhibitors (e.g. ciclosporin) and antimetabolites (e.g. azathioprine). In transplant recipients with malignancies, immunosuppression is often reduced to minimal levels as part of their treatment. Other risk factors are the presence of keratotic skin lesions (actinic keratoses and viral warts) and the male sex. Interestingly recipients of heart transplants are more at risk of developing NMSC than kidney recipients, perhaps owing to their increased level of immunosuppression and increased age at transplantation. There is increasing evidence that human papillomavirus (HPV) may be implicated in the pathogenesis of SCC and it has been shown that the spectrum and prevalence of HPV infection are much greater in the immunosuppressed patient.

Interestingly sirolimus (Rapamune) – a mammalian target of rapamycin inhibitor which inhibits T cells and is occasionally used as an immunosuppressive agent in renal transplant recipients – has been shown to inhibit rather than promote cancers in these patients. Switching immunosuppression from a calcineurin inhibitor to a mammalion target of rapamycin inhibitor may be included as part of the treatment of patients with squamous cell carcinoma.

Zwald FO, Brown M. Skin cancer in solid organ transplant recipients. J Am Acad Dermatol 2011; 65(2); 253–280.
Campistol, JM et al. Sirolimus therapy after early cyclosporine withdrawal reduces the risk for cancer in adult renal transplantation. J Am Soc Nephrol 2006; 17(2):581–589.

9. C Mixed cryoglobulinaemia

This hepatitis C-positive patient is presenting with a small vessel vasculitic rash over his lower limbs. This has been caused by a mixed cryoglobulinaemia, a well-documented association of hepatitis C. Cryoglobulinaemia can be associated with other conditions and if the antecedent history of hepatitis C had not been documented further investigations for these should be done:

Infection:
>   Hepatitis A, B and C; HIV; Epstein–Barr virus; cytomegalovirus
>   Endocarditis; streptococcal infections; syphilis
>   Malaria; toxoplasmosis

Autoimmune:
>   Systemic lupus erythematosus (SLE); rheumatoid arthritis; Sjögren's syndrome; polyarteritis nodosa; Henoch–Schönlein purpura

Haemoproliferative:
>   Waldenström's macroglobulinaemia; multiple myeloma; lymphoma; chronic lymphocytic leukaemia

Investigation of cryoglobulinaemia requires some planning – venepuncture for a blood sample without anticoagulants should be undertaken and the sample must be taken promptly to the laboratory while maintaining the sample temperature at 37°C. Management is with NSAIDs for simple arthralgia, but immunomodulatory drugs and plasmapheresis may be indicated for renal, neurological or other organ involvement. For cryoglobulinaemia associated with hepatitis C pegylated interferon-α and ribavirin have demonstrated efficacy.

Livedoid vasculitis is a hyalinising vascular disease characterised by ulceration of the lower limbs. It can appear as livedo reticularis but frequently with ulceration and often with thrombus. It is of unknown aetiology but has been found to occur in those with multiple myeloma and with SLE. Livedo reticularis refers to reddish-violet reticular discoloration of the skin typically affecting the lower limbs. It is caused by an interruption of blood flow in the dermal arteries, due to vascular obstruction, inflammation or vasospasm.

Tedeschi A, et al. Cryoglobulinaemia. Blood Rev 2007; 21(4):183–200.

10. D Herpes simplex

This man has a herpetic whitlow on his thumb, likely to have been acquired through direct contact with an individual with herpes virus in his role as a healthcare professional. It can, however, also be transmitted though contact with genitalia with herpetic ulcers. It can be caused by either herpes virus 1 or 2 and symptoms typically include swelling, reddening and tenderness of the skin of the infected finger. There may be axillary adenopathy but other systemic manifestations are rare. The vesicle or vesicles contain clear fluid and are painful, typically disproportionately so. The infection is self-limiting, but topical aciclovir can be applied to the infected skin and has been shown to be effective in decreasing symptom duration. Lancing may lead to bacterial superinfection and so should be avoided.

Syphilis causes a painless chancre at the site of inoculation of the treponemes. This appears as a painless ulcer that lasts for a period of time before healing rather than as a painful vesicle as in this case. Secondary syphilis is typified by a diffuse maculopapular rash potentially affecting many body surfaces, including the palms and soles. Disseminated gonococcal infection can cause a macular or a pustular rash, and this can on occasion manifest with a single pustule that could be mistaken for a herpetic vesicle. Disseminated gonococcal infection usually manifests in ways other than cutaneous lesions; however, as in this cases, the absence of other symptoms such as fever or arthralgia/arthritis make disseminated gonococcal infection unlikely. Chancroid is a sexually transmitted infection caused by *Haemophilus ducreyi* that can cause a painful ulcer at the site of inoculation. Similar to syphilis, however, it is an ulcer and not a vesicle as in this case. Behçet's disease is an immune-mediated systemic vasculitis that can cause orogenital ulceration. Ulcers rarely occur outside of these areas and finger vesicles are not part of the presenting picture.

Usatine RP, Tinitigan R. Nongenital herpes simplex virus. Am Fam Physician 2010; 82(9):1075–1082.
Drago F, Rampini E, Rebora A. Atypical exanthems: morphology and laboratory investigations may lead to an aetiological diagnosis in about 70% of cases. Br J Dermatol 2002; 147(2):255–260.

11. E Porphyria cutanea tarda

Porphyria cutanea tarda is an acquired condition caused by deficient activity of the uroporphyrinogen decarboxylase enzyme in the liver. It is associated with hereditary haemochromatosis, hepatitis C virus infection and alcohol. It presents with skin fragility and bullae on sun-exposed areas of skin. It can also present with scarring alopecia on the scalp and facial hypertrichosis. It can present identically to variegate porphyria, and porphyrin quantification needs to be undertaken to distinguish the two. The other diagnoses can all cause blistering but they do not have a photosensitive distribution, and are not associated with hepatitis C virus infection.

Cicatricial pemphigoid and pemphigus vulgaris are frequently associated with mucocutaneous lesions. Bullous pemphigoid classically has a distribution on the flexor surfaces and is not associated with scarring. Epidermolysis bullosa is associated with blistering lesions at sites of trauma and is not necessarily in a photosensitive distribution.

Sarkany RPE. The management of porphyria cutanea tarda. Clin Exp Dermatol 2001; 26:225–232.

12. A Calciphylaxis

This patient has a rare, but increasingly recognised, condition known as calciphylaxis, or calcific uraemic arteriolopathy. It is mainly seen in patients with end-stage or advanced chronic kidney disease, but not exclusively so. It is characterised by small vessel vasculopathy with mural calcification, intimal proliferation, fibrosis and thrombosis, with resultant tissue necrosis. It is thought to affect around 4% of haemodialysis patients with a mortality rate of between 60 and 80%.

The pathophysiology is poorly understood but its development thought to be related to a raised calcium phosphate product [corrected calcium (2.71 mmol/L) × phosphate (1.95 mmol/L) = 5.28; in this case guidelines suggest aim <4.0], hyperparathyroidism and vitamin D supplementation. Other risk factors include obesity, warfarin, type 1 diabetes, recent weight loss and steroids, many of which feature in this patient.

Although the differential diagnosis should include cholesterol emboli and vasculitis there is nothing in the history that would point to either of these. He is otherwise generally well and has many risk factors pointing towards calciphylaxis. The picture is not typical of malignant melanoma and he is well with no recent illnesses that would rule out disseminated intravascular coagulopathy.

Diagnosis is made on clinical suspicion and can be confirmed with biopsy. Treatment is often ineffective but includes optimising calcium load with withdrawal of calcium-containing phosphate binders, daily dialysis against a low calcium dialysate, withdrawal of vitamin D analogues, consideration of cinacalcet (a calcimimetic agent), and supportive treatment in terms of nutrition and prevention/treatment of infection. Other treatments such as hyperbaric oxygen and sodium thiosulphate have been used, but there is little evidence of their efficacy.

Bhambri A, Del Rosso JQ. Calciphylaxis – A review. J Clin Aesthet Dermatol 2008; 1(2):38–41.

13. D Send rubella and parvovirus serology

This woman presents with a viral exanthem. The cause is unclear but given her pregnant status rubella and parvovirus B19 must be excluded. Antepartum acquisition of rubella can lead to congenital deafness, ophthalmic complications and on occasion congenital heart defects. Antepartum parvovirus can lead to fetal anaemia, cardiac failure and hydrops. In the mother, parvovirus may cause an isolated transient microcytosis several weeks after the infection but this rarely causes a true anaemia. Very clear guidelines exist on management of viral exanthems in pregnancy and in this case the next step should be to send serology for rubella and parvovirus to enable appropriate referral to fetal medicine specialists.

The rash is not vesicular so varicella-zoster is not a differential diagnosis, and therefore neither serology nor aciclovir is indicated here. Varicella-zoster immunoglobulin can be given in cases of varicella-zoster IgG negative-exposed pregnant women but is not indicated in this case. Similarly human normal immunoglobulin can be given to non-immune pregnant women exposed to measles but is not relevant. The presentation is not one of a bacterial infection, and therefore there is no indication for intravenous ceftriaxone.

Health Protection Agency. HPA Rash Guidance Working Group. Guidance of viral rash during pregnancy. London: HPA, 2011 http://www.hpa.org.uk/webc/HPAwebFile/HPAweb_C/1294740918985 (last accessed May 2012)

14. D Tazocin

This patient has a widespread maculopapular rash which has several potential causes, but from the history and investigations given the most likely cause is a drug reaction to the tazocin she has been prescribed.

The diagnosis is unlikely to be due to cryoglobulins as the vast majority (around 90%) of cases are associated with hepatitis C (or B) infection which this woman does not have. In addition, her urine dipstick, rheumatoid factor and complements are normal, making a cryoglobulinaemia unlikely. The rash of cryoglobulinaemia is typically seen in dependent areas (e.g. lower limbs) and can include purpuric papules, erythematous macules and sometimes ulcerations.

GPA (Wegener's granulomatosis) is also unlikely; the immunological findings, particularly antineutrophil cytoplasm antibody which has 95% specificity in this condition, are negative and her urine dipstick is also negative. The rash of Wegener's is typically also seen on the lower limbs and is often described as palpable purpura.

Henoch–Schönlein syndrome is an IgA-mediated small vessel vasculitis, which predominantly affects children but can be seen in adults. The syndrome is characterised by a rash, abdominal pain, arthralgia and glomerulonephritis, of which the latter two are not seen here. In addition IgA is often raised in adults (>50% of cases). The rash is typically seen on the thighs and buttocks, although can be seen in the lower leg and ankles, and is also typically a palpable purpura.

Toxic shock syndrome due to *Staphylococcus aureus* is very rare in men and non-menstruating or postpartum women. It can present with a variety of skin manifestations varying from diffuse, red, macular rash similar to sunburn to more severe cases involving ulcerations, petechiae, vesicles and bullae, usually with associated oedema. Pruritus is not a feature.

Many different antibiotics are responsible for drug rashes and typically the rash is maculopapular, as here, and of symmetrical distribution. Tazocin is not an uncommon cause of drug rash and this can often be seen up to 7–10 days after starting the drug.

15. B It may progress to squamous cell carcinoma

This man has presented with actinic keratoses. These are lesions as described in the question which typically present in elderly fair-skinned patients. They are more common in men than in women, presumably because of increased sun exposure. They are often seen on areas that have been exposed to most sunlight over the years, typically the face, ears, scalp of bald men, dorsum of forearms and hands. They may also be seen on the shoulders and backs, particularly in those who have worked outdoors. The lesions usually start as rough 'sandpaper' spots which change over time to become scalier and larger.

Actinic keratoses may remain unchanged, regress or progress. It is thought that up to 25% will spontaneously regress within a year. It is also clear, however, that a significant proportion of actinic keratoses (although exact figures are unknown it is thought to be around 10%) will progress to invasive squamous cell carcinoma and should thus be regularly followed up. As patients often have multiple actinic keratoses, this risk can therefore be significantly higher.

Patients who are immunosuppressed (such as transplant recipients), particularly using azathioprine, are at significantly higher risk for many skin lesions and malignancies, including actinic keratosis, and should be regularly followed up in a dermatology clinic.

As there is a chance of progression to squamous cell carcinoma (SCC) the aim of treating actinic keratosis is to prevent this. Cryotherapy with liquid nitrogen is most common. Curettage is also used. There is some role for topical chemotherapeutic agents (such as 5-fluorouracil and imiquimod cream) also. Those at risk should use strict sun-protection measures.

Supplement on Actinic Keratoses. J Am Acad Dermatol 2000; 42:S1–S30.

16. B Intravenous fluids

This man has erythroderma likely to be secondary to his erythropoietin injection. He is shocked and intensive fluid resuscitation is urgently needed.

Erythroderma is a syndrome of intense and widespread erythema associated with exfoliation (also known as exfoliative dermatitis). Erythroderma can arise from a variety of causes, although most frequently as an extension of a pre-existing skin disorder such as eczema or psoriasis. Erythroderma may also be due to an adverse drug reaction and can on occasion be a dermatological manifestation of a systemic disease such as: HIV, lymphoma and certain malignancies including those of the rectum, lung and fallopian tube. Up to 30% of all cases of erythroderma are idiopathic. The visible cutaneous presentation is often accompanied by thermo-dysregulation and shock as in this case.

Management focuses on supportive therapy and identifying the underlying cause in order to remove the precipitant where possible. Restoration of fluid and electrolyte balance is a key objective and body temperature should be maintained. Wet wraps can be used to maintain skin moisture and emollients and mild topical steroids should be used. If secondary infection is present antibiotics should be given to cover predominantly staphylococci and streptococci. If pruritus is a feature antihistamines can be given. If a cause can be identified then specific treatment should be started including steroids for atopic dermatitis and acitretin or methotrexate for psoriasis.

Rothe MJ, Bernstein ML, Grant-Kels JM. Life-threatening erythroderma: diagnosing and treating the 'red man'. Clin Dermatol 2005; 23(2):206–217.

17. A Nodal status at diagnosis is the most important factor in prognosis

Malignant melanoma accounts for only a small proportion of skin cancers (around 4%) but is associated with significant mortality. There are various different factors that help predict prognosis. The main factors are the thickness of tumour at presentation, ulceration of the primary tumour, mitotic rate and nodal involvement at presentation.

The Breslow thickness is a measurement of the vertical height of the tumour in the skin. The greater the Breslow thickness, the more likely it is that the tumour will invade lymphatic or blood vessels; thus deeper tumours are associated with poorer survival. It has been shown that an ulcerated primary tumour is likely to be more aggressive and will behave like a tumour of greater depth. Studies suggest that an ulcerated tumour, as compared with a non-ulcerated tumour, will behave as one in the next category of Breslow thickness.

Revised American Joint Committee on Cancer staging in 2010 categorises the disease into four stages, with several subcategories. In keeping with other staging systems it is based on the depth of the tumour (T), the presence and number of lymph nodes (N), and the presence of metastases (M):

Stage I refers to patients with melanomas (T1a through T2a), without evidence of lymph node involvement and without regional or distant metastases. Stage I is subdivided into stages IA and IB, based upon the thickness of the melanoma (<2 mm), its mitotic rate, and the absence (a) or presence (b) of ulceration. The 5-year survival rate is >90%.

Stage II refers to tumours that have a higher risk of recurrence (T2b through T4b), but do not have any evidence of lymph node involvement or metastases. Stage II is subdivided into stages IIA, IIB, and IIC, depending upon tumour thickness (>1 mm) and the absence (a) or presence (b) of ulceration. It has a 5-year survival rate of 50–80%.

Stage III refers to tumours where there is involvement of regional lymph nodes or the presence of satellite metastases and no primary tumour is found (N1–N3). Patients with stage III disease are subdivided as having stage IIIA, IIIB or IIIC disease, depending upon the number of regional lymph nodes involved. The 5-year-survival rate is 40–70%.

Stage IV refers to the presence of distant metastases (M1a–M1c). There are no subgroups and prognosis is poor with 5-year survival <20%.

Tumours on the head and neck or trunk are associated with a worse survival than those on the limbs owing to their lymphatic drainage.

Balch CM, et al. Final version of 2009 AJCC melanoma staging and classification. J Clin Oncol 2009; 27(36):6199.
Edge SB, Byrd DR, Compton CC, et al. (eds) Melanoma of the skin. In: American Joint Committee on Cancer Staging Manual, 7th edn. New York: Springer, 2010: 325.

18. C Epstein–Barr virus infection

The oropharynx shows red patches on the surface of the tongue bordered with greyish-white areas. This can be differentiated from oral thrush as the white areas cannot be scraped off with a tongue depressor and form oral hairy leukoplakia, as they manifest over the ventral surface as well as the sides of the tongue. Geographic tongue is most commonly painless, whereas the ulcers of Behçet's disease are painful. Geographic tongue itself is not pathognomonic of any particular disease process and occurs in up to 2% of the population during periods of physiological stress.

Lymphadenopathy, mild hepatitis, lymphopenia and rash following amoxicillin are typical of infectious mononucleosis, the causative agent of which is Epstein–Barr virus (EBV). Cytomegalovirus can cause an infectious mononucleosis-like illness but the monospot and Paul Bunnell tests are usually negative. In this case the differential positivity in the heterophile tests is probably due to being tested early in the course of this illness. A repeat test in several weeks time should return as both monospot and Paul Bunnell positive if this were EBV. It should be noted that all five of the answers listed can cause a false-positive heterophile test, but that the definitive laboratory investigation would be serology for EBV with a raised IgM a confirmed diagnosis.

Odumade OA, Hogquist KA, Balfour HH Jr. Progress and problems in understanding and managing primary Epstein-Barr virus infections. Clin Microbiol Rev 2011; 24(1):193–209.

19. D Protein electrophoresis and urinary Bence Jones protein

This woman has pyoderma gangrenosum, an ulcerating necrotic process that most frequently affects the legs, although atypical forms that affect the hands and arms and also a peristomal form can occur. Pyoderma gangrenosum is commonly mistaken for other infective or vascular causes of ulcers on the lower limbs but does not resolve with antimicrobials and vascular studies are frequently normal. The pyoderma gangrenosum itself can cause pain and disfiguration but rarely causes greater morbidity. The condition is associated with various other conditions, however, and when pyoderma gangrenosum is diagnosed further investigation for these may be indicated. These associated conditions include:

Gastroenterological: ulcerative colitis, Crohn's disease, chronic active hepatitis
Rheumatological: rheumatoid arthritis, Wegener's granulomatosis
Haematological: multiple myeloma

The constipation mentioned in this case with the raised plasma globulins (note the marked difference between the total protein and albumin), thrombocythaemia and hypercalcaemia make multiple myeloma a distinct possibility. As a malignant condition, investigations for this, with protein electrophoresis and Bence Jones protein, should be carried out promptly. Colonoscopy is not indicated in this case, but if pyoderma gangrenosum is diagnosed in the context of symptoms consistent with inflammatory bowel disease then this would be the next step. The diagnosis of pyoderma gangrenosum is typically a clinical one although if confirmation is required a skin biopsy may show a neutrophilic inflammatory infiltrate which is not always present. Further antimicrobials are not indicated – the clinical picture shows no signs of super added infection around the ulcer. Empirical steroids are not yet indicated in this case until diagnosis of any underlying condition has been made.

Wollina U. Clinical management of pyoderma gangrenosum. Am J Clin Dermatol 2002; 3(3):149–158.

20. E Tinea pedis

This woman presents with a pruritic, contagious, lower limb rash typical of a fungal skin infection – tinea pedis in this case. This is a common presentation in those who visit the gym or public swimming pools and can be passed within households through direct contact and fomites. Clinical presentation is with a pruritic, circumscribed, erythematous, often scaly lesion that is often nearly circular in nature. In the toe web spaces it may appear as just an erythematous discoloration, sometimes with an exudate or flaky scaling. The causative organisms vary in their antifungal sensitivities and so skin scrapings for culture are advisable. Empirical therapy can then be trialled while cultures incubate – topical agents such as miconazole or clotrimazole are appropriate first-line agents. In some cases oral terbinafine or itraconazole is necessary.

Bacterial causes of this rash such as cellulitis and erysipelas are unlikely given the more indolent presentation over several weeks and the absence of a C-reactive protein or white cell response. Cutaneous larva migrans is acquired through environmental exposure to canine hookworm and cannot be transmitted from human to human. It leaves a serpiginous trail that slowly progresses over several weeks. Larva currens is the term used to describe the cutaneous manifestations of strongyloides and presents as intensely pruritic lesions anywhere on the body which appear, track for several centimetres and disappear again, all within several hours.

Field LA, Adams BB. Tinea pedis in athletes. Int J Dermatol 2008; 47(5):485–492.

21. E Ischaemic heart disease

This is perforating collagenosis, a rare skin condition in which there is transepidermal elimination of altered collagen through the epidermis. It may be either inherited, and manifest in childhood, or acquired. Most commonly the acquired form is associated with chronic kidney disease (particularly dialysis requiring) and with diabetes. It has also been associated with malignancies [hepatocellular carcinoma (HCC), lymphoma and thyroid cancer], liver disease and hypothyroidism. It is frequently associated with pruritus and so superficial trauma and the Koebner phenomenon may play a part in the development of the disease.

Small lesions begin after minor trauma and then develop into larger papules or nodules over a few weeks. They are typically intensely itchy.

The lesions are often self-limiting and topical emollients may help with pruritus. There may also be a role for phototherapy and topical steroids.

22. E Pemphigus vulgaris

Pemphigus vulgaris is an autoimmune blistering disease which is caused by autoantibodies directed against antigens on keratinocytes, leading to the formation of blisters within the epidermis. It typically presents with oral lesions followed by cutaneous blisters, which are usually distributed on the face, scalp and upper torso. The blisters are usually flaccid and rupture easily. Affected skin is often painful. Oral lesions present as persistent oral mucosal ulceration. Nikolsky's sign is positive – this is characterised by gentle rubbing of the skin surface producing erosion. Under direct immunofluorescence IgG deposits can be seen on the surface of keratinocytes.

Behçet's disease is suspected when oral ulceration is seen in the presence of two of the following: genital ulceration, skin lesions (papulo-pustules), ocular inflammation or a positive pathergy reaction. Bullous pemphigoid presents with tense blisters and rarely affects the oral cavity. Dermatitis herpetiformis presents as a papular, vesicular eruption and epidermolysis bullosa is an inherited blistering disorder where blisters often form at sites of mechanical trauma.

Bystryn JC, Rudolph JL. Pemphigus. Lancet 2005; 366:61–73.

Chapter 3

Endocrinology

Questions

1. A 20-year-old man was seen in the outpatient clinic for an annual review of type 1 diabetes. He was on a multi-dose insulin regimen with long-acting and rapid-acting insulin analogues. At the last review, his HbA1c was 6.6% (3.8–5.5) and he reported no hypoglycaemic episodes.

   Currently his HbA1c is 6.4% and he reported several episodes of dizziness. He felt generally run down and tired. He had checked his blood sugars at the time of dizziness and they were mostly in the range of 4–5 mmol/L and at other times he was frankly hypoglycaemic. He was a second year university student and reported no recent changes in activity level or food intake; he denied any alcohol or illicit drug use.

   What is the most appropriate diagnostic test?

   A   Continuous glucose monitoring to check glycaemic control throughout the day
   B   Serum insulin and C-peptide levels
   C   Serum iron and ferritin levels
   D   Short Synacthen test
   E   Thyroid function tests

2. A 69-year-old woman was seen in the emergency department complaining of tiredness and dizziness. She gave a history of increased thirst and polyuria.

   On examination, her pulse was 110 beats per minute and regular, blood pressure 90/60 mmHg and respiratory rate 24 breaths per minute. Examination of the chest revealed dullness in the right mid-zone and reduced air entry in the same area.

   Investigations:

sodium 137 mmol/L (135–145)	corrected calcium 3.9 mmol/L (2.2–2.6)
potassium 4.2 mmol/L (3.5–5.0)	phosphate 0.8 mmol/L (0.8–1.4)
urea 15 mmol/L (2.5–7.5)	albumin 40 g/L (37–49)
creatinine 190 µmol/L (45–90)	

   Chest X-ray: mass lesion in right mid-zone

   What is the next most appropriate management step?

   A   Calcitonin
   B   Furosemide
   C   Intravenous fluids
   D   Pamidronate
   E   Prednisolone

3. A 43-year-old woman was seen in the clinic with a history of a neck lump. She did not have any symptoms and the lump was pointed out by her friend. There was no relevant past medical history or family history. She was not on any medications.

Examination revealed a palpable nodule in the right lobe of the thyroid gland. Clinically she was euthyroid.

Investigations:

thyroid-stimulating hormone 3.85 mU/L (0.4–5.0)	corrected calcium 2.45 mmol/L (2.2–2.6)
free thyroxine 15.8 pmol/L (10–25)	
Ultrasound: 1.5 × 1.75 cm solid lesion in the right lobe of thyroid with microcalcifications	

What is the next most appropriate management step?

A   Fine-needle aspiration cytology
B   Radio-iodine uptake scan
C   Right lobectomy with removal of isthmus
D   Serum calcitonin estimation
E   Serum thyroglobulin estimation

4.   A 52-year-old man with type 2 diabetes and hyperlipidaemia had his annual review. He had no other medical problems. He is currently on metformin, gliclazide and atorvastatin.
        Physical examination was unremarkable except that he had a body mass index of 32 kg/m^2 and his blood pressure was 140/90 mmHg.

Investigations:

total cholesterol 4.9 mmol/L (3–5)	potassium 3.5 mmol/L (3.5–5.0)
low-density lipoprotein-cholesterol 2.6 mmol/L (2–3)	urea 5.5 mmol/L (2.5–7.5)
	creatinine 102 µmol/L (60–110)
triglyceride 2.9 mmol/L (0.6–1.69)	HbA1c 7.8% (3.8–5.5)
sodium 135 mmol/L (135–145)	

He was started on ramipril and exenatide GLP-1 (glucagon-like peptide-1) analogue injections for better hypertension and diabetic control. To improve his lipid control, he was started on bezafibrate in addition to atorvastatin. Three weeks later he was admitted to the emergency department with epigastric pain and vomiting.

sodium 139 mmol/L (135–145)	creatinine 152 µmol/L (60–110)
potassium 3.9 mmol/L (3.5–5.0)	amylase 380 U/L (60–180)
urea 12 mmol/L (2.5–7.5)	creatine kinase 348 U/L (25–195)

What is the most likely cause of his symptoms?

A   Acute kidney injury due to dehydration and ramipril/bezafibrate
B   Acute pancreatitis resulting from hypertriglyceridaemia
C   Acute peptic ulcer induced by bezafibrate
D   Acute rhabdomyolysis due to bezafibrate and atorvastatin combination
E   Exenatide-induced acute pancreatitis

5.   A 38-year-old woman was seen in the clinic after she developed a wedge compression fracture in her thoracic spine. She also complained of vague aches and pains as well as difficulty climbing stairs and getting up from sofas.
        Her past history was remarkable only for a roux-en-Y gastric bypass for obesity 8 years earlier. She was on the oral contraceptive pill and also took over-the-counter multi-vitamin supplements.

Investigations:

haemoglobin 10.1 g/dL (11.5–16.5)	creatinine 78 μmol/L (45–90)
mean corpuscular volume 82 fL (80–96)	bilirubin 3 mmol/L (1–22)
white cell count 9 × 10⁹/L (4–11)	albumin 45 g/L (37–49)
platelets 180 × 10⁹/L (150–400)	alanine aminotransferase 23 U/L (5–35)
sodium 140 mmol/L (135–145)	alkaline phosphatase 450 U/L (45–105)
potassium 3.8 mmol/L (3.5–5.0)	

What is the most useful diagnostic test?

A   Calcitonin
B   Parathyroid hormone
C   1,25-Dihydroxy-vitamin D
D   25(OH)-Vitamin D
E   Urinary 24-hour calcium excretion

6.   A 53-year-old man was referred by his general practitioner with a 2-month history of decreased libido and erectile dysfunction. He had a past history of type 2 diabetes mellitus and depression and was on metformin, ramipril, fluoxetine and simvastatin. He has had diabetes for the last 5 years and did not have any evidence of diabetic nephropathy, retinopathy or neuropathy.
      Physical examination was unremarkable and he had normal testicular volume.

Investigations:

sodium 139 mmol/L (135–145)	serum free testosterone 170 pmol/L (105–830)
potassium 4.2 mmol/L (3.5–5.0)	luteinising hormone (LH) 4 IU/mL (1–9)
urea 4.4 mmol/L (2.5–7.5)	follicle-stimulating hormone 3 IU/mL (1–13)
creatinine 78 μmol/L (60–110)	prolactin 2690 mU/L (<360)
Pituitary MRI: normal	

What is the most likely cause of his symptoms?

A   Depression-related erectile dysfunction
B   Diabetes-related erectile dysfunction
C   Fluoxetine-induced hyperprolactinaemia
D   Hypogonadotrophic hypogonadism
E   Metformin-induced hyperprolactinaemia

7.   A 39-year-old woman was referred with a history of weight gain, secondary amenorrhoea and weakness on getting up from a sitting position. There was no significant past medical history. She was on the combined oral contraceptive pill.
      On examination, she was obese, had proximal muscle weakness and central fat distribution with a rounded face. Pulse was 90 beats per minute and blood pressure 150/90 mmHg.

Investigations:

sodium 142 mmol/L (135–145)	thyroid-stimulating hormone 2.0 mU/L (0.4–5.0)
potassium 3.3 mmol/L (3.5–5.0)	free thyroxine 12 pmol/L (10–25)
urea 5.0 mmol/L (2.5–7.5)	corrected calcium 2.32 mmol/L (2.2–2.6)
creatinine 76 μmol/L (60–110)	

What is the most appropriate diagnostic investigation?

A   High-dose dexamethasone suppression test
B   Insulin tolerance test
C   Plasma adrenocorticotrophic hormone (ACTH) level
D   Two 24-hour urine collections for free cortisol
E   Short Synacthen test

8. A 35-year-old woman was bought into the emergency department with reduced consciousness. While in the emergency department she had a seizure and was found to have a glucose level of 1.5 mmol/L. She was treated with intravenous dextrose.
    She had no past history of note and was not on any medications. Her mother died of a medullary thyroid cancer and her father was diabetic.

Investigations:

| plasma insulin 140 pmol/L (fasting 20–140) | C-peptide 0.15 nmol/L (0.25–0.65) |

What is the most likely diagnosis?

A   Exogenous insulin use
B   Insulinoma
C   Liver dysfunction
D   Neuroendocrine tumour
E   Sulphonylurea abuse

9. A 52-year-old man was referred with a history of headaches, decreased libido, malaise and obstructive sleep apnoea. His wife mentioned that her husband's appearance had changed from family photos and now he had prominent eyebrows and chin. He was being treated with ramipril 10 mg and amlodipine 10 mg once daily for hypertension, but the blood pressure control was poor.
    On examination, he had prominent supraorbital ridges and large hands.

Investigations:

sodium 138 mmol/L (135–145)	creatinine 97 µmol/L (60–110)
potassium 4.3 mmol/L (3.5–5.0)	fasting glucose 6.3 mmol/L (4–6)
urea 5.8 mmol/L (2.5–7.5)	

What is the most appropriate diagnostic investigation?

A   Growth hormone level
B   Insulin tolerance test
C   Low-dose dexamethasone suppression test
D   Oral glucose tolerance test with growth hormone levels
E   Pituitary MRI

10. A 45-year-old man was seen in the emergency department after having fainted. He also gave a history of general tiredness, malaise, decreased libido and increased weight. He did not have any significant past medical history apart from an admission to the intensive care unit a year ago with head injury because of a road traffic accident.
    His general practitioner had recently diagnosed hypothyroidism and had started 50 µg levothyroxine 2 weeks ago. On examination, his pulse was 70 beats per minute and regular, blood pressure 96/50 mmHg and respiratory rate 24 breaths per minute.
    He had slight pallor and delayed relaxation of ankle reflexes.

Investigations:

haemoglobin 12.0 g/dL (13.0–18.0)	sodium 132 mmol/L (135–145)
mean corpuscular volume 80 fL (80–96)	potassium 5.7 mmol/L (3.5–5.0)
white cell count 6×10^9/L (4–11)	creatinine 76 µmol/L (60–110)
platelets 160×10^9/L (150–400)	glucose 4.2 mmol/L (4.0–7.8)

What is the most appropriate next step in management?

A   Insulin–dextrose infusion (8 units of regular insulin with 50 mL 50% dextrose over 30 minutes)
B   Intravenous dextrose (50 mL of 25% dextrose)
C   Intravenous hydrocortisone (100 mg every 8 hours)
D   Intravenous levothyroxine (500 mg loading dose then 50–100 mg daily)
E   Intravenous liothyronine (25 mg every 8 hours)

11. A 23-year-old woman was involved in a road traffic accident. Subsequently she had a subdural haematoma evacuated. She had a basal skull fracture as well. Postoperatively she had been doing well but 48 hours later developed nausea, headache and vomiting.
    On examination, her temperature was 37.6°C, pulse 110 beats per minute and regular, blood pressure 130/85 mmHg, and respiratory rate 18 breaths per minute.
    Her total fluid intake was 3 L during the past 24 hours and output was 1.2 L.

Investigations:

sodium 123 mmol/L (135–145)	creatinine 69 µmol/L (45–90)
potassium 3.5 mmol/L (3.5–5.0)	plasma osmolality 258 mosmol/kg (275–295)
urea 4.3 mmol/L (2.5–7.5)	urine osmolality 450 mosmol/kg (50–1400)

What is the most appropriate next step in management?

A   Aldosterone
B   Carbamazepine
C   Demeclocycline
D   Desmopressin
E   Fluid restriction

12. A 56-year-old man with type 2 diabetes was seen in the clinic for annual review. He was on 12 units of regular insulin three times a day and on 24 units of NPH (neutral protamine Hagedorn) insulin at bedtime. He was also on metformin 850 mg twice a day. His other medications included ramipril 5 mg once daily and simvastatin 40 mg at night. He did not report any hypoglycaemic events but said that occasionally, on waking up, the bed sheets were drenched in sweat and that he had headaches in the morning.
    Home glucose monitoring showed (normal random glucose 4.0–7.8 mmol/L):

Investigations:

Pre-breakfast: 8–11 mmol/L	Pre-bedtime: 4.5–6.0 mmol/L
Pre-lunch: 5–6 mmol/L	2-hour post-lunch: 8–11 mmol/L
Pre-evening meal: 4.5–7.0 mmol/L	HbA1c 6.9% (3.8–5.5)

What is the most appropriate next step in management?

A   Increase lunchtime regular insulin
B   Increase metformin to 850 mg three times daily

C   Increase morning regular insulin
D   Increase night-time NPH insulin
E   Reduce night-time NPH insulin

13. A 68-year-old woman was admitted with worsening shortness of breath and ankle swelling. Over the past 2 months she could walk only a few metres. She also complained of palpitations, sweating, diarrhoea, losing weight and grittiness in her eyes. All these symptoms had got worse following a recent lower respiratory tract infection.

On examination, she was sweating and had a temperature of 38.1°C. She had tremor in both hands, a small goitre and bilateral exophthalmos. Her pulse was 140 beats per minute and irregular, blood pressure 170/90 mmHg jugular venous pressure was elevated +9 cm but there were no bruits or murmurs. Respiratory rate was 24 breaths per minute, oxygen saturation 96% on air and chest was clear.

Investigations:

Electrocardiogram: atrial fibrillation rate 140 beats per minute
Chest X-ray: mild cardiomegaly

What is the most appropriate next step in management?

A   Aspirin and hydrocortisone first then propranolol and potassium iodide 1 hour later
B   Carbimazole and propranolol first, potassium iodide and hydrocortisone 1 hour later
C   Hydrocortisone first, then propranolol and carbimazole; potassium iodide 1 hour later
D   Potassium iodide first then propranolol and carbimazole and hydrocortisone 1 hour later
E   Propranolol first then potassium iodide and hydrocortisone; carbimazole 1 hour later

14. A 45-year-old woman was admitted with nausea and vomiting. Two months prior to admission, she had undergone a roux-en-Y gastric bypass operation for obesity. Her postoperative period was uneventful and she was discharged with nutritional advice. She had lost about 10 kg of body weight postoperatively.

She was treated on admission with intravenous 0.9% saline and dextrose. On the second day of admission, the nurses noticed that she was confused and unsteady on her feet. She also complained of tingling and numbness in her legs.

On examination, her temperature was 37.2°C, pulse 94 beats per minute and regular, blood pressure 110/70 mmHg and respiratory rate 18 breaths per minute. She was alert but confused in time and place. Neurological examination revealed horizontal nystagmus and reduced fine touch and joint position sense in her legs.

Investigations:

sodium 139 mmol/L (135–145)	haemoglobin 12 g/dL (11.5–16.5)
potassium 3.8 mmol/L (3.5–5.0)	white cell count 10 × 10⁹/L (4–11)
urea 10 mmol/L (2.5–7.5)	platelets 156 × 10⁹/L (150–400)
creatinine 102 μmol/L (45–90)	
Chest X-ray: normal	

What is the most appropriate next step in management?

A   Intramuscular hydroxocobalamin supplementation
B   Intravenous magnesium supplementation
C   Intravenous niacin supplementation
D   Intravenous thiamine supplementation
E   Oral zinc supplementation

15. A 59-year-old man was referred with a 2-year history of difficult-to-control hypertension. He was on amlodipine 10 mg once daily, ramipril 10 mg once daily and doxazosin 4 mg once daily. However, clinic and home readings were still in the range of 160/90 mmHg. He did not give any significant past medical history apart from hypertension.

    On examination, his pulse was 78 beats per minute and regular, blood pressure 172/88 mmHg and respiratory rate 14 breaths per minute. His body mass index was 24.8 kg/m^2 (20–25), body habitus normal; heart sounds normal and there were no bruits.

    Investigations:

sodium 138 mmol/L (135–145)	haemoglobin 12.8 g/dL (13.0–18.0)
potassium 3.4 mmol/L (3.5–5.0)	white cell count 9 × 10^9/L (4–11)
urea 7 mmol/L (2.5–7.5)	platelets 126 × 10^9/L (150–400)
creatinine 124 µmol/L (60–110)	
Chest X-ray: normal	

    What is the most appropriate next investigation?

    A   CT of the adrenals
    B   MIBG (*meta*-iodobenzylguanidine) scan
    C   Plasma aldosterone:renin ratio
    D   Plasma metanephrine level
    E   Plasma renin activity

16. A 23-year-old man was admitted with a history of vomiting and tiredness. He was being treated for type 1 diabetes and was on a basal bolus regime with insulin lispro (fast-acting insulin) and insulin glargine (long-acting insulin). He gave a history of vomiting and abdominal pain for the last 3 days. He had omitted the insulin doses for the last day as he had not eaten anything.

    On examination, his weight was 80 kg and mucous membranes were dry. Temperature was 37.6°C, pulse 120 beats per minute and regular, blood pressure 100/60 mmHg and respiratory rate 30 breaths per minute. Heart sounds were normal and chest was clear. Apart from mild epigastric tenderness, abdominal examination was normal.

    Investigations:

sodium 142 mmol/L (135–145)	creatinine 89 µmol/L (60–110)
potassium 3.8 mmol/L (3.5–5.0)	glucose 30 mmol/L (4.0–7.8)
urea 11 mmol/L (2.5–7.5)	amylase 33 U/L (60–180)
Urine dipstick: glucose ++, ketones +++	
Arterial blood gases on air:	
pH 6.99 (7.34–7.44)	
PaO_2 13 кРа (10–13)	
$PaCO_2$ 2.2 кРа (4.4–5.9)	
bicarbonate 10 mmol/L (18–24)	

    He was admitted and started on 0.9% saline infusion intravenously with regular intravenous infusion of insulin 8 units per hour. Two hours later repeat blood gas analysis showed:

pH 7.2 (7.34–7.44)	sodium 139 mmol/L (135–145)
PaO_2 12 кРа (10–13)	potassium 3.5 mmol/L (3.5–5.0)
$PaCO_2$ 3 кРа (4.4–5.9)	glucose 11 mmol/L (4.0–7.8)
bicarbonate 10 mmol/L (18–24)	

What is the most appropriate next step in management?

A   Continue 8 units/h insulin infusion, add potassium 40 mmol/L to the 0.9% saline infused at 0.5 L/h and add 10% dextrose infused at 125 mL/h

B   Continue insulin at 8 units/h and switch from 0.9% saline infusion to 5% dextrose infusion with 40 mmol/L potassium added and infused at 0.5 L/h

C   Reduce insulin to 4 units/h, add potassium 20 mmol/L to the 0.9% saline infusion and repeat glucose in the next half hour

D   Reduce insulin to 6 units/h and switch from 0.9% saline infusion to 5% dextrose infusion with 40 mmol/L potassium added, infused at 0.5 L/h

E   Reduce insulin to 6 units/h and switch to dextrose–saline with 20 mmol/L of potassium added and infused at 0.5 L/h

17. A 56-year-old man was admitted with increasing lethargy, weight gain and constipation. He had been diagnosed with hypothyroidism 2 years ago, but had not been taking the levothyroxine regularly. He also complained of loss of libido.

On examination, his body mass index was 34 kg/m². He had coarse skin, scalp alopecia, loss of the lateral third of the eyebrows and gynaecomastia. His temperature was 36.4°C, pulse 58 beats per minute, blood pressure 170/104 mmHg and respiratory rate 14 breaths per minute.

Investigations:

haemoglobin 10.2 g/dL (13.0–18.0)	thyroid-stimulating hormone 98 mU/L (0.4–5.0)
mean corpuscular volume 88 fL (80–96)	free thyroxine (T$_4$) 1.2 pmol/L (10–25)
white cell count 10 × 10⁹/L (4–11)	free triidothyronine (T$_3$) 0.2 pmol/L (5–10)
platelets 162 × 10⁹/L (150–400)	9 am cortisol 200 nmol/L (200–700)
sodium 135 mmol/L (135–145)	prolactin 1597 U/L (75–375)
potassium 5 mmol/L (3.5–5.0)	luteinising hormone 3 U/L (1–9)
creatinine 112 µmol/L (60–110)	

What is the most appropriate management?

A   Oral levothyroxine and oral bromocriptine

B   Oral levothyroxine replacement

C   Oral levothyroxine, intravenous hydrocortisone and intravenous triiodothyronine

D   Triiodothyronine intravenously with fluids and hydrocortisone

E   Triiodothyronine intravenously and oral bromocriptine

18. A 50-year-old man was referred to the hypertension clinic with a 5-year history of hypertension that was difficult to control. He was on ramipril 10 mg once daily, bendrofluazide 2.5 mg once daily, amlodipine 10 mg once daily and doxazosin extended release 16 mg once daily. There was no other past history or family history of note. He denied excessive salt intake and had made dietary and lifestyle adjustments.

On examination, his temperature was 37.2°C, pulse 90 beats per minute and regular, blood pressure 180/100 mmHg with no significant difference between the arms, and respiratory rate 14 breaths per minute. The rest of the physical examination was unremarkable.

After withdrawing and substituting the interfering drugs, the following tests were done:

Investigations:

sodium 145 mmol/L (135–145)	haemoglobin 14.8 g/dL (13.0–18.0)
potassium 3.8 mmol/L (3.5–5.0)	white cell count 6×10^9/L (4–11)
urea 8 mmol/L (2.5–7.5)	platelets 150×10^9/L (150–400)
creatinine 97 µmol/L (60–110)	

Electrocardiogram: left ventricular hypertrophy

$2 \times$ urine metanephrines: normal

plasma aldosterone 90 (aldosterone, pmol/L: upright 100–800, supine 100–450)

direct plasma renin 0.5 (renin, mU/L: upright 5.4–60, supine 5.4–30)

aldosterone:renin ratio 180 (aldosterone:renin ratio – normal <100)

9 am cortisol after overnight 1 mg dexamethasone – 40 mmol/L (<50)

CT of the abdomen: no abnormalities detected

What is the next step in management?

A   Add spironolactone
B   High-dose dexamethasone suppression test
C   MIBG (*meta*-iodobenzylguanidine) scan
D   Pituitary MRI
E   Selective adrenal vein sampling

19. A 43-year-old man was referred to the emergency department after a fall. He sustained a fracture and dislocation of his left ankle, but could not remember how the fall had happened. In the past he had had a few episodes of palpitations. The dislocation was reduced under opiate analgesia. His only other significant past medical history was hypertension for which he was on amlodipine 10 mg once daily.

On examination, his pulse was 80 beats per minute, blood pressure 150/90 mmHg and respiratory rate 16 breaths per minute. The rest of the physical examination was normal.

Investigations:

haemoglobin 13.4 g/dL (13.0–18.0)	sodium 141 mmol/L (135–145)
white cell count 8×10^9/L (4–11)	potassium 4.5 mmol/L (3.5–5.0)
neutrophils 5×10^9/L (1.5–7.0)	urea 9 mmol/L (2.5–7.5)
platelets 295×10^9/L (150–400)	creatinine 78 µmol/L (60–110)

Electrocardiogram: left ventricular hypertrophy and sinus rhythm

Later on in the evening, he was taken to the theatre for an open reduction and internal fixation of the fracture. However, on induction of anaesthesia, his blood pressure rose up to 280/150 mmHg and the operation was abandoned.

What is the most appropriate next investigation?

A   24-hour urine free cortisol
B   24-hour urine metanephrines
C   Plasma aldosterone:renin ratio
D   Thyroid function tests
E   Urine porphobilinogen

20. A 29-year-old woman was referred for suspected hyperthyroidism. Four weeks ago, she had a sore throat followed by palpitations, excessive sweating, diarrhoea and heat intolerance. She had also lost weight. She went to her general practitioner who ordered thyroid function tests which showed:

Investigations:

free thyroxine (T$_4$) 37.4 pmol/L (10–25)	thyroid-stimulating hormone 0.01 mU/L (0.4–5.0)

She was started on carbimazole 20 mg daily and propranolol 10 mg three times a day by her general practitioner. Two weeks after starting the drugs she was seen in the clinic where she said that her symptoms had subsided and her weight had steadily increased.
     Physical examination showed a pulse of 70 beats per minute and regular, and she was clinically euthyroid. There was a small smooth firm goitre with no bruit.

Repeat blood tests showed:	thyroid peroxidase antibodies 4 IU/mL (<50)
free thyroxine (T$_4$) 8 pmol/L (10–25)	thyroid-stimulating antibodies: negative
thyroid-stimulating hormone 6 mU/L (0.4–5.0)	

What is the most appropriate next step in management?

A   Reduce propranolol to 5 mg three times a day and carbimazole to 5 mg daily and recheck thyroid function
B   Stop carbimazole and propranolol and monitor thyroid function tests in 6 weeks
C   Stop carbimazole and propranolol and order thyroid ultrasound to assess the goitre
D   Stop carbimazole and propranolol and start levothyroxine replacement at 25 µg daily
E   Stop propranolol and reduce carbimazole to 10 mg daily and monitor thyroid function tests

21. A 45-year-woman was seen in the clinic for a follow-up visit. She had been diagnosed with hyperparathyroidism secondary to parathyroid hyperplasia and had had a parathyroidectomy 2 years ago. She was maintained on calcium and α-calcidiol. During the clinic visit she complained of burning abdominal pain as well as diarrhoea and occasionally she passed large amounts of foul-smelling faeces which floated in the toilet.
     Physical examination was normal apart from mild epigastric tenderness. Steatorrhoea was confirmed by Sudan III staining of the stool.

Investigations:

Gastroscopy: two small gastric ulcers and oesophagitis

What is the next most appropriate investigation?

A   d-Xylose test
B   Faecal elastase and chymotrypsin
C   Fasting gastrin and chromogranin A level in serum

D   24-hour urinary 5-HIAA (5–hydroxyindoleacetic acid)
E   Vasoactive intestinal peptide (VIP) (serum)

22. A 46-year-old woman was seen in the clinic with a history of palpitations and weight loss. She had been diagnosed with hyperthyroidism and started on carbimazole which was titrated accordingly. After 6 months, she complained of grittiness in the eyes and watering.
      On examination, she had exophthalmos, diplopia and corneal ulceration with oedema of the optic discs.

Investigations:

Thyroid function tests showed:	free triiodothyronine (T$_3$) 4 pmol/L (5–10)
free thyroxine (T$_4$) 11 pmol/L (10–25)	thyroid-stimulating hormone 4.9 mU/L (0.4–5.0)

What would be the most appropriate treatment?

A   Ablation of thyroid gland with radio-iodine [131]I
B   Increase the dose of carbimazole
C   Radiotherapy to the eye
D   Systemic steroids
E   Total thyroidectomy

23. A 49-year-old woman was being reviewed at the clinic for primary hypothyroidism. Blood tests at the time showed that she was euthyroid. However, her corrected serum calcium was 2.7 mmol/L.
      Further questioning showed that she did not have a history of renal stones, depression, constipation, back pain, other mental health problems or abdominal pain. She did not have any recent history of fractures.

Investigations:

Further tests showed:	corrected calcium 2.71 mmol/L (2.2–2.6)
sodium 134 mmol/L (135–145)	phosphate 0.7 mmol/L (0.8–1.4)
potassium 5.4 mmol/L (3.5–5.0)	parathyroid hormone 8.2 pmol/L (0.9–5.4) 25 (OH)
urea 6 mmol/L (2.5–7.5)	vitamin D$_2$ + vitamin D$_3$ 70 nmol/L (75–150)
creatinine 86 µmol/L (45–90)	
Urine calcium:creatinine clearance ratio 0.008 (>0.01)	

What is the next step in management?

A   CT of the neck
B   DXA (dual-energy X-ray absorptiometry) scan for bone mineral density
C   Reassure the patient
D   Refer for parathyroid surgery
E   ^{99m}Tc-sestamibi scan for parathyroid

24. A 49-year-old man was seen in the diabetes clinic for his annual review. He has had type 2 diabetes for the past 6 years and was on metformin 1000 mg twice daily and gliclazide 80 mg twice daily. He was also on simvastatin 40 mg once daily and ramipril 5 mg once daily. He did not report any hypoglycaemic episodes. His home blood sugar monitoring showed the following levels (normal random glucose level 4.0–7.8 mmol/L).

Investigations:

pre-meal level (mmol/L) to 2-h post-meal level (mmol/L):	dinner 8.1–15.1
breakfast 7.8–14.1	His body mass index was 26 and his blood pressure 132/84 mmHg
lunch 7.1–10.1	
HbA1c 9.8% (3.8–5.5)	creatinine 86 µmol/L (60–110)
haemoglobin 13.5 g/dL (13.0–18.0)	total cholesterol 3.8 mmol/L (3–5)
sodium 138 mmol/L (135–145)	low-density lipoprotein 1.6 mmol/L (<3)
potassium 3.6 mmol/L (3.5–5.0)	
Urine dipstick: normal	

What is the most appropriate next step in management?

A   Add basal insulin glargine in the morning
B   Add exenatide 10 µg twice daily
C   Add mixed insulin (short and intermediate acting) twice a day
D   Add pioglitazone 15 mg once daily
E   Add sitagliptin 100 mg once daily

25. A 22-year-old man was admitted to the intensive therapy unit after being involved in a motor vehicle accident. He was the driver and had been involved in a head-on collision with another car. He had sustained a basal skull fracture, and fractures of the right maxilla, left sphenoid sinus, left humerus and femur, as well as multiple rib fractures.

   The femoral and humerus fractures were operated on the same day and the rib fractures taped. He was noted to have cerebrospinal fluid rhinorrhoea and the torn dura mater was also repaired.

Investigations:

sodium 134 mmol/L (135–145)	creatinine 105 µmol/L (60–110)
potassium 3.4 mmol/L (3.5–5.0)	glucose 4.5 mmol/L (4.0–7.8)
urea 3.4 mmol/L (2.5–7.5)	

   He received a total of 2.5 L of intravenous fluids over the next 24 hours. By day 3, his Glasgow Coma Scale score was 14, temperature 36.7°C, pulse 90 beats per minute and blood pressure 120/60 mmHg.

sodium 163 mmol/L (135–145)	creatinine 73 µmol/L (60–110)
potassium 4.1 mmol/L (3.5–5.0)	glucose 5.2 mmol/L (4.0–7.8)
urea 4 mmol/L (2.5–7.5)	chloride 130 mmol/L (95–107)
Urine volume: 360 mL/h (30–70)	
Urine specific gravity: 1.000–1.005 (1.002–1.030)	

What is the next most appropriate step in management?

A   Fluid restrict to 1.5 L/day
B   Demeclocycline 150 mg four times daily
C   Desmopressin 100 µg three times daily
D   Intravenous infusion of 0.45% saline at a rate of 1 L/6 hours
E   Tolvaptan 15 mg once daily

26. A 42-year-old man was admitted with severe central abdominal pain, worse on lying down. He also had episodes of vomiting. His only past medical history was of inguinal hernia repair at the age of 28 years.

On examination, his temperature was 37.8°C, pulse 110 beats per minute, blood pressure 160/96 mmHg and respiratory rate 24 breaths per minute. Abdominal examination revealed tenderness in the epigastric region. CT showed evidence of acute pancreatitis for which he was treated conservatively and discharged a week later.

On the subsequent outpatient visit 3 months later, fasting blood tests showed the following picture:

Investigations:

haemoglobin 14.5 g/dL (13.0–18.0)	corrected calcium 2.56 mmol/L (2.2–2.6)
white cell count 8.5 × 10⁹/L (4–11)	phosphate 0.8 mmol/L (0.8–1.4)
neutrophils 5 × 10⁹/L (1.5–7.0)	fasting glucose 6.2 mmol/L (4–6)
platelets 213 × 10⁹/L (150–400)	HbA1c 5.9% (3.8–5.5)
sodium 135 mmol/L (135–145)	cholesterol 9.5 mmol/L (3–5)
potassium 3.6 mmol/L (3.5–5.0)	high-density lipoprotein 1.2 mmol/L (>1)
urea 4 mmol/L (2.5–7.5)	triglycerides 7.5 mmol/L (0.6–1.69)
creatinine 77 µmol/L (60–110)	

What would be the most appropriate treatment?

A Bezafibrate
B Nicotinic acid
C Pamidronate
D Rosuvastatin
E Simvastatin

27. A 56-year-old white man was recently found to have type 2 diabetes on an incidental blood test and was started on metformin 1000 mg twice daily.

Six months later, on review, his blood tests were:

Investigations:

HbA1c 7.1% (3.8–5.5)	low-density lipoprotein-cholesterol 3.1 mmol/L (<3)
haemoglobin 14.2 g/dL (13.0–18.0)	triglycerides 1.4 mmol/L (0.6–1.69)
creatinine 78 µmol/L (60–110)	bilirubin 3 mmol/L (1–22)
total cholesterol 4.9 mmol/L (3–5)	alanine transaminase 38 U/L (5–35)
high-density lipoprotein-cholesterol 1.0 mmol/L (>1)	alkaline phosphatase 65 U/L (45–105)

He was started on simvastatin 40 mg at night. Two months later, he came back with diffuse muscle aches, especially in the thighs and upper arms.

Repeat investigations showed: creatine kinase (CK) 1628 U/L (25–195)

What is the most appropriate next step in management?

A Continue simvastatin and monitor CK levels and symptoms after 4 weeks
B Continue simvastatin and start coenzyme Q supplementation
C Stop simvastatin and later switch to bezafibrate
D Stop simvastatin and later switch to ezetimibe
E Stop simvastatin and later switch to a lower dose of a more potent statin

28. A 34-year-old man of Taiwanese origin presented to the emergency department with severe weakness of all four limbs of 6 hours' duration.

On further questioning, he has had some muscle aches over the past 2 days. The day of presentation, he had woken up with muscle aches, especially in the thigh and around the shoulders. By midday he found it difficult walking or climbing stairs and could not get up from the chair and called the ambulance. He had no visual, sensory or bladder/bowel symptoms. He did, however, give a history of increased sweating, tremulousness, anxiety and palpitations over the last 2 months. He had no significant past history of note and was not on any medications.

On examination, he had hypotonia, grade 3 power proximally and grade 4 power distally with reduced reflexes in all four limbs. Sensory examination was normal and plantar reflex was flexor.

Investigations:

sodium 138 mmol/L (135–145)	bilirubin 4 mmol/L (1–22)
potassium 2.8 mmol/L (3.5–5.0)	alanine aminotransferase 21 U/L (5–35)
urea 4 mmol/L (2.5–7.5)	aspartate transaminase 32 U/L (5–35)
creatinine 76 µmol/L (60–110)	corrected calcium 2.39 mmol/L (2.2–2.6)
albumin 43 g/L (37–49)	creatine kinase 155 U/L (25–195)

He was started on potassium infusion and his symptoms improved.

Which test would confirm the diagnosis?

A   HIV serology
B   Lumbar puncture and protein analysis with microscopy
C   MRI of cervical spine
D   Nerve conduction studies
E   Thyroid function tests

29. A 19-year-old woman with type 1 diabetes and recently diagnosed hypothyroidism was seen in the clinic. Normally her glycaemic control was very good with HbA1c between 6.5 and 7% and very few hypoglycaemic episodes. She was maintained on a basal bolus regimen with rapid-acting analogue insulin and the basal insulin glargine. She was also on levothyroxine 50 µg. However, recently she had been having several episodes of hypoglycaemia along with increased fatigue.

Examination was normal.

What is the most appropriate diagnostic investigation?

A   C-peptide level
B   Nocturnal oxygen saturations
C   Serum calcium, vitamin D and parathyroid hormone level
D   Serum vitamin B_{12} level
E   Short Synacthen test

30. A 45-year-old woman of Middle Eastern origin was referred to the clinic because of a fractured right humerus after minimal trauma. She mentioned that she had had diffuse body aches for several years. She also had noticed difficulty in getting up from sitting position as well as climbing stairs. She did not exercise much and seldom went out, other than for shopping. She took no supplements and had no other significant past history.

Dual-energy X-ray absorptiometry scan showed T-scores of –3 in the vertebrae and –2.5 in the femur (> –1).

Investigations:

corrected calcium 2.06 mmol/L (2.2–2.6)	parathyroid hormone 11.8 pmol/L (0.9–5.4)
phosphate 0.5 mmol/L (0.8–1.4)	25(OH)-vitamin D_2 + vitamin D_3 <10 nmol/L (75–150)
alkaline phosphatase 585 U/L (45–105)	creatinine 75 µmol/L (60–110)

^{99m}Tc-sestamibi scan: four-gland hyperplasia

What would be the most appropriate next step in management?

A   Parathyroidectomy
B   Start cholecalciferol/ergocalciferol supplementation
C   Start cinacalcet
D   Start metyrapone
E   Start pamidronate therapy

31. A 38-year-old man went to the general practitioner with a history of burning sensation while passing urine. Physical examination was unremarkable. His body mass index was 21 kg/m². Urine analysis was positive for glucose, nitrites and white blood cells.

    He was treated with antibiotics and later an oral glucose tolerance test showed a fasting glucose of 9.2 mmol/L and 2-hour postprandial glucose of 16 mmol/L. He was started on gliclazide 40 mg once daily with variable control. This was later increased to 80 mg twice daily. HbA1c (glycated haemoglobin) measured 6 months later was 8.9%.

    What is the most appropriate next step in management?

    A   Add metformin 500 mg twice daily
    B   Add pioglitazone 15 mg once daily
    C   Increase gliclazide to 160 mg twice daily
    D   Measure fructosamine levels
    E   Measure glutamic acid decarboxylase (GAD) antibodies

32. A 24-year-old woman was referred with a history of secondary amenorrhoea, 6 months after stopping the oral contraceptive pill. She also complained of occasional headache and that she stumbled sometimes when climbing stairs. She had no other significant past medical history. She was not on any medications. She had noticed that her blouses were slightly damp.

    On examination, milk could be expressed from her breasts. Visual field examination showed a field defect in the upper outer quadrants of both eyes.

    Investigations:

haemoglobin 11.0 g/dL (11.5–16.5)	prolactin 1080 mU/L (normal < 360) (serial dilutions done)
white cell count 4 × 10⁹/L (4–11)	
platelets 125 × 10⁹/L (150–400)	follicle-stimulating hormone 0.1 U/mL (1–13)
sodium 138 mmol/L (135–145)	luteinising hormone 0.2 U/mL (1–9)
potassium 3.9 mmol/L (3.5–5.0)	thyroid-stimulating hormone 0.1 mU/L (0.4–5.0)
urea 3.9 mmol/L (2.5–7.5)	free thyroxine (T_4) 8 pmol/L (10–25)
creatinine 67 µmol/L (45–90)	9 am cortisol 22 nmol/L (200–700)
	insulin-like growth factor 186 ng/mL (110–360)

    Pituitary MRI: 3-cm pituitary mass with a slight tenting of the optic chiasma
    No evidence of parasellar extension

    What is the most appropriate next step in management?

    A   Bromocriptine
    B   Octreotide
    C   Stereotactic radiosurgery
    D   Transcranial hypophysectomy
    E   Trans-sphenoidal surgery

33. A 28-year-old woman was seen in the clinic for a review of type 1 diabetes. She has had type 1 diabetes for the last 16 years and was on a basal bolus regimen with a long-acting analogue insulin glargine and short-acting insulin analogue lispro. Her only other medication was occasional paracetamol for headaches.

Over the past few months, she had had three hypoglycaemic episodes, one of which required external assistance. On looking at her glucose diary, there were several readings between 3 and 4 mmol/L which were asymptomatic. She has had recently started a fitness regime. She did not have any other past medical history. For the last 7 years she has had good glycaemic control with HbA1c between 6.0 and 6.5% (3.8–5.5). She tested blood sugars four times a day and took regular exercise.

On examination, her body mass index was 21 kg/m² and blood pressure 140/85 mmHg.

Investigations:

fasting glucose 4.1 mmol/L (4–6)	low-density lipoprotein 2.5 mmol/L (<3)
HbA1c 6.1% (3.8–5.5)	high-density lipoprotein 1.3 mmol/L (>1.3)
cholesterol 4.5 mmol/L (3–5)	

What is the most appropriate next step in management?

A   Add ramipril 5 mg once daily and titrate the dose to target blood pressure of <130/80 mmHg
B   Add simvastatin 40 mg at night
C   Reduce basal insulin and pre-exercise rapid-acting insulin and avoid hypoglycaemia for the next 2 months
D   Switch from basal bolus to continuous subcutaneous insulin infusion therapy (insulin pump)
E   Switch from once daily glargine to twice daily detemir to improve glycaemic control

34. A 21-year-old woman was referred to the clinic with acne and hirsuitism. She had attained menarche at the age of 11 years and had occasional irregular periods. She had noticed increasing hirsuitism over the last few years. There was no other relevant history or family history.

On examination, her body mass index was 28 kg/m², pulse 76 beats per minute and blood pressure 130/85 mmHg.

She had hirsutism and acanthosis nigricans. Breast development was normal. Vaginal examination was normal apart from mild clitoromegaly.

Blood tests taken on the fifth day after menstruation showed:

Investigations:

estradiol 300 pmol/L (early follicular <300)	luteinising hormone 4 U/L (1–9)
17OH-progesterone 20 nmol/L (<10)	follicle-stimulating hormone 3 U/L (1–13)
free testosterone 3 nmol/L (<3)	cortisol (9 am) 150 nmol/L (200–700)

What is the single most useful diagnostic test?

A   CT of the adrenals
B   Karyotyping
C   MRI of the pituitary
D   Short Synacthen test
E   Ultrasound of the pelvis

35. A 58-year-old man was referred because of watery diarrhoea and 6-kg weight loss over the past 2 months. There was no history of bleeding or abdominal pain. He also felt weak and lethargic, and had increased thirst and reduced urine output. He had a previous history of hypertension for which he was taking ramipril. There was no relevant family history.

On examination, he looked thin and mildly dehydrated. The rest of the examination was normal.

Investigations:

sodium 139 mmol/L (135–145)	pH 7.20 (7.34–7.44)
potassium 2.6 mmol/L (3.5–5.0)	bicarbonate 8 mmol/L (18–24)
creatinine 135 µmol/L (60–110)	urinary 5HIAA (5-hydroxyindoleacetic acid) – normal
corrected calcium 2.75 mmol/L (2.2–2.6)	faecal fat 2 g/24 h (<7 g/24 h)
fasting glucose 6.5 mmol/L (4–6)	stool volume 1.5 L/24 h

Stool culture: no ova, cysts or pathogens isolated

What is the most useful diagnostic test?

A   Glucagon
B   Faecal elastase
C   Plasma vasoactive intestinal peptide (VIP)
D   Secretin stimulation test
E   Somatostatin test

36. A 67-year-old man was seen in the neurology clinic with a 6-month history of severe pain in the right thigh. He also had difficulty getting up from squatting position and had noticed wasting in the legs. Pain was more severe at night. He had a past history of type 2 diabetes for 11 years and hypertension for 14 years. He was on metformin and gliclazide for diabetes and lisinopril for hypertension. He was also on simvastatin and ezetimibe for hyperlipidemia.

On examination, he was haemodynamically stable. Neurological examination of the lower limbs showed quadriceps wasting bilaterally with weakness in knee extension bilaterally and absent knee reflexes. Plantar reflex was flexor bilaterally. Sensations were intact.

Investigations:

haemoglobin 12.8 g/dL (13.0–18.0)	potassium 4.5 mmol/L (3.5–5.0)
white cell count 9×10^9/L (4–11)	urea 7 mmol/L (2.5–7.5)
neutrophils 6×10^9/L (1.5–7.0)	creatinine 98 µmol/L (60–110)
platelets 178×10^9/L (150–400)	HbA1c 8.7% (3.8–5.5)
sodium 137 mmol/L (135–145)	

Chest X-ray: normal

Cerebrospinal fluid: clear, protein 0.52 g/L (0.2–0.4), white cell count 2×10^9/L (lymphocytes only)

What is the most likely diagnosis?

A   Amyotrophic lateral sclerosis
B   Diabetic lumbosacral plexopathy
C   Guillain–Barré syndrome
D   Meralgia paraesthetica
E   Mononeuritis multiplex

37. A 55-year-old man was admitted with a history of nausea and vomiting. He had a past history of diabetes for which he was on gliclazide 160 mg twice daily and metformin 850 mg three times daily. His last HbA1c was 8.8% (3.8–5.5). He was also on simvastatin 40 mg at night and ramipril 10 mg once daily.

On examination, he was haemodynamically stable and had some epigastric tenderness. He also had eruptive xanthomas on his trunk and upper arms.

Investigations:

haemoglobin 13.1 g/dL (13.0–18.0)	bilirubin 3 mmol/L (1–22)
mean corpuscular volume 82 fL (80–96)	albumin 45 g/L (37–49)
white cell count 12 × 10⁹/L (4–11)	alanine transaminase 78 U/L (5–35)
platelets 180 × 10⁹/L (150–400)	alkaline phosphatase 290 U/L (45–105)
sodium 140 mmol/L (135–145)	total cholesterol 17 mmol/L (3–5)
potassium 3.8 mmol/L (3.5–5.0)	triglycerides 22 mmol/L (0.6–1.69)
creatinine 110 µmol/L (60–110)	high-density lipoprotein 1.2 mmol/L (>1.0)
glucose 21 mmol/L (4.0–7.8)	

What is the most appropriate next step in management?

A   Atorvastatin
B   Dextrose–insulin infusion
C   Gemfibrozil
D   Heparin infusion
E   Niacin

38. A 65-year-old woman was admitted with chest pain, cough and fever. She had a past history of diabetes for which she was on metformin 850 mg twice daily. She was also on simvastatin 40 mg at night and ramipril 10 mg once daily.
    Chest X-ray showed left lower lobe consolidation and she was started on intravenous amoxicillin and gentamicin.
    Blood tests 3 days after admission showed:

Investigations:

haemoglobin 13.1 g/dL (11.5–16.5)	glucose 15 mmol/L (4–7.8)
mean corpuscular volume 82 fL (80–96)	bilirubin 3 mmol/L (1–22)
white cell count 21 × 10⁹/L (4–11)	albumin 35 g/L (37–49)
neutrophils 16 × 10⁹/L (1.5–7.0)	alanine transaminase 45 U/L (5–35)
platelets 180 × 10⁹/L (150–400)	alkaline phosphatase 110 U/L (45–105)
sodium 140 mmol/L (135–145)	thyroid-stimulating hormone 0.6 mU/L (0.4–5.0)
potassium 3.8 mmol/L (3.5–5.0)	free thyroxine (T_4) 9.1 pmol/L (10–25)
creatinine 110 µmol/L (45–90)	free triiodothyronine (T_3) 2.3 pmol/L (5–10)

What is the most appropriate investigation?

A   Radio-iodine uptake scan
B   Repeat thyroid function tests in a week and then in 2–3 months
C   Thyroid-binding globulin measurement
D   Thyroid peroxidase antibody measurement
E   Thyroid ultrasound

39. A 38-year-old man with a 2-year history of type 2 diabetes had his annual review. He was taking metformin and pioglitazone.
    His blood pressure was 145/88 mmHg on ramipril.

Investigations:

HbA1c 7.2% (3.8–5.5)	total cholesterol 5.3 mmol/L (3–5)
creatinine 97 μmol/L (60–110)	high-density lipoprotein 0.9 mmol/L (>1.0)
estimated glomerular filtration rate (eGFR) 80 mL/min (>90)	low-density lipoprotein 3 mmol/L (2–3)
	triglycerides 2.8 mmol/L (0.6–1.69)
alanine transaminase 45 U/L (5–35)	

Urine albumin: creatinine ratio 0.9 (<2.5)

What is the most appropriate management?

A   Lifestyle advice and recheck in 3 months time
B   Start bezafibrate
C   Start nicotinic acid
D   Start omega 3 fatty acids
E   Start simvastatin

40. A 65-year-old man with a 12-year history of type 2 diabetes was seen for an annual review. He was on metformin, gliclazide and pioglitazone, along with ramipril for hypertension and microalbuminuria. He had previous proliferative retinopathy treated with laser photocoagulation. He also mentioned that he had a deep aching pain in his left forefoot.

On examination, the left foot was hot to touch and there was swelling and redness over the left forefoot, but no tenderness over the tarsal bones. He also had bilateral peripheral sensory neuropathy up to the mid-shin level.

Investigations:

haemoglobin 12.9 g/dL (13.0–18.0)	creatinine 107 μmol/L (60–110)
white cell count 8.2 × 10⁹/L (4–11)	estimated glomerular filtration rate (eGFR) 58 mL/min (>90)
C-reactive protein 10 mg/L (<10)	
erythrocyte sedimentation rate 32 mm/1st h (0–20)	alanine transaminase 45 U/L (5–35)
	uric acid 0.28 mmol/L (0.23–0.46)

Urine albumin:creatinine ratio – 21.9 (<2.5)

X-ray of left foot: soft tissue oedema over the tarsal bones as well as joint space widening

MRI of left foot: soft tissue swelling and stretching of ligaments

What is the most likely diagnosis?

A   Cellulitis due to diabetic foot
B   Charcot's foot affecting the forefoot bones
C   Diffuse interstitial skeletal hyperostosis (DISH) of diabetes
D   Gouty arthritis
E   Osteomyelitis of the forefoot

41. A 17-year-old girl was referred to the clinic with a history of primary amenorrhoea. She had always been athletic and had attributed this amenorrhoea to her lifestyle. There was no family history of delayed menarche.

On examination, she had normal breasts with pale areolae and scanty pubic hair development. Pelvic examination revealed that the vagina was short and ended blindly.
        Karyotyping showed XY genotype.

What is the most appropriate next step in management?

A   Day 21 progesterone measurement
B   Gonadotrophin-releasing hormone therapy
C   Human chorionic gonadotrophin (hCG) therapy
D   Orchidectomy
E   Transvaginal ultrasound

42. A 57-year-old woman was referred to the clinic with a history of fatigue, decreased libido and malaise. She was diagnosed with hypothyroidism 3 years ago by her general practitioner and was on thyroxine. However, despite thyroxine replacement, her symptoms did not subside. She had her menopause 5 years ago. She took her medicines regularly. There was no other past history of significance.

Investigations:

haemoglobin 10.9 g/dL (11.5–16.5)	potassium 5.5 mmol/L (3.5–5.0)
white cell count 5.4 × 10⁹/L (4–11)	creatinine 65 µmol/L (45–90)
platelets 158 × 10⁹/L (150–400)	thyroid-stimulating hormone 0.3 mU/L (0.4–5.0)
mean corpuscular volume 82 fL (80–96)	free thyroxine (T_4) 15.8 pmol/L (10–25)
sodium 132 mmol/L (135–145)	free triiodothyronine (T_3) 3.1 pmol/L (5–10)

What is the most appropriate investigation?

A   Assay for interfering antibodies to thyroid-stimulating hormone (TSH)
B   Iodine-131 uptake scan
C   Insulin tolerance test
D   Serum thyroid-binding globulin measurement
E   Thyroid-stimulating hormone receptor-stimulating antibody measurement

43. A 32-year-old man was seen in the clinic along with his wife for primary infertility. She previously has had one child and had a gynaecology review which was normal.
        He had no significant past medical history and was a non-smoker. Alcohol intake was <10 units/week and he did not report any recreational drug use. He had normal onset of puberty. However, he had a 'weak' libido. On questioning he shaved only once a week.
        On examination: height 183 cm, weight 81 kg, heart rate 69 beats per minute, blood pressure 108/66 mmHg, temperature 37.1°C. He had mild gynaecomastia. Testicular volume was 4 mL (15–25).

Investigations:

testosterone 5 nmol/L (10–28)	estradiol 350 pmol/l (<250)
luteinising hormone 20 U/L (1–9)	thyroid-stimulating hormone 2 mU/L (0.4–5.0)
sex hormone-binding globulin 28 nmol/L (20–40)	cortisol (9 am) 290 nmol/L (200–700)
follicle-stimulating hormone 14 U/L (1–13)	prolactin 140 mU/L (<360)

What is the most useful diagnostic investigation?

A   CT of the adrenal gland
B   Karyotyping
C   MRI pituitary
D   Short Synacthen test
E   Testicular ultrasound

Answers

1. D Short Synacthen test

Type 1 diabetes is due to absolute lack of insulin; >95% of type 1 diabetes is due to autoimmune destruction of islet cells. People with one autoimmune disease are often more at risk of developing another. Hence people with type 1 diabetes have an increased risk of getting other autoimmune diseases such as Addison's disease, hypothyroidism and pernicious anaemia.

Given his symptoms of increased episodes of hypoglycaemia, lethargy and tiredness, the most likely diagnosis is primary autoimmune hypoadrenalism (Addison's disease). Unexplained increase in the frequency of hypoglycaemic episodes, lethargy and tiredness in a person with type 1 diabetes should prompt the search for hypoadrenalism. The diagnostic test for hypoadrenalism is a short synacthen test.

Short Synacthen test (SST) is done by injecting (intramuscularly or intravenously) a synthetic analogue of adrenocorticotrophic hormone (250 mg Synacthen), with blood withdrawn for serum cortisol estimation prior to and at 30 and 60 minutes afterwards. If the adrenal response is intact, the cortisol level rises post-administration.

Although continuous glucose monitoring might be useful in elucidating the pattern of hypoglycaemic episodes and in tailoring the insulin regimen, it would not provide a diagnosis in this instance.

Serum insulin and C-peptide levels would not be useful in this instance as neither insulinoma nor factitious hyperinsulinism is the first diagnostic possibility here.

Thyroid function tests are useful as polyglandular autoimmune syndrome is a possibility, but the symptoms suggest primary hypoadrenalism rather than thyroid dysfunction. Hence the first priority would be to rule out hypoadrenalism.

2. C Intravenous fluids

The clinical picture is suggestive of a lung cancer with hypercalcaemia. Her symptoms are primarily due to hypercalcaemia. Calcium levels >3.75 mmol/L suggest severe hypercalcaemia.

Symptoms of severe hypercalcaemia include polyuria, polydipsia, dehydration, nausea, vomiting, pancreatitis and cardiac arrhythmias. ECG changes include shortened QT interval and widened T wave.

Initial treatment is adequate fluid replacement. This alone may be enough to bring the calcium levels down. After adequate fluid replacement, diuresis with loop diuretics may enhance calcium excretion. For cancer-related hypercalcaemia, bisphosphonates such as pamidronate would be the next step, though the effect on calcium levels is usually a delayed one. Prednisolone can be also used in the treatment of hypercalcaemia, but the initial treatment is intravenous fluid.

Mechanism of hypercalcaemia, in this instance, is most likely to be paraneoplastic secretion of PTHrP (parathyroid hormone-related peptide) by the carcinoma. Parathyroid hormone levels would be low or undetectable in this instance. The other mechanism of hypercalcaemia in this case could be lytic metastases in the bones.

Demshar R, Vanek R, Mazanec P. Oncologic emergencies: new decade, new perspectives. AACN Adv Crit Care 2011; 22(4):337–348.

3. A Fine-needle aspiration cytology

This question concerns the management of a single nodule in the thyroid. She is clinically and biochemically euthyroid and the ultrasound reveals some microcalcifications which point towards a neoplastic process.

Sonographically suggestive features are microcalcifications, hypoechoic solid lesions, irregular margins, increased vascularity within nodule and signs of extracapsular spread.

In this instance, the initial step is fine-needle aspiration (FNA) of the nodule (**Figure 3.1**), if the nodule can be clearly palpated, it can be done in the clinic; if not an ultrasound-guided FNA should be done.

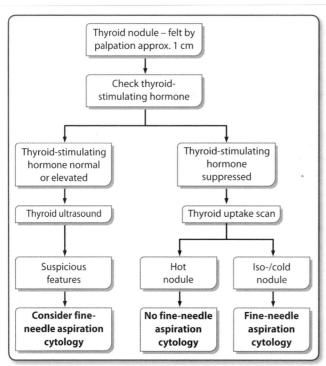

Figure 3.1 Evaluation of a solitary thyroid nodule.

The histology determines further management. The Royal College of Pathologists' classification is used for thyroid FNA reporting.

The RCPath classification:
Thy 1 – non-diagnostic
Thy 2 – benign
Thy 3 – atypia/non-diagnostic or follicular neoplasm
Thy 4 – suspicious of malignancy
Thy 5 – malignancy

Royal College of Pathologists G089. – Guidance on the reporting of thyroid cytology. London: Royal College of Pathologists, 2009.

4. E Exenatide-induced acute pancreatitis

Exenatide is a GLP-1 (glucagon-like peptide-1) analogue, which is known to increase the risk of developing acute pancreatitis. The risk is increased if the person has hypertriglyceridaemia or a previous history of pancreatitis. On starting exenatide injections patients are warned to contact their doctor and stop exenatide if they develop abdominal pain.

Exenatide is often given as a second- or third-line agent in type 2 diabetes prior to insulin therapy. It tends to produce some weight loss as well, which is advantageous in a person with high body mass index. GLP-1 is an incretin hormone which is produced by the gut in response to food intake and increases food-related insulin release.

Although hypertriglyceridaemia can induce acute pancreatitis this is mainly seen in severe cases with triglyceride levels >11.3 mmol/L. Bezafibrate does not increase the incidence or worsen the symptoms of peptic ulcer disease.

Combination therapy with a fibrate and a statin is known to increase the incidence of myalgia and rhabdomyolysis. However, the creatine kinase level is only modestly elevated whereas in rhabdomyolysis it is usually elevated five times above the upper limit. Also hyperkalaemia is a feature of rhabdomyolysis which is not seen here.

Acute kidney injury can be worsened by ramipril; however, the symptoms and elevated amylase level in this case points towards pancreatitis rather than renal injury as the cause.

Elashoff M, et al. Pancreatitis, pancreatic, and thyroid cancer with glucagon-like peptide-1-based therapies. Gastroenterol 2011; 141(1):150–156.

5. D 25(OH)-Vitamin D

The gastric bypass procedure can result in malabsorption of micronutrients including vitamin D. This results in osteomalacia and proximal muscle weakness which this person has. The main circulating form of vitamin D is the 25(OH)-vitamin D, which would be the single best test here. Since there is no indication of renal issues, measurement of $1,25(OH)_2$-vitamin D (the bioactive form) is not indicated.

6. C Fluoxetine-induced hyperprolactinaemia

Selective serotonin reuptake inhibitors (SSRIs) such as fluoxetine activate serotoninergic pathways (via type 2A serotonin receptors) and stimulate prolactin release. They are much more likely to produce hyperprolactinaemia compared with tricyclic antidepressants or monoamine oxidase inhibitors.

Although depression and diabetes can cause erectile dysfunction, given the high prolactin level, this has to be considered as the most important factor.

Follicle-stimulating hormone and luteinising hormone levels are both normal and hence the patient does not have hypogonadotrophic hypogonadism. Metformin does not cause hyperprolactinaemia.

Treatment of SSRI-related sexual dysfunction consists of switching the drug (in consultation with a psychiatrist), adding small amounts of dopamine agonist (such as bromocriptine) cautiously, phosphodiesterase-5 inhibitors and other drugs.

Papakostas GI et al. Serum prolactin levels among outpatients with major depressive disorder during the acute phase of treatment with fluoxetine. J Clin Psychiatry 2006; 67(6):952–957.

7. D Two 24-hour urine collections for free cortisol

The history and physical examination is suggestive of Cushing's syndrome. The next step is a screening test for Cushing's syndrome. The currently acceptable screening tests for Cushing's syndrome are: overnight 1 mg dexamethasone suppression test, urinary free cortisol levels and salivary cortisol level. Of these, because she is on combined oral contraceptive pills, urine collection for free cortisol is more appropriate because oestrogen can interfere with the overnight suppression test, unless it is stopped a few weeks prior to the test.

The low-dose dexamethasone suppression test is often used as a screening test in those with high pretest probability of Cushing's syndrome and also to confirm the diagnosis.

The high-dose dexamethasone suppression test is used to identify the source of the cortisol hypersecretion.

Insulin tolerance testing is used to diagnose ACTH/cortisol and growth hormone reserve and short Synacthen test is for hypoadrenalism.

Plasma adrenocorticotrophic hormone (ACTH) levels are useful for identifying the source of hypercortisolism. High ACTH levels suggest either pituitary or ectopic ACTH secretion and low levels suggest primary adrenal hypersecretion. However, ACTH levels are not useful as a screening test.

Nieman LK, et al. The diagnosis of Cushing's syndrome: an Endocrine Society Clinical Practice Guideline. J Clin Endocrinol Metab 2008; 93:1526–1540.

8. A Exogenous insulin use

The combination of reduced blood sugar, low C-peptide and high insulin level suggests exogenous insulin use. In the case of both insulinoma and sulphonylurea abuse, C-peptide levels would be high. A blood level for sulphonylurea would clarify the diagnosis in that case.

The insulin mRNA is translated as a single chain precursor called pre-proinsulin, and removal of its signal peptide during insertion into the endoplasmic reticulum generates proinsulin. Within the endoplasmic reticulum, proinsulin is cleaved by endopeptidases into insulin and C-peptide. Insulin and free C-peptide are stored in secretory granules within the cytoplasm. When the beta cell is stimulated, insulin and C-peptide are secreted into the islet capillary blood.

Hence both sulphonylurea compounds, which stimulate insulin release and insulinoma (which oversecretes insulin), both produce elevated insulin and C-peptide levels. Insulinoma is a type of neuroendocrine tumour.

In liver dysfunction with hypoglycaemia, the insulin level would not be high with a suppressed C-peptide level.

Cryer PE, et al. Evaluation and management of adult hypoglycemic disorders: an Endocrine Society Clinical Practice Guideline. J Clin Endocrinol Metab 2009; 94(3):709–728.

9. D Oral glucose tolerance test with growth hormone levels

The clinical scenario described is suggestive of acromegaly. This is strengthened by the difficult to control hypertension and impaired glucose tolerance.

To screen for the presence of acromegaly, IGF-1 (insulin-like growth factor-1) level can be used and, to confirm, an oral glucose tolerance test with serial measurement of growth hormone is commonly used.

Isolated growth hormone levels are less useful as the secretion tends to be episodic. IGF-1 levels are more useful for screening. Measurement of IGF-1 should be followed by an oral glucose tolerance test. Serial measurement of glucose and growth hormone levels are done 30, 60 and 120 minutes after a 75 g oral glucose load. In normal people growth hormone level will be suppressed to <1 ng/mL after a 75 g oral glucose load. If there is still doubt then a thyroid-stimulating hormone-releasing hormone test may be useful.

Pituitary MRI is done after biochemical confirmation of acromegaly as incidental pituitary masses are seen in approximately 10% of normal volunteers.

The low-dose dexamethasone suppression test is used in Cushing's syndrome and the insulin tolerance test in hypoadrenalism.

Hall WA. Pituitary magnetic resonance imaging in normal human volunteers: occult adenomas in the general population. Ann Intern Med 1994; 120(10):817–820.

10. C Intravenous hydrocortisone (100 mg every 8 hours)

The history of possible previous traumatic brain injury followed by malaise, decreased libido and increased weight suggest the development of hypopituitarism due to head injury. Traumatic brain injury can cause pituitary dysfunction in up to a third of cases. Most commonly this is manifested acutely as diabetes insipidus. However, later on panhypopituitarism may develop insidiously.

Supplementing thyroxine alone in this situation may precipitate an adrenal crisis since thyroxine can accelerate the catabolism of cortisol. Treatment of adrenal crisis is primarily fluid replacement, hydrocortisone and treatment of the precipitating condition such as an infection. Before starting treatment blood sample for cortisol and adrenocorticotrophic hormone estimation are sent off. Once the crisis is over, tests of pituitary reserve are carried out such as short Synacthen test, luteinising hormone or follicle-stimulating hormone levels, thyroid function tests, testosterone, prolactin and insulin-like growth factor-1 levels. Urine and plasma osmolality should be measured to assess posterior pituitary function.

Schneider M, et al. Anterior pituitary hormone abnormalities following traumatic brain injury. J Neurotrauma 2005; 22(9):937–46.
Behan LA, Agha A. Endocrine consequences of adult traumatic brain injury. Horm Res 2007; 68(5):18–21.

11. E Fluid restriction

The clinical picture is suggestive of the syndrome of inappropriate antidiuretic hormone (SIADH) release due to release of stored vasopressin from the hypothalamopituitary axons because of neural trauma from the basal skull fracture. The released vasopressin causes excess retention of free water, especially if fluids are administered, as in this case. This leads to plasma hypo-osmolality and urine hyperosmolality; hyponatraemia may also result.

The initial management is fluid restriction. Demeclocycline can be tried if fluid restriction is not effective. In severe cases hyponatraemia may lead to convulsions and altered state of consciousness. Treatment in severe cases is with hypertonic saline, but this must be used very cautiously. Serum sodium must be monitored carefully and rate of rise of sodium must be slow.

Injury to the pituitary stalk produces a classic triphasic response – an initial phase of reduced vasopressin secretion leading to diabetes insipidus, followed by a phase of release of stored vasopressin leading to SIADH; this is followed by a phase of diabetes insipidus again while the neural damage recovers. The final phase of diabetes insipidus may result in only partial or no recovery.

12. E Reduce night-time NPH insulin

The history of night sweats and headache points towards nocturnal hypoglycaemia. The pre-bed glucose levels are low which again points towards nocturnal hypoglycaemia. The high morning glucose levels point towards 'Somogyi's effect' – i.e. nocturnal hypoglycaemia causes anti-insulin hormones such as cortisol, glucagon and adrenaline to be secreted, which drives the blood sugar up. This results in nocturnal hypoglycaemic episodes followed by early morning hyperglycaemia.

Since the neutral protamine Hagedorn (NPH) insulin given at bedtime is the most likely cause of the nocturnal hypoglycaemia, dose reduction is the most logical step. Also as pre-bed blood glucose values are low normal, depending on when the evening meals are, the evening dose of regular insulin might need to be reduced.

It is vital to consider possible 'Somogyi's effects' prior to increasing the night-time insulin dose. Nocturnal hypoglycaemia is often asymptomatic but can result in night sweats, nightmares, headache and sudden death (increased risk of cardiac arrhythmias). A 2 am capillary blood glucose levels often helps to diagnose this problem. Continuous blood glucose monitoring may also be helpful. This should be contrasted with the 'Dawn effect' where there is a morning rise in blood sugar in response to waning insulin and a growth hormone surge which antagonises the action of insulin.

13. B Carbimazole and propranolol first, potassium iodide and hydrocortisone 1 hour later

This patient has a thyroid storm which if left untreated thyroid storm has significant morbidity and mortality (~30%). It is a multi-system disorder. Previously, it was usually seen after surgery for thyrotoxicosis but this is now uncommon as most instances of thyrotoxicosis are better controlled prior to surgery. The most common causes are intercurrent illnesses especially infections. Surgery in the presence of unrecognised thyrotoxicosis and trauma is also a cause, but in rare cases. It can occasionally occur without any precipitating factors in untreated or partially treated thyrotoxicosis. Graves' disease is the most common underlying cause, followed by toxic nodular goitre.

Clinical features include tachycardia and tachyarrhythmias, especially with heart failure, fever, tremour, nausea and vomiting as well as diarrhoea. These can result in dehydration. Central nervous system features such as agitation, delirium and coma can be seen. In elderly people, apathetic form can be seen with weakness, apathy, confusion and no fever. Signs include fever, tremors, features of congestive cardiac failure such as oedema, raised jugular venous pressure, congestive hepatomegaly and dyspnoea.

Diagnosis is made clinically. Free thyroxine (T_4) and triiodothyronine (T_3) should ideally be measured. T_3 levels may be decreased because of general ill-health (non-thyroidal illness syndrome).

The diagnostic criteria used include the Burch and Wartofsky scale which looks at heart rate, temperature, congestive cardiac failure, atrial fibrillation, liver function test abnormalities, central nervous system dysfunction and presence of precipitating events. A score of >45 suggests thyroid storm.

Thyroid storm is a medical emergency and ideally should be treated in an high dependency unit or intensive therapy unit setting.

Supportive measures include rest, fluid and electrolyte management, oxygen, antibiotics (if indicated), nutritional supplementation, paracetamol, tepid sponging and other cooling aids, as well as cardiovascular support. Specific measures include propranolol, carbimazole, potassium iodide (1 hour after carbimazole) and glucocorticoids such as hydrocortisone.

This patient is haemodynamically stable. Hence propranolol is a reasonable choice as the first-line drug. In more unstable patients, esmolol infusion can be used. Propranolol has the additional benefit of blocking the peripheral conversion of T_4 to T_3. The therapy depends on sequential blocking of the thyroid hormone synthesis. Carbimazole blocks thyroid hormone synthesis and hence should be administered first. An hour later iodides (either Lugol's solution or potassium iodide) may be given. Hydrocortisone may be given as the adrenal glands are often unable to increase the output of glucocorticoids in thyrotoxicosis. Fluids are often indicated but must be given cautiously depending on the degree of congestive cardiac failure. Cooling measures may be undertaken if the temperature is high; this includes paracetamol and other local measures.

Propylthiouracil may also be used instead of carbimazole. It has the additional advantage of peripheral blockade of T_4 to T_3 conversion. However, it also has a higher incidence of fatal liver necrosis.

Other measures that could be used include plasmapheresis, cholestyramine or colestipol (to prevent enterohepatic recirculation) and dialysis.

Burch HB, Wartofsky L. Life-threatening thyrotoxicosis. Thyroid storm. Endocrinol Metab Clin North Am 1993; 22:263.

Bahn Chair RS, et al. Hyperthyroidism and other causes of thyrotoxicosis: management guidelines of the American Thyroid Association and American Association of Clinical Endocrinologists. Thyroid 2011; 21(6):593–646.

Bartalena L, Henneman G. Graves' disease complications. www.thyroidmanager.org (last accessed May 2012).

14. D Intravenous thiamine supplementation

Thiamine is a water-soluble vitamin with low body stores that can be depleted in around 10–20 days. Its active metabolite is thiamine pyrophosphate, which is important for carbohydrate metabolism.

Prolonged starvation leads to thiamine depletion. In such a situation, sudden carbohydrate load without accompanying thiamine would lead to Wernicke's encephalopathy (WE) and peripheral neuropathy (dry beri-beri).

The classic triad of WE is confusion, ocular problems and ataxia. Delirium, ophthalmoplegia and nystagmus are the common manifestations. Peripheral neuropathy is also seen. Chronic alcoholism is the most common cause due to reduced intake of thiamine and reduced absorption from the gut.

Diagnosis is by measuring thiamine levels in blood or red cell transketolase activity. Both are difficult to perform and are not entirely specific. Other methods that have recently come into play include measuring thiamine and its metabolites in red cells by high-performance liquid chromatography.

MRI is specific but not sensitive. Typically there is involvement of periventricular areas bilaterally. These include the medial aspect of the thalamus, hypothalamus and mamillary bodies, the periaqueductal region and the floor of the fourth ventricle where an increased T2 signal is seen.

Korsakoff's syndrome with loss of short-term memory and variable cognitive problems may develop subacutely, often after WE.

Treatment is intravenous thiamine. This should be done upon suspecting the condition and should not wait for biochemical or radiological confirmation. In this case rapid weight loss due to bariatric surgery and vomiting followed by intravenous dextrose precipitated the condition. Recently more than 200 cases of WE have been reported after bariatric surgery.

Post-bariatric surgery, patients are also prone to vitamin B_{12}, zinc, vitamin D and magnesium deficiencies, and hence these should also be monitored. Here the clinical picture is clearly that of WE.

Sechi G, Serra A. Wernicke's encephalopathy: new clinical settings and recent advances in diagnosis and management. Lancet Neurol 2007; 6:442–455.

15. C Plasma aldosterone:renin ratio

In the presence of difficult to control hypertension, a low potassium concentration in the serum (despite being on ramipril) should raise the suspicion of primary hyperaldosteronism (PA). The screening test for this is plasma aldosterone:renin ratio. The ratio is more sensitive than plasma renin activity or plasma aldosterone levels on their own.

Many drugs, especially spironolactone, amiloride, diuretics and angiotensin-converting enzyme inhibitors, affect the test. Most guidelines recommend a morning (2 hours after waking up and after 15–30 minutes rest) plasma aldosterone:renin ratio measurement (off spironolactone and diuretics) as a screening test, followed by a confirmatory test.

One of four confirmatory tests used involves measuring plasma aldosterone after doing one of the following:
1. Oral salt load
2. Saline infusion
3. After fludrocortisone suppression
4. Captopril challenge test

Once biochemically confirmed, then a CT/MRI of the adrenals would be helpful to distinguish between adenoma (Conn's syndrome) and hyperplasia. If there is still any doubt, selective adrenal vein sampling may be required.

Plasma metanephrine level and *meta*-iodobenzylguanidine scan are used to diagnose phaeochromocytomas rather than primary hyperaldosteronism.

Funder JW, et al. Case detection, diagnosis, and treatment of patients with primary aldosteronism: an Endocrine Society clinical practice guideline. J Clin Endocrinol Metab 2008; 93:3266–3281.

16. A Continue 8 units/h insulin infusion, add potassium 40 mmol/L to the 0.9% saline infused at 0.5 L/h and add 10% dextrose infused at 125 mL/h

Current guidelines for diabetic ketoacidosis have progressed from a sliding scale to fixed dose insulin infusion at 0.1 unit/kg per-hour infusion. If blood glucose falls below 14 mmol/L, instead of reducing the insulin infusion, it is recommended that the insulin infusion remain the same, but add 10% dextrose infusion at 125 mL/h. The 0.9% saline infusion is separate and continues.

Potassium supplementation is added to the 0.9% saline infusion depending on the potassium concentrations.

If serum potassium >5.5 mmol/L – do not add potassium
If serum potassium 3.5–5.5 mmol/L – add 40 mmol to every litre of 0.9% saline
If serum potassium <3.5 mmol/L – consult with seniors regarding the best delivery mechanism and concentration.

In general, long-acting insulins such as glargine or NPH (neutral protamine Hagedorn) should be continued while the patient is on the intravenous insulin infusion. This prevents hyperglycaemia and ketosis from recurring.

Similarly the glucose infusion should continue if the blood glucose is <14 mmol/L until the patient is eating and drinking.

Savage MW, et al. Joint British Diabetes Societies guideline for the management of diabetic ketoacidosis. Diabetic Med 2011; 28:508–515.

17. B Oral levothyroxine replacement

The clinical features and the lab data are suggestive of severe primary hypothyroidism with low free thyroxine and free triiodothyronine, and high thyroid-stimulating hormone. There is also the history of poor concordance with medication. The clinical features are not suggestive of myxoedema coma, and so intravenous triiodothyronine is not necessary in this instance. Oral levothyroxine therapy is sufficient.

Severe hypothyroidism by itself causes hyperprolactinaemia. Bromocriptine is not necessary; correction of the hypothyroidism would bring the level of prolactin down.

Severe hypothyroidism can occasionally result in significant thyrotroph, hyperplasia, causing a secondary thyrotroph adenoma in the pituitary. This thyrotroph hyperplasia usually resolves with thyroxine replacement.

Hekimsoy Z, et al. The prevalence of hyperprolactinaemia in overt and subclinical hypothyroidism. Endocr J 2010; 57(12):1011–1015.

18. A Add spironolactone

Though the aldosterone:renin ratio is high, both aldosterone and renin levels are low in this instance. In this case effective treatment would be to add a small dose of spironolactone.

Given the low aldosterone level the suspicion of primary aldosteronism (Conn's syndrome and other causes of high aldosterone level) is less here. The most likely diagnosis is low renin essential hypertension and, given that the patient is already on bendrofluazide, the best course is adding a mineralocorticoid antagonist such as spironolactone. The other possibilities are extremely rare such as Liddle's syndrome, rare mutations in steroidogenesis pathway and congenital adrenal hyperplasia (CAH). Another rare cause is excessive liquorice ingestion. These possibilities are entertained if spironolactone fails to control the blood pressure.

Selective adrenal vein sampling is the current gold standard for Conn's syndrome and, as described above, is not indicated here.

The urine metanephrine level is normal twice and hence there is no need to do an MIBG (*meta*-iodobenzylguanidine) scan. Similarly pituitary MRI and high-dose dexamethasone suppression tests are not indicated here, since the screening test (overnight dexamethasone suppression test) is negative and the index of suspicion is low.

Mulatero P, et al. Diagnosis and treatment of low-renin hypertension. Clin Endocrinol 2007; 67: 324–334.

19. B 24-hour urine metanephrines

His past history of hypertension, palpitations, left ventricular hypertrophy (LVH) on the ECG and syncopal episodes, together with the hypertensive episode on anaesthesia, is suggestive of phaeochromocytoma, and hence a 24-hour urine metanephrine is the best investigation among the options. The other screening test would be plasma metanephrine level.

Although Conn's syndrome would result in hypertension and LVH on the ECG, hypertensive crisis with anaesthesia is not common. Also serum potassium was normal, which makes Conn's syndrome unlikely. Similarly Cushing's syndrome does not commonly produce crisis on anaesthesia induction.

Although hypertension is known to occur with a thyroid storm, and surgery on the thyroid can precipitate it, the symptom complex here favours a catecholamine-related tumour rather than thyroid dysfunction. Though there is history of episodic palpitations, other history suggestive of thyrotoxicosis, such as fever, diarrhoea and weight loss, is absent. Resting ECG did not show sinus tachycardia or abnormal rhythms and physical examination did not reveal any signs of thyrotoxicosis.

Acute intermittent porphyria presents more with abdominal pain and neuropsychiatric symptoms rather than syncopal episodes.

Terzolo M, et al. AME position statement on adrenal incidentaloma. Eur J Endocrinol 2011; 164(6):851–870. Chen H, et al. The North American Neuroendocrine Tumor Society consensus guideline for the diagnosis and management of neuroendocrine tumors: pheochromocytoma, paraganglioma, and medullary thyroid cancer. Pancreas 2010 39(6):775–783.

20. B Stop carbimazole and propranolol and monitor thyroid function tests in 6 weeks

The clinical and biochemical picture is suggestive of subacute thyroiditis (de Quervain's thyroiditis). The aetiology is unknown, but immune alteration following a viral illness in susceptible individuals is suspected.

Initial presentation is with sore throat and flu-like symptoms, followed by transient hyperthyroidism (because of release of preformed thyroid hormones from follicles due to follicular disruption). Four to six weeks later there may be a phase of hypothyroidism (because of glandular destruction) in about 25% of those affected followed by return of normal thyroid function (due to regeneration from the edges of the areas of destruction). In the initial phase a thyroid gland is often enlarged and tender.

Treatment is mainly supportive. For pain and sore throat non-steroidal anti-inflammatory drugs can be used. For the hyperthyroid phase propranolol is useful for symptomatic control. In severe cases prednisolone may be useful. Recurrences are common.

Watchful monitoring is all that is required during the hypothyroid phase. In 10% of cases hypothyroidism may be prolonged and require levothyroxine supplementation.

Carbimazole is not useful as the primary pathology is not overproduction of thyroid hormones but release of preformed hormones from follicular disruption.

Propranolol can be stopped as she does not have any hyperthyroid symptoms.

Thyroid ultrasound is not indicated as the clinical and biochemical picture is suggestive of subacute thyroiditis. An iodine-131 uptake scan during the hyperthyroid phase may be useful as it would show decreased uptake of iodine [whereas Graves' disease or thyroid nodule causing hyperthyroidism would show increased uptake either diffusely (Graves' disease) or as a hot spot (nodule)].

Other causes of subacute thyroiditis include interferon-α therapy, radiation, renal cell carcinoma (paraneoplastic) and amiodarone.

Bindra A, Braunstein GD. Thyroiditis. Am Fam Physician 2006; 73(10):1769–1776.

21. C Fasting gastrin and chromogranin A level in serum

The clinical picture described here is suggestive of multiple endocrine neoplasia 1 (MEN1) or Wermer's syndrome. This comes from a history of parathyroid involvement (nearly all of those with MEN1 develop hyperparathyroidism by the age of 50) and gastrinoma, which is suggested by the gastric ulcers. Up to 40% of those with MEN1 may develop gastrinoma. Zollinger–Ellison syndrome (ZES) is the manifestation of excess gastric acid due to gastrinoma. Twenty-five per cent of cases of ZES are due to MEN1. Less commonly, insulinomas and glucagonomas may develop.

In MEN1 this is more likely to be due to multiple intraduodenal tumours rather than a pancreatic tumour. These are also more likely to be malignant than the sporadic tumours and more likely to metastasise. The presence of steatorrhoea in this case suggests inactivation of pancreatic lipase due to the high gastrin and acid levels. In the case of neuroendocrine tumours, chromogranin A, a storage vesicle protein, is a good marker and can be elevated in up to 46% of cases of gastrinoma. Fasting gastrin level is usually elevated in gastrinomas. Care must be taken to exclude conditions which cause hypergastrinaemia such as atrophic gastritis and PPI (proton pump inhibitor) treatment.

MEN1 as mentioned presents with parathyroid, pancreatic and pituitary tumours. Prolactinomas and growth hormone-secreting adenomas are the common pituitary lesions. Monitoring consists of measuring serum calcium, prolactin, insulin-like growth factor-1 and chromogranin A levels periodically. Somatostatin receptor scintigraphy is used to image the neuroendocrine tumours such as gastrinomas.

Surgical management is difficult in gastrinomas due to MEN1 and total cure is seldom achieved because of the multiplicity of tumours. Hence medical treatment with PPIs and H$_2$ receptor blockers such as ranitidine is preferred.

Gagel RF, Marx SJ. Chapter 40. Multiple endocrine neoplasia. In: Kronenberg HM, et al. (eds), Williams Textbook of Endocrinology, 11th edn. Philadelphia, PA: Saunders, 2008.

22. D Systemic steroids

Graves' ophthalmopathy can develop before or after the thyroid disease manifests. Management is dependent on the severity of the disease. Many classifications including NOSPECS have been used for assessing the severity of Graves' disease. Most also look at the level of inflammatory activity.

The treatment depends on the severity and activity. She is euthyroid after antithyroid drug therapy. At this point in time neither radio-iodine nor surgery would be the treatments of choice. There are reports that radio-iodine treatment in patients with active hyperthyroidism can worsen the eye disease. Smoking can also worsen eye disease in Graves' disease.

For mild eye disease, observation is the best policy supplemented by artificial tears.

With moderate eye disease, the first treatment option would be steroids. In severe eye disease the first treatment choice would be intravenous steroids such as pulsed methylprednisolone. Other methods that have been used include radiotherapy to the orbits, surgical decompression of the orbit and rituximab.

In this instance with euthyroid status achieved by antithyroid drugs, the best therapeutic option would be pulsed intravenous steroid therapy.

Soeters MR, et al. Optimal management of Graves' orbitopathy: a multidisciplinary approach. Neth J Med 2011; 69(7):302–308.
Bahn RS et al. Hyperthyroidism and other causes of thyrotoxicosis: management guidelines of the American Thyroid Association and American Association of Clinical Endocrinologists. Endocr Pract 2011; 17(3):456–520.

23. C Reassure the patient

This person has mildly elevated serum calcium and parathyroid hormone (PTH) levels. She also has a normal phosphate and vitamin D levels. However, the urine calcium:creatinine clearance ratio is reduced, suggesting that she has relative hypocalciuria in the presence of hypercalcaemia. PTH is also not suppressed in the presence of hypercalcaemia. The combination of these suggests familial hypocalciuric hypercalcaemia (FHH). In primary hyperparathyroidism, the urine calcium:creatinine clearance ratio would be higher than 0.01, suggesting that urine calcium excretion in normal or increased.

Most of FHH is caused by autosomal dominant loss-of-function mutations in the calcium-sensing receptor (*CaSR*) gene, which encodes the *CaSR*. Elevations in serum calcium concentration stimulate the *CaSR*, which promotes calcitonin production and urinary calcium excretion while suppressing the synthesis and secretion of PTH, thereby lowering the calcium concentration. Mutations in *CaSR* impair the feedback inhibition of PTH with rising serum calcium. Hence higher than normal serum calcium levels are needed to inhibit the release of PTH, thus leading to either normal or slightly elevated PTH levels despite hypercalcaemia. The degree of hypercalcaemia depends on how severely the mutation affects the function of the *CaSR* molecule. In effect the mutation resets the calcium homeostasis to a slightly higher serum calcium level.

In the kidneys, *CaSR* is involved in the feedback inhibition of PTH-independent calcium reabsorption. Mutations in the *CaSR* gene prevent this feedback inhibition of calcium which helps lower serum calcium in the presence of hypercalcaemia. Since calcium is reabsorbed despite hypercalcaemia, the calcium concentration in the urine is low despite high serum calcium (relative hypocalciuria).

FHH is a benign disorder and does not usually need treatment. Genetic testing for mutations in *CaSR* can be carried out to confirm the diagnosis. More than 200 different mutations in *CaSR* have been identified to date.

Rarely there is an autoimmune version of this with autoantibodies against *CaSR*.

Varghese J, et al. Benign familial hypocalciuric hypercalcemia. Endocr Pract 2010: 1–16.

24. C Add mixed insulin (short and intermediate acting) twice a day

This patient has significant hyperglycaemia with high, fasting, postprandial, blood sugar levels and a very high HbA1c. In particular his postprandial blood sugars are high. The target HbA1c in this individual is 7% (or lower, if it can be safely achieved without hypoglycaemic episodes).

Addition of pioglitazone and sitagliptin would each only bring the HbA1c down by < 1%. Addition of a glucagon-like peptide-1 (GLP-1) agonist such as exenatide would bring the HbA1c down by 1–1.7% and in addition would benefit the weight. However, in this instance the HbA1c is >9% and there is significant hyperglycaemia. Insulin therapy is usually initiated in type 2 diabetes mellitus when combination oral agent therapy, with or without GLP-1 receptor agonist therapy, fails to achieve the glycaemic goal or when a patient, whether drug naïve or on a treatment regimen, presents with a HbA1c level >9.0% and symptomatic hyperglycaemia.

Since the HbA1c is 9.8% and the person is already on metformin and gliclazide, only the addition of insulin would bring about adequate control. The ideal regimen would be a basal bolus one, since his home monitoring indicates both pre-meal and post-meal hyperglycaemia. The options given here are basal insulin and twice a day insulin. Of these, basal insulin is unlikely to do be fully effective, especially for the postprandial hyperglycaemia, and hence the most effective technique among the options would be twice a day mixed insulin. Once the insulin regimen has been established, insulin secretagogues such as sulphonylureas should ideally be tapered and stopped. Guidelines on the optimal drug to be used and optimal time to start each class of drugs as well as optimal combinations of various drugs are evolving.

Nathan DM, et al. Medical management of hyperglycemia in type 2 diabetes: a consensus algorithm for the initiation and adjustment of therapy: a consensus statement of the American Diabetes Association and the European Association for the Study of Diabetes. Diabetes Care 2009; 32(1):193–203.
Handelsman Y, et al. American Association of Clinical Endocrinologists Medical Guidelines for Clinical Practice for developing a diabetes mellitus comprehensive care plan. Endocr Pract 2011; 17 (2):1–53.

25. C Desmopressin 100 µg three times daily

This young man has diabetes insipidus secondary to severe cranial trauma. He has hypernatraemia, with increased output of dilute urine, suggesting diabetes insipidus. Since he has extensive facial trauma as evidenced by cranial sinus fractures, the correct treatment here would be either subcutaneous or oral desmopressin. The diagnostic test to be used would be a water deprivation test; however, given his clinical history, this is not indicated here.

Trauma to the head, especially with basal skull fracture, is likely to damage the pituitary gland and especially the pituitary stalk. Classically a triphasic pattern of antidiuretic hormone (ADH) abnormalities is described:

- Initial phase of diabetes insipidus due to stunning of the neurons and subsequent decreased release of ADHs lasts 24 hours or so.
- Second phase of excess ADH due to the release of all the stored ADH, producing an SIADH (syndrome of inappropriate release ADH)-like picture.
- Third phase of more prolonged central diabetes insipidus which may be permanent. Partial or complete recovery is seen as well.

Fluid restriction, demeclocycline and tolvaptan are used for the management of SIADH; 0.45% saline is not indicated as the primary problem here is failure of the kidneys to retain water.

Robinson AG, Verbalis JG. Chapter 9, Posterior pituitary. In: Kronenberg HM et al. (eds), Williams Textbook of Endocrinology, 11th edn. Philadelphia, PA: Saunders, 2008.

26. A Bezafibrate

This patient has pre-diabetes and hypertriglyceridaemia. Though type 2 diabetes itself can lead to hypertriglyceridaemia, in this instance one has to think about other conditions that raise triglyceride levels as well, such as familial hypertriglyceridaemia (FHT). High levels of triglycerides are seen in uncontrolled diabetes, especially in conditions of insulin deficiency. However, it is unlikely that pre-diabetes would lead to such high levels of triglycerides in the absence of another abnormality in the lipid metabolism.

It is likely that the hypertriglyceridaemia itself induced the acute pancreatitis. FHT is relatively common with an incidence of 1 in 500. Aetiology is unknown and it causes an elevated VLDL (very-low-density lipoprotein) level.

Complications include acute pancreatitis and premature coronary heart disease.

Treatment includes dietary fat restriction, alcohol restriction and, in conditions with very high triglyceride levels, drugs such as nicotinic acid, gemfibrozil, fenofibrate and bezafibrate. Statins also lower the triglyceride level, but to a much lesser extent than fibrates or nicotinic acid. The drug of choice in this instance would be fibrates. Nicotinic acid, even in the long-acting formulations, has a high rate of producing flushing and diarrhoea. It also worsens glycaemic control, and therefore fibrates would be the drug of choice.

Treatment with fibrates does lead to an increase in incidence of abnormalities in the liver function tests. Hence monitoring the liver function is important. The other issue with fibrates is increased incidence of muscle aches (myalgia) and rarely myositis and rhabdomyolysis. Statins have the same adverse effect and if combined, there is a higher risk of myalgia and myositis.

The other therapy that has been shown to be effective is omega-3 fatty acids.

Mahley RW, et al. Disorders of lipid metabolism. In: Kronenberg HM et al (eds), Williams Textbook of Endocrinology, 11th edn. Philadelphia, PA: Saunders Elsevier, 2008: 36.

27. E Stop simvastatin and later switch to a lower dose of more potent statin

Statin therapy has been associated with myalgia, myositis and rhabdomyolysis. Often cases of myositis are not accompanied by creatine kinase (CK) elevations. In most instances, however, symptomatic myalgias are accompanied by CK elevation. The mechanism of myalgia/myositis with statins has not been fully elucidated. Complicating this picture are studies suggesting that CK levels vary widely within the population and with activity and exercise. CK levels also have ethnic variations. Many centres suggest obtaining a baseline CK level prior to starting statins to reduce the effect of this variability. Some guidelines do not recommend this for the general population but do so for ethnic minorities and people at risk of myopathy. Routine later monitoring of statins is not recommended. Measure CK levels later only if the patient is symptomatic.

Always rule out hepatic problems, alcoholism and hypothyroidism because all of these can increase the incidence of statin-induced muscle damage.

Strategies to manage statin-related myopathies generally suggest:
- If asymptomatic and CK elevations <5–10 times the upper limit then continue the statin and monitor.
- If symptomatic (mild muscle aches and tolerable symptoms) and CK levels <5–10 times the upper limit, then continue statin at same or reduced dose and monitor.
- If tolerable symptoms and CK levels >5 times upper limit then stop statin and allow time for muscle to recover. Then alternative strategies for restarting statins – see below.
- If significant symptoms/rhabdomyolysis develops then stop statin and carefully consider the risk of restarting statins. Think of alternatives to statins.

Alternative strategies:
1. Use a lower dose of a more potent statin, e.g. atorvastatin or rosuvastatin
2. Use a statin with less impact on cytochrome P450 such as pravastatin or fluvastatin
3. Use alternate-day dosage of longer-acting statin such as atorvastatin
4. Use combination of lower-dose statin with ezetimibe.

In general, combining fibrates with statins increases the risk of myopathy. Ezetimibe by itself does not have clinical trial evidence to indicate lower cardiovascular risk. Coenzyme Q10 has been shown in some trials to mitigate the effect of statin-induced myopathy; however, larger trials have failed to replicate the effect.

Hence, in this instance, the correct strategy would be to stop simvastatin and allow time for recovery and then switch to a lower dose of a more potent statin.

Arca M, Pigna G. Treating statin-intolerant patients. Diabetes Metab Syndr Obes 2011; 4:155–166.
McKenney JM, et al. Final conclusions and recommendations of the National Lipid Association Statin Safety Assessment Task Force. Am J Cardiol 2006; 97(8A):89C–94C.

28. E Thyroid function tests

The presentation is suggestive of hypokalaemic periodic paralysis. The features are hypotonia, reduced power and reflexes as well as intact sensorium, allied with a low potassium and improvement with potassium supplementation. Patients also have muscle cramps and aches.

The main differential diagnosis here would be Guillain–Barré syndrome and transverse myelitis apart from myasthenia gravis and polymyositis. However, the low potassium level would suggest that the diagnosis is hypokalaemic periodic paralysis. Most cases of hypokalaemic periodic paralysis are familial. In males of Chinese and Latin American origin, hyperthyroidism can lead to hypokalaemic periodic paralysis.

In thyrotoxic periodic paralysis the hypokalaemia is due to an intracellular shift of potassium rather than absolute deficiency. Other causes of potassium depletion such as diarrhoea must be ruled out first. Heavy physical activity and stress can precipitate the attack, as can carbohydrate-rich meals.

There are two aspects to the treatment: immediate restoration of normal serum potassium level and later attainment of euthyroid status.

Oral or intravenous potassium can be used. However, it is important to remember that the hypokalaemia is due to intracellular shift. Hence aggressive treatment could lead to hyperkalaemia. Beta-blockers can be effective in preventing episodes.

Once the acute treatment is done, attaining euthyroid status would be important in preventing future episodes.

Pothiwala P, Levine SN. Analytic review: thyrotoxic periodic paralysis: a review. J Intensive Care Med 2010; 25(2):71–77.

29. E Short Synacthen test

A person with a history of multiple autoimmune problems (type 1 diabetes and hypothyroidism) is at risk of developing other autoimmune problems and should raise the suspicion of polyglandular autoimmune syndrome (PAI) type 2.

The symptoms of fatigue and recurrent hypoglycaemia in a person with type 1 diabetes should raise the suspicion of Addison's disease. In the presence of Addison's disease, adding levothyroxine without replacing hydrocortisone could potentially exacerbate the symptoms.

PAI type 2 is characterised by Addison's disease plus one of the other autoimmune diseases such as type 1 diabetes, hypothyroidism, pernicious anaemia and myasthenia gravis.

Women have a higher risk than men. Polygenic inheritance associated with HLA-DR3 and HLA-DR4 and non-HLA genes (MICA5.1, PTPN22, CTLA4, VNTR).

The standard diagnostic test for hypoadrenalism is the short Synacthen test.

Michels AW, Gottlieb PA. Autoimmune polyglandular syndromes. Nat Rev Endocrinol 2010; 6(5):270–277.

30. B Start cholecalciferol/ergocalciferol supplementation

The most likely explanation of this woman's symptoms is severe vitamin D deficiency. Prolonged vitamin D deficiency would result in persistent hypocalcaemia and raised parathyroid hormone (PTH). This rise in PTH is called secondary hyperparathyroidism.

The initial therapy would be replacement of vitamin D either as cholecalciferol/ergocalciferol or as calcitriol. She should also be evaluated for malabsorption syndromes such as coeliac disease, though in this case lack of adequate sun exposure is more likely to the reason.

Proximal myopathy is very common in severe vitamin D deficiency.

Fraser WD. Hyperparathyroidism. Lancet 2009; 374:145–158.

31. E Measure glutamic acid decarboxylase (GAD) antibodies

The clinical picture of normal body mass index (BMI), young age and difficult to control blood sugars with oral hypoglycaemic agents soon after diagnosis points towards 'latent autoimmune diabetes of adulthood' (LADA).

In this instance a positive GAD antibody result would suggest that the person probably has LADA. A C-peptide level would also give additional information regarding beta-cell reserve.

However, there is controversy on the management of LADA; some authorities advocate early insulin therapy whereas others prefer oral agents first and insulin later.

Given his BMI, metformin may not be the first choice here. Pioglitazone has shown some benefit in small clinical trials; however, early insulin therapy in LADA is known to preserve beta-cell function better. Immunomodulatory agents are undergoing trials in LADA.

Fructosamine levels are measured in instances where HbA1c results may not be reliable – for instance in anaemia, pregnancy, haemoglobinopathies.

Cernea S, et al. Beta-cell protection and therapy for latent autoimmune diabetes in adults. Diabetes Care 2009; 32(2):S246–S252.

32. E Trans-sphenoidal surgery

Trans-sphenoidal removal of the adenoma is appropriate for a non-functioning macroadenoma resulting in visual field defects. The raised prolactin level is most probably due to stalk compression and subsequent reduction in dopamine reaching the pituitary. Lack of dopamine results in disinhibition of the pituitary lactotrophs, resulting in hyperprolactinaemia.

The symptoms are suggestive of hyperprolactinaemia with galactorrhoea and amenorrhoea. Her visual field symptoms are suggestive of optic chiasma involvement.

Pituitary MRI shows a 3-cm lesion which suggests that it is a macroadenoma (>1 cm). Prolactin-secreting macroadenomas (macroprolactinomas) generally secrete large quantities of prolactin – usually >8000 mU/mL. Since the prolactin level is <2000 mU/mL, it is more likely that the prolactin secretion is from disinhibition rather than from the adenoma itself. Treatment for a prolactinoma is medical therapy initially with dopamine agonists such as bromocriptine or cabergoline.

Octreotide is useful as medical therapy in acromegaly to reduce growth hormone levels. Stereotactic radiosurgery is useful in situations where surgery is contraindicated or if there is residual tumour after surgery. Transcranial surgery is generally reserved for large tumours where full resection may not be possible with trans-sphenoidal approach.

Melmed S et al. Diagnosis and treatment of hyperprolactinemia: an Endocrine Society clinical practice guideline. J Clin Endocrinol Metab 2011; 96(2):273–288.

33. C Reduce basal insulin and pre-exercise rapid-acting insulin and avoid hypoglycaemia for the next 2 months

This young woman had very good glycaemic control with low HbA1c. Since she started her exercise regimen without altering her insulin doses, she has had several episodes of severe hypoglycaemia. More worryingly, she has hypoglycaemia unawareness with several hypoglycaemic episodes being asymptomatic. In general, hypoglycaemia tends to provoke hypoglycaemia unawareness, with the threshold of blood sugar at which symptoms arise getting lower with prolonged low blood sugar levels. Restoration of hypoglycaemia awareness is best brought about by avoiding hypoglycaemia for 6–8 weeks. Conversely prolonged hyperglycaemia would lead to symptoms occurring at higher blood sugar levels.

At the age of 28 years there is no compelling rationale to start simvastatin with a single raised cholesterol level. Dietary and lifestyle adjustment would be the first step. Similarly for high blood pressure, the reading should be interpreted cautiously and the test repeated. Again initial management would be lifestyle modification, but the drug of choice, if that does not work, would be ramipril. In the child-bearing age group, warning must be given about the teratogenic potential.

Although insulin pump would alleviate the recurrent hypoglycaemia, simpler measures should be tried first. Similarly, whereas twice a day detemir might offer some beneficial effect, advice on exercise and a modification of the current regimen should be tried first.

Bakatselos SO. Hypoglycemia unawareness. Diabetes Res Clin Pract 2011; 93(1):S92–96.

34. D Short Synacthen test

This woman has features of hyperandrogenism such as acne and hirsuitism as well as high levels of 17OH-progesterone. The combination would suggest 'non-classic' congenital adrenal hyperplasia (CAH).

Congenital adrenal hyperplasia is most commonly due to mutations in 21-hydroxylase (cytochrome P450 CYP21A2) enzyme. This is an important enzyme in the steroid biosynthetic pathway which mediates the conversion of 17OH-progesterone to 11-deoxycortisol (precursor of cortisol) and of progesterone to deoxycorticosterone (precursor of aldosterone). If there is loss of function of this enzyme, cortisol production is affected, the adrenocorticotrophic hormone (ACTH) level goes up because of lack of feedback and hence there is over-stimulation of the adrenal cortex with excess production of cortisol precursors. These precursors are then diverted into sex hormone synthesis. This may lead to androgen excess and ambiguous genitalia in girls. Aldosterone deficiency may lead to salt wasting, hypovolaemia and shock. Approximately, 90% of CAH is due to mutations in this enzyme. The phenotype varies depending on the severity of the deletion/

mutation. Rarer forms of CAH are associated with mutations in 11β-hydroxylase and 3β-steroid dehydrogenase.

Classically there are three phenotypes with CYP21A2 involvement: classic type with either salt wasting or simple virilising without aldosterone deficiency and non-classic. Classic salt wasting CAH is apparent in the neonatal period with failure to thrive, hypovolaemia and shock. The simple virilising form may present with ambiguous genitalia in girls.

Non-classic CAH is often asymptomatic and may be apparent only in adulthood with androgen excess. In late childhood, it may present with premature pubarche, accelerated bone age and acne. In women, this may present with hirsutism, oligomenorrhoea, subfertility and acne, and can be mistaken for polycystic ovarian syndrome.

Non-classic CAH usually presents with signs of hyperandrogenism such as acne and hirsuitism. Some women also have irregular cycles and subfertility.

In the classic forms, basal 17OH-progesterone levels are high; in non-classic CAH, the elevation in 17OH-progesterone level may be modest and hence a more confirmatory test is needed. This is the Synacthen test, performed by measuring 17OH-progesterone prior to and 60 minutes after 250 µg synthetic adrenocorticotrophic hormone (ACTH). Stimulated values are elevated in patients with classic and non-classic varieties (in excess of 35 nmol/L usually).

In adult women with non-classic CAH, glucocorticoid treatment does not bring additional benefit for hyperandrogenism. Hirsuitism in these individuals can be treated with eflornithine locally, spironolactone, cyproterone acetate and oral contraceptives systemically.

Subfertility, however, may benefit from glucocorticoid therapy to reduce ACTH levels.

Similarly adult males with non-classic CAH require treatment only in cases of subfertility.

Stewart PM. In: Kronenberg HM, et al. Williams Textbook of Endocrinology, 11th edn. Saunders; 2008.

35. C Plasma vasoactive intestinal peptide (VIP)

Symptoms of large-volume watery diarrhoea, metabolic acidosis and hypokalaemia suggest a VIPoma. A serum VIP level >200 pmol/L would establish the diagnosis. It is also called WDHA (watery diarrhoea, hypokalaemia and achlorhydria) syndrome. Hypercalcaemia can be seen with this presentation. Raised creatinine is most likely because of the dehydration. Hyperglycaemia is seen in a third of cases because of increased glycogenolysis in liver.

Localisation of the tumour can be achieved by CT of the abdomen and for small tumours by endoscopic ultrasound and radiolabelled octreotide scanning. The last can also be used for looking for local recurrence and metastases. Most of these tumours are located in the pancreas. VIP is involved in smooth muscle relaxation, secretion of water and bicarbonate from the intestine and pancreas, and also inhibits gastric acid secretion and colonic reabsorption of potassium.

Immediate treatment is to correct the fluid loss, hypokalaemia and metabolic acidosis. Somatostatin analogues such as octreotide are effective in controlling the diarrhoea. Surgical resection is the only curative treatment. Debate persists as to whether somatostatin analogues can shrink the tumour.

With gastrinomas, abdominal pain, heart burn and diarrhoea are the common symptoms. Diarrhoea is partly due to the fat malabsorption because of lack of pancreatic lipase (degraded by the excess gastric acid) and partly due to small bowel inflammation. Very high serum gastrin level and gastric acid hypersecretion would clinch the diagnosis. In cases of intermediate gastrin levels, a secretin stimulation test should be performed.

Song S, et al. Diagnosis and treatment of pancreatic vasoactive intestinal peptide endocrine tumors. Pancreas 2009; 38(7):811–814.
Batcher E, et al. Pancreatic neuroendocrine tumors. Endocr Res 2011; 36(1):35–43.

36. B Diabetic lumbosaccral plexopathy

The clinical picture of severe pain in the proximal legs with wasting, weakness and loss of knee jerk, and minimal sensory involvement is typical of diabetic lumbosacral plexopathy or diabetic amyotrophy.

It is usually seen with poorly controlled diabetes and the aetiology has not been fully elucidated. It is thought to be an immune-mediated vascular radiculopathy.

Treatment is essentially symptomatic, with physiotherapy and occupational therapy. Good control of diabetes is essential. Intravenous immunoglobulin and pulse glucocorticoid such as methylprednisolone have been tried, but neither has an extensive evidence base.

Tricyclic antidepressants may improve the pain as do pregabalin and gabapentin.

Little AA, et al. Diabetic neuropathies. Pract Neurol 2007; 7:82–92.

37. B Dextrose–insulin infusion

This patient has severe triglyceridaemia, probably due to insulin deficiency from longstanding, poorly controlled diabetes and diet/alcohol and genetic factors. Both VLDL (very-low-density lipoprotein) and chylomicrons would be raised. At such high triglyceride (TG) levels, the VLDL and chylomicron removal mechanisms would be saturated.

The priority here would be to get the triglyceride level under control to avoid complications such as pancreatitis.

Though niacin and gemfibrozil would bring the TG level under control, in such an acute setting a better option needs to be adopted. Heparin has the issue that, although it causes the release of endothelial lipoprotein lipase (LPL) early on, later the LPL level decreases, so monotherapy with heparin is not advocated.

Insulin–dextrose infusion would correct the insulin deficiency, which brought this on as well as reduce the triglyceride level. It will also provide calories for the patient and allow him to remain nil by mouth, reducing the dietary lipids temporarily.

Once the TG level comes down, gemfibrozil or other alternatives may be considered. Also a low-fat diet should be advised.

Ewald N, et al. Severe hypertriglyceridemia and pancreatitis: presentation and management. Curr Opin Lipidol 2009; 20(6):497–504.

38. B Repeat thyroid function tests in a week and then in 2–3 months

This patient has sick euthyroid syndrome (non-thyroidal illness syndrome). In this condition, the thyroid function tests may be variable. No treatment or investigations are required at this stage. Once she has recovered from the acute illness, the thyroid function can be reassessed. The thyroid function should be monitored during the illness and 1–2 months after recovery.

The conditions to exclude include primary thyroid illness, other medications affecting the thyroid and pituitary–hypothalamic illness. Drugs that affect the thyroid include glucocorticoids, dobutamine, amiodarone, salicylates, beta-blockers and anticonvulsants.

Adler SM, Wartofsky L. The nonthyroidal illness syndrome. Endocrinol Metab Clin North Am 2007; 36(3):657–672, vi.

39. E Start simvastatin

The patient has risk factors for coronary vessel disease: nearly 40 years old, 2-year history of type 2 diabetes, hypertension, and total cholesterol and low-density lipoprotein (LDL) are high. The National Institute for Health and Clinical Excellence (NICE) recommends simvastatin for those with type 2 diabetes and aged above 40 years. For people below 40 years, if cardiovascular disease risk is high then statins are recommended. Since he has significant risk, statin is the best initial therapy.

If the triglycerides continue to be high despite optimal statin therapy then addition of a fibrate may be considered especially when other factors such as alcohol, liver disease and poor control are ruled out. Given his raised LDL, omega-3 fatty acids may not be the best choice.

Though lifestyle advice may be given, the high-risk profile means that, in addition to lifestyle changes, pharmaceuticals may be needed.

National Collaborating Centre for Chronic Conditions. Type 2 diabetes: national clinical guideline for management in primary and secondary care (update). London: Royal College of Physicians, 2008.

40. B Charcot's foot affecting the forefoot bones

This presentation is typical of Charcot's foot (neuropathic arthropathy). This patient has diabetes and peripheral neuropathy. He has non-tender swelling over the forefoot with increased temperature and redness. Erythrocyte sedimentation rate is elevated but C-reactive protein and white cell count are normal.

Charcot's foot develops over a background of neurological impairment in the foot. There are two main contributors: the neuropathy results in increased likelihood of trauma and sympathetic denervation results in increased blood supply. This hyperaemia increases bone resorption and renders the foot more vulnerable to micro- and macro-fractures during weight bearing. Normal walking may result in micro-fractures and dislocations, and these fail to heal properly eventually resulting in architectural changes in the foot. Continued walking would result in abnormal weight bearing, leading to ulcers and other complications. The most common areas affected are the mid- and forefoot.

The condition is self-limiting with treatment mainly consisting of avoiding weight bearing on the foot.

Rogers LC, et al. The Charcot foot in diabetes. Diabetes Care 2011; 34(9):2123–2129.

41. D Orchidectomy

Karyotyping shows a XY genotype, but phenotypically she is female from birth with well-developed secondary sexual characteristics.

This suggests androgen insensitivity syndrome (AIS), previously called testicular feminisation syndrome (this term was considered pejorative and is no longer used).

AIS is a diverse syndrome of many causes and has many phenotypes, ranging from mild to partial to complete.

This girl probably has complete AIS. In partial AIS, the external genitalia are not fully feminised and, in mild AIS, the external genitalia are those of a male.

In AIS due to androgen receptor mutations, the tissues are insensitive to the androgens and hence wolffian duct structures do not develop. In the absence of testosterone action on tissues, oestrogen causes unopposed development of female external genitalia. However, the tests still produce anti-müllerian hormone which inhibits the development of müllerian duct structures such as the uterus and the fallopian tubes. Hence in complete AIS, the vagina ends blindly.

The other conditions resembling AIS with an XY genotype are:
- 3β-Hydroxysteroid dehydrogenase 2 deficiency
- Leydig cell hypoplasia or aplasia
- Smith–Lemli–Opitz syndrome (associated with learning disability)
- Lipoid congenital adrenal hyperplasia
- Swyer's syndrome
- 5α-Reductase deficiency
- Luteinising hormone receptor mutations
- 17α-Hydroxylase deficiency
- 17,20-Lyase deficiency
- 7β-Hydroxysteroid dehydrogenase deficiency.

Other lab findings in complete AIS include elevated testosterone levels; genetic sequencing of the androgen receptor gene can identify the mutation responsible.

In complete AIS, since the testes could be found in the labia, inguinal ring or intra-abdominally, the incidence of testicular malignancy is high (4–9%) and hence, after attaining puberty, the testes should be removed. Since the testes are genetically normal, the rate of malignancy prior to puberty is very low. However, they should be removed earlier if there are concerns about carcinoma *in situ* and puberty induced hormonally.

Oakes MB, et al. Complete androgen insensitivity syndrome – a review. J Pediatr Adolesc Gynecol 2008; 21(6):305–310.

42. C Insulin tolerance test

This woman has been adequately replaced with thyroxine (T_4) as indicated by the free T_4 and triiodothyronine (T_3) levels. Additional measurement of thyroid-binding globulins is not necessary since the free hormone levels are already given. Her symptoms are not suggestive of thyrotoxicosis; hence radio-iodine uptake scan and thyroid-stimulating hormone (TSH) receptor antibody measurement are not required. Her symptoms are persistent, hence hypopituitarism should be ruled out first.

In the set of options given, insulin tolerance test showing failure of growth hormone and cortisol levels to increase with hypoglycaemia would suggest hypopituitarism. Indeed a low TSH level in the presence of low thyroid hormone levels (normal in this case due to supplementation) should raise suspicion of a pituitary problem.

Luteinising hormone and follicle-stimulating hormone should be high in postmenopausal women; absence of this or reduction in adrenocorticotrophic hormone level or TSH-releasing hormone stimulation test could also be used to diagnose hypopituitarism.

43. B Karyotyping

Klinefelter's syndrome (KS) is one of the most common genetic forms of male hypogonadism affecting up to 1 in 600 adult males. This is classically because of meiotic non-disjunction. The phenotype becomes clear only after puberty. In the early years of life, the gonadal function as well as the pituitary function is normal and the phenotype is not apparent. However, during puberty, the follicle-stimulating hormone and luteinising hormone levels rise whereas the inhibin B concentrations become undetectable. Testosterone levels do not rise much and, typically in adulthood, the testosterone levels are low or low–normal. Estradiol levels are high–normal or high. The reason for hypogonadism in KS is likely to be abnormalities in the steroidogenic enzyme pathway or due to elevated estradiol levels within the testes.

Adults with KS show a varying degree of androgenisation with androgen deficiency and hypergonadotrophism. Testes show extensive fibrosis and hyalinisation of the seminiferous tubules and hyperplasia of the interstitium. The tubules show scanty areas of preserved spermatogenesis.

Typically adults with KS have hypergonadotrophic hypogonadism with small testes, increased height, gynaecomastia, narrow shoulders, broad hips, and a tendency towards insulin resistance and metabolic syndrome. If not treated adequately, there may be loss of muscle mass, redistribution of body fat and osteoporosis. However, it must be emphasised that the phenotype is widely variable and men with KS may be completely asymptomatic and commonly have no intellectual impairment.

These individuals have a higher than normal incidence of autoimmune disorders.

Karyotyping will show the extra X chromosome and will confirm the diagnosis. Of patients 80–90% are the non-mosaic 47 XXY genotype; 5–10% have a mosaic form, the most common being 47 XXY/46 XY mosaicism. The rest are due to 48 XXXY, 48 XXYY and 49 XXXXY abnormalities.

Androgen replacement is the treatment of choice to maintain muscle mass, prevent metabolic complications and restore libido.

Men with KS generally have azoospermia; however, some individuals, especially those with mosaicism, may have areas of spermatogenesis and have occasionally been found to have spermatozoa in the ejaculate, and rare cases of spontaneous fertility have been described. Fertility can be restored in up to 50% of these individuals especially in mosaicism with intracytoplasmic sperm injection (ICSI) when spermatozoa can be retrieved by testicular exploration (TESE – testicular sperm extraction).

Children with KS have preserved spermatogonia which undergo massive apoptosis around the early pubertal stage. Cryopreservation of sperm in adolescence is therefore of importance.

Paduch DA, et al. New concepts in Klinefelter syndrome. Curr Opin Urol 2008; 18(6):621–627.

Chapter 4

Gastroenterology

Questions

1. A 56-year-old man with a history of chronic pancreatitis presented to the emergency department with epigastric pain. Five weeks ago, he had suffered from a very severe episode of epigastric pain that lasted for 2 days, which had been precipitated by an alcohol binge. After the initial episode the pain reduced, but over the past 4 weeks had been gradually increasing in severity. His appetite had been reduced and he had had early satiety and nausea. He had lost 3 kg in weight.

   On examination, he had a body mass index of 23 kg/m², and looked comfortable at rest. He was not icteric. His cardiovascular and respiratory examinations were normal but he had a tender epigastric mass. Murphy's sign was negative.

   Investigations:

haemoglobin 13.6 g/dL (13.0–18.0)	alkaline phosphatase 168 U/L (45–105)
white cell count 12.1 × 10⁹/L (4–11)	alanine transaminase 26 U/L (5–35)
platelets 187 × 10⁹/L (150–400)	albumin 34 g/L (37–49)
bilirubin 15 mmol/L (1–22)	amylase 220 U/L (60–180)

   What is the most likely diagnosis?

   A   Adenocarcinoma of the pancreas
   B   Biliary stricture
   C   Intraductal papillary mucinous neoplasm
   D   Pancreatic pseudocyst
   E   Splenic vein thrombosis

2. A 54-year-old woman was referred by her general practitioner with a 6-week history of gradual onset abdominal pain and distension. She had no previous medical history, did not drink and was not taking any medication.

   On examination, she had tender hepatomegaly and obvious shifting dullness. The rest of her physical examination was normal.

   Investigations:

haemoglobin 17.3 g/dL (11.5–16.5)	bilirubin 37 mmol/L (1–22)
white cell count 5.8 × 10⁹/L (4–11)	alkaline phosphatase 138 U/L (45–105)
platelets 362 × 10⁹/L (150–400)	alanine transaminase 120 U/L (5–35)
haematocrit 74% (36–46)	albumin 29 g/L (37–49)
international normalised ratio 1.6 (<1.4)	

   What is the most likely diagnosis?

   A   Budd–Chiari syndrome
   B   Constrictive pericarditis

C   Hepatocellular carcinoma
D   Portal vein thrombosis
E   Tricuspid regurgitation

3. A 38-year-old man presented with a 6-hour history of haematemesis and melaena. He had been diagnosed with alcohol-related cirrhosis 3 years ago, after a variceal haemorrhage but had been lost to follow-up. He had no other past medical history, and currently took no medications.

    On examination, he was agitated with a Glasgow Coma Scale score of 14/15, pulse 114 beats per minute and blood pressure 83/40 mmHg. He had pale conjunctivae, icteric sclera and an obvious asterixis. There were multiple spider naevi on his anterior chest wall, moderate ascites and splenomegaly.

    He was resuscitated with blood products and an upper gastrointestinal endoscopy was requested.

Investigations:

haemoglobin 7.6 g/dL (13.0–18.0)	urea 16 mmol/L (2.5–7.5)
white cell count 7 × 10⁹/L (4–11)	creatinine 76 µmol/L (60–110)
platelets 101 × 10⁹/L (150–400)	bilirubin 86 mmol/L (1–22)
international normalised ratio 1.9 (<1.4)	alkaline phosphatase 453 U/L (45–105)
sodium 132 mmol/L (135–145)	alanine transaminase 44 U/L (5–35)
potassium 4.2 mmol/L (3.5–5.0)	albumin 28 g/L (37–49)

What is the appropriate first-line pharmacological therapy prior to endoscopy?

A   Antibiotics, propranolol and terlipressin
B   Antibiotics and terlipressin
C   Antibiotics, propranolol and octreotide
D   Propranolol and octreotide
E   Propranolol and terlipressin

4. A 56-year-old homeless and alcohol-dependent man was admitted to hospital with haematemesis and persistent vomiting at a weekend. He was kept nil by mouth while awaiting an endoscopy. He finally had his endoscopy on his third day of admission.

    Endoscopy revealed erosive gastritis. Following the endoscopy he was allowed to eat but the next day he still felt unwell.

Investigations:

haemoglobin 13.2 g/dL (13.0–18.0)	urea 6.9 mmol/L (2.5–7.5)
white cell count 6 × 10⁹/L (4–11)	creatinine 76 µmol/L (60–110)
platelets 189 × 10⁹/L (150–400)	glucose 4.2 mmol/L (3.0–6.0)
sodium 138 mmol/L (135–145)	phosphate 0.23 mmol/L (0.8–1.4)
potassium 3.1 mmol/L (3.5–5.0)	magnesium 0.5 mmol/L (0.75–1.05)

What is the most appropriate next step in management?

A   Replace magnesium
B   Replace potassium
C   Replace phosphate
D   Start nasogastric (NG) feeding at a reduced rate
E   Thiamine administration

5. A 67-year-old man presented to the emergency department with a 1-day history of right upper quadrant pain associated with shivering. He also complained of nausea and anorexia. He had no past medical history and was not taking any medications.

On examination, he was icteric and had a temperature of 38.3°C. Abdominal examination revealed right upper quadrant tenderness and negative Murphy's sign.

Investigations:

haemoglobin 13.2 g/dL (13.0–18.0)

white cell count 14.8 × 10⁹/L (4–11)

platelets 546 × 10⁹/L (150–400)

bilirubin 56 mmol/L (1–22)

alanine transaminase 45 U/L (5–35)

alkaline phosphatase 489 U/L (45–105)

albumin 34 g/L (37–49)

What is the most likely diagnosis?

A   Acalculous cholecystitis
B   Acute cholecystitis
C   Acute pancreatitis
D   Alcoholic hepatitis
E   Ascending cholangitis

6. A 29-year-old woman was referred for colonoscopic screening for a hereditary polyposis syndrome. Her maternal grandfather was diagnosed with colorectal cancer at the age of 65 years, and her maternal aunt was diagnosed with colorectal cancer at the age of 52 years. Her mother was diagnosed with endometrial cancer at the age of 48 years.

DNA testing had shown a mutation in the mismatch repair (*MMR*) gene. Her colonoscopy showed colonic polyps.

What is the most likely syndrome?

A   Familial adenomatous polyposis (FAP)
B   Juvenile polyposis
C   Lynch's syndrome (hereditary non-polyposis colorectal cancer)
D   MUTYH-associated polyposis
E   Peutz–Jeghers syndrome

7. A 54-year-old woman presented with a longstanding history of diarrhoea. This was not associated with bleeding but she had recently suffered some weight loss and pruritus ani.

Examination was normal.

Colonoscopy: the following was seen (see **Figure 4.1**).

Figure 4.1 *See colour plate section.*

What is the most appropriate management?

A   Endoscopic removal
B   Ivermectin

    C   Mebendazole
    D   Praziquantel
    E   Steroids and albendazole

8. A 56-year-old man presented to the emergency department with severe epigastric pain radiating to his back which had been increasing in severity for the last 6 hours. He had also developed nausea and vomiting. He had no past medical history, took no medications and did not drink alcohol. There was no family history of note.

    On examination, he appeared unwell and was icteric. His body mass index was 27 kg/m². His pulse was 130 beats per minute and blood pressure 104/76 mmHg. Capillary refill time was 3 seconds. He had reduced air entry and a dull percussion note at the base of the right lung. Cardiovascular examination was normal. Abdominal examination revealed a tender epigastrium with no guarding or rigidity. Murphy's sign was negative.

Investigations:

haemoglobin 12.4 g/dL (13.0–18.0)	amylase 1780 U/L (60–180)
white cell count 16 × 10⁹/L (4–11)	corrected calcium 2.4 mmol/L (2.2–2.6)
platelets 489 × 10⁹/L (150–400)	lactate dehydrogenase 456 U/L (10–250)
sodium 142 mmol/L (135–145)	bilirubin 19 mmol/L (1–22)
potassium 3.8 mmol/L (3.5–5.0)	alanine transaminase 36 U/L (5–35)
urea 18 mmol/L (2.5–7.5)	alkaline phosphatase 167 U/L (45–105)
creatinine 167 µmol/L (60–110)	albumin 36 g/L (37–49)
C-reactive protein 167 mg/L (<10)	

Chest X-ray: right-sided pleural effusion

Which of the following features, when present on admission, would predict a severe attack of pancreatitis?

    A   Acute Physiology and Chronic Health Evaluation II (APACHE II) score >5
    B   Amylase >1000 U/L (60–180)
    C   C-reactive protein >150 mg/L (<10)
    D   Glasgow Coma Scale score >3
    E   Pleural effusion

9. A 35-year-old man presented to the hepatology clinic with a new diagnosis of hepatitis B virus infection.

Hepatitis B surface antigen (HBsAg): positive	
Hepatitis B e antigen (HBeAg): negative	
Hepatitis B e antibody (HBeAb): positive	

HBV DNA 564 IU/mL	alanine transaminase 18 U/L (5–35)

Liver biopsy: fibrosis score 0/6

What is the most appropriate management?

    A   Adefovir
    B   Lamivudine
    C   Pegylated interferon-α
    D   Tenofovir
    E   Watch and wait

10. A 25-year-old man was referred to the gastroenterology clinic with abnormal liver function tests and right upper quadrant pain. He had a 2-month history of intermittent diarrhoea, associated with episodes of rectal bleeding. He had no past medical history and took no medications. He drank occasional alcohol.

Investigations:

haemoglobin 12 g/dL (13.0–18.0)	bilirubin 35 mmol/L (1–22)
white cell count 7 × 10⁹/L (4–11)	alkaline phosphatase 280 U/L (45–105)
platelets 167 × 10⁹/L (150–400)	alanine transaminase 23 U/L (5–35)
ferritin 56 g/L (15–300)	albumin 36 g/L (37–49)

Hepatitis B and C serology: negative
HIV: negative
Antimitochondrial antibodies: negative
Antinuclear antibodies: negative

Perinuclear antineutrophil cytoplasmic antibodies (pANCAs) 1:160 <5

Ultrasound of abdomen: normal

What is the most appropriate next investigation?

A   Endoscopic retrograde cholangiopancreatography (ERCP)
B   Fibroscan
C   Liver biopsy
D   Magnetic resonance cholangiopancreatography (MRCP)
E   Triple-phase CT of the liver

11. A 64-year-old woman presented with symptoms of pain on swallowing over the last 2 weeks. There was no history of dysphagia or reflux. She had previously been fit and well, except for a recent urinary tract infection for which she received a short course of antibiotics. She took no other medications.
    Examination was normal.

What is the most likely diagnosis?

A   Cytomegalovirus
B   Eosinophilic oesophagitis
C   Oesophageal candidiasis
D   Oesophageal carcinoma
E   Achalasia

12. A 44-year-old man presented with abnormal liver function tests. He had type 2 diabetes. He drank 40 units of alcohol per week but was on no other medication.
    On examination he had a 3-cm hepatomegaly but no other signs of chronic liver disease.

Investigations:

haemoglobin 14.3 g/dL (13.0–18.0)	alanine transaminase 58 U/L (5–35)
white cell count 6.8 × 10⁹/L (4–11)	albumin 35 g/L (37–49)
platelets 189 × 10⁹/L (150–400)	ferritin 742 g/L (15–300)
haematocrit 60% (40–52)	transferrin saturation 35% (20–50)
bilirubin 24 mmol/L (1–22)	random glucose 8.1 mmol/L (3.0–6.0)
alkaline phosphatase 134 U/L (45–105)	

Hepatitis C virus IgG: positive   Hepatitis C virus RNA 0 IU/mL

Liver ultrasound: mild hepatomegaly with bright echotexture.

Liver biopsy: haemosiderosis

What is the most likely cause of his iron overload?

A   Alcoholic fatty liver disease
B   Diabetic hepatosteatosis
C   Hepatitis C virus
D   Hereditary haemochromatosis
E   Thalassaemia

13. A 54-year-old man presented with a 6-month history of loose stools, 12-kg weight loss and non-specific abdominal pain. There was no blood or mucus in the stools. Two years ago, he was investigated by the rheumatologists for arthralgia affecting a number of joints. He had no other past medical or surgical history. There was no family history of note. He attended with his son who was concerned that he had been become more forgetful recently.

    On examination, he was thin. He had angular stomatitis. Neurological, cardiovascular and respiratory examinations were normal. His Mini-Mental State Examination score was 16/30.

Investigations:

haemoglobin 11.2 g/dL (13.0–18.0)	platelets 567 × 10⁹/L (150–400)
white cell count 5.6 × 10⁹/L (4–11)	C-reactive protein 13 mg/L (<10)

Chest X-ray: normal

Duodenal biopsies: non-specific granulomas

What is the most likely diagnosis?

A   Abdominal tuberculosis
B   Crohn's disease
C   Sarcoidosis with small bowel involvement
D   Small intestinal lymphoma
E   Whipple's disease

14. A 60-year-old woman was referred with symptoms of fatigue, right upper quadrant pain, pruritus and abnormal liver function tests. She was generally fit and well, but had been treated for Graves' disease 10 years ago. Her current medications were thyroxine and hormone replacement therapy.

    On examination, she had a 3-cm tender hepatomegaly.

Investigations:

bilirubin 9 mmol/L (1–22)	alanine transaminase 350 U/L (5–35)
alkaline phosphatase 100 U/L (45–105)	albumin 37 g/L (37–49)

Antinuclear antibody 1: 160
Anti-smooth muscle 1: 80
Anti-LKM1: negative
Antimitochondrial antibody: negative

IgA 3.2 g/L (0.8–3.0)	IgM 1.2 g/L (0.4–2.5)
IgG 34 g/L (6.0–13.0)	

Histology:
interface hepatitis and portal plasma cell infiltration, with bridging necrosis
normal biliary histology

What is the most appropriate treatment?

A   Azathioprine
B   Ciclosporin
C   Methotrexate
D   Prednisolone
E   Ursodeoxycholic acid

15. A 57-year-old woman presented with a 6-month history of worsening abdominal pain that occurred after eating. The pain had been so severe that she had not wanted to eat and she had lost around 4 kg in weight. She had no history of dysphagia, early satiety, nausea or vomiting. Her past medical history included transient ischaemic attack, hypertension and hypercholesterolaemia. Her current medications were simvastatin, ramipril, aspirin and dipyridamole. There was no relevant family history.

She had a regular pulse rate of 68 beats per minute and a blood pressure 146/84 mmHg. Her cardiovascular and respiratory examinations were normal. On abdominal examination, she had mild central abdominal tenderness, with no abdominal masses or organomegaly.

What is the most likely diagnosis?

A   Biliary colic
B   Chronic mesenteric ischaemia
C   Duodenal ulcer
D   Gastric carcinoma
E   Gastric ulcer

16. A 48-year-old woman presented to her general practitioner after an episode of right upper quadrant pain 3 weeks previously. The pain was constant in nature, occurred after eating and was associated with nausea. It lasted for 6 hours in total. She had no fever at the time, and had been well since this episode. She had never had symptoms like this previously. She had no past medical history and took no medications.

On examination, she looked well and her observations were normal. She was not jaundiced. Her abdomen was soft and non-tender with no organomegaly.

Investigations:

Ultrasound of the abdomen:
gallstones in the gallbladder
normal gallbladder wall thickness
no common bile duct dilatation or intrahepatic biliary dilatation

What is the most appropriate treatment?

A   Endoscopic retrograde cholangiopancreatography (ERCP)
B   Laparoscopic cholecystectomy after 6 weeks
C   Lithotripsy of gallbladder stones
D   Open cholecystectomy after 6 weeks
E   Watchful waiting

17. A 28-year-old man with known ulcerative colitis (UC) was admitted to hospital with symptoms of bloody diarrhoea and abdominal pain for the preceding 4 days. He was opening his bowels 16 times per day, and complained of severe central abdominal pain. His UC was normally well controlled on 5-aminosalicylate treatment.

On examination, he was pale and had a pulse of 100 beats per minute and blood pressure of 118/68 mmHg. Abdominal examination revealed a generally tender abdomen, with no guarding or rigidity.

Investigations:

haemoglobin 10.4 g/dL (13.0–18.0)	urea 9 mmol/L (2.5–7.5)
white cell count 5 × 10⁹/L (4–11)	creatinine 110 µmol/L (60–110)
platelets 489 × 10⁹/L (150–400)	erythrocyte sedimentation rate 68 mm/1st h (0–20)
sodium 136 mmol/L (135–145)	C-reactive protein 74 mg/L (<10)
potassium 4 mmol/L (3.5–5.0)	

Abdominal X-ray: large bowel diameter within normal limits

What is the next most appropriate step in management?

A   Ciclosporin, intravenous hydrocortisone, subcutaneous heparin and calcium supplementation
B   Intravenous hydrocortisone 100 mg four times daily, oral metronidazole, subcutaneous heparin, calcium supplementation
C   Intravenous hydrocortisone 100 mg four times daily, subcutaneous heparin, calcium supplementation
D   Oral prednisolone 40 mg once daily, calcium supplementation, oral metronidazole
E   Oral prednisolone 40 mg once daily, calcium supplementation and mesalazine enemas

18. A 45-year-old man was admitted to hospital with confusion and jaundice. He had a history of alcohol dependence, and drank 10 cans of strong lager per day. He had developed vomiting and diarrhoea 2 days ago and had been unable to eat or drink anything since. He had no other medical history and no relevant family history.

On examination, he was icteric and had palmar erythema. Temperature was 38.0°C. There was no asterixis. Abdominal examination revealed tender 4-cm hepatomegaly, with no splenomegaly or ascites.

Investigations:

haemoglobin 13.2 g/dL (13.0–18.0)	urea 9.7 mmol/L (2.5–7.5)
white cell count 14.5 × 10⁹/L (4–11)	creatinine 136 µmol/L (60–110)
platelets 156 × 10⁹/L (150–400)	bilirubin 170 mmol/L (1–22)
prothrombin time 18 s (11.5–15.5)	alkaline phosphatase 189 U/L (45–105)
sodium 143 mmol/L (135–145)	alanine transaminase 67 U/L (5–35)
potassium 3.3 mmol/L (3.3–5.0)	albumin 34 g/L (37–49)

Maddrey discriminant function: 38
Chest X-ray, blood cultures and urine cultures were negative

What is the most appropriate treatment?

A   *N*-Acetylcysteine
B   Nutritional supplementation
C   Pentoxifylline
D   Prednisolone
E   Supportive care

19. A 57-year-old woman with known ulcerative colitis (UC) attended the outpatient clinic. Her UC had previously been refractory to steroids but since starting on azathioprine 6 months ago her symptoms had been well controlled and she was opening her bowels two times per day with no blood and no abdominal pain.

On examination, she was thin and abdominal examination was unremarkable.

Investigations:

Flexible sigmoidoscopy – quiescent colitis
Histology: quiescent ulcerative colitis with inclusion cell bodies   C-reactive protein 5 (<10 mg/L)
Serum cytomegalovirus IgG: positive   Serum cytomegalovirus DNA: positive

What is the next most appropriate step in management?

A   Continue current treatment
B   Intravenous ganciclovir for 3 weeks
C   Intravenous ganciclovir for 2–3 days followed by oral valganciclovir for 3 weeks in total
D   Oral valganciclovir for 3 weeks
E   Stop azathioprine

20. A 64-year-old woman presented to the emergency department with three episodes of haematemesis and melaena. She had a past medical history of ischaemic heart disease. Her admission medications consisted of aspirin 75 mg once daily. She did not drink alcohol or smoke.
    On examination, she was pale, her pulse was 90 beats per minute and blood pressure 134/78 mmHg. She underwent a gastroscopy which showed a gastric ulcer with a non-bleeding visible vessel and altered blood in the upper gastrointestinal tract. The ulcer was injected with 10 mL of adrenaline and a clip was applied to the visible vessel. Haemostasis was achieved.

What is the most appropriate next step in management?

A   40 mg twice daily intravenous omeprazole for 3 days then convert to 40 mg twice daily oral omeprazole, and repeat endoscopy in 24 hours
B   40 mg twice daily oral omeprazole and *Helicobacter pylori* eradication and repeat endoscopy in 6–8 weeks
C   80 mg intravenous omeprazole bolus followed by a 72-hour protein pump inhibitor infusion at 8 mg/h and repeat endoscopy in 6–8 weeks
D   80 mg intravenous omeprazole bolus followed by a 72-hour protein pump inhibitor infusion at 8 mg/h, tranexamic acid and *Helicobacter pylori* eradication therapy and repeat endoscopy in 24 hours
E   80 mg twice daily intravenous omeprazole, tranexamic acid and *Helicobacter pylori* eradication and repeat endoscopy in 24 hours

21. A 54-year-old woman presented to hospital with a 3-day history of abdominal pain and nausea. She had also developed a generalised, pruritic rash. There was a history of epilepsy, atrial fibrillation and osteoarthritis, for which she was on carbamazepine, phenytoin, amiodarone, warfarin and diclofenac. She took no other medications and did not smoke or drink.
    On examination, she had a widespread urticarial rash, cervical lymphadenopathy and right upper quadrant tenderness.

Investigations:

haemoglobin 13.2 g/dL (13.0–18.0)	eosinophils 1.5 × 10⁹/L (0.04–0.4)
white cell count 6.4 × 10⁹/L (4–11)	bilirubin 30 mmol/L (1–22)
platelets 189 × 10⁹/L (150–400)	alkaline phosphatase 486 U/L (45–105)
international normalised ratio 1.2 (<1.4)	alanine transaminase 846 U/L (5–35)
neutrophils 3.6 × 10⁹/L (1.5–7.0)	albumin 37 g/L (37–49)
lymphocytes 1.4 × 10⁹/L (1.5–4.0)	
Paracetamol levels: normal	

What is the most likely cause?

A   Amiodarone
B   Carbamazepine
C   Diclofenac
D   Phenytoin
E   Warfarin

22. A 56-year-old woman presented with abdominal distension, which she first noticed 6 months ago.

On examination, she was thin with gross abdominal distension and shifting dullness. There were no palpable masses or organomegaly.

An ascitic tap was performed:

Investigations:

white cell count 17 polymorphonuclear leukocytes (PMNs)/mm³ (<250)	
culture – no organisms seen	fluid albumin 22 g/L
fluid protein 27 g/L	serum albumin 35 g/L (37–49)

What is the most likely cause of her ascites?

A   Carcinomatosis peritonei
B   Liver cirrhosis
C   Ovarian cancer
D   Nephrotic syndrome
E   Tuberculosis peritonitis

23. A 43-year-old man presented with a history of gastro-oesophageal reflux symptoms. He underwent an upper gastrointestinal endoscopy and the following abnormalities were seen (see **Figure 4.2**).

Figure 4.2 *See colour plate section.*

Which one of the following is a risk factor for progression to adenocarcinoma in this disease?

A   Duration of reflux history
B   Female sex

C   Heavy alcohol use
D   Expression of p53
E   Previous Nissen fundoplication

24. A 35-year-old woman presented to her general practitioner with symptoms of fatigue, for the preceding 12 months. She reported intermittent loose stools and bloating, associated with a 3-kg weight loss. She also complained of a skin rash on her arms. She had no past medical history and was on no medications.
     On examination, she looked thin and was pale. She had a blistering skin eruption covering both elbows. The rest of the examination was normal. She was referred for a skin biopsy.
     Skin biopsy – granular IgA at dermoepidermal junction

What is the most useful diagnostic investigation?

A   Colonoscopy and ileal biopsies
B   Gastroscopy and distal small bowel biopsies
C   Gastroscopy and small bowel biopsies with periodic acid–Schiff (PAS) staining
D   Serum acetylcholinesterase (ACE) levels
E   Tissue transglutaminase antibodies

25. A 21-year-old, white, male medical student presented with jaundice. One week ago, he returned from his elective to the Indian subcontinent where he had visited India, Bangladesh and Pakistan. Four days before, he arrived back in the UK and he felt mildly unwell with a fever. Three days ago, he developed abdominal pain, vomiting, fever and pale stools. Today he noticed that he had yellow sclera, and came to hospital. He was not sexually active. During his elective he had not undertaken any exposure-prone procedures and had not had any transfusions, operations or needle-stick injuries. He had no previous medical problems, did not drink alcohol and was not on any medication.
     On examination, he had a soft abdomen with tender hepatomegaly. He had tender posterior cervical lymphadenopathy.
     An ultrasound of his liver was normal.

What is the most useful diagnostic investigation?

A   Anti-HAV IgM
B   HBsAg
C   Epstein–Barr virus IgM antibody
D   HEV RNA
E   HIV antibody

26. A 54-year-old man was reviewed in the hepatology clinic with a new diagnosis of alcohol-induced cirrhosis, with no evidence of hepatic decompensation. He had no previous medical history.
     He underwent a gastroscopy which showed three columns of medium-sized oesophageal varices and portal hypertensive gastropathy in the stomach. There were no gastric varices or evidence of bleeding.

What is the next most appropriate management step?

A   Combination therapy with isosorbide mononitrate and propranolol
B   Combination therapy with propranolol and endoscopic variceal band ligation
C   Endoscopic variceal band ligation
D   Isosorbide mononitrate therapy
E   Propranolol therapy

27. A 54-year-old man presented to his general practitioner with right upper quadrant pain that had been present for approximately 2 months. He was not jaundiced and had no weight loss. He had emigrated to the UK from Iran 23 years ago.

On examination, there was tenderness in the right upper quadrant with no organomegaly or masses.

Investigations:

haemoglobin 12.8 g/dL (13.0–18.0)	eosinophils 2.3 × 10⁹/L (0.04–0.4)
white cell count 7.8 × 10⁹/L (4–11)	bilirubin 18 mmol/L (1–22)
platelets 413 × 10⁹/L (150–400)	alkaline phosphatase 134 U/L (45–105)
neutrophils 3.2 × 10⁹/L (1.5–7.0)	alanine transaminase 28 U/L (5–35)
lymphocytes 0.5 × 10⁹/L (1.5–4.0)	albumin 36 g/L (37–49)

Liver ultrasound: 4.5 × 5 cm cystic lesion with an irregular cyst wall and a 3 × 3 cm cystic lesion with daughter cyst in right lobe of liver

What is the most likely diagnosis?

A Amoebiasis
B Cystadenoma
C Echinococcal cyst
D Polycystic liver disease
E Simple cyst

28. A 38-year-old man presented for assessment of abnormal liver function tests. He had recently been diagnosed with emphysema and evaluation at that point indicated that he had α_1-antitrypsin deficiency.

Investigations:

bilirubin 24 mmol/L (1–22)	alanine transaminase 48 U/L (5–35)
alkaline phosphatase 189 U/L (45–105)	albumin 36 g/L (37–49)

What is the most likely genotype of his α_1-antitrypsin deficiency?

A *PIMZ*
B *PIMM*
C *PISZ*
D *PISS*
E *PIZZ*

29. A 78-year-old man was referred for percutaneous endoscopic gastrostomy (PEG) insertion due to reduced nutritional intake secondary to a chronic disease.

In which of the following situations should PEG insertion NOT be used?

A Cystic fibrosis
B Motor neuron disease
C Oesophageal carcinoma – T1N0M0
D Peritoneal dialysis
E Systemic sclerosis

30. A 48-year-old man presented to the emergency department with a 2-day history of right upper quadrant pain associated with shivering, nausea and anorexia. He has no past medical history and was not taking any medications.

On examination, he was icteric and had a temperature of 38.3°C. His pulse was 106 beats per minute and blood pressure 110/73 mmHg. Abdominal examination revealed right upper quadrant tenderness and negative Murphy's sign.

Investigations:

haemoglobin 13.2 g/dL (13.0–18.0)	alanine transaminase 45 U/L (5–35)
white cell count 14.8 × 10⁹/L (4–11)	alkaline phosphatase 489 U/L (45–105)
platelets 546 × 10⁹/L (150–400)	albumin 34 g/L (37–49)
bilirubin 56 mmol/L (1–22)	

What is the most likely causative organism?

A   *Enterobacter* species
B   *Enterococcus faecalis*
C   *Escherichia coli*
D   *Klebsiella* species
E   *Streptococcus* species

31. A 19-year-old woman presented to the gastroenterology clinic with a 6-month history of 4-kg weight loss and diarrhoea. She opened her bowels six times per day with no blood in the stools; she had right iliac fossa abdominal pain. She had recently returned from a gap year travelling in south east Asia and Africa. She had complained of painful red eyes in the past. There was no family history of note. She had no past medical history and took no medications.
    On examination, she looked thin with aphthous mouth ulcers. She was haemodynamically stable. Ophthalmological examination was normal. Abdominal examination was normal except for tenderness of the right iliac fossa.

Investigations:

haemoglobin 11.3 g/dL (13.0–18.0 g/dL)	platelets 456 × 10⁹/L (150–400)
white cell count 7 × 10⁹/L (4–11)	C-reactive protein 8 mg/L (<10)

What is the most likely diagnosis?

A   Behçet's disease
B   Coeliac disease
C   Crohn's disease
D   Small bowel bacterial overgrowth
E   Tropical sprue

32. A 46-year-old woman presented with a 6-month history of difficulty swallowing foods and liquids. She reported occasional regurgitation of foods, and chest pain.
    She underwent a barium swallow (see **Figure 4.3**).

What is the most likely diagnosis?

A   Achalasia
B   Diffuse oesophageal spasm
C   Hiatus hernia
D   Nutcracker oesophagus
E   Oesophageal carcinoma

Figure 4.3

33. A 67-year-old man presented with a history of bright red rectal bleeding mixed in with his stool. He had had no change in his bowel habit, and had not suffered any weight loss. He had a previous medical history of atrial fibrillation and prostate cancer.

Investigations:

haemoglobin 8.8 g/dL (13.0–18.0)   platelets 187 × 10⁹/L (150–400)
white cell count 4.6 × 10⁹/L (4–11)

Colonoscopy: showed the following (see **Figure 4.4**).

Figure 4.4 *See colour plate section.*

What is the most appropriate first-line treatment?

A Argon photocoagulation
B Prednisolone enemas
C Sucralfate enemas
D Topical 5-aminosalicylic acid (5ASA) treatment
E Hyperbaric oxygen therapy

34. A 45-year-old woman presented to the clinic with abnormal liver function tests, which had been discovered on routine blood tests. She was asymptomatic.
    Investigations were performed which showed the following:

Investigations:

HBsAg: positive
HBeAg: negative
Total anti-HBc: positive
HBV DNA: 320 IU/mL
HCV IgG: positive
HCV RNA: 0 IU/mL
Total anti-HDV: positive
HDAg: negative
HDV RNA: positive

What is the most likely diagnosis?

A Acute hepatitis B virus (HBV), chronic hepatitis C virus (HCV), previous hepatitis D virus (HDV)
B Acute HBV, previous HCV, acute HDV
C Chronic HBV, chronic HCV, previous HDV
D Chronic HBV, previous HCV, chronic HDV
E Previous HBV, chronic HCV, previous HDV

35. A 33-year-old man with known ulcerative colitis (UC) was seen in the outpatient clinic. Over the last year he had required two courses of steroids for his UC. Over the past 3 weeks he had been having bloody diarrhoea and some associated abdominal pain. Two weeks ago, he had been given another reducing course of prednisolone. He was currently opening his bowels four times per day. He had no other medical problems. His current medications were 30 mg prednisolone once daily, Calcichew D$_3$ and mesalazine 800 mg three times daily.
    Examination was unremarkable:

Investigations:

C-reactive protein 12 (<10 mg/L)	thiopurine methyltransferase (TPMT) 50 pmol/h (26–50)
Abdominal X-ray: no toxic dilatation	
Flexible sigmoidoscopy: mild – moderate colitis	
Histology: mild – moderate colitis	
Stool culture: no ova, cysts or parasites	
Clostridium difficile: negative	

What is the most appropriate next management step?

A   Azathioprine
B   Infliximab
C   Intravenous hydrocortisone
D   6-Mercaptopurine
E   Methotrexate

36. A 45-year-old woman with a history of cirrhosis presented with worsening abdominal distension, which was causing her discomfort. She had no other past medical history and was currently taking propranolol as primary prophylaxis against variceal haemorrhage.
    On examination, she had a distended abdomen with shifting dullness indicating moderate ascites. Her abdomen was not tense. There was no evidence of encephalopathy and she was haemodynamically stable.

What is the most appropriate initial therapy?

A   Dietary salt reduction and combination therapy with spironolactone 100 mg once daily and furosemide 40 mg once daily
B   Dietary salt reduction and spironolactone 100 mg once daily
C   Dietary salt reduction and furosemide 40 mg once daily
D   Large-volume paracentesis with albumin cover
E   Large-volume paracentesis with albumin cover and spironolactone 100 mg once daily

37. A 79-year-old woman presented with symptoms of severe heartburn occurring at night, and associated with nausea but no vomiting. She had no symptoms of dysphagia or weight loss. She had never had these symptoms previously. Her past medical history consisted of hypertension, hypercholesterolaemia, depression and osteoporosis.

Which medication is the most likely cause of her symptoms?

A   Alendronate
B   Amlodipine
C   Citalopram
D   Ramipril
E   Simvastatin

38. A 28-year-old woman with colonic Crohn's disease presented with perianal pain associated with a discharge from her perineal region. She felt unwell and had a reduced appetite. She was on mesalazine 800 mg three times daily and the oral contraceptive pill.
    On examination, she had mild left-sided abdominal tenderness, and examination of her perineum revealed a perianal fistula with perianal tenderness on palpation.

What is the most appropriate next investigation?

A   Anorectal ultrasound
B   Examination under anaesthetic (EUA)
C   Fistulography
D   Pelvic MRI
E   Pelvic CT

39. A 41-year-old man was admitted with symptoms of colicky abdominal pain and vomiting. He had also been passing stools mixed with blood and mucus. He had had similar symptoms on four previous occasions, which had spontaneously resolved. He had no known medical problems.
    On examination, he was haemodynamically stable. There was a soft 'sausage-shaped' mass in the right iliac fossa but no other abnormalities.

Investigations:

haemoglobin 10.1 g/dL (13.0–18.0)	platelets 163 × 10⁹/L (150–400)
white cell count 4.3 × 10⁹/L (4–11)	C-reactive protein <5 mg/L (<10)

Abdominal X-ray: intussusception
[Technetium-99m] pertechnetate scan: positive

What is the most likely diagnosis?

A   Crohn's disease
B   Henoch–Schönlein purpura
C   Meckel's diverticulum
D   Peutz–Jeghers syndrome
E   Small bowel lymphoma

40. A 45-year-old woman presented to the emergency department with severe right upper quadrant abdominal pain. She had a 2-year history of intermittent right upper quadrant pain, which occurred approximately once a month, usually after eating, and lasted approximately 40 minutes. She had no past medical history and took no medications.
    Examination was normal except for tenderness in her right upper quadrant.

Investigations:

bilirubin 16 mmol/L (1–22)	amylase 356 U/L (60–180)
alkaline phosphatase 804 U/L (45–105)	IgA 2.4 g/L (0.8–3.0)
alanine transaminase 84 U/L (5–35)	IgG 7 g/L (6.0–13.0)
albumin 38 g/L (37–49)	IgM 4 g/L (4.0–2.5)

Antinuclear antibody: negative

Ultrasound of the abdomen:
dilated common bile duct to 12 mm
no intrahepatic duct dilatation
no gallstones in the gallbladder and no filling defects in the bile ducts

Endoscopic retrograde cholangiopancreatography:
dilated 12-mm common bile duct
no filling defects seen

What is the most likely diagnosis?

A   Acute acalculous cholecystitis
B   Autoimmune cholangitis
C   Chronic pancreatitis
D   Primary sclerosing cholangitis
E   Sphincter of Oddi dysfunction (type 1)

41. A 45-year-old woman with known coeliac disease was reviewed in the clinic. She complained of increased frequency of loose stools and some weight loss over the past 2 months. She had been diagnosed with coeliac disease aged 23 years, and had been fully compliant with a gluten-free diet.
    Examination revealed a body mass index of 18 kg/m² with a pulse of 96 beats per minute. Physical examination was normal and there was no lymphadenopathy.

Investigations:

Full blood count: normal

Duodenal biopsies: normal

Small bowel barium follow-through: ulcerated area in the jejunum

---

CT of the chest/abdomen/pelvis:

normal lungs, liver, kidneys, pancreas and pelvic appearances

no lymphadenopathy

no intestinal obstruction

What is the most likely cause of her symptoms?

A   Microscopic colitis
B   Relapse of coeliac disease
C   Small bowel lymphoma
D   Small bowel adenocarcinoma
E   Ulcerative jejunoileitis

42. A 66-year-old man presented with a 3-day history of worsening abdominal pain and distension. He felt nauseous and had been intermittently vomiting. He had not opened his bowels for 3 days, and had passed flatus only intermittently.

On examination, his pulse was 104 beats per minute and blood pressure 112/68 mmHg. Abdomen was soft, distended, with some generalised tenderness and the percussion note was tympanic.

A provisional diagnosis of small bowel obstruction was made and an abdominal CT was performed (see **Figure 4.5**).

Figure 4.5

What is the most likely cause of the obstruction?

A   Adhesions
B   Crohn's disease
C   Gallstone ileus
D   Inguinal hernia
E   Small bowel lymphoma

43. A 54-year-old man presented with vomiting, retrosternal pain and an inability to swallow his saliva. He underwent an endoscopy and was found to have a food bolus which was successfully removed. Twelve hours later, he became acutely unwell, with chest pain and shortness of breath.

   On examination, his temperature was 37.1°C, pulse 98 beats per minute, blood pressure 110/70 mmHg, respiratory rate 22 beats per minute and oxygen saturation 92% on air.

Investigations:

Chest X-ray: (see **Figure 4.6**)

Electrocardiogram: sinus tachycardia

Figure 4.6

What is the most appropriate next step in management?

A   Co-amoxiclav and metronidazole
B   Furosemide
C   Low-molecular-weight heparin
D   Omeprazole
E   Salbutamol

44. A 44-year-old man presented with jaundice and abdominal pain in association with lethargy. He first noticed the jaundice 2 weeks ago, and his abdominal pain started 3 days ago and had worsened considerably since. He had no past medical history, took no medications and there was no family history of note. He had a history of heavy alcohol intake of over 100 units a week for the past 6 years.

   On examination, he was icteric, and had visible scratch marks on his upper body. He had pale conjunctivae. Abdominal examination revealed a tender epigastrium and 4-cm tender, hepatomegaly. There was no splenomegaly or ascites. Rectal examination was normal.

Investigations:

haemoglobin 8.8 g/dL (13.0–18.0)	albumin 34 g/L (37–49)
mean corpuscular volume 108 fL (80–96)	bilirubin 167 mmol/L (1–22)
white cell count 7.4 × 10⁹/L (4–11)	alanine transaminase 56 U/L (5–35)
platelets 256 × 10⁹/L (150–400)	aspartate transaminase 64 U/L (1–31)
reticulocytes 10% (0.5–2.5)	alkaline phosphatase 168 U/L (45–105)
international normalised ratio 1.6 (<1.4)	

Antinuclear antibody – negative
Anti-smooth muscle antibody – negative
Antimitochondrial antibody – negative
HCV Ab – negative
HBsAg – negative

cholesterol 8.5 mmol/L (<5.2)   triglycerides 4.3 mmol/L (0.45–1.69)

Ultrasound of the liver:
smooth hepatomegaly
no intra- or extrahepatic duct dilatation, no cirrhosis, no ascites

What is the most likely diagnosis?

A   Caroli's disease
B   Crigler–Najjar syndrome
C   Gilbert's syndrome
D   Mirizzi's syndrome
E   Zieve's syndrome

45. A 72-year-old woman with a history of systemic sclerosis presented with melaena and an associated haemoglobin drop. She underwent appropriate resuscitation with blood products, fluids and a proton pump inhibitor, and had an upper gastrointestinal endoscopy.

Investigations:

Upper gastrointestinal endoscopy: multiple lesions in stomach (see **Figure 4.7**).

Figure 4.7 *See colour plate section.*

What is the most appropriate management?

A   Adrenaline injection sclerotherapy
B   Argon photocoagulation (APC)
C   Beta-blocker
D   Corticosteroids
E   Endoscopic band ligation

Answers

1. D Pancreatic pseudocyst

Chronic pancreatitis is a chronic inflammatory condition of the pancreas and has a number of long-term complications, including an increased incidence of pancreatic cancer, biliary stricturing, pancreatic pseudocyst formation and splenic vein thrombosis. The most common of these is pancreatic pseudocyst which occurs in 10–25% of patients with chronic pancreatitis. Pancreatic pseudocysts are localised pancreatic fluid collections. Raised pressure within the pancreatic ducts causes damage to the ducts, leading to leakage of pancreatic enzymes which become enclosed by a fibrotic reaction, leading to pseudocyst formation. Most will resolve spontaneously. The patient's symptoms of worsening abdominal pain, early satiety (as a consequence of the pseudocyst compressing the stomach) and nausea are classic signs of pancreatic pseudocyst formation. Adenocarcinoma of the pancreas is a complication of chronic pancreatitis. The risk is small but the incidence is estimated to be 16.5 times higher in patients with chronic pancreatitis than in age-matched controls. In adenocarcinoma of the pancreas a longer time period of symptoms would be expected and early satiety is uncommon. The absence of jaundice makes a biliary stricture unlikely. Splenic vein thrombosis commonly presents with upper gastrointestinal bleeding from ruptured fundal varices, and would not usually present with abdominal pain. Intraductal papillary mucinous neoplasms of the pancreas are not associated with chronic pancreatitis, and usually present with type 2 diabetes.

Tandon RK, et al. Chronic pancreatitis: Asia–Pacific consensus report. J Gastroenterol Hepatol 2002; 17:508–518.
Habashi S, Draganov P. Pancreatic pseudocyst. World J Gastroenterol 2009; 15(1):38–47.

2. A Budd–Chiari syndrome

Budd–Chiari syndrome is characterised by hepatic venous outflow obstruction. It presents with a triad of abdominal pain, hepatomegaly and ascites. The amount of ascites present is dependent upon the extent and rapidity of the hepatic vein occlusion. Factors that predispose to the development of Budd–Chiari syndrome are acquired and inherited hypercoagulable states. Polycythaemia rubra vera (PRV) accounts for between 10% and 40% of cases. Paroxysmal nocturnal haemoglobinuria, the antiphospholipid syndrome and protein C, protein S and antithrombin III deficiency are also causes. Tumoral invasion, aspergillosis and Behçet's syndrome are rare causes.

Constrictive pericarditis manifests with tender hepatomegaly and may cause ascites, but a raised jugular venous pressure (JVP) would also be present, along with Kussmaul's sign (a raised JVP on inspiration) and a pericardial knock in 50% of cases. Hepatocellular carcinoma does not usually manifest with ascites, and is very uncommon (<2%) in those who do not have liver cirrhosis. Portal vein thrombosis does not give tender hepatomegaly as it is usually presinusoidal/prehepatic. Often the liver biochemistry and clotting will be normal and there may be splenomegaly because of portal hypertension. In tricuspid regurgitation, pulsatile hepatomegaly and a raised JVP would be present.

Menon KV, Shah V, Kamath PS. The Budd–Chiari Syndrome. N Engl J Med 2004; 350:578–585.

3. B Antibiotics and terlipressin

The patient has had an acute variceal haemorrhage, with evidence of significant haemodynamic instability. American and British guidelines have been developed on the management of acute variceal bleed and both recommend a short course of broad-spectrum antibiotics (norfloxacin is recommended in the American guidelines; in the UK there may be local variations but current practice is to use broad-spectrum antibiotics such as ciprofloxacin and tazocin) and terlipressin. A recent meta-analysis has shown that antibiotics significantly reduce mortality in upper gastrointestinal bleeding in patients with chronic liver disease, and so they are recommended in all patients. Terlipressin is a synthetic analogue of vasopressin, and acts as a splanchnic vasoconstrictor. A systematic review has shown it to be effective in controlling acute variceal haemorrhage, and reducing mortality. A systemic review of somatostatin and its analogues (such as octreotide) showed an improvement in haemostasis but no reduction in mortality, and so terlipressin is recommended over somatostatin analogues. Beta-blockers (such as propranolol) are not recommended in acute variceal haemorrhage, as they reduce blood pressure and blunt the physiological increase in heart rate associated with bleeding. Beta-blockers are recommended as primary and secondary prophylaxis for variceal bleeding.

Garcia-Tsao, et al. AASLD practice guidelines. Prevention and Management of Gastroesophageal Varices and Variceal Hemorrhage in Cirrhosis. Hepatology 2007; 46(3):922–938.
Scottish Intercollegiate Guidelines Network. SIGN guideline 105: Management of acute upper and lower gastrointestinal bleeding, A national clinical guideline. Edinburgh: SIGN, 2008.

4. E Thiamine administration

The patient has refeeding syndrome caused by prolonged fasting followed by rapid re-administration of a normal diet. Refeeding syndrome occurs because of the body's adaptive changes to prolonged fasting, which are designed to preserve protein and muscle. During starvation the principal adaptive changes are a reduction in the body's basal metabolic rate and a shift from carbohydrate to protein and fat use to fulfil the body's energy requirements. During prolonged starvation (in this particular case it is due to his poor intake and alcohol diet followed by a hospital fast) severe depletion of intracellular phosphate, potassium and magnesium also occurs. Serum levels remain normal and so this intracellular loss is often not apparent during the fasting state. When feeding occurs after a prolonged fast, insulin levels become raised as a result of glucose absorption. Elevated insulin levels cause magnesium, glucose, phosphate and potassium to be absorbed intracellularly which can lead to a dramatic drop in serum levels of these minerals. Hyperinsulinaemia also leads to the breakdown of fat, protein and glycogen, a process that requires magnesium and phosphate which further deplete serum levels. The first step in treatment consists of thiamine replacement, and then slow feeding at less than 50% of the body's requirements should be instigated. Potassium, magnesium and phosphate should all be replaced, but thiamine administration is the first step. Without treatment refeeding syndrome can cause rhabdomyolysis and arrhythmias, and may prove fatal.

Hisham M, et al. Refeeding syndrome: What is it, and how to prevent and treat it? BMJ 2008; 336:1495–1498.

5. E Ascending cholangitis

This patient has Charcot's triad – fever, abdominal pain and jaundice – which indicates the diagnosis of ascending cholangitis. The triad is seen in 50–70% of patients with ascending cholangitis. Acute cholecystitis typically presents with right upper abdominal pain, nausea, vomiting and fever. The usual examination findings are tenderness in the right upper abdomen, a palpable gallbladder and Murphy's sign. A positive Murphy's sign has a specificity of 79–96% for the diagnosis, so the negative Murphy's sign strongly rules against acute cholecystitis. Acalculous cholecystitis is cholecystitis that occurs without any gallstones present. It causes 5–10% of cases of cholecystitis. It presents similarly to acute cholecystitis and is therefore unlikely. Acute pancreatitis does not present with jaundice or rigors. Alcoholic hepatitis presents with cholestatic abnormalities of the liver function tests; however, it is not associated with rigors and there is no history to suggest excessive alcohol consumption.

Flowcharts for the diagnosis and treatment of acute cholangitis and cholecystitis: Tokyo Guidelines. J Hepatobiliary Pancreat Surg 2007; 14:27–34.

6. C Lynch's syndrome

The answers given are all syndromes that can cause colonic polyps.

Lynch's syndrome (hereditary non-polyposis syndrome) is a genetic disorder that is associated with a significantly increased risk of certain types of cancer (colorectal, small bowel, endometrial, renal pelvis or ureteric). It is autosomally dominantly inherited, and is due to a mismatch repair (*MMR*) gene mutation. Prior to the identification of the *MMR* gene diagnosis was made using with the modified Amsterdam criteria.

Modified Amsterdam criteria:

- Colorectal cancer, or another Lynch's syndrome cancer, which affects three or more relatives, in at least two generations of the same family.
- One affected family member has to be a first-degree relative of the other two.
- One affected relative must be aged younger than 50 at diagnosis.

Although it is named hereditary non-polyposis syndrome, Lynch's syndrome can cause colonic polyposis. These polyps occur at a younger age, and are more likely to become cancerous than colonic polyps in patients without Lynch's syndrome.

Familial adenomatous polyposis (FAP) is an autosomally dominantly inherited syndrome. It is caused by mutations of the adenomatous polyposis coli (*APC*) gene on chromosome 5, and has a very high penetrance. On colonoscopy it is suspected when over 100 adenomatous colonic polyps are observed.

Juvenile polyposis is characterised by the presence of multiple hamartomatous, as opposed to adenomatous, colonic polyps. It is distinguished from Peutz–Jeghers syndrome, in which hamartomatous polyps are also seen, by histological differences. As its name would suggest, it typically manifests during childhood, and polyps are usually present in affected individuals before they reach the age of 20 years. MUTYH-associated polyposis is an autosomal recessive disorder which is caused by mutations in the *MUTYH* gene. The polyps are adenomatous or mixed adenomatous/hyperplastic.

Peutz–Jeghers syndrome is a syndrome in which pigmentation of the mucocutaneous surfaces is seen in combination with hamartomatous gastrointestinal polyps. It is inherited in an autosomal dominant fashion. There is an associated increase risk of oesophageal, gastric, pancreatic, small bowel and colorectal cancer, and a 50% lifetime risk of breast cancer.

Cairns SR, et al. Guidelines for colorectal cancer screening and surveillance in moderate and high risk groups (update from 2002). Gut 2010; 59:666–690.

7. C Mebendazole

The endoscopic image shows pinworm, or *Enterobius vermicularis*. The treatment for this is a single dose of mebendazole. It usually presents with intense pruritus ani, but can cause weight loss, irritability, diarrhoea, abdominal pain or colitis with eosinophilia. In rare cases it can colonise the female genital tract causing vaginal discharge. It is usually diagnosed via the 'Sellotape test' where the sticky side of Sellotape is placed onto the perianal skin and then examined under a microscope for ova. It has a worldwide distribution and particularly affects children.

Endoscopic removal is the treatment of choice for anisakiasis – a helminth infection. Ivermectin is used in the treatment of strongyloides infestation. Praziquantel is used to treat schistosomiasis, and steroids and albendazole are used where there is a suspicion of neurocysticercosis, or in the treatment of severe trichinellosis.

Clinical Guidelines of the British Infection Society. Eosinophilia in returning travellers and migrants from the tropics: UK recommendations for investigation and management. J Infect 2010; 60:1–20.

8. E Pleural effusion

Acute pancreatitis is an acute inflammatory process of the pancreas, with variable involvement of other organs. It has a mortality rate in the region of 10–15% of proven cases, which increases in necrotising pancreatitis to 30–40%. Given the substantial mortality associated with severe pancreatitis it is important to be able to risk stratify patients early in admission who are at high risk of developing severe pancreatitis, as these patients should be managed in a high dependency or intensive care unit. There are a variety of ways of predicting severity, which can be used at different time periods. On admission the only answer given that predicts severity is the presence of a pleural effusion. The APACHE II score is a severity of illness score that is principally used on intensive care units. It is measured in the first 24 hours of admission and predicts the likelihood of death. The APACHE II score needs to be over 8 on admission to predict severe pancreatitis, and the Glasgow Coma Scale (GCS) score and C-reactive protein should be used only after 24 hours. The amylase value is not a predictor of severity of pancreatitis.

The parameters that predict severity at different time points are shown in **Table 4.1**.

UK guidelines for the management of acute pancreatitis. Gut 2005; 54:1–9.

Table 4.1 Features that may predict a severe attack of acute pancreatitis	
Time point	**Features that may predict severity**
Initial assessment	Clinical impression of severity
	Body mass index >30 kg/m^2
	Pleural effusion on chest radiograph
	APACHE II score >8
24 hours after admission	Clinical impression of severity
	APACHE II score >8
	GCS score ≥3
	Persisting organ failure, especially if multiple
	C-reactive protein >150 mg/L
48 hours after admission	Clinical impression of severity
	Multiple or progressive organ failure
	GCS score ≥3
	Persisting organ failure for 48 hours
	C-reactive protein >150 mg/L

9. E Watch and wait

Chronic hepatitis B (CHB) is divided into five main phases which may not always occur sequentially:

Immunotolerent phase – patients tend to be HBeAg positive, have high HBV DNA levels, normal or low levels of aminotransaminases, little or no liver necroinflammation, and virtually no or slow progression of fibrosis. Patients are highly contagious in this phase. Individuals infected as adults do not usually go through this phase.

Immunoreactive phase – patients are HBeAg positive, have elevated HBV DNA levels (but lower than the immunotolerant phase), increased or fluctuating levels of aminotransferases, moderate or severe liver necroinflammation, and more rapid progression of fibrosis. This phase may last for several weeks to several years. During this phase there is a higher chance of spontaneous loss of HBeAg.

Inactive carrier state – patients may follow seroconversion from HBeAg to anti-HBe antibodies. During this phase HBV DNA levels can be low or even undetectable and aminotransferases are often normal. Progression of the disease to cirrhosis does not happen and HBsAg loss and seroconversion to anti-HBs antibodies may occur spontaneously in 1–3% of cases per year.

HBeAg-negative state – patients are HBeAg negative and have episodic reactivation of infection with fluctuating levels of HBV DNA and aminotransferases. They have an active hepatitis which can lead to a worsening of liver fibrosis. This is due to the development of a mutation in the virus that leads to the virus failing to produce HBeAg.

HBsAg-negative phase – this occurs with loss of HBsAg. They are HBsAg negative, anti-HBc positive and anti-HBs may be detectable. HBV DNA is usually not detectable in the serum; however, low-level HBV replication may persist with detectable HBV DNA in the liver. Immunosuppression may lead to reactivation in these patients.

Patients should be considered for treatment when HBV DNA levels are above 2000 IU/mL, and/or the serum alanine aminotransferase is above the upper limit of normal, and/or liver biopsy shows moderate or severe necroinflammation and/or fibrosis.

This patient does not fulfil criteria for treatment at present but he should be monitored closely. The patient is most likely in the 'HBV inactive carrier state'. If the HBV DNA levels and/or the aminotransferases rise then it is likely that the patient has progressed to the 'HBeAg negative CHB' and treatment should be considered.

EASL clinical practice guidelines: Management of chronic hepatitis B virus. J Hepatol 2009; 50:227–242.

10. D Magnetic resonance cholangiopancreatography (MRCP)

The patient has primary sclerosing cholangitis (PSC). PSC is a cholestatic liver disease that is characterised by multiple intra- and extrahepatic biliary strictures. These occur as a result of chronic inflammatory changes leading to fibrosis of the bile ducts. It is diagnosed in patients with cholestatic abnormalities of their liver function tests in whom cholangiography shows segmental dilatation and multifocal strictures of the intra- and extrahepatic bile ducts, and in whom there has been exclusion of secondary causes of sclerosing cholangitis.

Cholangiography is essential for the diagnosis, and the gold standard used to be endoscopic retrograde cholangiopancreatography (ERCP); however, this procedure is complicated by pancreatitis and sepsis in 5% of cases. MRCP and ERCP have been shown to have similar diagnostic accuracy in the diagnosis of PSC, and therefore MRCP is the next appropriate step, especially in the non-jaundiced patient. ERCP still has an important role in equivocal cases, as MRCP can miss early cases without bile duct dilatation, and for therapeutic intervention such as stent insertion.

European Association for the Study of the Liver. EASL Clinical Practice Guidelines: Management of cholestatic liver diseases. J Hepatol 2009; 51:237–267.

11. C Oesophageal candidiasis

Odynophagia (pain on swallowing) is a classic symptom of oesophageal candidiasis. Patients are often able to pinpoint the pain to a very specific retrosternal point. The main risk factor for oesophageal candidiasis is immunosuppression, one of the causes of which is broad-spectrum antibiotic treatment. Other common causes of immunosuppression leading to oesophageal candidiasis are HIV infection (where it is an AIDS-defining illness), diabetes and haematological malignancies. Cytomegalovirus can cause oesophagitis, but it is usually seen only in advanced AIDS and there is nothing in this woman's history to indicate this diagnosis. Eosinophilic oesophagitis commonly affects men in their 20s to 30s and usually presents with dysphagia and/or food impaction. Presentation with odynophagia is uncommon. Oesophageal carcinoma is usually painless and presents with dysphagia. Achalasia does not present with odynophagia but presents with dysphagia and reflux of food.

Pappas PG, Kauffman CA, Andes D, et al. Clinical practice guidelines for the management of candidiasis: 2009 update by the Infections Diseases Society of America. Clin Infect Dis 2009; 48:503.

12. A Alcoholic fatty liver disease

There are a number of causes of hepatic iron overload, the most clinically significant of which is hereditary haemochromatosis (HH). The diagnosis of HH is made in patients with evidence of clinical iron overload. The transferrin saturation is over 50% in the majority of patients, and the ferritin is usually over 1000. Confirmation of the diagnosis is achieved by *HFE* (human haemochromatosis gene) genotyping and finding homozygosity for *C282Y*, or heterozygosity for *C282Y/H63*. This patient has a transferrin saturation and ferritin level that are too low for HH, and the most likely diagnosis is haemosiderosis secondary to alcoholic fatty liver disease. The appropriate management is reduction of alcohol intake. Hepatitis C virus (HCV) can cause hepatic iron overload but this patient does not have chronic HCV, having cleared the virus spontaneously. Thalassaemia also causes iron overload, but this patient has a normal full blood count, ruling out this diagnosis.

AASLD practice guidelines. Diagnosis and management of haemochromatosis. Hepatology 2001; 33(5):1321–1328.

13. E Whipple's disease

This man has presented with symptoms of malabsorption (weight loss and diarrhoea) associated with some cognitive impairment. His investigations reveal granulomas on duodenal biopsy. With this combination of signs and symptoms, the only diagnosis that could be the cause is Whipple's disease. Although Crohn's disease can present with malabsorption and granulomas it does not usually manifest symptoms of neurological involvement. Sarcoidosis can rarely cause small bowel disease, and can have neurological and rheumatological involvement. Granulomas will also be present on biopsy, but the absence of skin or lung manifestations makes this unlikely. Small bowel lymphoma is rare and can present with malabsorption. Neurological involvement can occur but it is very unlikely in the absence of lymphadenopathy, and it does not present with arthralgia. Abdominal tuberculosis can cause small bowel granulomas, malabsorption and neurological involvement, but it does not cause a migratory polyarthritis.

Whipple's disease is a rare disorder caused by the organism *Tropheryma whipplei*. It classically presents with diarrhoea, weight loss and a migratory polyarthritis. Neurological changes are seen in up to 50%, with the most common change being cognitive impairment, and cardiac involvement manifests clinically in 17–55%. The most common cardiac manifestation is pericarditis which occurs in around 50% of affected patients. Whipple's disease is diagnosed by periodic acid–Schiff (PAS) staining of small bowel biopsy specimens which on light microscopic examination show magenta-stained inclusions within macrophages of the lamina propria.

Fenollar F, Puéchal X, Raoult D. Whipple's disease. N Engl J Med 2007; 356:55–66.

14. D Prednisolone

This patient has classic clinical, biochemical and histological features of autoimmune hepatitis, with evidence of bridging fibrosis on liver biopsy. This is not primary biliary cirrhosis (PBC) or an overlap syndrome, as antimitochondrial antibodies (AMAs) are negative and there is no evidence of the florid histological biliary changes seen in PBC on liver biopsy. Therefore neither methotrexate nor ursodeoxycholic acid would be an appropriate first-line treatment for this patient.

The criteria for treatment of autoimmune hepatitis are: (a) AST /ALT (asparate transaminase/alanine transaminase) >5 × upper limit of normal (ULN), (b) IgG >2 × ULN, and (c) features of bridging necrosis, multilobular necrosis or cirrhosis on liver biopsy. Initial treatment should be with corticosteroids, either prednisolone or budesonide. Combination treatment with steroids and azathioprine from the beginning is an option but azathioprine monotherapy is not appropriate as it takes up to 12 weeks to have therapeutic effect and thus will not treat her acute inflammation. If patients are intolerant of steroids then ciclosporin can be considered, and it is also an option in children where the effects of steroids on growth may be an issue.

Manns MP, et al. Diagnosis and management of autoimmune hepatitis. Hepatology 2010; 51(6):2193.

15. B Chronic mesenteric ischaemia

This woman has the classic features of chronic mesenteric ischaemia. This usually presents with postprandial abdominal pain that is so severe that those affected develop a fear of eating and subsequently lose weight. The classic examination finding is of mild abdominal tenderness which is disproportionately mild in comparison to the reported pain. Patients with chronic mesenteric ischaemia usually have evidence of previous atherosclerotic disease such as ischaemic heart disease, cerebrovascular disease or peripheral vascular disease. Biliary colic can present with postprandial pain, but is rarely associated with weight loss. Duodenal ulcer pain typically occurs 2–3 hours after eating and in 50–80% of patients pain occurs at night. Gastric ulcers present with pain that is precipitated by food, but are not associated with weight loss. Gastric carcinoma rarely presents with postprandial abdominal pain, commonly presenting with anaemia or weight loss.

White CJ. Chronic mesenteric ischaemia: Diagnosis and management. Prog Cardiovasc Dis 2011; 54:36–40.

16. E Watchful waiting

The patient has symptoms suggestive of a single uncomplicated episode of biliary colic. Current guidelines recommend watchful waiting in patients with gallstones who are asymptomatic or who have had only one episode of biliary pain. Asymptomatic gallstones are common in the general population (10%, rising to 60% by the age of 80 years), as are upper gastrointestinal symptoms, which can result in an incorrect attribution of symptoms from another cause to gallstones. In one study a group of 252 cholecystectomy cases were reviewed by 9 surgeons, who were able to agree in only 52% of cases that the cholecystectomy was required, and who disagreed in 44% of cases. Therefore distinguishing patients whose pain is related to gallstones and will benefit from cholecystectomy is difficult. Cholecystectomy has a mortality risk of 0.14–0.5%, with the mortality risk from complications of gallstones being lower than this, and therefore in asymptomatic patients or those who have only had one episode of biliary type pain the benefits of watchful waiting outweigh the risks of cholecystectomy.

World Gastroenterology Organisation. WGO Practice Guideline: Asymptomatic Gallstone Disease. World Gastroenterology Organisation; 2008.

17. C Intravenous hydrocortisone 100 mg four times daily, subcutaneous heparin, calcium supplementation

The patient has acute, severe ulcerative colitis (UC) based on the Truelove and Witts criteria. These are a combination of a stool frequency of more than six per day combined with signs of systemic toxicity: (a) pulse >90 beats per minute, (b) erythrocyte sedimentation rate >30 mm/h, (c) haemoglobin <10.5 g/dL or (d) temperature >37.8°C. Patients who fulfil these criteria should be admitted to hospital for intravenous hydrocortisone therapy, with a starting dose of 100 mg four times daily. Oral prednisolone is not appropriate management in colitis of this severity. Ciclosporin is as effective as methylprednisolone as a first-line therapy for acute, severe UC but it is currently recommended only in patients in whom steroids are best avoided, and this is not applicable here. Antibiotic therapy should not routinely be given in acute UC and should be started only when there is a reasonable suspicion of infection, such as recent admission to hospital, a first attack of short duration or when stool cultures are positive. Subcutaneous heparin should be given to all patients with acute, severe UC to prevent venous thromboembolism, and calcium supplementation should be given to all patients expected to have a course of steroids of over 6 weeks – this will include all patients with acute UC.

Truelove SC, Witts LJ. Cortisone in ulcerative colitis; final report on a therapeutic trial. BMJ 1955; 2:1041e8. Travis SL, et al. European evidence-based Consensus on the management of ulcerative colitis: Current management. J Crohn's Colitis 2008; 2:24–62.

18. D Prednisolone

The patient has alcoholic hepatitis (AH). AH is not easy to define but has certain characteristic features:
- History of excessive alcohol intake
- Jaundice with bilirubin >80
- Hepatomegaly
- Mild fever but no infective cause found.

There are a number of scoring systems used to diagnose AH but one of the most common is the Maddrey discriminant function (MDF) to assess the severity of AH. A score of >32 indicates a severe alcoholic hepatitis and is an indication for treatment with steroids.

MDF = (bilirubin (in µL/17) + [(PT − control PT) × 4.6]
In this case the MDF = (170/17) + [(18 − 12) × 4.6] = 38

Where PT is prothrombin time (in seconds).

Patients with a MDF of over 32 have a predicted mortality rate of 30–50%. There is evidence that prednisolone therapy reduces mortality in this group, and therefore steroids are considered first-line treatment in patients with alcoholic hepatitis. The standard treatment is prednisolone 40 mg once daily for 28 days. Nutritional supplementation appears to improve mortality in certain subgroups of patients, and improves biochemical parameters, but has not shown an overall survival benefit and should not be used as initial monotherapy. Supportive care would be the appropriate treatment if this was a mild or moderate alcoholic hepatitis. Pentoxifylline has shown some promise in reducing deaths from hepatorenal syndrome in severe alcoholic hepatitis, but it is recommended as first-line therapy only if there is the presence of early renal failure or contraindications to steroid use, neither of which is the case with this patient.

O'Shea RS, et al. Alcoholic liver disease. Hepatology 2010; 51(1):307.

19. A Continue current treatment

Cytomegalovirus (CMV) infection has a worldwide distribution but is most common in developing countries where prevalence can be very high (almost 100% in adults). CMV infection is usually asymptomatic, and immunosuppressive therapy only rarely causes the development of severe CMV-related disease. It more usually causes latent CMV infection to undergo a subclinical reactivation. This is usually mild and self-limiting and therefore screening for latent infection is not recommended on patients commencing immunosuppressant therapy with inflammatory bowel disease. In this patient's case although there is evidence of CMV infection, with CMV IgG (indicating a risk for reactivation) and CMV DNA, and inclusion bodies within the colonic mucosa, the patient is asymptomatic and has no overt clinical disease so no specific antiviral treatment is required and the azathioprine can be continued. In severe CMV colitis, treatment with intravenous ganciclovir should be commenced, with a switch to oral valganciclovir after 2–3 days if appropriate clinically.

Rahier JF, et al. European evidence based Consensus on the prevention, diagnosis and management of opportunistic infections in inflammatory bowel disease. J Crohn's Colitis 2009; 3(2):47–91.

20. C 80 mg intravenous omeprazole bolus followed by a 72-hour protein pump inhibitor infusion at 8 mg/h and repeat endoscopy in 6–8 weeks

Her endoscopic finding of a non-bleeding visible vessel indicates a high risk of re-bleeding, and therefore treatment with an 80 mg bolus of omeprazole (or other comparable protein pump inhibitor), followed by an 8 mg/h omeprazole infusion for 72 hours and repeat endoscopy in 6–8 weeks is the appropriate post-endoscopy management. Haemostasis is achieved with endoscopic intervention. Two endoscopic modalities should be used to reduce the risk of re-bleeding which would include injection with adrenaline, plus one of heater probe coagulation, clipping or argon beam diathermy. The aim of additional acid suppression therapy is to maintain intragastric pH above 6 to stabilise clots and prevent re-bleeding. There is no evidence to support the use of tranexamic acid in non-variceal upper gastrointestinal bleeding. If *Helicobacter pylori* is present then eradication therapy should be started; however, in this patient a result is not given and so eradication therapy should not be started until the *Helicobacter pylori* result is known. All patients with gastric ulcers should have a repeat endoscopy in 6–8 weeks to ensure ulcer healing and exclude gastric carcinoma. There is no requirement for repeat endoscopy within 24 hours if there is no further gastrointestinal bleeding.

Scottish Intercollegiate Guidelines Network. SIGN Guidelines. Management of acute upper and lower gastrointestinal bleeding: A national clinical guideline. Edinburgh: SIGN, 2008.

21. D Phenytoin

With the exception of warfarin all of the drugs listed can result in idiosyncratic drug reactions causing hepatotoxicity. The answer in this scenario is phenytoin as this is the only drug listed that causes an immunoallergic hepatotoxicity. This is characterised by fever, lymphadenopathy, rash and severe hepatocyte injury, and can cause raised eosinophils. Sulfa drugs and halothane can also cause an immunoallergic reaction. The mechanism by which this occurs is by enzyme–drug adduction on the cell surface causing IgE release. Amiodarone causes a dose-dependent hepatotoxicity and typically causes steatohepatitis. Carbamazepine causes a mixed reaction with bile duct injury. Diclofenac causes a direct hepatotoxic reaction. With all idiosyncratic drug reactions the most important management step is identifying and stopping the causative drug. With the exception of *N*-acetylcysteine in paracetamol overdose there are no specific antidotes for drug-induced hepatotoxicity. Liver transplantation can be required if acute liver failure occurs, defined by jaundice followed by encephalopathy within 12 weeks, and all patients who develop this should be managed in a liver transplantation centre.

Lee WE. Drug induced hepatotoxicity. N Engl J Med 2003; 349:474–485.

22. B Liver cirrhosis

The differential diagnosis of new-onset ascites includes cirrhosis of the liver (the cause in 85% of cases), carcinomatosis peritonei, massive liver metastases, tuberculosis peritonitis, and rarer causes such as nephrotic syndrome and heart failure.

The serum–ascites albumin gradient (SAAG) is the most accurate measure for determining the cause of ascites, with a 97% accuracy in diagnosing ascites secondary to portal hypertension when a SAAG of >11 g/L is present.

The SAAG is calculated by the following equation:
SAAG = Serum albumin – Ascitic fluid albumin

This is more accurate than the previously favoured transudate (fluid protein <25 g/L) and exudate (fluid protein >25 g/L) because in 25% of cases patients with cirrhosis can have a fluid protein >25 g/L. For causes of ascites classified by the SAAG see **Table 4.2**

Table 4.2 Causes of ascites by SAAG	
SAAG >11	**SAAG <11**
Cirrhosis	Carcinomatosis peritonei
Nephrotic syndrome	Tuberculous peritonitis
Heart failure	Pancreatitis

The only two answers given that could cause a SAAG >11 are cirrhosis and nephrotic syndrome. The patient has a normal albumin level and no peripheral oedema, which makes nephrotic syndrome highly unlikely, and therefore liver cirrhosis is the correct answer.

Moore KP, Aithal GP. BSG Guidelines on the management of ascites in cirrhosis. Gut 2006; 55:1–12.

23. A Duration of reflux history

The picture shows Barrett's oesophagus, more accurately known as columnar lined oesophagus (CLO). This occurs when the normal oesophageal squamous lining has been replaced by a metaplastic columnar epithelium. A diagnosis of Barrett's oesophagus is made when a segment of columnar metaplasia is seen above the gastro-oesophageal junction during endoscopy, and has been confirmed histologically. The principal clinical concern in Barrett's oesophagus is the risk for progression to oesophageal adenocarcinoma.

The factors that have been associated with progression to adenocarcinoma are:
- Age >45 years
- Duodenogastro-oesophageal reflux
- Early onset of reflux disease
- Length of reflux history
- Male gender
- Oesophageal mucosal damage (ulceration or stricturing) >8 cm length of Barrett's oesophagus (extended disease)

Molecular markers such as p53 expression are sometimes used in research as surrogate markers of adenocarcinoma risk, but their usefulness clinically has not been ascertained and so they should be used only for research purposes. Smoking and alcohol are associated with gastro-oesophageal reflux disease but they do not appear to be associated with Barrett's oesophagus.

BSG Guidelines: Guidelines for the diagnosis and management of Barrett's columnar-lined oesophagus. A Report of the Working Party of the British Society of Gastroenterology, 2005.

24. B Gastroscopy and distal small bowel biopsies

This patient has coeliac disease, as evidenced by the symptoms of fatigue, diarrhoea and bloating, and dermatitis herpetiformis. The gold standard diagnostic test is gastroscopy and D2 biopsies. Small intestinal biopsy shows certain characteristic histological changes. These are crypt hyperplasia and loss of height of small intestinal villi, an inflammatory infiltrate into the lamina propria and epithelium.

Tissue transglutaminase (TTG) antibodies are highly sensitive, being present in over 90% of patients with untreated disease, but are less specific. They are best used for serological screening for coeliac disease. Immunoglobulin A levels should always be requested when TTG antibodies are tested, as false negatives can occur in IgA deficiency. Periodic acid–Schiff staining is required to diagnose Whipple's disease. Serum angiotensin-converting enzyme levels are used to diagnose sarcoidosis, which can occasionally present with small bowel involvement; however, the rash described is not typical of sarcoidosis. A colonoscopy and ileal biopsies would be appropriate if Crohn's disease was suspected. The malabsorptive symptoms could indicate Crohn's disease, but dermatitis herpetiformis is not associated with Crohn's disease.

British Society of Gastroenterology. BSG guidelines. Guidelines for the management of patients with coeliac disease. London: British Society of Gestroenterology, 2010.

25. A Anti-HAV IgM

This patient has the classic clinical features of hepatitis A virus (HAV). This is diagnosed in the acute phase by the presence of anti-HAV IgM, which is present for 14 days to 6 months after infection. Anti-HAV IgG develops later, approximately 5–6 weeks after the onset of acute infection, and is present in serum for many years. The presence of anti-HAV IgG confers protective immunity against further infection with hepatitis A virus. HAV infection consists of four stages. The first stage is an asymptomatic incubation period, lasting on average 28 days (although it varies from 10 days to 50 days) when viral shedding takes place. The second phase is the prodromal phase, during which symptoms of fever, dark urine, pale stools, malaise, headache and gastrointestinal upset occur. This is followed within 10 days by the development of jaundice (the icteric phase). The final phase is the convalescent phase when recovery from the infection occurs. On examination jaundice, cervical lymphadenopathy and tender hepatosplenomegaly may be seen, but examination is usually normal.

Hepatitis E virus presents in a similar way to HAV, but it has a longer incubation period of 15–60 days, with an average of 40 days from exposure to symptoms, and posterior cervical lymphadenopathy has not been reported. Hepatitis B virus (HBV) can be very difficult to exclude from acute HAV clinically. However, medical students in the UK are screened for HBV prior to medical school entry and vaccinated if not already immune. Even if this did not happen, this patient has no risk for contracting HBV. The classic presentation of Epstein–Barr virus (EBV) is with a triad of fever, lymphadenopathy and sore throat, which is not present in this patient. Jaundice is uncommon in EBV occurring in less than 5% of cases. HIV seroconversion can present with generalised lymphadenopathy but not really jaundice. Similar to HBV, this patient has no obvious risk factors for contracting this illness.

World Health Organization Department of Communicable Disease Surveillance and Response. Hepatitis A. 2000. WHO/CDS/CSR/EDC/2000.7.
Cohen JI. Epstein–Barr virus infection. N Engl J Med 2000; 343:481–492.

26. E Propranolol therapy

Non-selective beta-blockers reduce portal pressure (the driver for varices formation) by decreasing cardiac output and acting as a splanchnic vasoconstrictor. The risk of a first variceal bleed in patients with medium or large varices is significantly reduced by beta-blocker therapy (30% in controls versus 14% in beta-blocker-treated patients) and provides a statistically significant reduction in mortality; they are recommended as first-line therapy for primary prophylaxis of variceal haemorrhage. Endoscopic variceal band ligation (EVL) is as effective as beta-blocker therapy at decreasing the risk of first variceal haemorrhage, and is recommended as a first-line alternative to beta-blockers in patients with a high risk of variceal bleeding (i.e. those with more advanced cirrhosis or decompensated liver disease). However, in low-risk patients, such as the man in the scenario, beta-blockers are the first-line recommendation as the side-effect profile is better, and they are more cost-effective.

Isosorbide mononitrate (ISMN) is not recommended as primary prophylaxis for variceal haemorrhage because studies have shown a higher mortality in patients over 50 years receiving ISMN therapy than in those taking placebo, and ISMN when compared with placebo for the prevention of variceal haemorrhage showed higher bleeding rates.

An unblinded trial has shown a significantly lower rate of haemorrhage in combination therapy with ISMN and nadolol, compared with nadolol alone; however, two more recent, large, double-blinded, controlled trials were unable to confirm this result, and significantly more side effects were noted in the combination group, so combination therapy is not recommended.

Endoscopic variceal ligation alone has been compared with EVL and beta-blocker therapy, but no differences in the incidence of bleeding or death were seen between groups, so this is not recommended for primary prophylaxis either.

Garcia-Tsao G, et al. AASLD Practice Guidelines. Prevention and Management of Gastroesophageal Varices and Variceal Hemorrhage in Cirrhosis. Hepatology 2007; 46(3):922–938.

27. C Echinococcal cyst

Echinococcal (hydatid) cystic disease is usually caused by *Echinococcus granulosus* in the UK. It is most frequently found in individuals returning from the Middle East, eastern Europe, north and east Africa and Asia. It has an incubation period of months to years, and is transmitted via ingestion of eggs from canine faeces. It commonly presents with asymptomatic cysts discovered on routine abdominal imaging, but it can present with right upper quadrant pain and fever if liver cysts leak or become infected, or with hepatomegaly, cholestasis, biliary cirrhosis, portal hypertension and ascites. The cysts can rupture into the peritoneal space, leading to anaphylaxis and secondary cyst formation. An eosinophilia is present usually only when the cyst is leaking. Cyst aspiration can be complicated by anaphylaxis and cyst dissemination and so should be carried out only in specialist centres. Treatment recommendations have been published by the World Health Organization and treatment is based on cyst size, location and stage. Treatment is albendazole ± praziquantel ± cyst aspiration with the puncture, aspiration, injection and re-aspiration technique. Of all the causes of liver cysts given, hydatid disease is the only one that will cause an eosinophilia and the only one where daughter cysts are seen. Amoebiasis may cause an eosinophilia but it causes liver abscesses not liver cysts.

Brunetti E, Kern P, Vuitton DA. Writing Panel for the WHO-IWGE. Expert consensus for the diagnosis and treatment of cystic and alveolar echinococcosis in humans. Acta Trop 2010; 114(1):1.

28. E PIZZ

α_1-Antitrypsin (AAT) deficiency is defined as the inheritance of two severe deficiency alleles at the locus encoding AAT. It has a prevalence of 1 case per 3000–5000 persons in the USA. AAT is a serine protease inhibitor encoded by SERPINA-1 (also known as PI). AAT deficiency classically presents with severe, early onset, panacinar emphysema with a basilar predominance. AAT deficiency presents with predominant lung or liver involvement or both dependent on the inherited allele as indicated in **Table 4.3**:

Table 4.3 α_1-Antitrypsin alleles and their phenotype		
Allele	**Risk of emphysema**	**Risk of liver disease**
PIZZ	Very high	High
MZ	Possibly increased	Possibly increased
SZ	Increased	Possibly increased

Those with the *PIZZ* allele are at high risk of lung and liver involvement, and therefore this man is most likely to have this allele. Patients with the *PIMZ* allele may be at increased risk for lung and liver disease but the evidence is not robust. There is an increased risk of chronic obstructive pulmonary disease in those with the *PISZ* allele, but it is not as high as in those with the *PIZZ* allele.

Silverman EK. Alpha 1-antitrypsin deficiency. N Engl J Med 2009; 360:2749–2757.

29. C Oesophageal carcinoma – T1N0M0

Percutaneous gastrostomy (PEG) insertion is an important tool for the maintenance of long-term enteral nutrition in those in whom oral access is reduced. It is performed endoscopically. The most common indication for PEG placement is acute ischaemic or haemorrhagic stroke. In certain situations PEG placement is not appropriate, and in others caution should be used.

In T1N0M0 oesophageal carcinoma PEG insertion should not be performed for two reasons. There is a potential risk of seeding of malignant cells leading to PEG stoma metastases and there is a danger that the placing of a PEG may mean that, should the patient require an oesophagectomy, the stomach would not be suitable for forming a gastric tube.

In patients with cystic fibrosis nutritional status is often poor and nutritional failure common. The placement of a PEG improves nutritional status, which can help respiratory function. Progressive neuromuscular diseases such as motor neuron disease are valid indications for PEG insertion, but when ventilatory function is compromised this should occur only after an anaesthetic assessment. PEG insertion improves nutritional status in peritoneal dialysis patients, improving the likelihood of survival and of receiving a kidney transplant, but it also increases the risk of fungal peritonitis. PEG insertion can be carried out but dialysis should not occur for 3 days prior to the procedure and prophylactic antifungal therapy should be given. In systemic sclerosis, although there is no specific outcome data, the procedure is considered safe and may reduce aspiration, and so it should be performed if clinically required.

Westaby D, et al. BSG guidelines. The provision of a percutaneously placed enteral tube feeding service. Gut 2010; 59: 1592–1605.

30. C *Escherichia coli*

This man has ascending cholangitis, as evidenced by Charcot's triad of fever, abdominal pain and rigors which is present in 50–70% of patient with ascending cholangitis.

The most likely causative organism is *Escherichia coli* which is cultured in the bile of 31–44% of patients with ascending cholangitis.

Other causative organisms are shown in **Table 4.4**:

Antimicrobial therapy for acute cholangitis: Tokyo Guidelines. J Hepatobiliary Pancreat Surg 2007; 14:59–67.

Table 4.4 Causative organisms of ascending cholangitis	
Organism	**Positive rate in bile (%)**
Escherichia coli	31–44
Klebsiella species	8.5–20
Enterobacter species	5–9.1
Proteus species	1–4.8
Salmonella typhi	0.8–2.6
Salmonella paratyphi	0.8–2.3
Citrobacter species	1.6–4.5
Pseudomonas species	0.5–7.0
Streptococcus species	2–10
Enterococcus faecalis	2.6–10
Clostridium species	3–12.7
Bacteroides species	0.5–8.0

31. C Crohn's disease

This woman has presented with malabsorption (weight loss and diarrhoea), abdominal pain and scleritis, a classic spectrum of symptoms and signs associated with Crohn's disease. Small bowel bacterial overgrowth and coeliac disease do not cause abdominal pain or scleritis, although they can cause malabsorption. Tropical sprue causes malabsorption and can cause glossitis, but not aphthous ulceration.

Behçet's disease can present in a similar way, but to diagnose Behçet's disease the following criteria must be met:
- Recurrent oral ulceration: this can consist of major or minor aphthous ulceration or herpetiform ulceration, which occurs at least three times in a year. It can be observed by a physician or the patient

AND two of the following:
- Eye lesions: anterior or posterior uveitis, retinal vasculitis or cells in the vitreous humour.
- Recurrent genital ulceration
- Skin lesions: erythema nodosum, papulopustular lesions, pseudofolliculitis or acneiform nodules in non-adolescents
- A positive skin pathergy test.

The second European evidence-based consensus on the diagnosis and management of Crohn's disease: Definitions and diagnosis. J Crohn's Colitis 2010; 4:7–27.
Kontogiannis V, Powell RJ. Behçet's disease. Postgrad Med J 2000; 76:629–637.

32. A Achalasia

The barium swallow shows the classic findings of achalasia. Achalasia is an oesophageal motor disorder that is characterised by a failure of relaxation of the lower oesophageal sphincter (LOS). Pathologically inflammatory changes are seen in the oesophageal myenteric (Auerbach's) plexus. This leads to selective loss of post-ganglionic inhibitory neurons, with the postganglionic neurons of the myenteric plexus being spared, leading to unopposed cholinergic stimulation, high basal pressures and a failure of relaxation of the LOS. The classic radiological finding on barium swallow is smooth tapering of the lower oesophagus, leading to the closed LOS, which resembles a bird's beak in appearance. Oesophageal carcinoma classically presents with a long area of irregular mucosal narrowing. A hiatus hernia appears as a widening below the LOS. Nutcracker oesophagus and diffuse oesophageal spasm are diagnoses that can be made only on oesophageal manometry.

Vaezi MF, et al. Practice guidelines diagnosis and management of achalasia. Am J Gastroenterol 1999; 94(12):3406–3412.

33. C Sucralfate enemas

The appearances in the endoscopic picture are of radiation enteritis. The most common cause for this is pelvic radiotherapy for prostate carcinoma. The first-line treatment for radiation enteritis is sucralfate enemas in those patients for whom it is causing a reduced quality of life, or who are anaemic. Argon photocoagulation and hyperbaric oxygen therapy are recommended as second-line therapies for the treatment of radiation proctitis but both have disadvantages which mean they are not recommended as first-line treatment. The appearances are not consistent with inflammatory bowel disease for which a topical 5ASA treatment would be given. Prednisolone enemas are not recommended in radiation enteritis.

British Society of Gastroenterology. BSG guidelines. Practice guidance on the management of acute and chronic gastrointestinal problems arising as a result of treatment for cancer. London: BSG, 2011.

34. D Chronic HBV, previous HCV, chronic HDV

With acute HBV infection, the first marker that goes up is HBV-DNA. This is followed by HBsAg, HBeAg and anti-HBc IgM. Although anti-HBc IgM is not given, it would be expected that a patient with acute HBV infection would have high HBV DNA levels and be HBeAg positive. Chronic HBV infection is characterised by the presence of HBsAg, for more than 6 months with or without symptoms and regardless of viral load.

This patient has had HCV in the past because she is HCV IgG positive and she will remain positive for the rest of her life. Her viral load is zero meaning that she has cleared the virus spontaneously.

Hepatitis delta is a defective RNA virus. It can occur only as a co-infection with hepatitis B, because it requires a hepadnavirus such as HBV for its own replication. It invariably causes a more severe form of hepatitis in those who are co-infected with HDV than those with just HBV. It can occur as an acute infection with HBV, sometimes leading to a fulminant hepatitis, or as a superinfection in those already chronically infected with HBV, where it can cause a severe chronic active hepatitis.

In acute HBV–HDV infection the following serological markers will be positive: HBsAg, HBeAg and HBV DNA, anti-HBc, IgM anti-HDV, HDV RNA and HDAg. The development of anti-HDV antibodies occurs late in the acute phase of infection, and after infection they decline to undetectable levels. As anti-HDV appears hepatitis D antigen (HDAg) disappears. IgG and IgM anti-HD take months to years to decline after recovery from acute infection.

In contrast in HBV–HDV superinfection, persistent infection occurs in 90% of cases and usually results in persistent HDV infection. HDV viraemia (detectable HDV RNA) appears in the preacute phase and with active liver disease. There may be high titres of IgM and IgG anti-HDV and these can persist indefinitely. HBsAg titres and HBV–DNA can decline to almost undetectable levels with HDV co-infection but there is still persistence of HBsAg. This patient has chronic HBV–HDV superinfection as shown by the positive markers of HDV replication in combination with positive HBsAg.

WHO, Department of Communicable Disease Surveillance and Response. Hepatitis Delta. WHO, 2001. http://www.who.int/csr/disease/hepatitis/HepatitisD_whocdscsrncs2001_1.pdf (last accessed May 2012)

35. A Azathioprine

This patient has steroid-refractory ulcerative colitis, having required three courses of steroids within the last year without adequate control of his symptoms. Other causes of a failure to respond to steroids, such as cytomegalovirus colitis or cancer, should be excluded, and once these have been ruled out thiopurine therapy with azathioprine should be added. Thiopurine methyltransferase (TPMT) is an enzyme that is involved with the metabolism of azathioprine (and 6-mercaptopurine).

A TPMT level should be checked prior to commencement of azathioprine therapy as very low levels (<10) indicate deficiency of the enzyme and an increased propensity to myelotoxicity from azathioprine. A full blood count should be monitored before and after treatment starts to monitor for myelotoxicity. 6-Mercaptapurine is a metabolite of azathioprine that is associated with fewer side effects. In the UK this is used in those who cannot tolerate azathioprine therapy. The patient described does not yet fulfil the Truelove and Witts criteria for acute severe colitis and so does not require intravenous steroids immediately; however, these should be considered if he does not improve. Infliximab can be considered in this situation, but thiopurines are the usual first-line management. There is not enough evidence regarding the use of methotrexate in steroid-refractory ulcerative colitis to recommend its use in this situation.

Truelove SC, Witts LJ. Cortisone in ulcerative colitis; final report on a therapeutic trial. BMJ 1955; 2:1041e8.
Travis SL, et al. European evidence-based Consensus on the management of ulcerative colitis: Current management. J Crohn's Colitis 2008; 2:24–62.

36. A Dietary salt reduction and combination therapy with spironolactone 100 mg once daily and furosemide 40 mg once daily

Cirrhosis is the most common cause of ascites, being present in 75% of cases. Cirrhosis causes portal hypertension, by obstructing flow through the portal vasculature. Portal hypertension has a variety of consequences including the development of portosystemic shunts and intestinal disturbances causing bacterial translocation and endotoxaemia. This leads to release of prostaglandins and nitric oxide, with subsequent vasodilatation, particularly in the splanchnic beds. The result of this is decreased renal blood flow and activation of the renin–angiotensin system leading to avid sodium and water retention and ascites. In patients with moderate, but not tense, ascites the American Association for the Study of Liver Diseases (AASLD) guidelines recommend initial dietary salt reduction, in combination with spironolactone and furosemide therapy. Spironolactone therapy is particularly useful as it works on the distal tubule of the kidney where most sodium retention occurs. The combination with furosemide is recommended to counteract the hyperkalaemia caused by spironolactone. In a patient with tense ascites large-volume paracentesis is recommended for symptomatic relief, but this is not recommended in patients with non-tense ascites due to the potential risk of infection associated with cannulation of the peritoneum. Monotherapy with spironolactone is not recommended due to the potential for hyperkalaemia, and monotherapy with furosemide is less effective than combination therapy and so is not recommended.

Runyon BA. AASLD practice guidelines. Management of adult patients with ascites due to cirrhosis: an update. Hepatology 2009; 49(6):2087.

37. A Alendronate

Bisphosphonates, and in particular alendronate, are well recognised to cause oesophageal ulceration and symptoms of heart burn. All patients taking alendronate should be advised to drink plenty of water when taking their medication and to stay upright for 30–60 minutes after taking it to try to prevent this complication. All patients complaining of dyspepsia should be questioned to see if they are taking the following medications that are well known to cause dyspeptic symptoms: bisphosphonates, calcium channel antagonists, steroids, non-steroidal anti-inflammatory drugs, nitrates and theophyllines. Calcium channel antagonists can cause dyspepsia, but do not cause symptoms of oesophagitis. Citalopram, ramipril and simvastatin do not cause oesophagitis.

National Institute for Health and Clinical Excellence. Dyspepsia. Clinical guideline CG17. London: NICE, 2004.

38. B Examination under anaesthetic (EUA)

Perianal disease complicates Crohn's disease in up to 54% of cases. The incidence varies dependent on the site of Crohn's disease, with 12% of patients with ileal disease, 15% with ileocolonic disease,

41% with colonic disease and rectal sparing, and 91% of those with colonic disease and rectal involvement being affected. The investigation of choice for fistulating Crohn's disease in the usual circumstances is pelvic MRI as this has a 76–100% accuracy for delineating the track of fistulae; the presence of perianal pain nearly always indicates an abscess, however, and so in those with perianal pain the initial investigation should by EUA plus drainage if required, performed by an experienced surgeon. This should not be delayed until MRI is performed. Anorectal ultrasound is highly operator dependent and is not recommended routinely at present, and CT and fistulography are not recommended for the investigation of fistulating Crohn's disease.

The Second European evidence-based consensus on the diagnosis and management of Crohn's disease: Special situations. J Crohn's Colitis 2010; 4:63–101.

39. C Meckel's diverticulum

Meckel's diverticulum is the most common congenital abnormality of the gastrointestinal tract occurring in 0.6–4.0% of people. It is caused by the failure of the omphalomesenteric duct to obliterate in infancy. It occurs in the small bowel, and is lined by ileal mucosa, with ectopic gastric mucosa within the diverticulum in up to 50% of cases. It presents with obstruction due to intussusception or adhesive band, ulceration, diverticulitis and perforation. Bleeding from the diverticulum can cause iron deficiency anaemia. Preoperative diagnosis is difficult but a positive [^{99m}Tc] pertechnetate scan is the most accurate diagnostic test. The tracer concentrates in ectopic gastric mucosa, hence its clinical utility. Although the other diagnoses could present with intussusception they would not cause a positive [^{99m}Tc] pertechnetate scan, and therefore the diagnosis is Meckel's diverticulum.

Sagar J, et al. Meckel's diverticulum: A systematic review. J R Soc Med 2006; 99:501–505.

40. E Sphincter of Oddi dysfunction (type 1)

Sphincter of Oddi dysfunction (SOD) is characterised by symptoms of pancreatobiliary obstruction in the absence of structural causes. For SOD to be diagnosed, a patient has to experience typical biliary pain lasting for more than half an hour which is severe enough to warrant presentation to a physician or to cause them to stop their daily activities, and has occurred at least twice in the previous 12 months with no evidence of structural abnormalities.

The Milwaukee criteria have been used to further categorise SOD:
Type I SOD: the presence of biliary pain with an alkaline phosphatase and ALT/AST (alanine transaminase/aspartate transaminase) more than twice normal on at least two separate occasions, and a dilated common bile duct (as is the case here).
Type II SOD: biliary pain and only one or two of the criteria for SOD type 1.
Type III SOD: biliary pain and no objective criteria.

Acute acalculous cholecystitis has a variable presentation but is unlikely without the presence of elevated leukocytes and a fever. Autoimmune cholangitis is characterised by an elevated IgG level a positive antinuclear antibody and negative antimitochondrial antibody. Chronic pancreatitis is unlikely to cause this pattern of elevated liver enzymes, and does not cause a dilated common bile duct in isolation. Primary sclerosing cholangitis is characterised by cholestatic abnormalities of liver function tests with multifocal strictures and segmental dilatations on cholangiopathy, which this patient does not have.

Bistritz L. Sphincter of Oddi dysfunction: Managing the patient with chronic biliary pain. World J Gastroenterol 2006; 12(24): 3793–3802.

41. E Ulcerative jejunoileitis

All of the five answers are possible complications in a patient with coeliac disease but ulcerative jejunoileitis is the most likely in the scenario given. The patient's compliance with the gluten-free diet makes a relapse of coeliac disease unlikely. Microscopic colitis can occur concomitantly with coeliac disease but is an unusual cause of weight loss. Small bowel lymphoma, although an important diagnosis to exclude, is unlikely to occur in patients who have been compliant with a gluten-free diet for over 5 years, and in the absence of intra-abdominal lymphadenopathy.

Small bowel adenocarcinoma is another potential complication of coeliac disease, but usually presents at an advanced stage with metastatic disease. Ulcerative jejunoileitis is not common but is a complication of coeliac disease that can result in ulceration and stricturing. It is difficult to distinguish it from small intestinal lymphoma clinically. It is usually treated by a gluten-free diet, but if this is not successful, then early surgery is recommended.

British Society of Gastroenterology. BSG guidelines. Guidelines for the management of patients with coeliac disease. London: BSG, 2010.

42. C Gallstone ileus

Gallstone ileus is responsible for around 1–4% of small bowel obstructions, but accounts for up to 25% in patients aged over 65 years. It classically presents with an insidious onset over a few days, with a waxing and waning of symptoms due to the 'tumbling phenomenon' of the gallstone lodging and dislodging at various levels of the bowel. This often leads to a delay in diagnosis. The CT shown clearly shows a gallstone in the small bowel, and therefore it is the only possible correct diagnosis. It is treated surgically, but may present on the medical take and thus is an important diagnosis to be aware of. It is caused by recurrent episodes of calculous cholecystitis, resulting in inflammation and adhesions between the gallbladder wall and gastrointestinal tract, which is then followed by the gallstone eroding through the gallbladder wall to form a cholecystenteric fistula with eventual erosion into the gastrointestinal tract, and then becoming impacted. Stones less than 2 cm in diameter seldom become impacted.

Ayantunde AA, Agrawal A. Gallstone ileus: Diagnosis and management. World J Surg 2007; 31:1292–1297.

43. A Co-amoxiclav and metronidazole

The chest X-ray shows a pneumomediastinum and the most likely cause of this in this case is oesophageal perforation post-endoscopy. This is a recognised iatrogenic complication of the procedure, and occurs in an estimated 0.03% of diagnostic gastroscopies. The incidence of oesophageal perforation increases when endoscopic interventions are performed, with a risk of 0.5% in oesophageal dilatation rising to up to 25% for oesophageal stent placement. The initial management of oesophageal perforation is identical to that of any other perforated viscus – intravenous fluid resuscitation, broad-spectrum intravenous antibiotics and keeping the patient nil by mouth. Opiate analgesics should be used for pain control and total parenteral nutrition should be instigated. Oesophageal perforation has a high morbidity and mortality because of the oesophagus's proximity to the mediastinum and complications of mediastinitis, empyema, sepsis and multi-organ dysfunction. The reported mortality rate varies from 10% to 60% dependent on when treatment is instigated. Further management can involve surgical repair or expandable polymesh stent placement.

Kaman L, et al. Management of esophageal perforation in adults. Gastroenterol Res 2010; 3(6):235–244.

44. E Zieve's syndrome

This patient has the classic features of Zieve's syndrome. This is a syndrome of jaundice, haemolysis, hyperlipidaemia and abdominal pain in patients with excess alcohol consumption. It was first described by Zieve in 1958. It has a good prognosis and is treated conservatively, with cessation of alcohol intake being the most important management step. There is rarely a need for blood transfusion. The other answers given can all cause jaundice but present very differently.

Caroli's disease is a congenital malformation of the biliary tree that causes segmental saccular dilatation of the biliary tree. It causes a non-obstructive jaundice and presents with recurrent ascending cholangitis. It does not cause haemolysis or hyperlipidaemia and ultrasound scan usually shows cystic dilatation of the biliary tree.

Crigler–Najjar syndrome and Gilbert's syndrome are congenital disorders due to a reduction in the enzyme uridine diphosphate glycosyltransferase (UGT). Crigler–Najjar syndrome is an autosomal recessive disorder, in which there is a complete absence of the UGT enzyme (type 1) or a markedly reduced level (type 2). This results in a severe unconjugated hyperbilirubinaemia. It presents soon after birth with persistent jaundice. Type 1 is always fatal before the age of 2 years due to kernicterus. Type 2 is less severe and can be treated with phenobarbital. Gilbert's syndrome is a mild illness and is much more common. It is due to reduced activity of the UGT enzyme and results in a mild unconjugated hyperbilirubinaemia which is commonly precipitated by stress, such as viral infections. It presents with normal liver function tests and no haemolysis.

Mirizzi's syndrome occurs when gallstones become impacted in the cystic duct or Hartmann's pouch and cause external compression of the common hepatic duct. This may present with abdominal pain and obstructive jaundice but the ultrasound scan classically shows a contracted gallbladder with dilated intra- and common hepatic ducts and a normal calibre common bile duct.

Gitlin N. Zieve syndrome and porphyrinuria in an alcoholic. BMJ 1969; 1:96–98.
Pemberton M, Wells AD. The Mirizzi syndrome. Postgrad Med J 1997; 73:487–490.

45. A Argon photocoagulation

The endoscopic appearances shown in Figure 4.7 are of gastric angiodysplasia. This is most commonly seen in gastric antral vascular ectasia (GAVE), also referred to as watermelon stomach (due to the appearance of columns of tortuous ectatic vessels following the longitudinal gastric folds which resemble the stripes on a watermelon). It is a rare condition but is the cause of bleeding in 4% of patients presenting with upper gastrointestinal haemorrhage. The most common presentation of GAVE is chronic gastrointestinal blood loss, usually presenting with iron deficiency anaemia. GAVE is usually associated with chronic medical conditions, most commonly cirrhosis, autoimmune connective tissue disorders, Raynaud's disease or sclerodactyly. Other conditions in which it has been described include scleroderma, bone marrow transplantation, chronic renal failure and hypertension. First-line treatment is ablation of the vascular lesions with argon photo-coagulation or laser therapy. These therapies have been reported to reduce the need for further blood transfusions in 12 of 13 and 77% of patients in separate studies, although repeat therapy is sometimes required. Argon photocoagulation is the most commonly used modality in the UK. Beta blockers to reduce portal pressure have been investigated as a treatment due to the possible association of GAVE with cirrhosis, but no significant benefit has been reported. Corticosteroids were used in the treatment of GAVE based on case reports that showed that 4 of 11 patients responded to treatment with them; however, systemic side effects limit their use. There is one case report showing effective treatment of GAVE with endoscopic variceal band ligation but this is not enough evidence to change practice. Antrectomy was the definitive treatment of choice prior to endoscopic therapy, but it has a high reported mortality rate of 50% in patients with cirrhosis.

Selinger CP, Ang YS. Gastric antral vascular ectasia (GAVE): An update on clinical presentation, pathophysiology and treatment. Digestion 2008; 77:131–137.

Chapter 5

Haematology and immunology

Questions

1. A 23-year-old woman was referred by her general practitioner with a short history of easy bruising, bleeding gums and menorrhagia. She had no past medical history and was taking no medication.

   On examination, there were numerous bruises, especially over her arms and legs. The rest of the examination was normal.

   Investigations:

haemoglobin 10.5 g/dL (11.5–16.5)	international normalised ratio 1.0 (<1.4)
mean corpuscular volume 89 fL (80–96)	activated partial thromboplastin time 28 s (30–40)
white blood cell 5 × 10⁹/L (4–11)	
platelets 35 × 10⁹/L (150–400)	

   Peripheral blood film (see **Figure 5.1**)

   Figure 5.1 *See colour plate section.*

   What is the most likely diagnosis?

   A   Aplastic anaemia
   B   Fanconi's anaemia
   C   Paroxysmal nocturnal haemoglobinuria
   D   Primary immune thrombocytopenia (idiopathic thrombocytopenic purpura)
   E   Thrombotic thrombocytopenic purpura

2.   A 24-year-old woman from Rwanda presented with a productive cough, weight loss and fever for the last 1 month. Other than a 6-month history of persistent diarrhoea she had no past medical history and took no regular medications.

On examination, she had a body mass index of 17 kg/m², but was otherwise well. Examination of her chest revealed right upper zone inspiratory crackles.

Investigations:

haemoglobin 11.4 g/dL (11.5–16.5)	IgA 2.9 g/L (0.8–3.0)
white cell count 2.1 × 10⁹/L (4–11)	IgG 8.3 g/L (6.0–13.0)
neutrophils 1.9 × 10⁹/L (1.5–7.0)	IgM 1.1 g/L (0.4–2.5)
platelets 459 × 10⁹/L (150–400)	

Chest X-ray: (see **Figure 5.2**)

Sputum: 1+ acid-fast bacilli seen

ELISpot: negative

Figure 5.2

What is the most likely explanation for these results?

A   Acquired immunodeficiency
B   Common variable immunodeficiency
C   Non-tuberculous mycobacterial infection
D   Severe combined immunodeficiency
E   Surreptitious steroid use

3. A 45-year-old man presented with fever, right upper quadrant pain and deranged liver function tests (LFTs). Radiography and subsequent endoscopic retrograde cholangiopancreatography and biopsy suggested primary sclerosing cholangitis with pancreatitis. Despite steroids his LFTs continued to deteriorate and on biopsy he was found to have an autoimmune hepatitis.

With increased immunosuppression his LFTs stabilised but he then developed renal impairment. Further imaging revealed marked retroperitoneal fibrosis.

Investigations:

haemoglobin 9.8 g/dL (13.0–18.0)	IgA 0.9 g/L (0.8–3.0)
white cell count 6.8 × 10⁹/L (4–11)	IgG 33.9 g/L (6.0–13.0)
neutrophils 4.6 × 10⁹/L (1.5–7.0)	IgM 2.5 g/L (0.4–2.5)
platelets 587 × 10⁹/L (150–400)	

Antinuclear antibody negative: antineutrophil cytoplasmic antibody weakly positive perinuclear pattern

What is the most likely diagnosis?

A   IgA deficiency
B   Wegener's granulomatosis
C   Polyarteritis nodosa
D   Hyper-IgG4 disease
E   Sarcoidosis

4. A 22-year-old Turkish woman was admitted to hospital with pneumonia. She reported no past medical history of note and was taking no regular medications.

Clinical examination was consistent with lobar pneumonia.

As part of her work-up she had routine blood tests:

Investigations:

haemoglobin 10.1 g/dL (11.5–16.5)	red cell count 6.7 × 10¹²/µL (4.6–6.0)
mean corpuscular volume 63 fL (80–96)	HbA₂ 5.3% (1.5–3.5)
mean corpuscular haemoglobin 18.7 pg (28–32)	

What is the most likely diagnosis?

A   Alpha (α)-thalassaemia trait
B   Beta (β)-thalassaemia trait
C   Delta beta (δβ)-thalassaemia
D   Thalassaemia intermedia
E   Zeta (ζ)-thalassaemia trait

5. A 24-year-old man, originally from Ghana, developed jaundice within 48 hours of admission to hospital for treatment of pneumonia. He had no past medical history of note except for diet-controlled type 2 diabetes. He had been treated with intravenous co-amoxiclav, fluids and oxygen.

General examination revealed conjunctival pallor and mild icterus. He was apyrexial and haemodynamically stable. Respiratory examination revealed reduced air entry and crepitations at the right lung base. There were no signs of chronic liver disease and abdominal examination was normal.

Investigations:

haemoglobin 7.8 g/dL (13.0–18.0)	albumin 32 g/L (37–49)
mean corpuscular volume 78 fL (80–96)	protein 72 g/L (60–76)
white cell count 12 × 10⁹/L (4–11)	alkaline phosphatase 105 U/L (45–105)
platelets 236 × 10⁹/L (150–400)	alanine transaminase 36 U/L (5–35)
international normalised ratio 1.0 (<1.4)	bilirubin 54 mmol/L (1–22)

Direct agglutination test: negative

Urine: haemoglobin +
Peripheral blood film (see **Figure 5.3**)

Figure 5.3 *See colour plate section.*

What is the most likely diagnosis?

A   Autoimmune haemolytic anaemia
B   Glucose-6-phosphate dehydrogenase deficiency
C   Microangiopathic haemolytic anaemia
D   Penicillin-induced haemolytic anaemia
E   Pyruvate kinase deficiency

6. A 21-year-old woman presented to the emergency department with a 6-hour history of light-headedness, severe abdominal pain, nausea and vomiting. The patient reported previous episodes of abdominal pain and swelling of the hands and feet. The episodes were becoming more frequent. She did not take any regular medications. Her father had a history of similar episodes.
    On examination, she was afebrile, with pulse 110 beats per minute and blood pressure 80/45 mmHg. There was generalised abdominal tenderness but no other abnormalities detected.

What is the most likely diagnosis?

A   Coeliac disease
B   Crohn's disease
C   Familial Mediterranean fever
D   Hereditary angio-oedema
E   Lactose intolerance

7. A 16-year-old boy presented with recurrent boils, furuncles and episodes of cellulitis for many years. Several of these had been incised and drained and had grown *Staphylococcus aureus*. He

had been seen by the infectious diseases team who had referred him to immunology for a further opinion.

Investigations:

haemoglobin 14.4 g/dL (13.0–18.0)	alanine transaminase 21 U/L (5–35)
white cell count 7.8 x 10⁹ /L (4–11)	alkaline phosphatase 79 U/L (45–105)
neutrophils 5.9 x 10⁹/L (1.5–7.0)	IgA 2.5 g/L (0.8–3.0)
platelets 241 x 10⁹/L (150–400)	IgG 9.3 g/L (6.0–13.0)
bilirubin 7 mmol/L (1–22)	IgM 2.1 g/L (0.4–2.5)
albumin 39 g/L (37–49)	

Staphylococcus aureus toxin testing: Panton–Valentine leukocidin negative

Neutrophil stain: fails to stain with nitroblue–tetrazolium dye

What is the most likely cause of his immunodeficiency?

A Chronic granulomatous disease
B Familial Mediterranean fever
C IgA deficiency
D Myeloperoxidase deficiency
E Nephrotic syndrome

8. A 59-year-old woman presented with several months' history of increasing abdominal discomfort, indigestion, weight loss, bone pain and night sweats. She had lost 7 kg over the past 3 months. She had no previous medical history and had not travelled abroad in the past 10 years.

On examination, she had massive hepatosplenomegaly. Respiratory, cardiovascular and neurological examinations were normal.

Investigations:

haemoglobin 10.4 g/dL (11.5–16.5)	platelets 408 × 10⁹/L (150–400)
white cell count 25 × 10⁹/L (4–11)	haematocrit 37% (36–46)

Blood film: leukoerythroblastic with 'tear-drop' poikilocytes

Trephine biopsy: hypercellular bone marrow

Cytogenetic analysis: positive for *JAK2* mutation

What is the most likely diagnosis?

A Chronic myeloid leukaemia
B Hodgkin's lymphoma
C Myelofibrosis
D Polycythaemia rubra vera
E Systemic mastocytosis

9. A 40-year-old woman presented to the emergency department with confusion and difficulty understanding. According to her partner she had been feeling unwell with fever for the past 2 days. She had a past medical history of systemic lupus erythematosus, and was taking hydroxychloroquine.

On examination, the patient was drowsy with a Glasgow Coma Scale score of 14/15 and a temperature of 37.7°C. She was pale and had numerous petechiae. Neurological examination revealed a receptive aphasia, but no other focal signs. The rest of her examination was normal.

Investigations:

haemoglobin 8.8 g/dL (11.5–16.5)	bilirubin 67 mmol/L (1–22)
mean corpuscular volume 81 fL (80–96)	albumin 36 g/L (37–49)
white cell count 5 × 10⁹/L (4–11)	alkaline phosphatase 114 U/L (45–105)
platelets 37 × 10⁹/L (150–400)	alanine transaminase 29 U/L (5–35)
sodium 135 mmol/L (135–145)	international normalised ratio 1.1 (<1.4)
potassium 4.8 mmol/L (3.5–5.0)	activated partial thromboplastin time 30 s (30–40)
urea 11.2 mmol/L (2.5–7.5)	fibrinogen 2.5 g/L (1.8–5.4)
creatinine 176 µmol/L (45–90)	lactate dehydrogenase 753 U/L (10–250)
protein 73 g/L (60–70)	

Direct antiglobulin test: negative

Anticardiolipin antibody: negative

Lupus anticoagulant: negative

Peripheral blood film: indicative of microangiopathic haemolytic anaemia

What is the most likely diagnosis?

A   Antiphospholipid syndrome (APS)
B   Disseminated intravascular coagulation (DIC)
C   Immune thrombocytopenia purpura (ITP)
D   Microangiopathic haemolytic anaemia (MAHA)
E   Thrombotic thrombocytopenia purpura (TTP)

10. A 20-year-old male student was referred for investigation after failing to achieve a protective hepatitis B surface antibody after a course of two hepatitis B vaccines and two booster vaccinations. He was known to have asthma, eczema and coeliac disease. He took salbutamol and Seretide inhalers and had had two courses of oral prednisolone in the last year for his asthma. He used daily topical emollients and had used six courses of topical steroids this year. He was not very compliant with his gluten-free diet.

Investigations:

haemoglobin 14.8 g/dL (13.0–18.0)	IgA 1.5 g/L (0.8–3.0)
white cell count 8.9 × 10⁹/L (4–11)	IgG 7.3 g/L (6.0–13.0)
neutrophils 5.4 × 10⁹/L (1.5–7.0)	IgM 3.1 g/L (0.4–2.5)
eosinophils 0.4 × 10⁹/L (0.04–0.4)	IgE 188 kU/L (<120)
platelets 148 × 10⁹/L (150–400)	

Hepatitis BsAg – negative
Hepatitis BcAb – negative
Hepatitis BsAb <10 IU

What is the most likely explanation for vaccine non-response?

A   Atopic phenotype
B   Coeliac disease
C   Inhaled steroid use
D   Systemic steroid use
E   Topical steroid use

11. A 33-year-old woman was referred to the allergy clinic. She reported itching of her lips and throat shortly after eating apples, nectarines and peaches, and so avoided these fruits. However, more recently she had experienced similar symptoms shortly after ingesting a salad. She was worried that she could not eat a balanced diet as she now avoided most fruit and vegetables. She suffered from mild allergic rhinitis in April and May. There was no other past medical history of note.

What is the most likely cause of her symptoms?

A   Atopic dermatitis
B   Fructose intolerance
C   Hereditary angio-oedema
D   Latex sensitivity
E   Oral allergy syndrome

12. A 54-year-old man attended the heart transplant clinic for routine review. He had a transplant 10 years previously. His medications include ciclosporin, azathioprine and a low dose of steroids.

Which of the following statements is correct regarding his immunosuppression medication?

A   Azathioprine acts on B cells
B   Ciclosporin acts on B cells
C   Ciclosporin can cause microangiopathy
D   Ciclosporin levels do not require to be monitored
E   Gingival hyperplasia is a common side effect of azathioprine

13. A 54-year-old man presented with a 5-month history of fatigue and abdominal discomfort. On examination, there was hepatosplenomegaly, but no significant lymphadenopathy. Numerous bruises were also noted.

Investigations:

haemoglobin 8.7 g/dL (13.0–18.0)	neutrophils 1.0 × 10⁹/L (1.5–7.0)
white blood cell 2 × 10⁹/L (4–11)	platelets 89 × 10⁹/L (150–400)
lymphocytes 1.0 × 10⁹/L (1.5–4.0)	

Trephine bone marrow biopsy: fibrosis

Peripheral blood film (see **Figure 5.4**): the cytoplasm of the abnormal cells is subsequently found to stain positive for tartrate-resistant acid phosphatase

Figure 5.4 *See colour plate section.*

What is the most likely diagnosis?

A   Aplastic anaemia

    B   Chronic lymphocytic leukaemia
    C   Hairy cell leukaemia
    D   Myelofibrosis
    E   Plasma cell leukaemia

14. A 23-year-old woman was referred by her general practitioner with refractory anaemia. Her only symptom was fatigue. She had no past medical history of note and was not taking any medications, although she was previously prescribed iron sulphate tablets for 2 months without benefit. She was a personal fitness instructor, and did not smoke or drink alcohol.

    The clinical examination was normal, except for mild angular cheilitis and conjunctival pallor.

Investigations:

haemoglobin 9.9 g/dL (11.5–16.5)	international normalised ratio 1.0 (< 1.4)
mean corpuscular volume 74 fL (80–96)	ferritin 7 g/L (15–300)
white cell count 3.5 × 10⁹/L (4–11)	vitamin B₁₂ 200 ng/L (160–760)
platelets 267 × 10⁹/L (150–400)	folate 7 ng/mL (2.0–11.0)

Peripheral blood film (see **Figure 5.5**):

Figure 5.5 *See colour plate section.*

What is the most likely diagnosis?

    A   Anaemia of chronic disease
    B   Aplastic anaemia
    C   Iron-deficiency anaemia
    D   Microangiopathic haemolytic anaemia (MAHA)
    E   Pernicious anaemia

15. A 28-year-old woman was referred to the allergy clinic complaining of a 2-year history of sneezing and itching of the nose and palate. She gained some symptomatic relief from taking chlorpheniramine at night. She reported that she had experienced similar symptoms when she visited a friend who kept cats. She did not keep pets or have regular contact with any animals. Her brother had asthma.

What is the most appropriate investigation?

    A   Cat-specific IgE serum
    B   CT of the sinuses
    C   Nasoendoscopy
    D   Peak flow diary monitoring
    E   Skin-prick testing for common aeroallergens

16. A 26-year-old woman was admitted to the emergency department with facial swelling and difficulty in breathing. She was well until 2 hours previously when she had felt some tingling in her lips and tongue. She had a similar episode around a year ago for which no cause was found. She also described recurrent episodes of abdominal pain, requiring admission but with negative investigations, as a teenager. She was taking no new or regular medication.

    On examination, her lips and tongue were swollen and there was some periorbital oedema.

Which one of the following is least likely regarding her diagnosis?

A   Danazol can be given to prevent attacks
B   Fresh frozen plasma can be given in an emergency
C   It can be triggered by angiotensin-converting enzyme inhibitors
D   It is highly responsive to antihistamines
E   Oestrogen should be avoided where possible

17. An18-year-old man presented to his general practitioner with sinusitis. He gave a history of a previous episode of sinusitis in the last year and two episodes of ear infections as a child. He was otherwise well, took no regular medication and did not require hospital treatment for any of his previous infections.

Investigations:

haemoglobin 11.5 g/dL (13.0–18.0)	IgG 14 g/L (6.0–13.0)
white cell count 12.1 × 10⁹/L (4–11)	IgM 1.9 g/L (0.4–2.5)
IgA <0.05 g/L (0.8–3.0)	

Which one of the following is not associated with this condition?

A   Anaphylaxis to blood products
B   Coeliac disease
C   Poor response to pneumococcal polysaccharide vaccines
D   Severe life-threatening infection with encapsulated bacteria in infancy
E   Systemic lupus erythematosus

18. A 29-year-old woman presented with several months' history of increasing fatigue and easy bruising.
    On examination, she appeared pale with numerous small bruises. The rest of her examination was normal.

Investigations:

haemoglobin 8.5 g/dL (11.5–16.5)	white cell count 23 × 10⁹/L (4–11)
mean corpuscular volume 84 fL (80–96)	platelets 8 × 10⁹/L (150–400)
Peripheral blood film (see **Figure 5.6**)	

What is the most likely diagnosis?

A   Acute lymphoblastic leukaemia
B   Acute myeloid leukaemia
C   Chronic lymphocytic leukaemia
D   Chronic myeloid leukaemia
E   Hairy cell leukaemia

19. A 19-year-old dental student presented with intermittent episodes of sneezing, chest tightness and shortness of breath. On direct questioning, she reported occasional itchy rashes on her hands. The symptoms had begun after she commenced her first clinical attachment and she

was worried that she would not be able to continue her studies. She had no previous history of allergies or atopy and was not taking any medications.

What is the most useful diagnostic investigation?

A   Peak flow monitoring diary
B   Sensitivity testing for common aeroallergens
C   Serum total IgE
D   Skin-prick testing for latex
E   Spirometry with bronchodilator reversibility testing

20. A 20-year-old male university student was admitted with meningitis. Prompt diagnosis and antimicrobial therapy led to a full recovery and following discharge the patient was referred to the immunology clinic.

Figure 5.6 *See colour plate section.*

On further questioning, he reported a history of recurrent ear, nose and throat attendances throughout childhood with tonsillitis, sinusitis and otitis media. He confirmed that he received a meningococcal C vaccine 3 years ago prior to commencing university.

Investigations:

haemoglobin 13.9 g/dL (13.0–18.0)	platelets 179 × 10⁹/L (150–400)
white cell count 7.8 × 10⁹/L (4–11)	IgA 0.8 g/L (0.8–3.0)
neutrophils 5.4 × 10⁹/L (1.5–7.0)	IgG 1.1 g/L (6.0–13.0)
lymphocytes 2.1 × 10⁹/L (1.5–4.0)	IgM 0.4 g/L (0.4–2.5)

HIV antibody test: negative

Reference laboratory typing of meningococcus from cerebrospinal fluid: meningococcus C

What is the most likely diagnosis?

A   Common variable immunodeficiency
B   Human immunodeficiency virus
C   Hyposplenism
D   Severe combined immunodeficiency
E   Surreptitious steroid use

21. A 23-year-old medical student presented to hospital with a 1-day history of fever and rigors. He also had headache and malaise but no neck stiffness or rash. Five days ago he returned from a 6-week elective in Thailand. He had no past medical history, and had been taking prophylactic doxycycline until a few days before his return.

On examination, the patient appeared unwell with a temperature of 38.5°C, pulse 100 beats per minute and blood pressure 90/50 mmHg.

Investigations:

haemoglobin 10.2 g/dL (13.0–18.0)	white cell count 7 × 10⁹/L (4–11)
mean corpuscular volume 86 fL (80–96)	platelets 178 × 10⁹/L (150–400)

haemoglobin 10.2 g/dL (13.0–18.0) white cell count 7×10^9/L (4–11)
mean corpuscular volume 86 fL (80–96) platelets 178×10^9/L (150–400)

Peripheral blood film (see **Figure 5.7**):

Figure 5.7 *See colour plate section.*

What is the most likely diagnosis?

A   Dengue fever
B   Dracunculiasis
C   Japanese encephalitis
D   *Plasmodium falciparum* malaria
E   Trypanosomiasis

22. A 58-year-old man was admitted with purulent cough, pleuritic chest pain and a fever. A left lower lobe pneumonia was diagnosed on chest X-ray. He also had evidence of oral candida infection. He had a similar admission 4 months ago with pneumonia. There was a history of recurrent sinusitis and he had had two urinary tract infections in the last year. He was a non-smoker.

In view of his recurrent pneumonia and abnormal chest X-ray he went on to have a chest CT which confirmed left lower lobe consolidation and also showed an anterior mediastinal mass.

Investigations:

haemoglobin 8.7 g/dL (13.0–18.0)	IgA 0.5 g/L (0.8–3.0)
white cell count 4.0 × 10⁹/L (4–11)	IgG 3 g/L (6.0–13.0)
platelets 90 × 10⁹/L (150–400)	IgM 0.2 g/L (0.4–2.5)
Human immunodeficiency virus: negative	

What is the most likely diagnosis?

A   Chronic granulomatous disease (CGD)
B   Common variable immunodeficiency (CVID)
C   Good's syndrome
D   Wiskott–Aldrich syndrome
E   X-linked agammaglobulinaemia (XLA)

23. A 68-year-old man with a history of severe chronic obstructive pulmonary disease (COPD) was referred to the allergy clinic by a respiratory specialist nurse. She recommended that he should receive the influenza vaccine; however, he was concerned that he may be allergic to eggs and wanted more advice. He reported that he had several episodes of lip swelling after ingesting eggs

as a child. However, he admitted that he would often eat cakes containing eggs and recently ate a chocolate mousse containing raw egg white with no adverse effects.

Investigations:

> Skin-prick testing was performed in the clinic:
>
> testing control 3 mm
>
> testing egg white 3 mm (<8 mm)

What is the most appropriate management step?

A   Avoid influenza vaccine
B   Perform oral challenge test to egg white
C   Perform specific egg-white IgE serum assay
D   Recommend influenza vaccine
E   Recommend *Echinacea*

24. A 36-year-old woman presented with fever and rigors following her return from a holiday in Kenya. Clinical examination was normal.
     A peripheral blood film was performed (see **Figure 5.8**):

Figure 5.8 *See colour plate section.*

What is the most likely cause?

A   Babesiosis
B   Filariasis
C   Leishmaniasis
D   Malaria
E   Trypanosomiasis

25. A 43-year-old woman returned for follow-up in the rheumatology clinic. She had a diagnosis of severe rheumatoid arthritis and had been receiving methotrexate and rituximab. She was concerned because she visited a friend the day previously who had shingles. The patient could not remember if she ever had chickenpox as a child and did not think she had had shingles before.

What is the most appropriate next step in management?

A   Give oral aciclovir
B   Give intravenous ganciclovir
C   Give varicella-zoster IgG
D   Review in 1 week for signs of infection
E   Urgently test varicella-zoster IgG titre

26. A 53-year-old man was referred by his general practitioner with persistently raised white blood cell count. His only complaint was of several months' history of fatigue. There was no past medical history of note.

On examination, he had some conjunctival pallor and moderate splenomegaly.

Investigations:

haemoglobin 10.7 g/dL (13.0–18.0)	white cell count 63 × 10⁹/L (4–11)
mean corpuscular volume 87 fL (80–96)	platelets 512 × 10⁹/L (150–400)

Peripheral blood film (see **Figure 5.9**)

Bone marrow: hypercellular with predominant granulopoiesis

Cytogenetic analysis: t(9:22) (q34;q11) detected

Figure 5.9 *See colour plate section.*

What is the most likely diagnosis?

A Acute lymphoblastic leukaemia
B Acute myeloid leukaemia
C Chronic lymphocytic leukaemia
D Chronic myeloid leukaemia
E Hairy cell leukaemia

Answers

1. D Primary immune thrombocytopenia

This patient most likely has primary immune thrombocytopenia (formerly known as idiopathic thrombocytopenic purpura), which is a common condition. It occurs in two forms, as an acute condition in children and a chronic condition in adults. It is due to increased destruction of platelets secondary to the formation of platelet autoantibodies, which reduce platelet lifespan from 10 days to a few hours.

Primary immune thrombocytopenia is usually idiopathic but it can be secondary to systemic disease, infection, drugs and other haematological disorders. The adult form is more common in women. Typical features at presentation include petechiae, easy bruising, gingival bleeding, epistaxis and menorrhagia. Splenomegaly is uncommon. In some cases patients are asymptomatic, having been identified as having an isolated thrombocytopenia on a routine blood test.

A full blood count and peripheral blood films confirm a thrombocytopenia. Haemoglobin, white cell count, international normalised ratio and activated partial thromboplastin time are usually normal. Bleeding time is usually prolonged. Bone marrow studies are often normal, but are important in excluding other causes.

Thrombotic thrombocytopenic purpura is typically associated with a microangiopathic haemolytic anaemia and is discussed in more detail elsewhere. Aplastic anaemia is characterised by a pancytopenia, and can therefore be discounted. Fanconi's anaemia is a rare autosomal recessive disorder that presents in childhood. It causes aplastic anaemia. Affected individuals are often born with congenital abnormalities and are at high risk of developing a wide range of neoplastic diseases, including acute myeloid leukaemia. Paroxysmal nocturnal haemoglobinopathy is associated with haemolytic anaemia, pancytopenia and thrombosis.

Hoffbrand V, Moss P, Pettit J. Bleeding disorders (Chapter 23) In: Essential Haematology, 5th edn. Oxford: Blackwell Publishing, 2006.
Provan D, et al. International consensus report on the investigation and management of primary immune thrombocytopenia. Blood 2010; 115:168–186.

2. A Acquired immunodeficiency

This woman has the clinical, radiographic and microbiological indicators of pulmonary tuberculosis and has a likely underlying immunodeficiency. The negative interferon-γ release assay (in this example the ELISpot test) should not detract from the diagnosis and is providing a false-negative result in the immunodeficient state. An interferon-γ release assay (IGRA) allows visualisation of the secretory product of individual activated T cells (i.e. those sensitised to tuberculosis from previous exposure) in a semi-quantitative manner. It does not give rise to false-positive results in those who have received the BCG vaccine, unlike the Mantoux test (the specific epitopes used in the IGRA are present only in *Mycobacterium tuberculosis* and not in the BCG strain of *M. bovis* used in vaccination). False-negative results can occur, however, and although IGRA is a sensitive test to detect latent tuberculosis infection it should be interpreted with caution in active tuberculosis and in immunocompromised individuals. In active tuberculosis (TB), particularly in miliary TB and TB meningitis, a false-negative result can occur. In those with immunodeficiency there may be false negatives due to a relative absence of circulating lymphocytes from which the IGRA can detect a response.

Severe combined immunodeficiency would not be compatible with this story as the condition is rapidly fatal in childhood without intervention. The normal/mildly raised immunoglobulins and the epidemiological history point away from common variable immunodeficiency which is often characterised by hypogammaglobulinaemia. The story is not consistent with surreptitious steroid use. This patient does not have a history consistent with non-tuberculous mycobacteria.

Herrera V, et al. Clinical application and limitations of interferon-gamma release assays for the diagnosis of latent tuberculosis infection. Clin Infect Dis 2011; 52(8):1031–1037.

3. D Hyper-IgG4 disease

This man is presenting with a multisystem disorder and a hypergammaglobulinaemia typical of hyper-IgG4 disease. This is a systemic disease characterised by infiltration of various organs by IgG4-positive plasma cells and T lymphocytes with subsequent sclerosis. Clinically this disease occurs predominantly in older men, and can cause inflammatory syndromes in the pancreas, biliary tree and retroperitoneum. Less frequently there can be renal, pulmonary and prostatic involvement. Typically one to two organ systems are involved but three to four systems can on occasion be affected. Most cases of hyper-IgG4 diseases have been found to be associated with autoimmune pancreatitis. Serum immunoglobulin elucidation and specific IgG4 levels and immunostaining of pathological specimens with anti-IgG4 antibody are diagnostic. The disease usually responds well to steroid therapy.

There is a relatively low IgA level in this case but the clinical picture does not fit with IgA deficiency. This disease is usually asymptomatic but where symptoms do occur there is typically a history of increased frequency of mucous membrane infections or of a severe blood transfusion reaction due to the presence of IgA in this product. Polyarteritis nodosa is a medium-vessel vasculitis that can cause multi-system inflammatory change and is associated with pANCA (perinuclear antisentrophil cytoplasmic antibody); however, the pancreatitis, hepatitis and retroperitoneal fibrosis in this case fit more with hyper-IgG4. Wegener's granulomatosis is again a multisystem vasculitis but it typically associated with pulmonary and renal involvement and usually has a cANCA (cytoplasmic ANCA) pattern. Sarcoidosis is a multi-system granulomatous condition that can be associated with pancreatitis, hepatitis, cholangitis and retroperitoneal fibrosis and although mildly elevated IgG levels can be found the profound high IgG levels in this case make hyper-IgG4 the more likely diagnosis.

Kamisawa T, Okamoto A. IgG4-related sclerosing disease. World J Gastroenterol 2008; 14(25):3948–3955.

4. B Beta (β)-thalassaemia trait

Prior to this admission, this patient was asymptomatic. She has mild anaemia, very low mean corpuscular volume and mean corpuscular haemoglobin, and elevated red blood cell count which could be in keeping with a thalassaemia trait. Critically, the analysis of haemoglobin reveals >3.5% HbA_2 $(\alpha_2\delta_2)$ which is indicative of a deficit in β-chain synthesis and is sufficient to make a diagnosis of β-thalassaemia trait.

The α-thalassaemia traits (caused by defective α-globin synthesis from one or two of the four α-globin genes) are also associated with microcytic red cells, and low mean corpuscular haemoglobin. However, anaemia is not usually present. Thalassaemia intermedia is a condition resulting from heterogeneous defects in chain synthesis; clinically, there may be extramedullary erythropoiesis, hepatosplenomegaly, bony deformities or evidence of iron overload. Homozygous δβ-thalassaemia results in 100% fetal haemoglobin HbF $(\alpha_2\gamma_2)$, due to the inability to synthesise the δ and β chains necessary for formation of HbA_2 and HbA, respectively. Zeta-globin is expressed during early embryonic development, although it may also be detected in adult patients with α-thalassaemias; its defective synthesis does not cause a thalassaemia trait in adults.

Hoffbrand V, Moss P, Pettit J. Genetic disorders of haemoglobin (Chapter 6). In: Essential Haematology, 5th edn. Oxford: Blackwell Publishing, 2006.
Chung SW, et al. Human embryonic zeta globin chains in adult patients with alpha thalassaemias. Proc Natl Acad Sci USA 1984; 81:6188–6191.

5. B Glucose-6-phosphate dehydrogenase deficiency

This patient, who is deficient in the enzyme glucose-6-phosphate dehydrogenase (G6PD), is suffering from an acute haemolytic episode secondary to infection.

Several hundred genetic variants of G6PD have been described to date, with variable levels of red cell susceptibility to oxidative stress. Normally, G6PD activity results in the reduction of NADP to NADPH, which in turn is necessary for the formation of reduced glutathione as a protective agent against red cell oxidants. In the absence of significant oxidant stress, patients with G6PD deficiency are usually asymptomatic. However, the condition is thought to be associated with a risk of developing diabetes. Recognised precipitants of acute haemolytic episodes include drugs (nitrofurantoin, primaquine, dapsone and others), fava beans and infection.

Intravascular haemolysis with jaundice and haemoglobinuria can develop very rapidly. Blood tests will reveal anaemia, raised bilirubin (unconjugated) and decreased levels of haptoglobin. The direct agglutination test will be negative, and the coagulation profile is also usually normal. The peripheral blood film usually exhibits 'bite' cells and 'blister' cells, as in this case, which arise as a result of splenic removal of Heinz bodies (deposits of oxidised, denatured DNA). Definitive diagnosis can be made by assaying enzyme activity; however, this is best performed once the acute phase has subsided (since the replacement immature red cells contain higher levels of enzyme, making a false negative more likely in the acute phase).

Treatment is by stopping precipitant medications and maintaining high urine output until haemoglobinuria has ceased. Transfusion may be indicated in severe anaemia. Autoimmune haemolytic anaemias may occur in different contexts, but are associated with a positive direct antiglobulin test. The peripheral blood film tends to exhibit microspherocytes.

Penicillin-induced haemolytic anaemias result from the generation of antibody to a penicillin-red cell membrane complex. The anaemia resolves with cessation of treatment. Microangiopathic haemolytic anaemia is discussed briefly in another question. Pyruvate kinase deficiency is autosomal recessive and associated with variable levels of anaemia. Jaundice is commonplace and many patients also suffer from gallstones. Peripheral blood film tends to show poikilocytes and 'prickle' cells. The diagnosis may be confirmed by enzyme assay. Splenectomy should be considered in transfusion-dependent patients.

Hoffbrand V, Moss P, Pettit J. Haemolytic anaemias (Chapter 5) In: Essential Haematology, 5th edn. Oxford: Blackwell Publishing, 2006.
Wan GH, et al. Decreased blood activity of glucose-6-phosphate dehydrogenase associates with increased risk for diabetes mellitus. Endocrine 2002; 19:191–195.

6. D Hereditary angio-oedema

Hereditary angio-oedema (HAE) is a rare autosomal dominant disease. It is caused by a deficiency in function C1 inhibitor and it has an estimated prevalence of 1 in 50,000. HAE is characterised by recurrent episodes of swelling involving the limbs, trunk, face, mouth, and sometimes genitalia and gut. It is not associated with urticaria. Symptoms typically begin in early childhood, deteriorate during puberty and persist throughout life. There is considerable variation in the severity and frequency of attacks. Delays in diagnosis are common and the diagnosis should be suspected in any patient who presents with recurrent angio-oedema or abdominal pain in the absence of associated urticaria. Most patients report a family history of angio-oedema; up to 25% cases occur anew.

The management of HAE includes treatment of acute attacks with purified C1-inhibitor replacement therapy and long-term prophylaxis to minimise the frequency and severity of recurrent attacks with agents such as danazol.

The other diagnoses may present with intermittent or relapsing and remitting symptoms, however, the history of the acute nature of the presenting complaint and the association with swelling of the hands and feet suggest that an allergic response and would be against the other diagnoses, including inflammatory bowel disease, malabsorption, angiotensin-converting enzyme inhibitor use or oestrogen therapy.

Zuraw BL. Hereditary angioedema. N Engl J Med 2008; 359:1027–1036.

7. A Chronic granulomatous disease

This man is presenting with an immunodeficiency predisposing him to recurrent bacterial infections most consistent with a neutrophil functional disorder. These are a diverse group of inherited diseases in which neutrophils have a disorder of phagocytosis or deficiency in the respiratory burst [including chronic granulomatous disease (CGD) and myeloperoxidase (MPO) deficiency]. Neutrophils produce reactive oxygen species which destroy bacteria after phagocytosis. Patients with these deficiencies are vulnerable to infections with catalase-positive organisms such as *Staphylococcus aureus*. The nitroblue–tetrazolium (NBT) test is the original and most widely known test for chronic granulomatous disease – it is negative in CGD, and positive in normal individuals. In MPO deficiency the majority of individuals show no signs of immunodeficiency but when they present often do so with *Candida albicans* infections. Patients with MPO deficiency have a respiratory burst with a normal NBT dye test but do not form bactericidal compounds due to their lack of peroxide. Treatment has historically been with long-term antimicrobial prophylaxis or in some cases stem cell transplant. Interferon-γ 1b has been trialled in the prevention of infection in CGD, having been shown to reduce infection frequency by 70% and to decrease its severity.

IgA deficiency is usually asymptomatic but patients can have increased frequency of mucous membrane infections including urinary tract and ear, nose and throat infections. IgA deficiency most frequently comes to light, however, after severe reactions to blood transfusions or on receiving intravenous immunoglobulin due to the presence of IgA in these products. Nephrotic syndrome can lead to a relatively immunocompromised state but the preserved immunoglobulins in this case mean that it is not the diagnosis here. Familial Mediterranean fever (FMF) is an autoinflammatory condition caused my mutations in the *MEFV* gene. Although it can cause period fevers, arthralgia, abdominal pain and serositis it does not present with recurrent staphylococcal infections. Confirmation of FMF is with the metaraminol provocative test.

Jones LB, et al. Special article: chronic granulomatous disease in the United Kingdom and Ireland: a comprehensive national patient-based registry. Clin Exp Immunol 2008; 152(2):211–218.

8. C Myelofibrosis

This is myelofibrosis, a clonal stem cell disease. Hyperplastic megakaryocytes result in progressive bone marrow fibrosis. Haematopoiesis then becomes increasingly active within both the spleen and the liver, clinically manifesting as splenomegaly (often massive) and hepatomegaly, respectively. Anaemia is common. Blood films are usually leukoerythroblastic with 'tear-drop' poikilocytes. The bone marrow aspirate is often unsuccessful owing to the hypercellularity of the marrow, therefore necessitating a trephine bone marrow biopsy. The *JAK2* mutation is present in approximately half, and some patients will also have a previous history of polycythaemia rubra vera. In up to one-fifth of patients the disease may transform to acute myeloid leukaemia.

The *JAK2* mutation is almost always detectable in polycythaemia rubra vera. These patients tend to present with symptoms of polycythaemia; massive splenomegaly would be quite unusual.

Chronic myeloid leukaemia is also a cause of massive splenomegaly, but tends to be associated with the Philadelphia chromosome t(9;22) (q34;q11). It may present with hypermetabolism, anaemia, easy bruising/increasing propensity to bleeding, etc., but it is often diagnosed incidentally following abnormal routine blood tests while the patient is asymptomatic or suffering from non-specific symptoms. Massive leukocytosis, low neutrophil alkaline phosphatase and raised uric acid levels are typical findings. The blood film exhibits increased numbers of cells throughout all stages of granulopoiesis. Bone marrow is usually hypercellular.

Hodgkin's disease tends to present in younger patients and is rarely associated with massive splenomegaly. It is not linked to the *JAK2* mutation.

Systemic mastocytosis is a rare myeloproliferative disorder typically characterised by haematological, gastrointestinal, cardiac and cutaneous involvement. It has a well-recognised association with recurrent anaphylaxis. Symptoms may include flushing, pruritus, abdominal pain, diarrhoea and bronchospasm. Examination may reveal hepatomegaly, splenomegaly, lymphadenopathy, signs of anaemia, urticaria and excoriations. Investigations may reveal anaemia, leukocytosis and thrombocytopenia. Bone marrow may be normo- or hypercellular. The *JAK2* mutation is rarely detected, whereas the c-*kit* mutation (A816V) is present in almost all cases.

Hoffbrand V, Moss P, Pettit J. Myeloproliferative disorders (Chapter 19) In: Essential Haematology, 5th edn. Oxford: Blackwell Publishing, 2006.

9. E Thrombotic thrombocytopenic purpura (TTP)

This patient is suffering from TTP, which can be familial or acquired. The condition is defined by five features: thrombocytopenia, microangiopathic haemolytic anaemia (MAHA), neurological abnormalities, renal failure and fever. All five need not be present for the diagnosis to be made. A typical clinical presentation is of fever, altered mental status, petechiae and symptoms of anaemia. Typical laboratory findings are of thrombocytopenia, normocytic anaemia, raised levels of unconjugated bilirubin (due to intravascular haemolysis), raised lactate dehydrogenase (LDH) (both from red cell lysis and tissue infarction), decreased haptoglobin and increased bleeding time. The peripheral blood film will be that of MAHA, showing schistocytes, helmet cells and thrombocytopenia. Further investigation may include neuroimaging.

Platelet transfusions are contraindicated as they are thought to fuel the process of thrombus formation and increase the risk of myocardial infarction and stroke, etc. There is said to be a 10–20% early mortality rate in treated patients, compared with a 90% mortality rate in untreated patients. Relapses are common following the acute treatment, and many patients will require maintenance treatment with steroids, immunosuppressants or biologics (e.g. rituximab). Response can be gauged by monitoring platelet and serum LDH levels. Ultimately, early treatment of the acute phase carries a good prognosis and most patients make a good recovery.

Antiphospholipid syndrome can occur as a primary condition or secondary to others such as systemic lupus erythematosus. It is associated with arterial and venous thromboses, and clinical complications may include stroke and renal impairment, among others. It is also a recognised cause of recurrent miscarriage. Laboratory investigations often reveal a haemolytic anaemia and thrombocytopenia. However, owing to the absence of anticardiolipin and lupus anticoagulant antibodies, it can be discounted as the cause in this patient.

Disseminated intravascular coagulation (DIC) occurs in response to many different underlying conditions including sepsis, malignancy and trauma. The clinical presentation may be that of the underlying condition, but in severe cases petechiae, ecchymoses and haemorrhage may be apparent. Hallmarks include thrombocytopenia, prolonged prothrombin time, activated partial thromboplastin time (APPT) and bleeding time, and depleted fibrinogen owing to the widespread coagulation and consumption of agents necessary for clotting.

Idiopathic thrombocytopaenic purpura is not characteristically associated with thrombosis and haemolytic anaemia.

MAHA alone does not explain this patient's presentation. It is diagnosed on the appearance of the peripheral blood film and has many causes including TTP, haemolytic uraemic syndrome, DIC and prolonged running/marching exercises.

Hoffbrand V, Moss P, Pettit J. Bleeding disorders (Chapter 23). In: Essential Haematology, 5th edn. Oxford: Blackwell Publishing, 2006.

10. B Coeliac disease

Approximately 4–10% of healthy individuals fail to elicit protective levels of hepatitis B antibodies after completing the standard HBV vaccination schedule. Factors suggested to contribute to non-response include: age, obesity, immunosuppression and route of vaccination but human leukocyte antigen (HLA) phenotype is considered the most important genetic marker of non-response. Coeliac disease is an HLA-associated disease and non-response to hepatitis B vaccine is well documented in undiagnosed coeliac disease and in those who adhere poorly to gluten-free diet. However, in adequately treated patients re-immunisation can lead to a satisfactory HBsAb response and should be recommended.

Topical administration of corticosteroids (to skin or eyes) or use through aerosol, or by intra-articular, bursal, or tendon injection is not a contraindication to immunisation. In asthma, including those on inhaled and short-course oral corticosteroids, hepatitis B immunisation has been specifically shown to elicit good antibody response. Systemic corticosteroid therapy usually does not contraindicate immunisation. Live-attenuated virus vaccines can still be administered when such therapy is short-term (i.e. less than 2 weeks) or when being prescribed for physiological maintenance doses. The exact amount of systemic corticosteroid and the duration of therapy needed to suppress the immune system sufficiently to potentiate adverse events in live vaccine use are not well defined, but greater than 20 mg/day for periods greater than 2 weeks is taken as a generally accepted level at which concern should be raised. Live vaccine administration should ideally not occur until the steroids have been discontinued and if possible a 3-month period should be left before live vaccine administration. There is currently little evidence either supporting or refuting an impact of corticosteroids in killed and sub-unit vaccinations (such as the hepatitis B vaccine). In this case the short and infrequent oral courses of steroids for the asthma cannot account for the vaccine non-response.

Ertem D, et al. The response to hepatitis B vaccine: does it differ in celiac disease? Eur J Gastroenterol Hepatol 2010; 22(7):787–793.

11. E Oral allergy syndrome

Oral allergy syndrome is a condition characterised by an IgE-mediated allergic response. The ingestion certain uncooked fruit and vegetables causes sudden onset of itching, irritation and swelling to the oropharynx. It is a form of contact allergy and may be occur in up to 50% of patients with allergic rhinitis to pollen. Birch allergy sufferers may have reactions to raw apples, pears, cherries, carrots and celery. The symptoms are generally self-limiting and resolve several minutes after stopping eating the food. Cooked foods do not typically cause this reaction because of the alteration of the protein complexes. Some patients with latex allergy may also have cross-sensitivity to certain foods that contain similar proteins, including: avocado, banana, chestnut and kiwi.

Atopic dermatitis (eczema) often occurs in early childhood and may be associated with asthma and allergic rhinitis.

The prevalence of fructose intolerance secondary to malabsorption may be increasing due to widespread use of high fructose corn syrups to sweeten many commercial food products. However, the degree to which fructose malabsorption contributes to gastrointestinal symptoms is not clearly established. Symptoms of fructose malabsorption appear to be more common in individuals who have an underlying functional bowel disorder such as irritable bowel syndrome.

Hereditary angio-oedema results from mutations in the C1-inhibitor gene and is associated with recurrent episodes of angio-oedema of the oropharynx and/or gut in the absence of urticaria.

Katelaris CH. Food allergy and oral allergy or pollen-food syndrome. Curr Opin Allergy Clin Immunol 2010; 10(3):246–251.

12. C Ciclosporin can cause microangiopathy

This patient is taking a combination of some of the most commonly prescribed immunosuppressants following solid organ transplantation.

Ciclosporin and tacrolimus are calcineurin inhibitors (CNIs) and work through disruption of T-cell signalling, namely inhibiting interleukin 2 (IL-2). It has a narrow therapeutic window and is variably metabolised. Trough levels must be closely monitored to ensure adequate immunosuppression and to limit long-term side effects, which include nephrotoxicity. Side effects of CNIs are many and varied but the most common ones include hypertension, hyperkalaemia (type 4 renal tubular acidosis), hirsutism, gum hypertrophy (particularly with ciclosporin), tremor and thrombotic microangiopathy. In addition, particularly tacrolimus is implicated in NODAT (new-onset diabetes after transplantation). Special care should be taken in co-prescribing enzyme inducers or inhibitors which can dramatically interfere with CNI levels, causing over-immunosuppression and toxicity or under-immunosuppression and rejection.

Azathioprine is an antiproliferative drug which inhibits purine synthesis, thus decreasing T-cell proliferation. Its main side effects include hepatotoxicity and myelosuppression. It is also strongly associated with long-term development of skin cancers.

Although the exact pathophysiology is unclear, thrombotic microangiopathy is a clearly recognised side effect of both ciclosporin and tacrolimus. It may resolve on switching from one drug to the other, lowering levels of the drug or with plasma exchange/plasma infusion.

13. C Hairy cell leukaemia

Hairy cell leukaemia is a malignancy of mature B cells of unknown aetiology which is phenotypically characterised by hair-like projections of cytoplasm at the cell surface. It is most common in middle age, and predominantly affects men. There seems to be some racial susceptibility to the disease, with white people (especially Ashkenazi Jews) being most likely to be affected.

The abnormal cells infiltrate the reticuloendothelial system, resulting in bone marrow failure. Most presenting symptoms and signs are secondary to anaemia, thrombocytopenia and neutropenia. Leukocytosis sometimes occurs. Splenomegaly is very common and may be massive. Hepatomegaly may also arise. Abdominal discomfort may of course result from organomegaly. However, lymphadenopathy is infrequently apparent at presentation.

Diagnosis is usually made on the appearance of the peripheral blood film, with lymphocytes exhibiting characteristic hair-like projections, hence the name hairy cell leukaemia. The cytoplasm of these cells stains positive for tartrate-resistant acid phosphatase. Bone marrow sampling is also important. However, attempts at aspirating bone marrow are not uncommonly unsuccessful, in which case a trephine biopsy may be necessary; mononuclear cells with a 'fried egg' appearance are typical.

Aplastic anaemia may present with clinical features resulting from pancytopenia. The blood film would not be expected to reveal abnormal cells. The bone marrow biopsy typically demonstrates loss of haematopoietic cells and increased fat content. Plasma cell leukaemia may present with clinical features of acute leukaemia or myeloma; typically, an excess of plasma cells would be expected on the peripheral blood film.

Hoffbrand V, Moss P, Pettit J. Chronic lymphoid leukaemias (Chapter 15). In: Essential Haematology, 5th edn. Oxford: Blackwell Publishing, 2006.
Cannon T, et al. Hairy cell leukaemia: current concepts. Cancer Invest 2008; 26(8):860–865.

14. C Iron-deficiency anaemia

This is a case of iron-deficiency anaemia as demonstrated by the full blood count, ferritin and peripheral blood film. The full blood count reveals a microcytic anaemia and there is reduced ferritin. Iron studies would be expected to reveal a low serum iron, raised total iron-binding capacity and reduced transferrin saturation. The peripheral blood film exhibits microcytic, hypochromic red blood cells. Poikilocytes or target cells may also be present.

Iron-deficiency anaemia is a common condition, and occurs only after the reticuloendothelial iron stores have become completely depleted. The most common causes include chronic blood loss (e.g. gastrointestinal or menstrual), increased demands (e.g. during infancy, adolescence, pregnancy, or lactation), chronic dietary insufficiency, malabsorption disorders (e.g. coeliac disease) or parasitic infiltration of the gastrointestinal tract (e.g. hookworm). Treatment is of the underlying cause as well as with supplementary oral iron, in the form of ferrous sulphate. Where chronic blood loss is identified, it is of course important to exclude an underlying bleeding diathesis.

In the case of a premenopausal woman with refractory iron-deficiency anaemia it is important to explore menorrhagia as a potential cause. It is also important to establish compliance with previously prescribed oral iron supplements, which should be reinstated and continued for long enough to correct the anaemia and replace iron stores.

Hoffbrand V, Moss P, Pettit J. Hypochromic anaemias (Chapter 3). In: Essential Haematology, 5th edn. Oxford: Blackwell Publishing, 2006.

15. E Skin-prick testing for common aeroallergens

Her symptoms are typical of rhinitis. Patients may also report nasal discharge, blockage or congestion. Rhinitis may be allergic, non-allergic or infective. Allergic rhinitis is increasing in prevalence and affects more than a fifth of the UK population. It is more common in children with a family history of atopy. Common causes include: house-dust mite, pollen (grass, tree) and animals (cats, dogs, horses); rarer causes include: moulds, occupational (flour, animal hair).

The diagnosis is confirmed by obtaining the relevant history and examination and is supported by specific allergy testing which may include skin-prick testing for common aeroallergens and/or specific IgE testing. Given her history suggestive of cat allergy the specific IgE for cats is likely to be positive and broader testing to include all common aeroallergens including house-dust mite, grass and pollen may be more useful. Management strategies include education of allergen avoidance, nasal corticosteroids and antihistamines. Control of rhinitis may improve asthma control and immunotherapy may be highly effective in selected cases.

Peak flow monitoring may be very useful in the diagnosis and management of asthma. Nasoendoscopy and CT scanning of the sinuses may be considered if there are clinical features suggesting alternative diagnoses, such as chronic infection, nasal polyposis, malignancy or foreign bodies.

Greiner AN, et al. Allergic rhinitis. Lancet 2011; 378:2112–2122.
Scadding GK, et al. BSACI guidelines for the management of allergic and non-allergic rhinitis. Clin Exper Allergy 2008; 38:19–42.

16. D It is highly responsive to antihistamines

This woman has presented with symptoms of hereditary angio-oedema, also known as C1-inhibitor (INH) deficiency. It is a rare condition, inherited in an autosomal dominant fashion, and typically presents with a combination of cutaneous, abdominal and respiratory symptoms. Patients often describe previous episodes of angio-oedema or unexplained abdominal pain either in childhood or in early adulthood. Attacks are often associated with a prodrome around 1–2 hours before an attack, with tingling and possible mood disturbance or sensory changes.

There are several common triggers which should be avoided where possible. These include angiotensin-converting enzyme inhibitors, because of their effect on the kallikrein–bradykinin pathway, and oestrogen (contraception and hormone replacement therapy). Other triggers include trauma, infections (particularly dental) and psychological stress. Several drugs have been used for disease prevention. These include danazol (attenuated androgen) and tranexamic acid for long-term prophylaxis. C1-inhibitor concentrate is now available for short-term prophylaxis for surgical and dental procedures.

Treatment of acute attacks depends on their severity. Peripheral oedema will usually settle spontaneously, although danazol can be given. Abdominal symptoms should also settle spontaneously and adequate analgesia should be offered. If there is any suspicion of airway obstruction C1-INH concentrate should be infused, or if this is not available fresh frozen plasma may be used. Symptoms typically do not respond to antihistamines or corticosteroids.

Gompels MM, et al. C1 inhibitor deficiency: consensus document. Clin Exper Immunol 2005; 139(3):379–394.

17. D Severe life-threatening infection with encapsulated bacteria in infancy

This patient has presented with selective IgA deficiency. It is the most common of the immune deficiency disorders and, depending on population, is thought to affect up to around 1 in 400 people, more frequently males. It is defined as undetectable IgA levels, with normal IgG and normal IgM levels (although a proportion of patients will also have an IgG subclass deficiency) seen persistently over the age of 4 years. Patients are often asymptomatic or not diagnosed until early adulthood and most frequently will present with recurrent upper respiratory tract infections or sinusitis. They may also present with various gastrointestinal infections and chronic diarrhoea or have a history of urinary tract infections.

Patients with selective IgA deficiency also show an increased prevalence of autoimmune conditions, such as systemic lupus erythematosus (usually without nephritis), rheumatoid arthritis and coeliac disease. They are more prone to various food allergies and atopic dermatitis. A poor response to pneumococcal polysaccharide vaccines is recognised. Because a large proportion of patients (up to about 40%) with selective IgA deficiency have anti-A antibodies they have an increased risk of reactions, including anaphylaxis, to blood transfusions and intravenous immunoglobulins. Severe infection with encapsulated bacteria in infancy is associated with some of the other immune deficiencies, in particular the much rarer IgM deficiency or those with complement deficiencies, but not with selective IgA deficiency. Many patients who have isolated IgA deficiency are asymptomatic and have a very benign course; others will suffer recurrent infections with long-term sequelae such as bronchiectasis.

18. B Acute myeloid leukaemia

This patient has acute myeloid leukaemia. Her peripheral blood film shows a myeloid cell containing an Auer rod in the cytoplasm, which is pathognomonic for acute myeloid leukaemia. Bone marrow sampling should be undertaken before treatment is commenced.

Chronic lymphocytic leukaemia, hairy cell leukaemia and chronic myeloid leukaemia are discussed elsewhere. Acute lymphoblastic leukaemia is the most common childhood leukaemia and may present with clinical features of bone marrow failure or organ infiltration. Lymphoblasts would be expected on the blood film.

Hoffbrand V, Moss P, Pettit J. Acute leukaemias (Chapter 12). In: Essential Haematology, 5th edn. Oxford: Blackwell Publishing, 2006.

19. D Skin-prick testing for latex

A dental student who develops skin rashes on her hands and respiratory symptoms soon after starting a clinical attachment is highly suggestive of latex allergy as she probably would have been wearing latex gloves. In most cases this is a type I- or IgE-mediated hypersensitivity reaction. Symptoms include a contact urticaria resulting in erythema, weals and pruritus, and occurring within minutes of skin contact. Other manifestations associated with airborne exposure of the allergens include rhinorrhoea, watery eyes and asthma. Powdered latex gloves are more likely to cause problems than powder-free gloves because of the increased amount of allergen.

The best diagnostic test is skin-prick testing which involves puncturing the skin with varying concentrations of latex extract. A positive result is when a weal develops with surrounding erythema that is equal to or greater in diameter than a histamine control (>3 mm in diameter). Skin-prick testing has a sensitivity of 65–96% and specificity of 88–94% but the results need to be correlated with clinical symptoms. Although it is a very safe test there is a possibility of developing anaphylaxis.

Peak flow monitoring and spirometry with bronchodilator testing are useful tests for the diagnosis of asthma and may be helpful in the further investigation of this patient, but the skin-prick test for latex allergy is more likely to clinch the diagnosis with the presented history. Total serum IgE may be useful in monitoring patient with chronic atopic conditions; however, it would not be diagnostic as a single investigation. Specific IgE antibody testing is a possible option and in certain countries, such as the USA, this is the preferred diagnostic test.

Royal College of Physicians. Latex allergy – Occupational aspects of management. A national guideline. London: RCP, 2008.
Cullinan P, et al. Latex allergy guideline. Clin Exp Allergy 2003; 33:1484–1499.

20. A Common variable immunodeficiency

This patient has had failure of his vaccination and subsequent meningococcal disease. The immunoglobulin panel shows a relative pan-hypogammaglobulinaemia with markedly low IgG levels. This fits with a diagnosis of common variable immunodeficiency (CVID).

Common variable immunodeficiency is the most commonly encountered primary immunodeficiency. CVID represents a group of over 150 primary immunodeficiencies from a number of inherited defects, in most of which the specific genetic abnormalities are still unknown. Presentation is varied and diagnosis is often delayed until the second or third decade of life, but is typified by a history of recurrent infections including those of the ear, nose, throat, skin, and respiratory infections. Failure to develop immunity from vaccinations is often a feature of the history. Diagnosis is difficult in those without a recognised genetic defect, and is often a diagnosis of exclusion. Low immunoglobulin levels do point to the diagnosis but nephrotic syndrome, X-linked agammaglobulinaemia and haematological malignancies must be ruled out. Treatment is with immunoglobulin therapy either intravenously or subcutaneously.

The two most common forms of severe combined immunodeficiency (SCID) are X-linked SCID and adenosine deaminase deficiency. SCID manifests in early childhood and is rapidly fatal without bone marrow transplantation and therefore does not fit with this case. HIV could potentially fit with the history of this case but hypogammaglobulinaemia is not a feature of this disease as HIV depletes T-helper cells not B cells. Hypo- or asplenism again does not fit with the laboratory indices presented in this cases although would be consistent with the history of recurrent infections. Surreptitious steroid use does not fit with the clinical or laboratory information presented.

Park MA, et al. Common variable immunodeficiency: a new look at an old disease. Lancet 2008; 372:489–502.

21. D *Plasmodium falciparum*

The Giemsa-stained thin peripheral blood film reveals the distinctive ring trophozoites of *Plasmodium falciparum* malaria, as well as acanthocytosis (crenated erythrocytes). Multidrug-resistant forms of *P. falciparum* malaria are present in the rural areas of northern Thailand, especially along the Myanmar border. Furthermore, the patient appears to have discontinued his malaria prophylaxis early; it is usually recommended that it should be continued for one week after return from endemic areas. Giemsa-stained thick and thin peripheral blood films are used in the investigation of cases of suspected malaria. Differentiation between malarial species by microscopy requires considerable expertise. **Table 5.1** indicates some of the blood film findings that may be helpful in this respect.

Table 5.1 Blood film results for malarial species				
	P. falciparum	*P. malariae*	*P. vivax*	*P. ovale*
Red cell size	Normal	Normal	Enlarged	Enlarged
Red cell appearance	Some acanthocytosis	Normal	Angular distortion	Oval or fimbriated distortion
No. of parasites/cell	Multiple	One	One	One
Trophozoites	Rings	Compact	Irregular and fragmented	Compact
Other features	Two chromatin dots	One chromatin dot	Two chromatin dots and Schüffner's dots	One chromatin dot and Schüffner's dots

Japanese encephalitis is a mosquito-borne viral disease which is common in parts of south-east Asia and the Far East. Dengue fever is also a mosquito-borne viral disease that is endemic to many tropical and subtropical countries. Neither of these conditions is diagnosed on the appearance of the peripheral blood film. They can, however, be diagnosed by isolation of the virus, serological tests or reverse-transcriptase polymerase chain reaction (RT-PCR). Dracunculiasis is a parasitic disease caused by the round worm, *Dracunculus medinensis*. It is confined to half-a-dozen African countries and is close to eradication. It usually presents as a painful blister that subsequently ruptures to form an ulcer, from which the adult worm emerges. The diagnosis is clinical.

Trypanosomiasis is a parasitic protozoal disease that can be diagnosed by detecting trypanosomes on the blood film. *Trypanosoma cruzi* causes American trypanosomiasis (aka Chagas' disease) and is spread by blood-sucking triatominae insects. *Trypanosoma brucei gambiense* and *Trypanosoma brucei rhodesiense* cause African trypanosomiasis (aka sleeping sickness) and these are spread by infected tsetse flies.

Basic Malaria Microscopy, Part I. Learner's Guide, 2nd edn. Geneva: World Health Organization Press, 2010.

22. C Good's syndrome

Good's syndrome is a rare adult-onset immunodeficiency disorder. It is characterised by hypogammaglobulinaemia and B-cell depletion in the presence of a thymoma. This patient clearly has low levels of all immunoglobulin subclasses and a CT of the chest that suggests a thymoma. Patients typically present around the fifth decade with recurrent respiratory and sinus infections secondary to encapsulated organisms, similar to X-linked agammaglobulinaemia (XLA) or common variable immunodeficiency (CVID), or with symptoms related to the thymoma itself. In contrast to XLA and CVID, however, patients with Good's syndrome may also present with disorders of cell-mediated immunity, in particular to cytomegalovirus (CMV – including CMV colitis) or mucocutaneous candida infections. In addition haematological abnormalities are common. Anaemia (including red cell aplasia and haemolytic anaemia) is seen in around 50% of cases. Many patients will also have leukopenia and some thrombocytopenia. Management of patients with Good's syndrome includes surgical removal of thymoma and immunoglobulin replacement.

Although this patient could have a CVID, the haematological disorders, the presence of *Candida* species and the findings consistent with a thymoma make the diagnosis of Good's syndrome more likely. Chronic granulomatous disease is a congenital defect of neutrophil killing and will present earlier in life, and is characterised by chronic suppurative granulomas or abscesses affecting the skin and lymph nodes, and osteomyelitis. The other two diagnoses listed are very much diseases of childhood and would not present as late as this. Wiskott–Aldrich is an X-linked condition that presents with cellular and humoral immunodeficiency, thrombocytopenia and other haematological abnormalities, and eczema. It typically presents after the first few months of life and survival beyond the second decade is rare. X-linked agammaglobulinaemia (Bruton's syndrome) typically manifests in childhood, particularly in boys owing to its X-linked nature, and also presents with recurrent bacterial infections, particularly secondary to encapsulated organisms. Treatment is with lifelong intravenous immunoglobulin.

Kelleher P, et al. What is Good's syndrome? Immunological abnormalities in patients with thymoma. J Clin Pathol 2003; 56:12–16.

23. D Recommend influenza vaccine

Influenza can be a very serious infection if it affects certain individuals such as those with asthma and chronic obstructive pulmonary disease. The vaccines are developed from chicken embryos and as a result patients with egg protein allergy have a theoretical risk of developing anaphylaxis when given it. Evidence suggests that in practice the risk of adverse effects is extremely rare. The current trivalent inactivated influenza vaccine has very low levels of ovalbumin and a number of international guidelines, including those of the Centers for Disease Control and Prevention, have deemed it safe to give to patients with egg allergy. Current recommendations are that skin-prick testing is no longer necessary as there is poor correlation between test result and development of adverse effects.

Egg allergy often resolves later in life and if the reaction is not too severe eggs may be cautiously re-introduced into the diet. There is interest in the use of dietary supplementation and alternative therapies to reduce the risk and duration of influenza infection. Some herbalists believe that *Echinacea* may treat common colds and other viral illnesses, but clinical trials have been inconsistent and overall do not support these claims.

Clark AT, et al. British Society for Allergy and Clinical Immunology guidelines for the management of egg allergy. Clin Exper Allergy; 40:1116–1129.
Centers for Disease Control and Prevention (CDC). Prevention and control of influenza with vaccines: recommendations of the Advisory Committee on Immunization Practices (ACIP) 2011. MMWR Morb Mortal Wkly Rep 2011; 60(33):1128.

24. B Filariasis

Filariasis refers to a parasitic infection caused by any nematode from the *Filariidae* group. Only eight of the many described filarial nematodes are known to cause disease in humans. These are broadly categorised according to their principal site of infestation within their host: cutaneous (caused by *Onchocerca volvulus*, *Loa loa* and *Mansonella streptocerca*), lymphatic (*Wuchereria bancrofti*, *Brugia malayi* and *Brugia timori*) and body cavity (*Mansonella perstans* and *Mansonella ozzardi*). Filarial diseases are spread by insect vectors, including flies and mosquitoes, and tend to be largely confined to Africa, Asia, the Pacific and South and Central America.

Perhaps the most striking clinical appearance is that of elephantiasis. This occurs as the result of untreated lymphatic filarial disease, which ultimately damages the lymphatic system and typically results in gross lymphoedema of the lower limbs and genitals.

Filarial worms are often detected in the thick end of the blood film, as in this case. Treatment is usually with anthelmintic agents, such as ivermectin and albendazole.

Babeosis, leishmaniasis, malaria and trypanosomiasis are all protozoal diseases.

Katiyar D, Singh LK. Filariasis: current status, treatment, and recent advances in drug development. Curr Med Chem 2011; 18:2174–2185.

25. E Urgently test varicella-zoster antibody titre

This patient is clearly immunosuppressed and has been in contact with someone with shingles, i.e. varicella-zoster virus (VZV). In patients who are at high risk of infection (e.g. transplant recipients, patients receiving chemotherapy, post-bone marrow transplantation, neonates, patients with immunodeficiencies, those taking high-dose steroids/other immunosuppression for other reasons) it is important to establish whether contact has definitely taken place and whether the contact was likely to have been infectious.

As this patient is unsure whether she has had chickenpox in the past, the most important next step is to urgently check her VZV antibody levels. If they are positive then no further action is required. If they are negative then she should be given VZV immunoglobulin. This should be given ideally within 7 days of exposure. If the result is still unknown by this point then treatment with VZV Ig should be given regardless.

There is no evidence to suggest a role for empirically treating with antivirals. As the risk of VZV infection is significant and immunosuppressed patients in particular can become very unwell with disseminated or haemorrhagic zoster, it is definitely not appropriate to do nothing or adopt a watch-and-wait policy. Ideally, even if an immunocompromised patient thinks that they have had previous exposure to VZV, their IgG levels should still be checked and the same protocol followed as above.

Department of Health. Varicella (Chapter 34). In: Immunisation against infectious disease 'The Green Book'. London: Department of Health, 2011.

26. D Chronic myeloid leukaemia

Chronic myeloid leukaemia (CML) constitutes approximately 15% of all leukaemias, and is strongly associated with the t(9;22)(q34;q11) abnormality which gives rise to the constitutively active chimeric tyrosine kinase, Bcr-Abl (note that the Philadelphia chromosome refers to the abnormal chromosome 22). CML is slightly more common in men than women and, although it can affect people of almost any age, it usually occurs in middle age.

The disease, if left untreated, progresses through chronic, accelerated and blast phases. In the chronic phase, when most patients are diagnosed, there is an abundance of mature myeloid cells. Many of these patients are diagnosed following the incidental observation of a persistently raised white blood cell count. The accelerated phase is associated with the development of anaemia and thrombocytopenia, and patients presenting at this stage are more likely to be symptomatic. At this stage, there is often an increase in basophils, eosinophils and blast cells. Finally, the blast phase, which may occur over days or weeks, is characterised by blast transformation and crisis.

Symptoms of disease may include those related to hypermetabolism, anaemia, platelet dysfunction and hyperuricaemia. Clinical examination typically reveals splenomegaly, which may be massive. Diagnosis can be made on the blood and bone marrow appearance and cytogenetic analysis. The peripheral blood film usually appears leukoerythroblastic, whereas the bone marrow is hypercellular with predominant granulopoiesis. Furthermore, the neutrophil alkaline phosphatase level is low in CML, in contrast to leukaemoid reactions in which it is high.

Acute lymphoblastic leukaemia is the most common childhood leukaemia and may present with clinical features of bone marrow failure or organ infiltration. Lymphoblasts would be expected on the blood film.

Hoffbrand V, Moss P, Pettit J. Chronic myeloid leukaemia (Chapter 13). In: Essential Haematology, 5th edn. Oxford: Blackwell Publishing, 2006.

Chapter 6

Infectious diseases and genitourinary medicine

Questions

1. A 31-year-old man presented with a 3-day history of fever, a papular rash on his chest and legs, a polyarthritis affecting his right knee and right hand–third and fourth digits. He is homosexual and, 4 weeks ago, he had an episode of unprotected sexual intercourse.

    Examination revealed a warm and swollen right knee with a detectable effusion and dactylitis in the right hand. There was no palpable lymphadenopathy. His temperature was 38.3°C.

    Investigations:

haemoglobin 13.5 g/dL (13.0–18.0)	C-reactive protein 178 mg/L (<5)
white cell count 13.2 × 10⁹/L (4–11)	erythrocyte sedimentation rate 95 mm/1st h (0–20)
neutrophils 11.2 × 10⁹/L (1.5–7)	
platelets 522 × 10⁹/L (150–400)	

    Urea and electrolytes and liver function tests: normal
    Syphilis serology: *Treponema pallidum* particle agglutination: positive
    Rapid plasma reagin: negative

    Right knee X-ray: soft tissue swelling but no periostitis

    Aspiration of the right knee effusion: 3+ white cells, no organisms seen

    Urinalysis: 1+ leukocytes, 1+ nitrites

    What is the most likely diagnosis?

    A Disseminated gonococcal infection (DGI)
    B HIV seroconversion
    C Reiter's syndrome
    D Secondary syphilis
    E Seronegative arthropathy

2. A 43-year-old Eritrean woman who had lived in the UK for the last 6 years presented with right-sided weakness and a 3-month history of unresolving diarrhoea. She reported losing 12 kg in weight over the last year. She took no regular medications.

    Examination revealed power 2/5 in her right arm and right leg with hyperreflexia and an equivocal right plantar reflex. Cranial nerve examination detected no abnormalities. The retina could not be visualised at dilated fundoscopy. The rest of the examination was unremarkable except for obvious oral thrush.

Investigations:

haemoglobin 11.2 g/dL (11.5–16.5)	C-reactive protein 32 mg/L (<5)
white cell count 3.3 × 10⁹/L (4–11)	erythrocyte sedimentation rate
neutrophils 2.9 × 10⁹/L (1.5–7)	84 mm/1st h (0–20)
platelets 252 × 10⁹/L (150–400)	

Urea and electrolytes and liver function tests: normal

CT of the brain: (see **Figure 6.1**)

Figure 6.1

What is the most likely diagnosis?

A   Cerebral cryptococcomas
B   Cerebral lymphoma
C   Cerebral toxoplasmosis
D   Cerebral tuberculomas
E   Progressive multifocal leukoencephalopathy

3.   A 56-year-old white man presented with a 1-month history of progressive back pain and a 1-week history of night sweats and fever. He had lost 19 kg in weight over the last 6 months and had intermittent bouts of diarrhoea and constipation. On occasion he had noted fresh blood in his stool.

His pulse was 95 beats per minute, blood pressure 115/63 mmHg, respiratory rate 18 beats per minute and temperature 38.4°C. Examination revealed focal tenderness at the T8 vertebra. In the right leg, power was 4/5 and the plantar reflex was up-going. Abdominal examination was unremarkable and rectal examination revealed no masses and a normal anal tone.

Investigations:

haemoglobin 10.2 g/dL (13.0–18.0)	platelets 622 × 10⁹/L (150–400)
white cell count 14.2 × 10⁹/L (4–11)	mean corpuscular volume 75.5 fL (80–96)
neutrophils 12.8 × 10⁹/L (1.5–7.0)	albumin 30 g/L (37–49)

Urea and electrolytes and liver function tests: normal

MRI (see **Figure 6.2**)

Blood cultures: Gram-positive cocci isolated from both bottles at 24 hours

Figure 6.2

What is the most appropriate immediate management?

A Intravenous ceftriaxone
B Intravenous ceftriaxone and neurosurgical opinion
C Intravenous ceftriaxone and colonoscopy with biopsies
D Intravenous ceftriaxone and antituberculous therapy until mycobacterial smear and culture results are known
E Intravenous vancomycin

4. A 34-year-old man, admitted with diabetic ketoacidosis, gave a 2-day history of headache, nasal congestion, periorbital swelling and a blood-stained nasal discharge.

Over the subsequent 48 hours he became drowsy and unresponsive despite correction of his hyperglycaemic state.

ENT examination revealed black, necrotic lesions on a perforated nasal septum.

Investigations:

haemoglobin 14.5 g/dL (13.0–18.0)	platelets 553 × 10⁹/L (150–400)
white cell count 9.4 × 10⁹/L (4–11)	serum glucose 6.4 mmol/L (3.0–6.0)
neutrophils 8.6 × 10⁹/L (1.5–7.0)	

Urea and electrolytes and liver function tests: normal

CT of the brain: no brain abnormality

marked paranasal sinus mucosal thickening

no bony destruction

Cerebrospinal fluid: white cell count 1 × 10⁶/L (<5)

red cell count 4 × 10⁶/L (<5)

protein 0.31 g/L (0.15–0.45)	glucose 5.2 mmol/L (3.3–4.4)

Nasal swab: *Streptococcus pneumoniae* and *Staphylococcus aureus*

What is the most likely diagnosis?

A   Dental abscess
B   Nasal diphtheria
C   Orbital cellulitis
D   Rhinocerebral mucormycosis
E   Severe maxillary sinusitis

5.   A 31-year-old man from Slovakia presented with a 24-hour history of pain and swelling below the left jaw line. This was preceded by a 3-day history of fever and myalgia.

His observations showed temperature 38.5°C, pulse 88 beats per minute, blood pressure 130/75 mmHg and oxygen saturation 99% on air. On examination, he had bilateral palpable small lymph nodes in both deep cervical chains and a palpable tender mass below the left jaw. Otherwise examination was unremarkable.

Investigations:

haemoglobin 13.8 g/dL (13.0–18.0)	platelets 235 × 10⁹/L (150–400)
white cell count 4.1 × 10⁹/L (4–11)	C-reactive protein 34 mg/L (<5)
neutrophils 3.1 × 10⁹/L (1.5–7.0)	

Urea and electrolytes and liver function tests: normal

Monospot: negative

What is the most likely diagnosis?

A   Infectious mononucleosis
B   Lemierre's disease
C   Mumps
D   Salivary calculi
E   Tuberculosis

6.   A 35-year-old male judo athlete presented to the emergency department with a 48-hour history of breathlessness, fever and a cough productive of yellow sputum with streaks of fresh blood.

He had had recurrent attendances to his general practitioner with boils and furuncles over the preceding 18 months.

His temperature was 38.7°C, pulse 120 beats per minute, blood pressure 105/55 mmHg with respiratory rate 24 breaths per minute and oxygen saturation 92% on air. Auscultation of his chest revealed coarse inspiratory crackles at the left base.

Investigations:

haemoglobin 14.7 g/dL (13.0–18.0)	urea 7.9 mmol/L (2.5–7.5)
white cell count 19.4 × 10⁹/L (4–11)	creatinine 89 μmol/L (60–110)
neutrophils 17.8 × 10⁹/L (1.5–7.0)	C-reactive protein 378 mg/L (<5)
platelets 769 × 10⁹/L (150–400)	

Liver function tests: normal

Chest X-ray: consolidation of left lower zone with an intraparenchymal abscess

What is the most likely pathogen?

A   Group A streptococcus
B   *Klebsiella pneumoniae*
C   *Streptococcus milleri*
D   *Staphylococcus aureus*
E   *Streptococcus pneumoniae*

7.   A 29-year-old woman presented with a 12-hour history of pain, swelling and redness of her left leg. She reported cutting her leg shaving the previous evening but denied any travel. Throughout the day she had reported chills and shaking and had vomited twice since arriving in the emergency department.

On examination, her left leg was red from the distal tibia to the mid-thigh, with the skin proximal to the erythema appearing mottled. Palpation of the mottled area exhibited surgical emphysema. She had a temperature of 38°C, blood pressure 95/55 mmHg, pulse 105 beats per minute, respiratory rate 22 breaths per minute and oxygen saturation 99% on air.

Investigations:

haemoglobin 9.5 g/dL (11.5–16.5)	urea 19 mmol/L (2.5–7.5)
white cell count 17.8 × 10⁹/L (4–11)	creatinine 135 μmol/L (45–90)
neutrophils 15.9 × 10⁹/L (1.5–7.0)	C-reactive protein 279 mg/L (<5)
platelets 45 × 10⁹/L (150–400)	creatine kinase 879 U/L (35–170)

Liver function tests: normal

What is the most likely diagnosis?

A   Cellulitis
B   Fournier's gangrene
C   Meleney's gangrene
D   Type 1 necrotising fasciitis
E   Type 2 necrotising fasciitis

8.   A 69-year-old woman presented with a 3-day history of progressive pain, erythema and swelling of the right hand, wrist and now forearm. Two days before these symptoms started she had been bitten by her cat on the thenar eminence of that hand. Over the last 24 hours she had had fevers.

Her right hand and forearm are depicted in the clinical photo (see **Figure 6.3**). Her temperature was 38.5°C, pulse 95 beats per minute, and blood pressure 115/60 mmHg. There was lymphadenopathy in the right axillae.

Figure 6.3 *See colour plate section.*

Investigations:

haemoglobin 11.6 g/dL (11.5–16.5)	urea 7.9 mmol/L (2.5–7.5)
white cell count 15.4 × 10⁹/L (4–11)	creatinine 82 µmol/L (45–90)
neutrophils 14.6 × 10⁹/L (1.5–7.0)	C-reactive protein 245 mg/L (<5)
platelets 210 × 10⁹/L (150–400)	creatine kinase 125 U/L (35–170)

Liver function tests: normal
Blood clotting: normal

Blood culture: Gram-negative rods in the aerobic bottle at 24 hours

What is the most likely pathogen?

A   *Capnocytophaga canimorsus*
B   *Eikenella corrodens*
C   Group A streptococcus
D   *Pasteurella multocida*
E   *Staphylococcus aureus*

9. A 17-year-old Australian girl presented to the emergency department with a 12-hour history of pain and redness spreading from her groin across her left lower abdominal wall. She had had high fever and rigors over the last few hours and had vomited twice.

On examination, her temperature was 38.1°C, pulse 125 beats per minute, blood pressure 85/55 mmHg, respiratory rate 26 breaths per minute and oxygen saturation 99% on room air. There was marked swelling and erythema extending from her pubic symphysis across the left inguinal region. The skin across her abdominal left lower quadrant was dusky and exquisitely tender.

Investigations:

haemoglobin 10.2 g/dL (11.5–16.5)	potassium 3.6 mmol/L (3.5–5.0)
white cell count 16.9 × 10⁹/L (4–11)	urea 28.6 mmol/L (2.5–7.5)
neutrophils 15.6 × 10⁹/L (1.5–7.0)	creatinine 378 µmol/L (45–90)
platelets 863 × 10⁹/L (150–400)	C-reactive protein 359 mg/L (<5)
sodium 131 mmol/L (135–145)	creatine kinase 3654 U/L (35–170)

Arterial blood gas on air:	PO_2 16.8 kPa (11.3–12.6)
pH 7.31 (7.35–7.45)	base excess 10 mmol/L (± 2)
PCO_2 2.8 kPa (4.7–6.0)	bicarbonate 13.6 mmol/L (22–30)

What is the most appropriate next step in management?

A   Immediate plastic surgery review
B   Intravenous high-dose benzylpenicillin and flucloxacillin
C   Intravenous high-dose benzylpenicillin, flucloxacillin and gentamicin
D   Intravenous immunoglobulin and high-dose benzylpenicillin and clindamycin
E   Urgent MRI of abdomen and pelvis followed by plastic surgery review

10. A 78-year-old man presented with a 2-month history of increasing pain in his right foot and
     great toe. He was now unable to weight bear. He had a past medical history of hypertension,
     dyslipidaemia and type 2 diabetes. He was taking gliclazide, metformin, simvastatin, ramipril and
     amlodipine.
         On examination, there was a 3-cm ulcer over the base of his right hallux/metatarsophalangeal
     joint that on probing was deep to bone. There were necrotic edges and an offensive exudate and
     some erythema around the ulcer. He was apyrexial and haemodynamically stable.

     Investigations:

haemoglobin 10.6 g/dL (13.0–18.0)	creatine kinase 134 U/L (25–195)
white cell count 10.5 × 10⁹/L (4–11)	bilirubin 6 mmol/L (1–22)
neutrophils 6.8 × 10⁹/L (1.5–7.0)	alanine transaminase 35 U/L (5–35)
platelets 289 × 10⁹/L (150–400)	alkaline phosphatase 456 U/L (45–105)
urea 5.8 mmol/L (2.5–7.5)	albumin 31 g/L (37–49)
creatinine 140 µmol/L (60–110)	HbA1c 11.8% (3.8–6.4)
C-reactive protein 23 mg/L (<5)	

     Foot X-ray (see **Figure 6.4**)

Figure 6.4

What is the most appropriate next step in management?

A   Intravenous co-amoxiclav
B   Intravenous flucloxacillin and benzylpenicillin
C   MRI of the foot and intravenous co-amoxiclav
D   MRI of the foot and intravenous flucloxacillin and benzylpenicillin
E   MRI of the foot and surgical debridement with biopsy

11. A 27-year-old white woman presented to the emergency department with a 3-day history of
     progressive confusion, photophobia and altered sensation on the left side of her face. She worked

as a business executive and frequently travelled back and forth to Europe and the USA, but had been off work for the last 8 weeks with polymyalgia rheumatica diagnosed by her general practitioner. She denied alcohol or illicit substance abuse. She denied any recent sexual relations.

On examination, there was no discernible meningism and no fever. Neurological examination showed a left trigeminal palsy. There was also a fading bruise on her upper outer thigh.

Investigations:

---

haemoglobin 13.1 g/dL (11.5–16.5)

white cell count 6.1 × 10⁹/L (4–11)

neutrophils 4.5 × 10⁹/L (1.5–7.0)

platelets 198 × 10⁹/L (150–400)

C-reactive protein 45 mg/L (<5)

serum glucose 5.8 mmol/L (3.0–6.0)

Urea and electrolytes and liver function tests: normal

HIV rapid diagnostic test: negative

Cerebrospinal fluid: white cell count 18 x 10⁹ g/L (<5)

95% mononuclear

5% polymorphonuclear

red cell count <1 × 10⁶/L (<5)

protein 0.52 g/L (0.15–0.45 g/L)

glucose 4.9 mmol/L (3.3–4.4 mmol/L)

Microscopy, culture and sensitivities: no growth

What is the most likely diagnosis?

A   Herpes simplex encephalomeningitis
B   *Mycobacterium tuberculosis* meningitis
C   Neuroborreliosis
D   Progressive multifocal leukoencephalopathy
E   *Streptococcus pneumoniae* meningitis

12. A 68-year-old Indian banker presented to the outpatient department with a 4-week history of painful red nodules over the anterior aspects of both shins. His past medical history included chronic obstructive pulmonary disease for which he had previously received six courses of steroids in the last 12 months and he had lost 8 kg in weight over this period. He continued to smoke tobacco and had a 50 pack-year history.

On examination, there were, tender, smooth, shiny, 4–8 cm nodules over both anterior shins. Auscultation of his chest showed decreased breath sounds throughout but no focal abnormality. His abdomen was soft with no palpable organomegaly. There was no peripheral lymphadenopathy.

Investigations:

---

haemoglobin 10.4 g/dL (13.0–18.0)

white cell count 5.9 × 10⁹/L (4–11)

neutrophils 6.8 × 10⁹/L (1.5–7.0)

platelets 364 × 10⁹/L (150–400)

Urea and electrolytes and liver function tests: normal

Antistreptolysin O titre <200 IU/mL (<200)

Hepatitis C antibody: negative

Human immunodeficiency virus antibody: negative

Epstein–Barr virus (VCA) antibody: negative

Serum angiotensin-converting enzyme 22 µg/L (<40 µg/L)

Chest X-ray: widened upper mediastinum, clear lung fields

What is the most appropriate next investigation?

A   Bronchoscopy and endobronchial ultrasound-guided biopsy
B   CT of the thorax
C   Mantoux test
D   QuantiFERON test
E   Sputum microscopy, culture and susceptibilities

13. A 21 year-old woman, who was 18 weeks' pregnant, presented with her son who had a cropping vesicular rash over his face and torso. The rash began yesterday. She was concerned over the health of her pregnancy. She was originally from Kuwait but had been in the UK for 3 years. She was asymptomatic.

On examination, she was apyrexial and examinations of her chest, abdomen and oropharynx were normal. Full dermatological examination revealed no rash.

Investigations:

haemoglobin 12.8 g/dL (11.5–16.5)	platelets 178 × 10⁹/L (150–400)
white cell count 6.5 × 10⁹/L (4–11)	C-reactive protein <5 mg/L (<5)
neutrophils 4.8 × 10⁹/L (1.5–7.0)	

Urea and electrolytes and liver function tests: normal

Urine dipstick: normal

What is the most appropriate next step in her management?

A   Intravenous aciclovir
B   Intravenous immunoglobulin
C   Oral aciclovir
D   Send rubella and parvovirus serology from mother
E   Send varicella-zoster serology from mother

14. A 43-year-old woman presented with a 7-day history of fever, breathlessness and a cough productive of sputum. Three days of co-amoxiclav from her general practitioner had not improved her symptoms. She had returned from Spain 2 weeks ago. She was a non-smoker.

Examination of her chest revealed left mid-zone bronchial breathing. Her temperature was 38.8°C, pulse 105 beats per minute, blood pressure 105/55 mmHg and oxygen saturation 95% on room air.

Investigations:

haemoglobin 12.8 g/dL (11.5–16.5)	potassium 4.3 mmol/L (3.5–5.0)
white cell count 14.9 × 10⁹/L (4–11)	urea 8.9 mmol/L (2.5–7.5)
neutrophils 12.1 × 10⁹/L (1.5–7.0)	creatinine 87 µmol/L (45–90)
platelets 368 × 10⁹/L (150–400)	C-reactive protein 179 mg/L (<5)
sodium 138 mmol/L (135–145)	

Liver function tests: normal

Chest X-ray (see **Figure 6.5**)

What is the most likely causative organism?

A   *Coxiella burnetii*
B   *Haemophilus influenzae*
C   *Pseudomonas aeruginosa*
D   *Staphylococcus aureus*
E   *Streptococcus pneumoniae*

Figure 6.5

15. A 26-year-old man from Somalia presented to the emergency department after a fifth episode of haemoptysis over the preceding 24 hours. The last episode was 200 mL of fresh blood. He had lost approximately 12 kg of weight over the last 2 months and had fever and night sweats over that period.

On examination, he had a temperature of 37.8°C with a blood pressure of 105/68 mmHg and pulse 110 beats per minute. Focal crackles were heard over the upper right thorax.

Investigations:

haemoglobin 8.2 g/dL (13.0–18.0)	potassium 3.2 mmol/L (3.5–5.0)
mean corpuscular volume 88 fL (80–96)	urea 6.4 mmol/L (2.5–7.5)
white cell count 8.6 × 10⁹/L (4–11)	creatinine 45 μmol/L (60–110)
platelets 287 × 10⁹/L (150–400)	C-reactive protein 32 mg/L (<5)
sodium 139 mmol/L (135–145)	

Chest X-ray (see **Figure 6.6**)

What is the next most appropriate management step?

A Bronchoalveolar lavage
B Commence intravenous co-amoxiclav and clarithromycin
C Commence oral rifampicin, isoniazid, pyrazinamide and ethambutol
D CT of the thorax
E Pulmonary angiography and embolisation

Figure 6.6

16. A 68-year-old man with bronchiectasis presented with a 7-day history of progressive dyspnoea, fever and a cough productive of foul-smelling green sputum. He had been taking azithromycin three times per week, inhaled steroids and beta-agonists.

His temperature was 38°C, blood pressure 90/65 mmHg, pulse 80 beats per minute and respiratory rate 20 breaths per minute. Examination revealed crackles throughout both lung fields with bronchial breathing at the left base.

Investigations:

haemoglobin 13.5 g/dL (13.0–18.0)	potassium 4.3 mmol/L (3.5–5.0)
white cell count 12.7 × 10⁹/L (4–11)	urea 9.8 mmol/L (2.5–7.5)
neutrophils 10.8 × 10⁹/L (1.5–7.0)	creatinine 90 µmol/L (60–110)
platelets 238 × 10⁹/L (150–400)	C-reactive protein 189 mg/L (<5)
sodium 145 mmol/L (135–145)	

Chest X-ray (see **Figure 6.7**)

What is the most appropriate treatment?

A   Co-amoxiclav
B   Co-amoxiclav and clarithromycin
C   Doxycycline
D   Meropenem
E   Piperacillin–tazobactam

Figure 6.7

17. A 27-year-old man with acute myeloid leukaemia developed febrile neutropenia while in protective isolation 18 days after a reduced intensity allogeneic stem cell transplantation. He was started on piperacillin–tazobactam, gentamicin and vancomycin. He continued to be febrile at 48 hours and he was changed to meropenem and vancomycin. After a further 48 hours he was still febrile (38.5°C).

   Examination revealed a Hickman line exiting the right anterior chest wall with a clean exit site but was otherwise unremarkable. His observations showed a blood pressure of 124/76 mmHg, pulse 90 beats per minute, respiratory rate 20 breaths per minute and oxygen saturation 98% on air.

Investigations:

haemoglobin 9.8 g/dL (13.0–18.0)	creatinine 45 µmol/L (60–110)
white cell count 1.2×10^9/L (4–11)	C-reactive protein 140 mg/L (<5)
neutrophils 0.0×10^9/L (1.5–7.0)	Trough vancomycin levels 16.0 mg/dL
platelets 25×10^9/L (150–400)	(in severe sepsis target range 15–20)
urea 6.7 mmol/L (2.5–7.5)	

Four sets of blood cultures showed no growth at 48 hours

What is the most appropriate next step in management?

A   Add co-trimoxazole
B   Give further dose of gentamicin
C   High-resolution CT of the thorax
D   Perform further set of blood cultures and observe
E   Remove Hickman line

18. A 24-year-old woman presented with a 24-hour history of coryza, myalgia, headache and fever. She denied breathlessness or sputum production. She was 24 weeks' pregnant but had no other past medical history.

    She had a fever of 39.5°C, blood pressure 110/68 mmHg, pulse 95 beats per minute, respiratory rate 16 breaths per minute and oxygen saturation 98% on air. Examination revealed a clear chest, pink tympanic membranes and tonsillar arches with no evidence of exudate.

Investigations:

haemoglobin 11.4 g/dL (11.5–16.5)	urea 6.7 mmol/L (2.5–7.5)
white cell count 6.8 × 10⁹/L (4–11)	creatinine 48 μmol/L (45–90)
neutrophils 1.6 × 10⁹/L (1.5–7.0)	C-reactive protein 54 mg/L (<5)
platelets 235 × 10⁹/L (150–400)	
Throat swab: normal oral flora	

What is the next step in management?

A Advice on rest and fluid rehydration
B Amoxicillin
C Co-amoxiclav and clarithromycin
D Intravenous zanamivir
E Oral oseltamivir

19. A 68-year-old man originally from Ghana presented with streaking haemoptysis in his sputum. He reported having a longstanding cough usually productive of grey sputum. This had previously been investigated and 2 years ago he was fully treated for a confirmed *Mycobacterium tuberculosis* infection. He was known to have chronic obstructive pulmonary disease and was taking Symbicort, tiotropium and salbutamol inhalers.

    On examination he was well, with respiratory examination revealing only a prolonged expiratory phase but no added sounds. He was apyrexial, blood pressure 135/68 mmHg, pulse 68 beats per minute, respiratory rate 16 breaths per minute and oxygen saturation 96% on air.

Investigations:

haemoglobin 13.5 g/dL (13.0–18.0)	urea 6.8 mmol/L (2.5–7.5)
white cell count 6.7 × 10⁹/L (4–11)	creatinine 68 μmol/L (60–110)
platelets 345 × 10⁹/L (150–400)	C-reactive protein 14 mg/L (<5)
Sputum microscopy, culture and sensitivities: normal oral flora	
Chest X-ray (see **Figure 6.8**)	

What is the next most appropriate step in management?

A Cardiothoracic surgery opinion
B CT of the thorax
C Start intravenous liposomal amphotericin
D Start oral fluconazole
E Start rifampicin, isoniazid, pyrazinamide and ethambutol

Figure 6.8

20. A 28-year-old Somali man presented with a 2-month history of weight loss, fever, night sweats and a cough productive of grey sputum. He entered the country as an asylum seeker 6 months ago. In the past he was partially treated for tuberculosis in Somalia twice previously – at the age of 24 years and again at the age of 26 years.

Observations showed a temperature of 38°C, blood pressure 128/72 mmHg, pulse 90 beats per minute, respiratory rate 18 breaths per minute and oxygen saturation 98% on air. His weight was 51 kg and his height 173 cm. Examination of his chest revealed inspiratory crackles in the right upper zone.

Investigations:

haemoglobin 10.8 g/dL (13.0–18.0)	urea 7.8 mmol/L (2.5–7.5)
white cell count 4.3 × 10⁹/L (4–11)	creatinine 45 µmol/L (60–110)
platelets 456 × 10⁹/L (150–400)	C-reactive protein 51 mg/L (<5)

Sputum microscopy, culture and sensitivities: normal oral flora
Sputum acid-fast bacilli: 3+

Chest X-ray: consolidation in right upper zone, calcified nodule in left upper zone

The patient was commenced on rifampicin, isoniazid, pyrazinamide, ethambutol, moxifloxacin and streptomycin.

What is next most appropriate management step?

A   Discharge home with directly observed therapy (DOT)
B   Discharge home with outpatient appointment in 2 weeks
C   Negative pressure side room admission for the first 2 weeks of therapy then DOT
D   Negative pressure side room admission until sputum culture negative
E   Side room admission for the first 2 weeks of therapy then DOT

21. A 21-year-old female student presented with a 4-day history of dysuria and a 24-hour history of fever, rigors and left loin pain. She attended the general practitioner several days ago and was prescribed oral cefuroxime but had had no relief. She reported having five to six episodes of urinary tract infections requiring antimicrobials over the last year.

    Observations showed a temperature of 38.5°C, blood pressure 95/55 mmHg, pulse 110 beats per minute, respiratory rate 16 breaths per minute and oxygen saturation 99% on air. Examination showed a clear chest and a soft abdomen but with tenderness in the left loin.

    Investigations:

haemoglobin 12.6 g/dL (11.5–16.5)	urea 5.6 mmol/L (2.5–7.5)
white cell count 15.8 × 10⁹/L (4–11)	creatinine 67 µmol/L (45–90)
neutrophils 13.1 × 10⁹/L (1.5–7.0)	C-reactive protein 308 mg/L (<5)
platelets 268 × 10⁹/L (150–400)	

    Urinalysis: 2+ leukocytes, 3+ nitrites, 1+ blood

    Urine sputum microscopy, culture and sensitivities: *E. coli* (extended-spectrum β-lactamase producer)

    What is the most appropriate management?

    A   Intravenous cefuroxime
    B   Intravenous co-amoxiclav
    C   Intravenous meropenem
    D   Intravenous piperacillin–tazobactam
    E   Oral nitrofurantoin

22. A 34-year-old businessman who recently moved to the UK from Mumbai presented with a 7-day history of progressively worsening headache and fever and a 24-hour history of neck stiffness and photophobia. He denied any relevant past medical history.

    He had a temperature of 38°C, blood pressure 160/88 mmHg, pulse 80 beats per minute, respiratory rate 20 breaths per minute and oxygen saturation 99% on air. On examination, his Glasgow Coma Scale score was 14/15 and he appeared confused. His cranial and peripheral neurological examination detected no abnormalities.

    Investigations:

haemoglobin 10.8 g/dL (13.0–18.0)	potassium 4.1 mmol/L (3.5–5.0)
white cell count 5.6 × 10⁹/L (4–11)	urea 7.6 mmol/L (2.5–7.5)
neutrophils 3.8 × 10⁹/L (1.5–7.0)	creatinine 68 µmol/L (60–110)
platelets 346 × 10⁹/L (150–400)	C-reactive protein 41 mg/L (<5)
sodium 131 mmol/L (135–145)	serum glucose 6.8 mmol/L (3.0–6.0)

    CT of the brain: no space-occupying lesions, no acute bleed. Evidence of occipital leptomeningeal enhancement

Cerebrospinal fluid:	red cell count 10 × 10⁶/L (<5)
white cell count 750 × 10⁶/L (<5)	glucose 1.5 mmol/L (3.3–4.4)
lymphocytes 100 × 10⁶/L	protein 1.8 g/L (0.15–0.45)

    Microscopy: no organisms seen

    Auramine and Ziehl–Neelsen smear: no organisms seen

What is the most appropriate next step in management?

A   Intravenous aciclovir
B   Intravenous ceftriaxone
C   Intravenous ceftriaxone and dexamethasone
D   Oral rifampicin, isoniazid, pyrazinamide and ethambutol
E   Oral rifampicin, isoniazid, pyrazinamide, ethambutol and dexamethasone

23. A 19-year-old male student presented with a 24-hour history of worsening headache, fever and photophobia. Over the last 2 hours he reported a rash appearing over his forearms. He denied any travel and was usually fit and well.

On examination, he was febrile at 38.2°C and was lying in a darkened room. His Glasgow Coma Scale score was 15/15 and full neurological examination revealed no focal deficits. He had a purpuric non-blanching rash over his arms and shins. Funduscopy showed clear disc margins bilaterally.

Investigations:

haemoglobin 15.6 g/dL (13.0–18.0)	urea 5.6 mmol/L (2.5–7.5)
white cell count 18.8 × 10⁹/L (4–11)	creatinine 88 µmol/L (60–110)
neutrophils 16.7 × 10⁹/L (1.5–7.0)	C-reactive protein 248 mg/L (<5)
platelets 450 × 10⁹/L (150–400)	

Liver function tests: normal
Blood clotting: normal

What is the most appropriate sequence of management?

A   Ceftriaxone, steroids, lumbar puncture, inform health protection unit
B   CT of the head, lumbar puncture, ceftriaxone, inform health protection unit
C   CT of the head, lumbar puncture, steroids, ceftriaxone
D   Lumbar puncture, ceftriaxone, steroids, inform health protection unit
E   Side room, lumbar puncture, steroids, ceftriaxone, inform health protection unit

24. A 27-year-old male triathlete presented with a 1-week history of fever and myalgia, and more recently a history of progressive breathlessness and cough.

On examination, he was febrile at 39°C, blood pressure 110/65 mmHg, pulse 95 beats per minute, respiratory rate 20 breaths per minute and oxygen saturation 92% on air. Auscultation of his thorax revealed focal crackles in his left lower zone. His abdomen was soft and non-tender.

Investigations:

haemoglobin 14.6 g/dL (13.0–18.0)	creatinine 160 µmol/L (60–110)
white cell count 14.5 × 10⁹/L (4–11)	C-reactive protein 320 mg/L (<5)
neutrophils 13.9 × 10⁹/L (1.5–7.0)	creatine kinase 6729 U/L (25–195)
platelets 360 × 10⁹/L (150–400)	bilirubin 57 mmol/L (1–22)
sodium 134 mmol/L (135–145)	alanine transaminase 159 U/L (5–35)
potassium 4.4 mmol/L (3.5–5.0)	alkaline phosphatase 143 U/L (45–105)
urea 12.8 mmol/L (2.5–7.5)	albumin 23 g/L (37–49)

Urinalysis: 2+ protein, 3+ blood,

Chest X-ray: consolidation of left lower zone

What is the most likely causative organism?

A   *Haemophilus influenzae*
B   *Legionella pneumophila*
C   *Leptospira interrogans*
D   *Mycoplasma pneumoniae*
E   *Streptococcus pneumoniae*

25. A 16-year-old boy with severe learning difficulties presented with nausea, vomiting and bloody diarrhoea. His mother reported that these symptoms had been progressing over the last 3–4 days, and he had no longer been able to go on his respite care group day trips. Other than his learning difficulties he had no medical history and took no regular medications.

    On examination, he was afebrile with blood pressure 95/55 mmHg, pulse 95 beats per minute, respiratory rate 32 breaths per minute and oxygen saturation 99% on air. His chest was clear and his abdomen soft and non-tender. He had no neck stiffness or rash.

Investigations:

haemoglobin 6.9 g/dL (13.0–18.0)	creatinine 325 µmol/L (60–110)
mean corpuscular volume 95 fL (80–96)	C-reactive protein 98 mg/L (<5)
white cell count 13.8 × 10⁹/L (4–11)	creatine kinase 105 U/L (25–195)
platelets 568 × 10⁹/L (150–400)	bilirubin 78 mmol/L (1–22)
sodium 143 mmol/L (135–145)	alanine transaminase 16 U/L (5–35)
potassium 4.3 mmol/L (3.5–5.0)	alkaline phosphatase 98 U/L (45–105)
urea 31 mmol/L (2.5–7.5)	albumin 35 g/L (37–49)

What is the most likely diagnosis?

A   *Clostridium difficile*
B   *E. coli* O157
C   Leptospirosis
D   Norovirus
E   *Shigella* species

26. An 86-year-old female inpatient developed liquid diarrhoea opening her bowels 15 times in the past 24 hours. Ten days ago, she had been admitted to the orthopaedic ward for a fractured neck of femur. She had received cefuroxime and metronidazole perioperatively. Her past medical history included a previous peptic ulcer for which she was on omeprazole.

    Her temperature was 37.8°C, blood pressure 90/55 mmHg, pulse 105 beats per minute, respiratory rate 22 breaths per minute and oxygen saturation 98% on air. On examination, her abdomen was soft with tenderness in the left iliac fossa but no rebound or guarding. Her bowel sounds were hyperactive.

Investigations:

haemoglobin 12.7 g/dL (11.5–16.5)	creatinine 78 µmol/L (45–90)
white cell count 16.8 × 10⁹/L (4–11)	C-reactive protein 142 mg/L (<5)
neutrophils 14.9 × 10⁹/L (1.5–7)	bilirubin 6 mmol/L (1–22)
platelets 374 × 10⁹/L (150–400)	alanine transaminase 21 U/L (5–35)
sodium 149 mmol/L (135–145)	alkaline phosphatase 97 U/L (45–105)
potassium 3.8 mmol/L (3.5–5.0)	albumin 20 g/L (37–49)
urea 12.8 mmol/L (2.5–7.5)	

Stool microscopy, culture and sensitivities: no pathogens identified

What is the next step in management?

A   Intravenous immunoglobulins
B   Intravenous vancomycin
C   Oral metronidazole
D   Oral rifampicin
E   Oral vancomycin

27. A 43-year-old female travel writer presented with episodic creeping eruptions that were intensely pruritic. They could occur at any site on her body and would migrate for several centimetres over the course of several hours with an area of erythema around a track. She had no other past medical history.

On examination her chest, abdomen and cardiovascular systems were normal. On her left calf there was a 4-cm serpiginous track with an area of 3–4 cm of erythema extending outwards. There were old excoriated areas in various locations on her body.

Investigations:

haemoglobin 13.2 g/dL (11.5-16.5)	platelets 213 × 10⁹/L (150–400)
white cell count 6.8 × 10⁹/L (4–11)	C-reactive protein 4 mg/L (<5)
neutrophils 4.9 × 10⁹/L (1.5–7.0)	creatine kinase 105 U/L (35–170)
eosinophils 1.2 × 10⁹/L (0.04–0.4)	
Urea and electrolytes and liver function tests: normal	

What is the most likely diagnosis?

A   Cutaneous larva migrans
B   Filariasis
C   Loaiasis (*Loa loa*)
D   Schistosomiasis
E   Strongyloidiasis

28. A 35-year-old woman presented with a 3-day history of fever 1 week after returning from safari in Kenya. She had no other focal symptoms.

Her temperature was 38.5°C, pulse 90 beats per minute, blood pressure 125/72 mmHg, respiratory rate 18 breaths per minute and oxygen saturation 99% on air. On examination she had no focal neurological deficit and chest and abdominal examination were normal.

Investigations:

haemoglobin 12.8 g/dL (11.5–16.5)	urea 6.8 mmol/L (2.5–7.5)
white cell count 8.9 × 10⁹/L (4–11)	creatinine 78 µmol/L (45–90)
platelets 98 × 10⁹/L (150–400)	C-reactive protein 12 mg/L (<5)
Liver function tests: normal	
Malaria film: 0.5% *P. falciparum* trophozoites with occasional schizonts	

What is the next step in management?

A   Intravenous quinine
B   Oral artemisinin
C   Oral clindamycin
D   Oral Malarone
E   Oral quinine

29. A 31-year-old male doctor presented with a 4-week history of excessive flatulence, offensive belching and intermittent diarrhoea. He had returned from a 2-week trip around southern India at the same time as his symptoms had begun.

      On examination, he was apyrexial and haemodynamically stable. His abdomen was soft and non-tender with no palpable organomegaly. The rest of his examination was normal.

Investigations:

haemoglobin 14.3 g/dL (13.0–18.0)	platelets 198 × 10⁹/L (150–400)
white cell count 4.5 × 10⁹/L (4–11)	C-reactive protein 5 mg/L (<5)
neutrophils 3.9 × 10⁹/L (1.5–7.0)	

Urea and electrolytes and liver function tests: normal

Abdominal ultrasound: no abnormalities detected

What is the most appropriate next step in management?

A   Empirical metronidazole therapy
B   Entero-Test (string test)
C   Flexible sigmoidoscopy
D   Giardia serology
E   Stool ova, cyst and parasite examination

30. A 24-year-old male student from Peru presented with a self-terminating seizure during which there was urinary incontinence. The post-ictal phase was short-lived and he rapidly returned to normal. He had no past medical history and took no regular medications.

      On examination, he was apyrexial and his observations were within normal parameters. Full neurological examination revealed no focal neurological deficits.

Investigations:

haemoglobin 12.8 g/dL (13.0–18.0)	platelets 136 × 10⁹/L (150–400)
white cell count 4.6 × 10⁹/L (4–11)	C-reactive protein 5 mg/L (<5)
neutrophils 3.6 × 10⁹/L (1.5–7.0)	creatine kinase 969 U/L (25–195)

Urea and electrolytes and liver function tests: normal

Human immunodeficiency virus: negative

MRI of the brain (T2 weighted): see **Figure 6.9**

Figure 6.9

What is the most likely diagnosis?

A   Cerebral toxoplasmosis
B   Glioma
C   Neurocysticercosis
D   Progressive multifocal leukoencephalopathy
E   Racemose cyst

31. A 26-year-old male travel writer returned from a 3-month trip from Cape Town to Cairo with frank haematuria. He denied any dysuria, frequency, penile discharge or fever. He reported taking part in various outdoor activities including swimming in Lake Malawi. He reported taking over-the-counter praziquantel after this.

   His observations showed a temperature of 36.8°C, blood pressure 120/65 mmHg, pulse 65 beats per minute, respiratory rate 16 breaths per minute and oxygen saturation 99% on air. Respiratory, cardiovascular, abdominal, genital and cutaneous examinations were normal.

   Investigations:

haemoglobin 11.9 g/dL (13.0–18.0)	eosinophils 1.0×10^9/L (0.04–0.4)
white cell count 5.3×10^9/L (4–11)	platelets 378×10^9/L (150–400)
neutrophils 3.7×10^9/L (1.5–7.0)	C-reactive protein 8 mg/L (<5)
Urea and electrolytes and liver function test: normal	

   What is the most appropriate next step in management?

   A   Flexible cystoscopy
   B   Mid-stream urine for microscopy, culture and susceptibilities
   C   Schistosomiasis serology
   D   Stool for ova, cysts and parasites
   E   Terminal stream urine for ultrafiltration and microscopy

32. A 16-year-old boy with sickle cell disease presented with bony pain in his left shin. This had been present for 1 week. He admitted to several episodes of fever over the preceding days. He had recently returned from a family trip to Nigeria.

His observations showed a temperature of 38.3°C, blood pressure 145/75 mmHg, pulse 95 beats per minute, respiratory rate 18 breaths per minute and oxygen saturation 98% on air. On examination his chest was clear and his abdomen was soft with a 1-cm palpable spleen. His left anterior tibial plateau was hot with some overlying erythema.

Investigations:

haemoglobin 7.6 g/dL (13.0–18.0)	potassium 4.1 mmol/L (3.5–5.0)
white cell count 17.8×10^9/L (4–11)	urea 9.8 mmol/L (2.5–7.5)
neutrophils 15.9×10^9/L (1.5–7.0)	creatinine 56 µmol/L (60–110)
platelets 687×10^9/L (150–400)	C-reactive protein 178 mg/L (<5)
sodium 138 mmol/L (135–145)	creatine kinase 96 U/L (25–195)

Plain X-ray of the left leg: soft tissue oedema left leg with tibial periostitis

Blood cultures: Gram-negative rod isolated at 12 hours

What is the most likely pathogen?

A   *Brucella abortus*
B   *Pseudomonas aeruginosa*
C   *Salmonella* species
D   *Staphylococcus aureus*
E   *Streptococcus pyogenes*

33. A 17-year-old male student from the Ukraine presented with a 24-hour history of fever, odynophagia and dysphagia 3 days after returning from visiting his relatives.

On examination, he was drooling and had a mucus discharge from his right nasal passage. Oropharyngeal examination revealed an adherent pseudomembrane on the tonsillar arch. There was cervical and submandibular lymphadenopathy. He had a temperature of 38.0°C, blood pressure 120/65 mmHg, pulse 55 beats per minute, respiratory rate 24 breaths per minute and oxygen saturation 98% on air.

Investigations:

haemoglobin 10.4 g/dL (13.0–18.0)	platelets 647×10^9/L (150–400)
white cell count 14.6×10^9/L (4–11)	C-reactive protein 235 mg/L (<5)
neutrophils 12.9×10^9/L (1.5–7.0)	

Chest X-ray: normal

Electrocardiogram: first-degree heart block

What is the most appropriate next step in management?

A   Benzylpenicillin
B   Diphtheria antitoxin
C   Erythromycin
D   Metronidazole
E   Tetanus antitoxin

34. A 26-year-old male doctor presented with a needle-stick injury. He had been assisting in a laparotomy for a perforated bowel in an 86-year-old woman when a surgical needle had penetrated his glove and drew blood. He washed it profusely with soap and water immediately after the injury.

On examination, he was anxious but otherwise well. There was a small puncture mark on his left thumb.

What is the most appropriate immediate management step for the doctor?

A   Administration of a hepatitis B booster vaccination
B   Administration of hepatitis B immunoglobulin
C   Baseline HIV, HBV and HCV testing
D   Hepatitis BsAb testing and a save serum sent from the doctor
E   The affected doctor should return to the 86-year-old woman and request permission to test her for HIV, HBV and HCV

35. A 26-year-old businessman returned from a 1-month trip to Thailand with a short history of fever, myalgia and a transient maculopapular rash. He admitted to spending the majority of his time in Bangkok frequenting brothels and only intermittently used condoms. His last sexual health screen just prior to this trip was normal.

His observations showed a temperature of 37.8°C, blood pressure 130/65 mmHg, pulse 68 beats per minute, respiratory rate 16 breaths per minute and oxygen saturation 99% on air. On examination, he had a clear chest and soft abdomen. He had cervical lymphadenopathy and inspection of his oropharynx revealed oral candidiasis.

Investigations:

haemoglobin 12.6 g/dL (13.0–18.0)	neutrophils 3.1 × 10⁹/L (1.5–7.0)
white cell count 3.2 × 10⁹/L (4–11)	platelets 120 × 10⁹/L (150–400)

Urea and electrolytes and liver function tests: normal

Malaria film and malarial antigen test: negative

Human immunodeficiency virus rapid diagnostic test: negative

What is the next most appropriate investigation?

A   CD4 count
B   HIV antibody testing
C   HIV p24 antigen
D   HIV resistance testing
E   HIV viral load quantification

36. A 36-year-old man presented with a 48-hour history of fever 7 days after return from visiting his relatives in Botswana. A full systems review revealed no other symptoms.

He had a temperature of 38.5°C, pulse 110 beats per minute, blood pressure 110/65 mmHg and oxygen saturation 99% on air. His chest was clear and his abdomen was soft with no organomegaly. He was cachectic and on inspection of the oropharynx had oral thrush. Examination of his skin revealed a large black skin lesion on his upper arm.

Investigations:

haemoglobin 14.5 g/dL (13.0–18.0)	C-reactive protein 31 mg/L (<5)
white cell count 16.9 × 10⁹/L (4–11)	bilirubin 7 mmol/L (1–22)
neutrophils 16.1 × 10⁹/L (1.5–7.0)	alanine transaminase 30 U/L (5–35)
lymphocytes 0.1 × 10⁹/L (1.5–4.0)	alkaline phosphatase 98 U/L (45–105)
platelets 389 × 10⁹/L (150–400)	albumin 32 g/L (37–49)

Contd...

Contd...

> Urea and electrolytes: normal
>
> Urine dip: 1+ protein
>
> First malaria film: no parasites seen
>
> Blood cultures: Gram-negative bacilli in both bottles at 12 hours

What is the most likely diagnosis?

A Enteric fever
B HIV seroconversion
C Malaria
D Non-typhi salmonellosis
E Urological sepsis

37. A 31-year-old man from Australia presented with a 2-month history of an ulcer on his left calf which had been steadily growing in size. It was not painful and not pruritic. He had not had any previous similar lesions. He arrived in the UK from Victoria, Australia 3 months ago.

On examination, there was a 3 × 4 cm deep ulcer with ragged undermined edges extending several centimetres beyond the visible wound. Probing the wound did not elicit pain. Otherwise examination was normal.

Investigations:

> haemoglobin 12.9 g/dL (13.0–18.0)   C-reactive protein 9 mg/L (<5)
>
> white cell count 6.7×10^9/L (4–11)   random glucose 5.6 mmol/L (3.0–6.0)
>
> platelets 256×10^9/L (150–400)
>
> Urea and electrolytes and liver function tests: normal

What is the most likely diagnosis?

A Buruli ulcer
B Diabetic ulcer
C Leishmaniasis
D Lepromatous leprosy
E *Mycobacterium marinum*

38. A 25-year-old woman presented 4 weeks after a trip to Belize with a non-healing lesion on her left forearm. She denied any fever or night sweats and had been otherwise well. She had tried topical over-the-counter emollients and had had two courses of antimicrobials from her general practitioner with no improvement.

On examination, there was a 3-cm-diameter, roughly circular lesion with rolled edges ulcerating through the dermis. There was a smaller 2 to 3-mm satellite lesion adjacent to the main ulcer. Inspection of the oropharynx was normal, as was abdominal examination.

Investigations:

> haemoglobin 13.5 g/dL (11.5–16.5)   C-reactive protein 14 mg/L (<5)
>
> white cell count 7.1×10^9/L (4–11)   glucose 4.9 mmol/L (3.0–6.0)
>
> platelets 281×10^9/L (150–400)
>
> Urea and electrolytes and liver function tests: normal

What is the most likely diagnosis?

A   Ecthyma
B   Erysipelas
C   Impetigo
D   Leishmaniasis
E   *Mycobacterium marinum*

39. A 41-year-old woman presented with a 5-day history of myalgia, fever and headache 7 days after return from her honeymoon in Sri Lanka. She took Malarone daily and was vaccinated for hepatitis A and typhoid fever before embarking on her trip.

    Her observations showed temperature 39°C, pulse 110 beats per minute, blood pressure 95/55 mmHg and oxygen saturation 99% on air. On examination, there was a fine, macular rash on her torso but otherwise chest, abdominal and neurological examination was normal.

Investigations:

haemoglobin 13.8 g/dL (11.5–16.5)	alkaline phosphatase 87 U/L (45–105)
white cell count 3.2 × 10⁹/L (4–11)	albumin 36 g/L (37–49)
neutrophils 1.1 × 10⁹/L (1.5–7.0)	serum glucose 6.1 mmol/L (3.0–6.0)
platelets 320 × 10⁹/L (150–400)	fibrinogen 2.8 g/L (1.8–5.4 g/L)
C-reactive protein 25 mg/L (<5)	prothrombin time 12 s (11.5–15.5)
bilirubin 8 mmol/L (1–22)	activated partial thromboplastin time 31 s (30–40)
alanine aminotransferase 59 U/L (5–35)	

First malaria film: negative

Cerebrospinal fluid:	protein 0.30 g/L (0.15–0.45)
white cell count <1 x 10⁶/L (<5)	glucose 5.2 mmol/L (3.3–4.4)
red cell count <1 × 10⁶/L (<5)	

What is the most appropriate next step in management?

A   Fresh frozen plasma
B   Intravenous ceftriaxone
C   Intravenous fluids
D   Intravenous quinine
E   Intravenous zanamivir

40. A 38-year-old woman returned from a 2-week honeymoon in the Seychelles with a 3-day history of fever and marked arthralgia of the knees and small joints of the hand. She stated that she took regular malaria prophylaxis and received the correct vaccinations.

    On examination, she had a faint macular rash predominantly over her torso. Examination of her hands revealed a good range of movements and no palpable pannus. There was no discernible joint effusion in either knee. Otherwise examination was normal.

Investigations:

haemoglobin 12.5 g/dL (11.5–16.5)	platelets 347 × 10⁹/L (150–400)
white cell count 4.1 × 10⁹/L (4–11)	C-reactive protein 21 mg/L (<5)

Urea and electrolytes and liver function tests: normal

What is the most likely diagnosis?

A   Chikungunya
B   HIV seroconversion

C Japanese encephalitis
D O'nyong-nyong
E Syphilis

41. A 32-year-old man originally from Brazil and recently arrived in the UK presented with a 48-hour history of a rash preceded by 4 days of myalgia, itchy eyes and fever. He described the rash as starting on his scalp before spreading to his thorax and limbs. He lived with his wife and 5-year-old son.

He had a temperature of 38.8°C, pulse 100 beats per minute, blood pressure 130/75 mmHg and oxygen saturation 99% on air. On examination, he had a diffuse maculopapular rash extending across his face, torso and proximal limbs. Inspection of his oropharynx was normal. There was no palpable adenopathy.

Investigations:

haemoglobin 16.8 g/dL (13.0–18.0)	platelets 378 × 10⁹/L (150–400)
white cell count 3.1 × 10⁹/L (4–11)	C-reactive protein 53 mg/L (<5)
Urea and electrolytes and liver function tests: normal	
Monospot: negative	

What is the most likely diagnosis?

A HIV seroconversion
B Infectious mononucleosis
C Measles
D Rubella
E Syphilis

42. A 68-year-old man presented with a 24-hour history of confusion. He had no past medical history and took no regular medications.

His temperature was 37.8°C, pulse 85 beats per minute, blood pressure 125/72 mmHg and oxygen saturation 99% on air. On examination his respiratory, cardiological and abdominal examination was normal. Neurological examination showed no cranial or peripheral signs. Abbreviated Mental Test Score was 4/10. Examination of the skin revealed healing scabs below the knee on the left lateral aspect.

Investigations:

haemoglobin 13.8 g/dL (13.0–18.0)	platelets 265 × 10⁹/L (150–400)
white cell count 6.8 × 10⁹/L (4–11)	C-reactive protein 21 mg/L (<5)
neutrophils 3.8 × 10⁹/L (1.5–7.0)	serum glucose 6.5 mmol/L (3.0–6.0)
Urea and electrolytes and liver function tests: normal	
Urine dipstick: negative	
CT of the brain with contrast: no acute haemorrhage. No infarct	
Cerebrospinal fluid:	red cell count 13 × 10⁶/L (<5)
white cell count 482 x 10⁶/L (<5)	protein 0.7 g/L (0.15–0.45)
mononuclear 90%	glucose 4.5 mmol/L (3.3–4.4)

What is the most likely diagnosis?

A Bacterial meningitis
B Herpes simplex virus (HSV) encephalitis

C   Neuroborreliosis
D   Tuberculous meningitis
E   Varicella-zoster virus (VZV) encephalitis

43. A 56-year-old man presented with a 1-week history of fever and a 1-day history of confusion. According to his next of kin he returned from a 2-month trip to Ghana 2 weeks ago, where he was visiting relatives.

He had a temperature of 38.7°C, pulse 110 beats per minute, blood pressure 140/85 mmHg, respiratory rate 24 beats per minute and oxygen saturation 99% on air. There was neck stiffness but no focal neurological deficit. His chest and abdominal examinations were normal. There was no rash and inspection of his oropharynx was normal.

Investigations:

haemoglobin 11.9 g/dL (13.0–18.0)	urea 10.5 mmol/L (2.5–7.5)
white cell count 5.4 × 10⁹/L (4–11)	creatinine 129 µmol/L (60–110)
platelets 56 × 10⁹/L (150–400)	C-reactive protein 13 mg/L (<5)
Liver function tests: normal	
Malaria film: 3% *P. falciparum* trophozoites	

What is the most appropriate next management step?

A   CT of the brain
B   Intravenous artesunate
C   Intravenous quinine
D   Lumbar puncture
E   Oral quinine

44. A National Health Service trust plans to introduce a new test for *Clostridium difficile*, which is cheaper than the test currently used. The ward is trialling this new test on samples sent from patients. There is concern about the validity of a negative result, since patients are being moved out of side rooms when they might still have *C. difficile*. This is discussed with the laboratory and data are collected comparing new and old (gold standard) tests. The data are depicted in the table below.

	Old test positive	Old test negative	
New test positive	3	1	75%
New test negative	3	15	83%
	50%	94%	

What is the calculated negative predictive value of the new test?

A   20%
B   50%
C   75%
D   83%
E   94%

45. A 21-year-old student from Laos presented with a 2-month history of a pruritic rash over his dominant right hand. He had tried several, topical, over-the-counter creams and two courses of oral antimicrobials from his general practitioner with no effect. He reported returning to Laos to help with his father's fishing business 4 months ago.

On examination, there was a contiguous red scaly eruption with nodules over both dorsum and palmar aspects of his right hand and extending to cover his right wrist. There was no visible lymphangitis and no palpable axillary adenopathy.

Investigations:

haemoglobin 13.9 g/dL (13.0–18.0)	platelets 198 × 10⁹/L (150–400)
white cell count 7.8 × 10⁹/L (4–11)	C-reactive protein <5 mg/L (<5)

Urea and electrolytes and liver function tests: normal
random glucose 4.8 mmol/L (3.0–6.0)

What is the most likely diagnosis?

A   Buruli ulcer
B   Leishmaniasis
C   *Mycobacterium marinum*
D   Staphylococcal cellulitis
E   Tuberculoid leprosy

Answers

1. A Disseminated gonococcal infection (DGI)

This presentation most likely indicates an infective or postinfective picture and of those listed Reiter's syndrome, DGI or HIV seroconversion would fit with the 4-week timeline. DGI occurs in 1–2% of gonococcal infections and is caused by haematogenous spread of the bacteria from the initially infected mucosal membranes. DGI presents with a migratory polyarthralgia, particularly affecting the knees, elbows and often more distal joints, and can be associated with a tenosynovitis commonly affecting the wrist or Achilles flexor tendon sheaths. The cutaneous manifestations consist of painful maculopapular through to pustular lesions, and are usually peripherally located. Culture of the gonococcus is rare, particularly after administration of antimicrobial agents and polymerase chain reaction-based techniques from either mucosal/genital swabs or joint aspirates are needed. DGI necessitates a 7- to 14-day course of a third- or fourth-generation cephalosporin.

Secondary syphilis usually manifests several months after the initial painless ulcer of primary disease. Positive TPPA (*Treponema pallidum* particle agglutination) and enzyme immunoassay represent exposure of the patient to syphilis, and will remain positive for life even if the disease is treated. RPR (rapid plasma reagin) or VDRL (Venereal Disease Reference Laboratory) is a non-treponemal test that represents a measure of activity and active disease usually gives a positive RPR/VDRL titre. Reiter's syndrome includes a triad of a large joint inflammatory arthritis (commonly affecting the knee or sacroiliac joint, less likely to affect the small joints of the hand), ocular inflammation (a uveitis or conjunctivitis), and either a urethritis in men or a cervicitis in women. HIV seroconversion can present with a rash (which may be papular or maculopapular), fever and although arthropathy can be associated with HIV this usually only becomes apparent with CD4 counts less than 200 rather than as part of a seroconversion complex.

Rice PA. Gonococcal arthritis (disseminated gonococcal infection). Infect Dis Clin North Am 2005; 19(4):853–861.

2. C Cerebral toxoplasmosis

The patient has presented with what appears to be advanced HIV disease and is likely to have a CD4 count of well below 200. In addition to the neurological diagnosis, the history suggests opportunistic infections of the gastrointestinal system (which include *Cyclospora*, *Isospora*, *Microsporidia* and *Cryptosporidium* species in HIV-positive patients), eyes (particularly cytomegalovirus, toxoplasmosis and tuberculosis) and there is significant oral candidiasis.

In patients with advanced HIV, neurological presentations have a wide differential diagnosis and all the answers listed must be considered. The MRI appearance of multiple, thin-walled, ring-enhancing lesions with little oedema strongly suggests a diagnosis of cerebral toxoplasmosis. Definitive diagnosis can be obtained only with a neurosurgical or stereotactic biopsy, although circumstantial evidence can be gathered less invasively. In this case toxoplasmosis serology would be useful (and likely to show a strong dye test reaction), and a serum cryptococcal antigen would be negative.

This patient needs referral to an HIV centre, pyramethamine–sulfadiazine antitoxoplasmosis therapy and a reducing course of steroids for her cerebral disease with an urgent ophthalmological review. Antiretroviral therapy must be considered once the opportunistic infections are diagnosed and treatment commenced.

Contini C. Clinical and diagnostic management of toxoplasmosis in the immunocompromised patient. Parasitologia 2008; 50(1-2):45–50.

3. B Intravenous ceftriaxone and neurosurgical opinion

This is likely to be a pyogenic spinal/paraspinal infection that needs broad-spectrum antimicrobial therapy and an urgent neurosurgical opinion both to consider drainage of the collection and for possible stabilisation of the spine.

Streptococcus bovis and the *milleri* group of streptococci (*S. anginosus, S. constellatus* and *S. intermedius*) are all Gram-positive cocci and are frequently associated with abscesses. When these bacteria are isolated from sources outside the lumen of the gut, a search for a gastrointestinal malignancy should also be initiated as their movement to distal tissues usually indicates a gut mucosal disruption.

The duration of the symptomatology and marked weight loss may well point to an underlying gut cancer warranting further investigation once the spine has been stabilised and the sepsis syndrome controlled. The alternative to a malignant process would be a mycobacterial infection, possibly ileal tuberculosis (TB). However, the short duration of fever is likely to represent cytokine activation by the pyogenic collection and goes against a tuberculous diagnosis. Initiation of antituberculous therapy is a considered intervention and the indications to start this in the acute setting without suggestive microbiology are limited to TB meningitis.

Gelfand MS, Bakhtian BJ, Simmons BP. Spinal sepsis due to *Streptococcus milleri*: two cases and review. Rev Infect Dis 1991; 13(4):559–563.

4. D Rhinocerebral mucormycosis

Rhinocerebral mucormycosis is an opportunistic infection of the sinuses and brain caused by saprophytic fungi. The infection can rapidly result in death if urgent surgical debridement is not available. CT recognition of mucormycosis is facilitated by a clinical story of rapid progression of sinofacial disease with a background of immunosuppression or diabetes. Evidence of bone destruction on CT, historically a strong pointer towards *Mucor/Zygomycetes* species, is considered a late finding. Swabs sent for microscopy, culture and sensitivities usually show mixed upper respiratory tract flora and only if the clinician asks for a fungal stain and culture will laboratory results be helpful. Aggressive urgent debridement by an ENT surgeon is the mainstay of therapy, and can result in marked disfigurement of the patient. Medical care should focus on reversal of the immunocompromising state where possible – or in this case normalisation of blood sugar, in conjunction with aggressive antifungal therapy.

Nasal diphtheria produces few symptoms other than a watery or bloody discharge. There is often a small membrane visible in the nasal passages.

Orbital cellulitis is an ophthalmic emergency and often presents with erythema and oedema of the eyelids, ophthalmoplegia, fever, pain and a pink eye. Severe infections can spread to adjacent posterior ethmoidal cells which lie close to the optic canal and hence orbital cellulitis can quickly threaten sight.

Safar A, et al. Early identification of rhinocerebral mucormycosis. J Otolaryngol 2005; 34(3):166–171.

5. C Mumps

Mumps is a respiratory droplet-transmitted virus that typically presents 2–3 weeks after exposure with a short prodrome culminating in parotitis. This can be unilateral but is more commonly bilateral. In men, orchitis can also feature and in adults occurs in a third of cases but testicular atrophy occurs in less than half of these and oligospermia is rare. Pancreatitis and encephalitis are also rare but meningitis can complicate up to 10% of cases although the course is usually mild. Diagnosis is typically through serology and treatment is supportive. There is a highly effective vaccination programme in the UK but coverage is not complete and those visiting from countries where vaccination is not the norm, who have no natural immunity, are at risk.

Infectious mononucleosis and mononucleosis-like syndromes are caused by the Epstein–Barr virus and cytomegalovirus respectively. Although they can present with a non-specific viral prodrome they typically cause marked cervical adenopathy and frequently a mild transaminitis. The monospot test detects heterophile antibodies and although reasonably specific for Epstein–Barr virus has only a 70–90% sensitivity – the negative test in this case makes infective mononucleosis less likely but does not exclude it. Lemierre's disease is a focal anaerobic pharyngitis with vascular extension (typically into the jugular veins) leading to infected thrombus formation. It is caused by the oropharyngeal commensal *Fusobacterium necrophorum*. It typically presents with systemic fever, anterior triangle neck swelling (rather than submandibular as in this case) and often sequelae of mycotic spread from the thrombus. It would typically cause a leukocytosis and a C-reactive protein response. Salivary duct calculi can cause a painful unilateral parotitis but would not explain the prodrome evident in this case. Tuberculosis can cause scrofula, particularly in children, and even when not that extensive frequently causes palpable adenopathy. Patients typically have a longer history of fever, weight loss and sweats that may have been evident for months.

Senanayake SN. Mumps: a resurgent disease with protean manifestations. Med J Aust 2008; 189(8):456– 459.

6. D *Staphylococcus aureus*

The most common causes of intraparenchymal lung abscesses in the UK are *Klebsiella pneumoniae*, the milleri streptococci and *Staphylococcus aureus*. In south-east Asia *Burkholderia pseudomallei*, the causative organism of malleoidosis, should also be considered. This organism is the second most common cause of pneumonia after *Streptococcus pneumoniae* and requires use of broader-spectrum antimicrobials for community-acquired pneumonia in this district. The preceding history of recurrent boils and furuncles, with the now rapid progression of respiratory symptoms, makes a Panton–Valentine leukocidin-producing strain of *Staphylococcus aureus* the most likely causative organism. These strains are well documented to be transmitted by close bodily contact, particularly in close contact sports (such as judo). Identifying Panton–Valentine leukocidin-producing *S. aureus* from clinical indicators early in the course of the presentation can markedly change antimicrobial management. The Health Protection Agency has released specific guidance on this matter as outlined in the further reading below.

The lung abscesses caused by *Klebsiella pneumonia* and the milleri streptococci are usually a little more indolent. The former is the cause of Friedlander's pneumonia, whereas the latter can occur in isolation from oropharyngeal aspiration or as part of a more disseminated abscess formation, often from a source further down the gastrointestinal tract.

Streptococcus pneumoniae most frequently causes a lobar pneumonia, rarely causing intraparenchymal abscesses. Group A streptococcus is a rare cause of lower respiratory tract infections, more commonly causing upper respiratory tract pathology and also skin and skin structure infections.

Health Protection Agency. Guidance on the diagnosis and management of PVL-associated *Staphylococcus aureus* infections (PVL-SA) in England, 2nd edn. London: Health Protection Agency, 2008.

7. E Type 2 necrotising fasciitis

The rapid soft tissue progression with systemic compromise suggests a diagnosis more severe than cellulitis. Necrotising infections can broadly be divided into three groups. Type 1 (or Meleney's) occurs following trauma or surgery and often begins as a simple periwound superficial infection before rapid subsequent systemic disturbance. Type 1 fasciitis is polymicrobial in nature with bacterial synergy propagating the disease process. This means that breadth of antimicrobial cover with urgent plastic surgical debridement is key.

Fournier's gangrene is similarly polymicrobial and is typically described as occurring in the anogenital area, arising most frequently in diabetic patients. Similar breadth of antimicrobial cover with early involvement of a urologist is necessary.

Type 2 necrotising fasciitis is typically monomicrobial and is most commonly caused by group A streptococci, although *Staphylococcus aureus* can also cause this process with toxin production causing the extensive local tissue damage. This commonly presents with rapid progression of skin erythema and disproportionate pain with or without surgical emphysema on examination. Antimicrobial therapy should be directed towards Gram-positive organisms with high-dose penicillin/flucloxacillin [unless MRSA (meticillin-resistant *S. aureus*) is suspected] with synergistic aminoglycoside use but importantly also with a toxin production-inhibiting antimicrobials such as high-dose clindamycin. Again early plastic surgical involvement is of high importance.

Type 3 necrotising fasciitis or gas gangrene is typically caused by *Clostridium perfringens* and is characterised by myonecrosis – predominantly at sites of trauma or recent surgery.

Levine EG, Manders SM. Life-threatening necrotising fasciitis. Clin Dermatol 2005; 23(2):144–147.

8. D *Pasteurella multocida*

Cat and dog bites can lead to both severe local soft tissue infections and systemic infective syndromes. This case describes a cellulitic process that is slowly developing systemic compromise and is due to a Gram-negative organism. *Pasteurella* species is the stereotypical pathogen from domesticated animal bites and is usually successfully treated with co-amoxiclav which in addition will cover a wealth of other pathogens that may also be present. On occasion *Pasteurella* species can cause a more deep-seated local infection including osteomyelitis and has been documented to cause endocarditis following animal bites.

Capnocytophaga canimorsus is also a commensal of cat and dog oropharynges but is a much rarer cause of human disease following bites. It usually causes a rapid systemic collapse, frequently complicated by disseminated intravascular coagulopathy.

Eikenella corrodens is a commensal of the human oropharynx and causes indolent infections following human bites and also in intravenous drug users who lick their needles. This pathogen is one of the HACEK group of organisms (*Haemophilus* species, *Aggregatibacter* species, *Cardiobacterium hominis*, *Eikenella corrodens* and *Kingella kingae*) and is well documented as a cause of endocarditis.

Staphylococcus aureus and group A streptococci are Gram-positive organisms and are well documented as causes of cellulitis. They most frequently enter the subcutaneous tissues though cuts, grazes, microabrasions or onychogryphotic nails. These two pathogens can cause infective processes following bites but are more commonly encountered following human rather than animal bites.

Oehler RL, et al. Bite-related and septic syndromes caused by cats and dogs. Lancet Infect Dis 2009; 9(7):439–447.

9. A Immediate plastic surgery review

The vignette describes a case of severe necrotising fasciitis most likely to be caused by group A streptococci, perhaps entering through a microabrasion/pubic shaving trauma. The marked metabolic acidosis, acute kidney injury and haemodynamic compromise make source control imperative in halting the toxic upset caused by this soft tissue infective process. Transfer to theatre and surgical incision should not be delayed pending an MRI – necrotising fasciitis is a surgical emergency and even small delays can increase the area of tissue needing to be debrided and the associated mortality rate.

Antimicrobials, although beneficial, will not reverse the metabolic upset and should be selected based upon whether the presentation is more in keeping with a type 1, 2 or 3 necrotising fasciitis picture. The addition of clindamycin to the regimen, particularly in high doses, aids in halting toxin production from the causative pathogens at a ribosomal level.

The Laboratory Risk Indicator for necrotising fasciitis is a well-validated scoring system for delineating necrotising infections from other soft tissue infective processes such as cellulitis, with appropriate cut-offs providing a positive predictive value of 92.0% and negative predictive value of 96.0%.

Wong CH, et al. The LRINEC (Laboratory Risk Indicator for Necrotizing Fasciitis) score: a tool for distinguishing necrotizing fasciitis from other soft tissue infections. Crit Care Med 2004; 32(7):1535–1541.

10. E MRI of the foot and surgical debridement with biopsy

The foot X-ray shows periosteal reaction at the base of the first metatarsophalangeal joint with marrow oedema. Diabetic foot ulcers should be managed by those with a specialist interest in a multidisciplinary team involving diabetologists, vascular surgeons, and infectious disease physicians or clinical microbiologists. Limb retention with local debridement and prolonged courses of antimicrobials can be attempted, but amputations are still sometimes necessary. Clarification of whether there is bone involvement is necessary and is most easily achieved through MRI. The polymicrobial nature of these wounds means that deep tissue samples (or preferably bone samples where there is an osteomyelitis) should have full culture and susceptibility performed to allow directed antimicrobial therapy. This increases both the effectiveness of the antimicrobial regimen but also reduces side effects and adverse events from unnecessary antibiotics, including development of resistant organisms and *Clostridium difficile* infections.

Where empirical antimicrobial therapy is indicated – i.e. in the case of presentation of diabetic foot with systemic compromise – the choice of antimicrobials should cover both Gram-positive and Gram-negative pathogens as well as anaerobes. Common regimens include ciprofloxacin and clindamycin or ceftriaxone and metronidazole.

Scottish Intercollegiate Guideline Network. Management of Diabetes. Guideline 116. Edinburgh: SIGN, 2010.

11. C Neuroborreliosis

Neuroborreliosis is one of the more severe presentations of Lyme disease. Lyme disease can broadly be divided into early local manifestations (such as the typical erythema migrans target-like lesions), early disseminated complications (including meningitis, facial nerve palsies and encephalitis) and late complications (including arthritis and acrodermatitis chronicum atrophicans). Meningitis typically results in a cellular cerebrospinal fluid (CSF) with mononuclear cells predominating and a raised CSF protein. CSF can be sent for western blotting to detect *Borrelia burgdorferi*-specific proteins, whereas serum may reveal an antibody response. The international epidemiological picture of infected tick prevalence and locations of documented human case changes and updates can be found on both the Public Health England and Centre for Communicable Disease Control websites. Guidelines on the treatment of Lyme disease and post-tick-bite prophylaxis have recently been published as outlined in the further reading sections.

Mycobacterium tuberculosis meningitis is a possibility but the isolated cranial nerve palsy does not quite fit and the CSF white cell count is less than that expected as is the CSF protein. CSF polymerase chain reaction for *M. tuberculosis* is available but lacks specificity and a large volume sample (6–8 mL) for mycobacterial culture is still the recommended diagnostic path.

Stanek G, et al. Lyme borreliosis: clinical case definitions for diagnosis and management in Europe. Clin Microbiol Infect 2011; 17(1):69–79.

12. A Bronchoscopy and endobronchial ultrasound-guided biopsy

The history presented suggests either malignancy – most likely to be primary lung cancer – or post-primary pulmonary tuberculosis (TB). The latter is probably more likely and may well have reactivated given the steroid use over the preceding few months. The examination indicates erythema nodosum, of which TB is a recognised cause – other causes are somewhat excluded by the other investigation results.

The key to diagnosis of TB is through biopsy, histology and microbiological culture. A bronchoscopy with endobronchial ultrasound-guided biopsy will facilitate this and provide a specimen for histopathology which will help to exclude malignancy. Bronchoalveolar lavage can be performed for mycobacterial culture.

Given that this patient is from an area of the world where TB is endemic a QuantiFERON test will undoubtedly return a positive result and not be helpful. Similarly a Mantoux test will be reactive and even if >15 mm would not provide enough evidence to avoid the need for bronchoscopy. A CT of the thorax in this patient is necessary but again will not provide a definitive diagnosis.

Amicosante M, Ciccozzi M, Markova R. Rational use of immunodiagnostic tools for tuberculosis infection: guidelines and cost effectiveness studies. New Microbiol 2010; 33(2):93–107.

13. E Send varicella-zoster serology from mother

The child in this case has a rash typical of varicella, a respiratory and contact-transmitted virus with a high secondary attack rate. In those born and brought up in northern Europe most will have encountered chickenpox as a child and will be immune, but in those from more equatorial regions the prevalence is lower and so adults often remain non-immune. Pregnant mothers and those with immunocompromised conditions with a significant exposure to varicella or a zoster rash must have their chickenpox history elucidated. Those who give a clear history of previous chickenpox can be considered to be immune – whether pregnant or otherwise immunocompromised. Those who do not give a clear history must have their varicella-zoster IgG sent urgently. If negative they may benefit from intravenous varicella immunoglobulin but if positive varicella-zoster IgG will not provide any additional benefit. Varicella-zoster IgG determination can be made and immunoglobulin given where necessary up to 10 days after the exposure.

Non-immune mothers who become infected and are not given immunoglobulin can develop fetal complications which are dependent upon gestation:
- Up to 20 weeks: risk of limb hypoplasia, microcephaly, cataracts, and fetal death.
- Second and third trimesters: ophthalmic complications, microcephaly, skin scaring.
- 1 week before to 1 week after gestation: neonatal varicella characterised by severe pneumonitis and hepatitis.

Oral aciclovir plays no role in pregnancy-associated varicella. Intravenous aciclovir may be indicated in neonatal varicella or if the mother develops complications of varicella disease. In non-vesicular rashes rubella and parvovirus should be considered but not in this case.

Department of Health. Immunisation against infectious disease. The Green Book. London: Department of Health, 2007.

14. E *Streptococcus pneumoniae*

This woman presents with a lobar pneumonia that has failed to respond to broad-spectrum antimicrobial therapy. This clinical presentation in the absence of structural lung disease or smoking makes *Streptococcus pneumoniae* the most likely cause. Possible causes for non-response to antimicrobials include:
- Intrinsic resistance of the pathogen to the choice of antimicrobial (e.g. *Pseudomonas aeruginosa* or *Coxiella burnetii*)
- Acquired resistance of the pathogen to the choice of antimicrobial (e.g. *Streptococcus pneumoniae*, *Staphylococcus aureus* or *Haemophilus influenzae*)
- Subtherapeutic dosing
- Ongoing source of sepsis (no discernible intraparenchymal abscess or empyema).

The failure of the co-amoxiclav to resolve this patient's pathology is most likely due to acquired resistance. Penicillin resistance is particularly prevalent in continental Europe and has been found in up to 40% of *S. pneumoniae* cases from some countries. Treatment of this requires changing to a quinolone, a macrolide or a glycopeptide.
     If the patient had an underlying structural lung disease *Pseudomonas* species would be the more likely pathogen and therapy would need to be switched to ciprofloxacin or piperacillin–tazobactam.

Cardozo DM, et al. Nasopharyngeal colonization and penicillin resistance among pneumococcal strains: a worldwide 2004 update. Braz J Infect Dis 2006; 10(4):293–304.

15. E Pulmonary angiography and embolisation

The weight loss, fever and night sweats in a patient from sub-Saharan Africa with right apical consolidation make pulmonary tuberculosis the most likely diagnosis in this case. This patient will need sputum samples forwarding for an auramine/Ziehl–Neelsen smear and mycobacterial culture, and, if sputum cannot be provided, a bronchoscopy and bronchoalveolar lavage will be needed. The patient may also need a CT of the thorax to establish the parenchymal architecture and whether there is any mediastinal lymphadenopathy that might be amenable to endobronchial ultrasound-guided biopsy. The patient should also receive broad-spectrum antimicrobial cover for standard community-acquired pneumonia and will probably need to commence antituberculous therapy.
     However, the large-volume haemoptysis, anaemia and haemodynamic compromise make pulmonary angiography and embolisation of any actively bleeding arterioles the most pressing

intervention. Tranexamic acid can be given to try to ameliorate the symptoms but, with the degree of haemoptysis presented in this case, an urgent interventional radiology opinion must be obtained, from the nearest tertiary referral centre if not available locally.

Andersen PE. Imaging and interventional radiological treatment of haemoptysis. Acta Radiol 2006; 47(8):780–792.

16. E Piperacillin–tazobactam

Patients with structural lung disease – particularly cystic fibrosis and bronchiectasis – often develop infective complications from pathogens not typically encountered in community-acquired infections. In this case the patient's foul smelling sputum, fever and focal chest signs indicated a pneumonic process and although *Streptococcus pneumoniae*, *Haemophilus influenzae* or *Mycoplasma pneumonia* may be the cause (i.e. co-amoxiclav and clarithromycin would be appropriate for this CURB65 3 pneumonia), *Pseudomonas* species must be considered and appropriately covered by the antimicrobial regimen. Of the options available this leaves piperacillin–tazobactam or meropenem. Ciprofloxacin would be an alternative antipseudomonal agent but its use is restricted in many hospitals because of concerns over *Clostridium difficile*-associated diarrhoea. Piperacillin–tazobactam has a narrower spectrum of activity over meropenem and as such would be the preferred option in this case.

Azithromycin, although having no antipseudomonal activity itself, has been recommended under specific circumstances to reduce the frequency of infective exacerbations of bronchiectasis – acting predominantly through immunomodulatory mechanisms. Use of azithromycin in this way should be instigated only by specialist physicians experienced in its use.

Amsden GW. Anti-inflammatory effects of macrolides--an underappreciated benefit in the treatment of community-acquired respiratory tract infections and chronic inflammatory pulmonary conditions? J Antimicrob Chemother 2005;55(1):10–21.

17. C High-resolution CT of the thorax

Patients with similar presentations to this are commonly encountered on the haematology wards and most hospitals have established neutropenic sepsis protocols. A neutropenic state predisposes patients to rapidly progressing infections – most commonly from gastrointestinal tract migration of native flora – but investigations to rule out common foci should be undertaken at the outset of a neutropenic fever, i.e. mid-stream urine, sputum microscopy culture and sensitivities, a plain chest X-ray and blood cultures both peripherally and from any indwelling lines that may be present. Broad-spectrum antimicrobials should be commenced and should include a β-lactam with antipseudomonal cover, an aminoglycoside and if an indwelling line is *in situ* it is advisable to include a glycopeptide. If there is no resolution of fever at 48 hours a reassessment should be made and the antibacterial spectrum increased. If after a further 48 hours there is still no resolution of the fever consideration of whether there is line sepsis, *Pneumocystis jiroveci* pneumonia or fungal infections must be made. Line sepsis may be indicated by positive blood cultures – even if positive for microbes considered contaminants in other circumstances (e.g. coagulase-negative staphylococci), or suggested by a red or weeping exit site. Where concerns exist about line sepsis the line should be removed. Pneumocystis pneumonia might be suggested by a marked hypoxia, or early desaturation on exercise, or by chest X-ray changes which may include bilateral parenchymal opacification with basal sparing. Treatment of pneumocystis pneumonia would include high-dose co-trimoxazole. Investigation for yeast forms of fungal disease is through blood cultures but the low sensitivity of these is well documented. High-resolution CT of the thorax allows indirect diagnosis of fungal lung disease caused both by yeasts and by filamentous fungi and where available galactomannan can be useful. Galactomannan assays detect fungal antigens – particularly from filamentous fungi – and so suggest invasive disease; however, they can produce false-positive results with piperacillin–tazobactam treatment. Fungal nodules on the CT or other changes consistent with fungal disease necessitate broad-spectrum antifungal therapy.

Goldberg E, et al. Empirical antifungal therapy for patients with neutropenia and persistent fever: Systematic review and meta-analysis. Eur J Cancer 2008;44(15):2192–2203.

18. E Oral oseltamivir

This patient presents with a probable influenza in the context of pregnancy. The National Institute for Health and Clinical Excellence (NICE) guidelines outline appropriate use of antiviral agents and define groups who are at risk of complications from influenza and hence should receive antiviral therapy. For endemic or seasonal influenza these include patients with chronic heart, liver, neurological and kidney disease. Patients who are pregnant and those with diabetes mellitus should also receive the vaccine, as should those with asthma and chronic obstructive pulmonary disease.

In epidemic or pandemic influenza outbreaks these guidelines may be altered and attempts at containment may be made – usually with the goal of delaying rather than preventing spread and allowing time for vaccine production.

In pregnancy the initial advice from the academic community and the manufacturers was that inhaled zanamivir should be given in preference to oral oseltamivir, but following from the 2009–2010 H1N1 pandemic advice has been revised such that either of these two agents can be considered for pregnant women.

Health Protection Agency. Updated advice for providers of maternity services. London: HPA, 2011.

19. B CT of the thorax

This patient presents with haemoptysis but is haemodynamically stable with normal haemoglobin. The clinical and laboratory findings make a bacterial pneumonic process as the cause for the haemoptysis unlikely, and the previous history of full treatment for pulmonary tuberculosis make this a less likely, but not impossible, cause for this presentation. The radiographic findings of an apical cavity with crescent sign strongly suggest a mycetoma. This should be further investigated with thoracic imaging – in the stable patient a CT would be most appropriate but angiographic studies with potential coiling of bleeding vessels would be more appropriate if there was on-going haemoptysis. Cardiothoracic review should occur in every case of massive haemoptysis, and may also be appropriate in this case but not before a diagnosis has been made. Bronchoscopic examination with washings may provide more information.

Systemic antifungals have only a limited role in management of pulmonary mycetomas, with poor penetration of the drug to the needed site of activity. Interventional instillation of antifungals into the cavity has also met with limited success. The mainstay of treatment remains angiographic or surgical. Where antifungals are started, *Aspergillus* species must be covered and the agents most frequently used are liposomal amphotericin or itraconazole. Fluconazole has no role in treatment of any filamentous fungi, its spectrum of activity being limited to *Candida albicans*.

There is no indication to start another course of antituberculous therapy in this patient. However, sputa should be submitted for mycobacterial culture and if a bronchoscopy is performed washings should similarly be cultured.

Kapur S, Louie BE. Haemoptysis and thoracic fungal infections. Surg Clin North Am 2010;90(5):985–1001.

20. D Negative pressure side room admission until sputum culture negative

The concern with this patient, who has previously been treated for tuberculosis twice and now is diagnosed for a third time, is that he may have multidrug-resistant tuberculosis (MDRTB). MDRTB is defined as tuberculosis that is resistant to both rifampicin and isoniazid. Extended drug-resistant tuberculosis (XDRTB) is defined as that which is resistant to rifampicin, isoniazid, a quinolone and a second-line injectable drug.

This patient's acid-fast bacilli smear-positive sputum could have a rifampicin polymerase chain reaction performed which could provide a rapid mode of detecting possible rifampicin resistance with approximately 95% confidence. However, true confirmation of whether this patient has true MDRTB will require the mycobacteria to grow (0–8 weeks – typically 1–3) and then have drug susceptibilities performed (2–4 weeks).

Patients with suspected or confirmed MDRTB should be managed in strict respiratory isolation. Patients may need to be transferred to a hospital with appropriate negative pressure facilities, under the care of a respiratory physician with a specialist interest in this field.

National Institute for Health and Clinical Excellence. NICE guideline CG117 Tuberculosis. Clinical diagnosis and management of tuberculosis, and measures for its prevention and control. London: NICE, 2011.

21. C Intravenous meropenem

This patient has a pyelonephritis caused by an extended-spectrum β-lactamase (ESBL)-producing *E. coli*. The most common cause of urinary tract infections is *E. coli*, accounting for around 70%. Resistance rates vary but in England and Wales community rates of ESBL-producing *E. coli* are generally <5%. Risk factors for community ESBL infection include:
- Genitourinary pathology
- Previous bacterial infection
- Previous intravenous antibiotic treatment
- Hospitalisation in the previous 12 months
- Previous exposure to oral second-generation cephalosporins.

ESBL-producing bacteria exhibit resistance to all cephalosporins and treatment with penicillin-inhibitor compounds is also not advised given the high risk of failure. The majority of ESBL-producing bacteria retain susceptibility to nitrofurantoin. However, it concentrates well in the urine, and is often effective for uncomplicated lower urinary tract infections; it has no discernible activity in parenchymal infections or bacteraemias. Carbapenems retain activity against ESBL-producing bacteria and are effective in treating pyelonephritis and any bacteraemia that may result.

Calbo E, et al. Risk factors for community-onset urinary tract infections due to *Escherichia coli* harbouring extended-spectrum β-lactamases. *J Antimicrob Chemother* 2006;57(4):780–783.

22. E Oral rifampicin, isoniazid, pyrazinamide, ethambutol and dexamethasone

This patient presents with an indolent meningitis and epidemiological risk factors for tuberculous disease. The finding of leptomeningeal enhancement supports a diagnosis of tuberculous meningitis but is not conclusive. The cerebrospinal fluid microscopy and biochemistry are also in keeping with this diagnosis – the lack of visualisation of acid-fast bacilli is not surprising and should not detract from the accumulated evidence that this is tuberculosis (TB).

Antituberculous therapy should be initiated as soon as possible with adjunctive corticosteroid treatment. A Cochrane meta-analysis looking at tuberculous meningitis in immunocompetent children and adults has found that corticosteroid use in this condition imbues a relative risk reduction of 0.69 (95% CI 0.52–0.92). Concerns over the potential for corticosteroids to adversely alter the pharmacokinetic properties of TB medications are unsubstantiated, and the incidence of gastrointestinal bleeding from the dexamethasone remains low.

Thwaites G, et al. British Infection Society guidelines for the diagnosis and treatment of tuberculosis of the central nervous system in adults and children. J Infect 2009;59:167–187.

23. E Side room, lumbar puncture, steroids, ceftriaxone, inform health protection unit

Bacterial meningitis is a medical emergency and management should be performed confidently and in a timely fashion. Isolation of the patient will reduce the risk of onward spread in the emergency department. In cases where there are no signs of raised intracranial pressure a lumbar puncture should not be delayed in order to perform a CT of the brain; however, in HIV-positive patients a CT should be performed as the risk of space-occupying lesions increases markedly. If the lumbar puncture is going to be delayed for more than 30 minutes ceftriaxone should be given and the lumbar puncture performed when possible. The continuing care of the patient should involve close and regular monitoring. The health protection unit should be informed by telephone to contact trace and give antibacterial prophylaxis to those considered at risk. Within the department those exposed to respiratory secretions from the patient should contact occupational health to be assessed for similar prophylaxis.

The role of steroids in bacterial meningitis is continuously under review. A recent Cochrane review found that corticosteroids significantly reduced hearing loss and neurological sequelae, but did not reduce overall mortality. Other randomised controlled trials have found that the benefit is found in those with streptococcal meningitis more than meningococcal. The steroids must be given before or with the antimicrobials, but not after.

British Infection Society Guidelines on meningitis. J Infect 2003; 46(2) http://www.britishinfection.org/drupal/sites/default/files/MeningitisAlgorithm03.pdf (last accessed May 2012).
Brouwer MC, et al. Corticosteroids for acute bacterial meningitis. Cochrane Database Syst Rev 2010; (9):CD004405.

24. C *Leptospira interrogans*

The patient in this vignette has liver derangement, acute kidney injury and a pneumonic process. He is young and has risk factors for exposure to water sources. Leptospirosis, or Weil's disease, is acquired from coming into contact with water that has been contaminated by urine from infected animals. Clinically it can occur 4–14 days after exposure and can manifest in a range of severities from a 'flu-like illness' through to pneumonia, meningitis, myocarditis, hepatitis and renal interstitial tubular necrosis.

Streptococcus pneumoniae is the most common cause of community-acquired pneumonia and, although renal impairment can occur, liver derangement is not common. *Haemophilus* species is another common cause of community-acquired pneumonia, more commonly occurring in those with structural lung disease. *Mycoplasma* species typically occurs in 3- to 4-yearly cycles although sporadic cases can occur. It should be considered where there are more diffuse bilateral pneumonic changes and is often associated with hyponatraemia and a mild transaminitis.

Legionella species abides in many water sources and aerosolisation can lead to inhalation and subsequently either a transient febrile illness (Pontiac fever) or a pneumonia. It is typically acquired from air conditioning but also from residential complexes and hospitals where the water supply is poorly maintained.

Vinetz JM. Leptospirosis. Curr Opin Infect Dis 2001;14(5):527–538.

25. B *E. coli* O157

This patient presents with non-specific complaints but laboratory findings that fit with haemolytic uraemic syndrome (HUS). *Escherichia coli* O157 is the commonest cause of this in the UK, usually occurring in defined outbreaks linked to breakdown in hand hygiene in those with close contact with animals – several high-profile cases recently have occurred in children on day trips to petting zoos. Diagnosis is through culture of stool samples but results can take up to 48 hours so empirical management must be based upon the clinic picture. Antibiotic therapy should be avoided if possible in HUS as death of the *E. coli* O157 can result in an increased toxaemia and worsening parameters. Management is predominantly supportive with blood products and dialysis – plasma exchange has been used in some cases with varying success.

Leptospirosis can present in a non-specific manner but would not typically manifest as acute kidney injury and blood dyscrasias without an apparent hepatitis. Norovirus can cause an acute vomiting syndrome but would be unlikely to cause the laboratory findings shown. Similarly *Clostridium difficile* can cause a colitis that typically presents as diarrhoea rather than vomiting and, although insipient renal failure can occur, the severity in this case is out of keeping with the history.

Shigella species can cause a dysenteric presentation and vomiting can be a feature. Shigella outbreaks are also not uncommon in schools and institutions and the history in this case could point to shigellosis; however, the laboratory indices are disproportionately deranged for this, in isolation, to account for the presentation.

Pennington H. *Escherichia coli* O157. Lancet 2010;376:1428–1435.

26. E Oral vancomycin

This patient presents with a picture consistent with *Clostridium difficile*-associated diarrhoea. *Clostridium difficile* is a commensal in less than 2% of the adult population, but has been noted in over 20% of the over 65-year-old population. When the luminal flora is disturbed by systemic antimicrobial therapy, *C. difficile* infection, resistant to most frequently used antimicrobials, can cause a clinical picture of diarrhoea that can develop into a fulminant colitis. Risk factors for acquisition of *C. difficile*-associated diarrhoea include:

- Increasing age
- Severity of underlying diseases
- Non-surgical gastrointestinal procedures
- Presence of a nasogastric tube
- Administration of antibiotics
- Stay on an intensive therapy unit
- Duration of antibiotic course
- Duration of hospital stay
- Antiulcer medications.

Standard therapy is oral metronidazole, but for severe disease oral vancomycin has been shown to have increased efficacy. Markers for severe disease include:

- White cell count >15 × 10^9/L
- Creatinine >50% above baseline
- Temperature >38.5°C
- Severe colitis (abdominal signs, radiology or on endoscopy).

In severe *C. difficile* infection cases not responding to oral vancomycin, addition of intravenous metronidazole is recommended. The addition of oral rifampicin or intravenous immunoglobulin may also be considered although there are no firm data to support this. Even with initial resolution relapse rates are approximately 20%. Some patients require colectomy and indicators for a surgical review include megacolon (dilatation >10 cm), perforation or septic shock.

Health Protection Agency. *Clostridium difficile* infection: How to deal with the problem. London: HPA, 2008.

27. E Strongyloidiasis

Strongyloides stercoralis is a soil-transmitted helminth that initially enters humans in its larval stage through dermal penetration. It then migrates to the lungs (and can cause an eosinophilic pneumonia) before establishing an intestinal luminal infestation. Once established in the bowel the infection is usually asymptomatic but can in some cases cause a change in bowel habit, bloating, anorexia and sometimes nausea. *Strongyloides* species that escape from the gut can migrate to various anatomical areas including the skin, where they cause a cutaneous reaction termed 'cutaneous larva currens' characterised by a rapidly moving serpiginous rash with local histamine release. Hyperinfection syndrome can occur in those with Th2-oriented immunosuppression. This includes those with human T-lymphotropic virus type-I (HTLV-1) infection, as well as those who have had some forms of chemotherapy for malignancy, high-dose corticosteroids, or who are on immunosuppressant therapy following solid organ or bone marrow transplantation. Hyperinfection syndrome is not particularly seen in those with HIV infection. Investigation is typically through stool examination for ova, cysts and parasites – three specimens should be submitted for examination as faecal concentration of the larvae is variable.

Schistosomiasis can cause a cercarial dermatitis where the metacercariae enter (i.e. in the parts of the body that enter the infested waters). This typically resolves several days to 2 weeks after inoculation. Filariasis can cause lymphatic sclerosis while lymphadenitis and nocardiasis can cause chronic cutaneous scarring. Cutaneous larva migrans causes a slowly progressive serpiginous rash. *Loa loa* can cause calabar swellings over bony prominences.

Moore LSP, Chiodini PL. Tropical helminths. Medicine 2010;38(1):47–51.

28. B Intravenous quinine

Malaria can present with various syndromes varying from isolated fever, a viral-type prodrome, confusion, acute renal failure, breathlessness and acute respiratory distress syndrome (ARDS). The presence of one of these last three features – confusion, renal failure or ARDS – necessitates treating the patient as having severe malaria; two further criteria are indicators to treat as severe malaria: these are an absolute parasitaemia of >2% or the presence of circulating schizonts. The latter is a facet of the pathophysiology of malaria – circulating trophozoites infect erythrocytes before multiplying in the cytoplasm to create a schizont, which then ruptures and releases further trophozoites. When schizonts are seen in a blood film, it can mean that the peripheral parasitaemia is unrepresentative of the total parasite burden because of sequestration and that a further cycle of replication is imminent.

In mild malarial disease oral agents can be used including oral quinine, oral artemisinin derivatives or oral Malarone. In severe disease intravenous quinine or, where available, intravenous artemisinin derivatives should be used. Clindamycin can be used as an adjunct to quinine therapy as an alternative to doxycycline or fansidar but should never be used alone as an antimalarial.

Trampuz A, et al. Clinical review: Severe malaria. Crit Care 2003;7(4):315–323.

29. E Stool ova cyst and parasite examination

This patient presents with typical symptoms of giardiasis. *Giardia lamblia* is a protozoa acquired through faeco-oral transmission and is prevalent in much of the tropics but particularly the Indian subcontinent. It causes offensive and frequent belching and flatulence, and can progress to diarrhoea and abdominal cramps. Giardiasis is usually self-limiting; however, prolonged symptoms do occur in some individuals. Treatment is with metronidazole in the first instance, although for those cases in which there is clinical failure re-treatment with tinidazole has been documented to have a higher efficacy.

Diagnosis is predominantly though stool examination for ova, cysts and parasites. Three stool specimens should be submitted as sensitivity is 50–70% with a single stool rising to 90% after three specimens. If cysts cannot be identified in stool but there is still a clinical suspicion of giardiasis the Entero-test can be used as a second-line investigation and is relatively non-invasive compared with oesophagogastroduodenoscopy and biopsy for parasitological examination. The Entero-test involves a string-containing capsule being swallowed where it sits in the upper gastrointestinal tract for several hours before being withdrawn and sent for microscopy. Serological tests are not readily available.

Empirical metronidazole therapy could be initiated in this case but a firm diagnosis should be sought in all cases and additionally parasites often coexist. Therefore in this case, where there are risk factors for acquisition of other helminths, stool examinations for ova cysts and parasites may enable identification of co-infection which may require therapy other than metronidazole.

Pawlowski SW, Warren CA, Guerrant R. Diagnosis and treatment of acute or persistent diarrhoea. Gastroenterology 2009;136(6):1874–1886.

30. C Neurocysticercosis

Neurocysticercosis is the leading cause of epilepsy in the developing world and is caused by the helminth *Taenia solium* (pork tape worm). This parasite is transmitted either through ingestion of infected raw or undercooked meat or through the faeco-oral route. When infected meat is ingested, intestinal taeniasis results. This is usually asymptomatic but on occasion results in a change of bowel habit or generalised abdominal discomfort. When transmission occurs through a human-to-human faeco-oral route cysticercosis can result. The cysticerci can disseminate to all tissues, including the central nervous system. The resulting clinical presentation depends upon the location of cysts, but focal neurological signs or seizures (focal partial or generalised tonic–clonic) can result. If the cysticerci lodge near the cerebral ventricular system, hydrocephalus can occur. Racemose cysts are particular manifestations of neurocysticercosis in which a cyst forms in the subarachnoid space which can cause marked occlusive and mass effects. Brain CT or MRI appearances in neurocysticerci can vary markedly. Younger cysticerci can appear as hypodense cysts which may or may not have associated oedema. In more established neurocysticercosis they can have the appearance of ring-enhancing lesions or become calcified. Managing neurocysticercosis should initially involve anticonvulsant therapy. Use of anthelmintic agents in neurocysticercosis should be managed with care as increased seizure activity can occur and advice on use of albendazole or praziquantel should occur only under expert guidance.

Cerebral toxoplasmosis is uncommon in immunocompetent individuals, as is progressive multifocal leukoencephalopathy caused by the John Cunningham virus. Multiple gliomas are a rare entity.

Abba K, Ramaratnam S, Ranganathan LN. Anti-helmintics for people with neurocysticercosis. Cochrane Database Syst Rev 2010;(3):CD000215.

31. E Terminal stream urine for ultrafiltration and microscopy

This patient presents with risk factors for schistosomiasis (bilharzia) and a clinical syndrome that would fit with urinary disease (*Schistosoma haematobium*) which is prevalent throughout the lakes and rivers of east Africa. Schistosomes live in water snails and enter the human through dermal penetration of water-exposed tissues – therefore, acquisition does not necessitate swimming but only wading in infested water sources. Following acquisition, the schistosomes migrate haematogenously to either the perivesicular vascular plexus (*Schistosoma haematobium* resulting in haematuria) or the mesenteric vascular system (*Schistosoma mansoni* and *Schistosoma japonicum,* presenting with abdominal pain, bloody stool or with sequelae from hepatomegaly or splenomegaly). Errant schistosomes can migrate to all areas, causing particular problems when they enter the cerebrum or paraspinal tissues.

Diagnosis is either through direct examination (terminal stream urine for *S. haematobium*; stool ova cyst and parasite examination for *S. mansoni* and *S. japonicum*) or through serology. In this case the on-going haematuria increases the probability of urine microscopy providing the diagnosis and will be considerably faster than serology. Serological tests should always be interpreted with caution as antibody positivity lasts for many years and remains positive even after treatment of the underlying disease.

Treatment is with praziquantel, but this is only active against the adult worms so when empirical treatment is used (as in this case – often self-administered by travellers) it should be taken 6 weeks after exposure to allow immature worms to become susceptible. Prolonged (years) untreated infection with *S. haematobium* can predispose to transition cell carcinoma of the bladder and urological referral for cystoscopy is indicated in these cases.

Moore LSP, Chiodini PL. Tropical helminths. Medicine 2010;38(1):47–51.

32. C *Salmonella* species

The clinical presentation here is one of osteomyelitis of a long bone with a documented Gram-negative bacteraemia. The Gram-positive organisms staphylococci and streptococci are the commonest causes of osteomyelitis. However, in patients with sickle cell disease *Salmonella* (non-*typhi*) species are a relatively common cause of osteomyelitis. Capillary occlusion secondary to intravascular sickling causes decreased gut mucosal integrity permitting salmonella invasion. Expanded bone marrow with sluggish blood flow leads to an ischaemic focus for *Salmonella* to sequester. Occasionally multiple sites which may be symmetrical are involved. Distinguishing salmonella osteomyelitis from bone infarctions in the absence of positive microbiology can be difficult and radionuclide bone studies and MRI are often needed. Treatment is with prolonged courses of antimicrobials – ceftriaxone is frequently used and the majority of *Salmonella* species remain susceptible.

Brucella species is a Gram-negative organism acquired from ruminants – particularly goats and cows – and can cause deep-seated infections including septic arthritis and osteomyelitis. The presentation is often more indolent, however, and fever and night sweats are often predominating symptoms. It is difficult to isolate from microbiological cultures and serology is useful. Treatment again needs to be for a prolonged duration but β-lactams are ineffective and treatment usually involves rifampicin, doxycycline and gentamicin.

Battersby AJ, Knox-Macaulay HH, Carrol ED. Susceptibility to invasive bacterial infections in children with sickle cell disease. Pediatr Blood Cancer 2010;55(3):401–406.

33. B Diphtheria antitoxin

This patient presents with a severe upper respiratory tract infection with evidence of a tonsillar pseudomembrane that fits with a diagnosis of diphtheria. There is evidence of toxin-related sequelae with first-degree heart block apparent on the ECG. Diphtheria is a droplet-spread bacteria which is very infrequently seen in countries with developed immunisation programmes but is becoming prevalent once again – particularly in eastern Europe and Russia. Two to five days after exposure upper respiratory tract symptoms develop and can progress rapidly to cause both local airway issues and systemic toxic pathology – including most importantly cardiac conduction defects. Diagnosis is through throat swab for microscopy, culture and susceptibility testing, but the rapid progression and severity of cardiac sequelae when they are apparent mean that empirical treatment must often be initiated.

Although the infection can be treated with any of the antimicrobials cited in the question, the cardiac conduction defect noted on the patient's ECG necessitates administration of diphtheria antitoxin as a matter of emergency. This patient should remain on a cardiac monitor until his rhythm returns to normal and his airway will need to be monitored in case of compromise.

The possibility of on-going spread to non-immunised people or those in whom vaccination has waned (immune response to vaccine is thought to last approximately 10 years) necessitates immunisation or booster vaccination for contacts.

Salisbury D, Ramsay M, Noakes K. Immunisation against infectious diseases. London: The Stationery Office, 2006. http://immunisation.dh.gov.uk/gb-individual-current-chapters (last accessed May 2012).

34. D Hepatitis BsAb testing and a save serum sent from the doctor

Needle-stick injuries do occur even when all safeguards are adopted. Three main blood-borne viruses can be transmitted – hepatitis B (transmission rate is up to 30% in unvaccinated individuals), hepatitis C (transmission is approximately 3%) and HIV (transmission is approximately 0.3%). All healthcare professionals should be vaccinated against hepatitis B although some are non-responders. For that reason all those who suffer a needle-stick injury from a contaminated needle should have their HBsAb titre checked and if <10 mLU/mL hepatitis B immunoglobulin is indicated. A review of vaccination history is also indicated and if necessary a hepatitis B booster vaccination should be administered. These two interventions should not occur without checking the HBsAb titre and obtaining a vaccine history.

There is no indication for baseline testing for HCV and HIV in the recipient of the needle-stick injury and this information may have consequences for the future if a healthcare professional. Therefore only a save serum is indicated in the first instance.

If the donor in the needle-stick injury is known (in this case the 86-year-old patient) the donor should be consented for testing for hepatitis B, hepatitis C and HIV, but this should be undertaken by another healthcare professional – not the individual who sustained the injury, in order to avoid conflict of interest.

NHS employer's guidelines. Needlestick Injury, 2010. http://www.nhsemployers.org/Aboutus/Publications/Documents/Needlestick%20injury.pdf (last accessed May 2012).

35. C HIV p24

Human immunodeficiency virus (HIV) seroconversion typically presents with fever, rash, headache, odynophagia, adenopathy, and often perioral ulcers and oropharyngeal or genital thrush. This syndrome usually occurs within 3 months of acquisition and often much sooner. In this case the haematological parameters suggest a lymphopenia (absolute lymphocyte count can be a maximum of 0.1×10^9/L given the total white cell count and the neutrophil count).

HIV rapid diagnostic tests measure antibodies and historically have a 'window' period of 3 months (12 weeks). The currently prevalent fourth-generation tests cut this 'window' period to just 4 weeks during which time they may give a false-negative result. Where early diagnosis needs to be made several different tests can be performed, but most guidelines now stipulate p24 antigen detection as being the most useful with a faster result available than requesting viral load quantification and a greater specificity than CD4 counts. Repeating HIV antibody testing is necessary but this should be done after the window period has elapsed and will not provide a timely result where one is necessary. All positive HIV test results need to be confirmed with a second test. HIV resistance testing should be performed in all newly diagnosed cases of HIV prior to commencement of highly active antiretroviral therapy.

UK National Guidelines for HIV Testing. British HIV Association British Association of Sexual Health and HIV British Infection Society, 2008.

36. D Non-*typhi* salmonellosis

This man presents with undifferentiated fever and HIV and as such the most likely diagnosis is non-*typhi* salmonellosis. In HIV-positive patients the incidence of non-typhi salmonella bacteraemia is 40–100 times that in immunocompetent individuals. It typically presents with a Gram-negative sepsis picture of fever, hypotension and a neutrophilia. Non-*typhi Salmonella* species do not cause the typical rose spots and relative bradycardia described in enteric fever, and although HIV-positive patients can get *S. typhi* or *S. paratyphi* A, B and C, the features of this presentation are more in keeping with non-*typhi* salmonellosis. The clinical indicators of oral candidiasis and what is likely to be Kaposi's sarcoma on this man's arm suggest that his absolute CD4 count is under 200 cells/mm³. The presence of this advanced pathology suggests that this is not a seroconversion presentation.

Although the diagnosis of urological sepsis is possible, the lack of lower urinary symptoms and absence of nitrites or leukocytes in the urine dipstick make this diagnosis less likely. The negative malaria film makes it unlikely that there is a dual infection and the absence of a thrombocytopenia also goes against malaria. However, the patient should still have two further malaria films to make sure that there is not a low level parasitaemia contributing to his presentation.

Fernández Guerrero ML, et al. Focal infections due to non-typhi *Salmonella* in patients with AIDS: report of 10 cases and review. Clin Infect Dis 1997;25(3):690–697.

37. A Buruli ulcer

Mycobacterium ulcerans is endemic in central Africa, South and Central America, south-east Asia and Australia – particularly in areas of the coast of Victoria. It is an environmental organism most often associated with water sources but the exact mechanism of transmission is unclear. The clinical appearance usually begins with a pruritic nodule but over a period of 1–2 months the nodule ulcerates. The action of the mycolactone toxin produced by *M. ulcerans* causes local tissue destruction but this is usually painless. The undermined edges around the ulcer often extend far beyond the edge of the visible ulcer – up to 15 cm have been recorded. Diagnosis is through tissue biopsy and mycobacterial culture. Treatment for small lesions can be with rifampicin with streptomycin/clarithromycin but medical treatment has a low success rate. Surgical debridement is the mainstay of therapy with skin grafting often necessary given the wide margins needed.

Leprosy does cause anaesthetic areas and although there are visible dermal lesions these are not ulcerated to the extent noted in this case. Leishmaniasis causes ulcers with rolled edges, not undermined, and is often painful. Diabetic ulcers can be painless in neuropathic patients and extensive in nature. However, this diagnosis is unlikely in this young man with no past medical history with a normal random glucose.

Walsh DS, Portaels F, Meyers WM. Buruli ulcer: Advances in understanding *Mycobacterium ulcerans* infection. Dermatol Clin 2011;29(1):1–8.

38. D Leishmaniasis

This woman presents with a skin lesion unresponsive to two courses of antimicrobial treatment, to which impetigo, erysipelas and ecthyma would have responded. Leishmaniasis is caused by a parasite transmitted through sandfly bites. It is prevalent in much of Central and South America and the Middle East as well as in sub-Saharan Africa and into South Asia. There are several different species of *Leishmania* and pathophysiology depends to some extent on the species acquired:

- Cutaneous (typically *L. major*): typically appears as a lesion at the site of the bite with an ulcer forming, often with rolled edges. Secondary bacterial infection can occur.
- Mucocutaneous (including *L. viannia*): begins with skin lesions spreading to mucous membrane areas – particularly the nose and mouth.
- Visceral (including *L. donovani*): progresses from skin lesions to splenomegaly and fever and is often fatal.

Diagnosis is by biopsy for histopathological examination. Samples can also be forwarded for polymerase chain reaction in an attempt to speciate the organism but this is available only in specialist areas. Treatment is of itself potentially toxic, with amphotericin or sodium stibogluconate. Intralesional therapy can be given for cutaneous lesions; systemic therapy is needed for the other forms.

Impetigo is a pustular bacterial skin infection (staphylococci or streptococci) often characterised by thick yellow crusts forming around the ruptured pustules. Ecthyma is a similar process to impetigo (also staphylococci or streptococci) but with deeper structures becoming ulcerated. Erysipelas describes a rapidly spreading soft tissue infectious process typically caused by group A streptococci. Historically the term was used to describe facial lesions associated with *Streptococcus pharyngitis*. *Mycobacterium marinum* causes fish tank granuloma; the absence of fish contact in the history makes this diagnosis unlikely.

Moore EM, Lockwood DN. Leishmaniasis. Clin Med 2011;11(5):492–497.

39. C Intravenous fluids

This patient has dengue fever presenting with the classic history of fever, myalgia, headache and rash with a transient leukopenia and a mild transaminitis. Dengue is an arthropod-borne virus transmitted by day-biting mosquitos. There are four serotypes spread across the tropics. Initial infection with dengue typically presents with fever/arthralgia/rash although retro-orbital headaches can feature as can myalgia. Second exposure to a different serotype to that first encountered can progress to dengue haemorrhagic fever – a phenomenon of antibody-mediated enhancement. This can result in clotting derangement and haemorrhage as well as tissue oedema, including the pulmonary parenchyma. In this patient there is a tachycardic, hypotensive response that warrants rehydration but no signs of dengue haemorrhagic fever which may necessitate blood products.

The good concordance with Malarone and the negative first malaria film indicate that, although malaria should be ruled out with two further malaria films, there is no evidence to warrant initiation of empirical intravenous quinine. The typhoid vaccination, tachycardic response to infection, relative neutropenia and absence of a C-reactive protein response would go against enteric fever necessitating ceftriaxone. The normal cerebrospinal fluid would also confirm that ceftriaxone is not needed to cover for meningitis. Although the presentation could fit with influenza, dengue is more likely, and even if construed as influenza the treatment of choice, in the absence of overwhelming ventilatory failure, would be oral oseltamivir.

Teixeira MG, Barreto ML. Diagnosis and management of dengue. BMJ 2009;339:b4338.

40. A Chikungunya

This patient has a fever–arthralgia–rash presentation with a relative neutropenia and a low-level C-reactive protein after returning from an area known to have endemic chikungunya and dengue. Chikungunya is an arthropod-borne virus prevalent across the Indian ocean with spread to Italy now reported. Presentation is with fever–arthralgia–rash, arthralgia being predominant; sometimes joint pain continues for several months after the inoculation. Treatment is supportive with analgesia and non-steroidal anti-inflammatory drugs for the arthralgia.

The rash of syphilis can be macular, papular or maculopapular but classically occurs all over the body, including the palms and soles, whereas in this case the rash was over her torso. HIV seroconversion can present with fever, arthralgia and a macular rash but is less likely given the timeline and travel history. Headache or confusion which would make one concerned about encephalitis is absent; although Japanese encephalitis is arthropod borne and is in south-east and south Asia the presentation is not consistent with this diagnosis. O'nyong-nyong presents similarly to other fever–arthralgia–rash viruses but is confined to the east of sub-Saharan Africa.

Hochedez P, et al. Management of travellers with fever and exanthema, notably dengue and chikungunya infections. Am J Trop Med Hyg 2008;78(5):710–713.

41. C Measles

This man comes from a country with a low rate of completed childhood vaccination schedules and his arrival in the UK with a child of school-age puts him at risk of what are typically considered childhood diseases. Measles is a respiratory droplet-spread virus that is highly contagious, with a 90% secondary attack rate in the non-immune. It typically presents 2 weeks after exposure with a viral prodrome followed by conjunctivitis, a descending maculopapular rash and fever. Koplik's spots are sometimes visible in the oral cavity from 24 hours prior to the rash appearing until 24–48 hours after the skin rash is visible, when they disappear. As such Koplik's spots, although pathognomonic when seen, should not detract from the diagnosis when absent. A relative lymphopenia and on occasion transient neutropenia can occur. Confirmation of the diagnosis is with a salivary swab for IgM or serology although the latter takes considerably longer. Treatment is supportive. Prognosis is good, with neurological sequelae of encephalitis or secondary bacterial pneumonia being rare in the UK. Subacute sclerosing panencephalitis can occur 5–10 years after acquisition in 1/25 000 cases and is untreatable. The mumps–measles–rubella (MMR) vaccine provides over 90% protection against measles and can be given as postexposure prophylaxis up to 72 hours after exposure.

Secondary syphilis usually presents with a diffuse, non-pruritic, maculopapular rash that can affect the palms and soles and does not demonstrate a descending progression. HIV seroconversion can present with a diffuse, maculopapular rash and, although the patient should have a HIV test, the social history, the presence of conjunctivitis and the absence of adenopathy are not typical. Infectious mononucleosis caused by the Epstein–Barr virus and infectious mononucleosis-like syndrome caused by cytomegalovirus can present with a rash, the former classically after amoxicillin. However, adenopathy is almost universally present and a mild transaminitis is frequent. The negative monospot does not rule out Epstein–Barr virus but does decrease the likelihood of this diagnosis. Rubella can also present with a descending rash but typically causes posterior occipital and postauricular adenopathy.

Muscat M. Who gets measles in Europe? J Infect Dis 2011; 204(1):S353–365.

42. E Varicella-zoster encephalitis

This man has evidence of a resolving left L5 dermatome zoster rash and a new confusional state; there is reactive lymphocytosis (mononuclear) in the cerebrospinal fluid. The most likely cause is varicella-zoster encephalitis. During the viraemia of primary varicella and of zoster, cerebrospinal fluid (CSF) can have low numbers of lymphocytes and there may be VZV DNA detectable by polymerase chain reaction. However, the clinical manifestations of encephalitis associated with this are rare, but serious when they do occur. The encephalitis is not only due to the presence of the virus but also because of a vasculopathic process in response to this. Treatment is therefore with intravenous aciclovir but also with consideration as to whether steroids are required.

Tuberculous meningitis presents with a more subacute history than here. The CSF would show a similar mononuclear white cell picture, but would have a higher protein and a low CSF glucose. Neuroborreliosis again typically presents with a more subacute history with lethargy and focal neurological deficits although confusion can be a feature; CSF shows mononuclear white cells predominating with a high protein and a low glucose. The scabbing rash described in this case should not be confused with a Lyme disease eschar which would occur longer before the neurological presentation and would not be evident at this stage. Herpes simplex virus encephalitis presents very similarly to varicella-zoster encephalitis and would be more likely if it were not for the dermatomal rash. Bacterial meningitis typically has a much higher CSF white cell count and polymorphonuclear cells predominate.

Steiner I, et al. Viral meningoencephalitis: a review of diagnostic methods and guidelines for management. Eur J Neurol 2010; 17(8):999–e57.

43. C Intravenous artesunate

Malaria is caused by one of five mosquito-transmitted parasites – *Plasmodium falciparum, P. vivax, P. ovale, P. malariae* and *P. knowlesi*. Of these *P. falciparum* is the most likely to cause fatal disease. In children the most common complications are renal failure, cerebral malaria and severe anaemia. In adults renal failure and cerebral malaria also occur but instead of anaemic complications acute respiratory distress syndrome can occur. Cerebral malaria, even when treated, has a fatality of up to 20%. This patient presents with confusion and a stiff neck and a high percentage parasitaemia of *P. falciparum* malaria. A CT of the brain and lumbar puncture should be performed to look for concomitant disease processes but the most important step in the management of this patient is to treat the malaria without delay.

Historically quinine has been the antimalarial treatment of choice: oral in non-severe cases and intravenously where necessary. However, quinine is associated with QT prolongation and hence cardiac rhythm abnormalities and also with hypoglycaemia (as is malaria itself). Patients receiving intravenous quinine should be on a cardiac monitor and have regular blood sugar measurements. Artemisinin derivatives such as artesunate have a far better safety profile than quinine with fewer serious side effects. A large multi-country, randomized clinical trial on the treatment of severe malaria including cerebral malaria definitively showed decreased mortality rates with artesunate (15%) compared with quinine (22%).

John CC, et al. Adjunctive therapy for cerebral malaria and other severe forms of *Plasmodium falciparum* malaria. Expert Rev Anti Infect Ther 2010; 8(9):997–1008.

44. D 83%

Defining a diagnosis by a test outcome is dependent upon the test providing the correct result. Assigning characteristics to a test can be done in several ways but must always be in reference to the true diagnosis. In conditions where there is a pre-existing gold standard tests must be compared with that standard. Typically four clinical aspects of a test are discussed: sensitivity, specificity, positive predictive value and negative predictive value.

Table 6.1

	Old test positive	Old test negative	
New test positive	a	b	PPV = $a/(a+b)$
New test negative	c	d	NPV = $d/(c+d)$
	Sensitivity = $a/(a+c)$	Specificity = $d/(d+b)$	

The negative predictive value is a summary statistic describing the proportion of individuals with a negative test result who truly do not have the condition.

The positive predictive value is a summary statistic describing the proportion of individuals with a positive test result who truly do have the condition.

Sensitivity relates to the test's ability to identify positive results.

Specificity relates to the ability of the test to identify negative results.

False positives, i.e. those in box 'b' in the table above, represent a type I error and can lead to inappropriate rejection of a true null hypothesis. A type II error is the wrong decision that is made when a test fails to reject a false null hypothesis. A type II error may be compared with a so-called *false negative* in other test situations and is represented by those in box 'c' in the table above.

Harris M, Taylor G. Medical Statistics Made Easy, 2nd edn. Banbury: Scion Publishing Ltd, 2008.

45. C *Mycobacterium marinum*

'Fish tank granuloma' is caused by the environmental mycobacterium – *Mycobacterium marinum*. It is well documented as an occupational hazard in those who work with fish including those in the UK who keep tropical fish tanks. It typically causes papular or nodular lesions that are often multiple and can become confluent. In some cases it causes plaque-like lesions. Lesions can be painful or painless but are often pruritic. Diagnosis is through biopsy and mycobacterial culture but the putative diagnosis does need to be relayed to the microbiology laboratory as the culture conditions are different for *M. marinum* compared with other mycobacteria. No formal guidelines on treatment are currently published but treatment is usually with rifampicin and a second agent (ethambutol, clarithromycin or minocycline has been used) with treatment courses being continued for 1–2 months after lesions clinically resolve.

Buruli ulcer is caused by a water-associated mycobacterium – *Mycobacterium ulcerans* – and causes painless ulcers with markedly undermined edges which are not evident in this case. Staphylococcal skin infections are very common and can affect a hand/wrist as in this case after trauma or microabrasions. However, the absence of a leukocytosis and a normal C-reactive protein go against a bacterial cause as does the failure to improve with two courses of antibiotics. Tuberculoid leprosy typically causes anaesthetic hypopigmented circumscribed lesions rather than nodular or plaque-like lesions. Lepromatous leprosy can cause these latter signs but lesions are more widely dispersed and often symmetrical. Leishmaniasis causes skin ulcers typically with rolled edges and would not usually spread to cover an entire hand.

Cheung JP, et al. *Mycobacterium marinum* infection of the hand and wrist. J Orthop Surg 2010;18(1):98–103.

Chapter 7

Neurology, ophthalmology and psychiatry

Questions

1. A 71-year-old widowed man, with a 2-month history of rapidly progressive cognitive decline and clumsiness, was admitted to hospital after concerns were raised by his neighbour. He was withdrawn, irritable, confused and unkempt.

    On examination, the patient was gaunt and inactive. He was easily startled and, despite making eye contact, was not engaging verbally. Cardiorespiratory and abdominal examinations were normal. Neurological examination was limited by poor compliance, but signs of myoclonus and ataxia were apparent.

    Investigations:

MRI of the brain: symmetrical hyperintensity within the striatum
Cerebrospinal fluid (CSF):   CSF white cell count 4/mm³ (100% lymphocytes)   CSF protein 0.4 g/L   glucose (CSF:blood ratio) 0.6   CSF culture and Gram stain: no organisms seen   CSF protein 14-3-3: positive
Electroencephalogram: generalised periodic spike–wave activity

    What is the most likely diagnosis?

    A   Corticobasal degeneration
    B   Isolated cerebral angiitis
    C   Limbic encephalitis
    D   Sporadic Creutzfeldt–Jakob disease
    E   Variant Creutzfeldt–Jakob disease

2. A 54-year-old man presented to the outpatient clinic with a 3-month history of worsening pain radiating from neck to the posterolateral aspect of the left arm and forearm. It was a constant deep ache, with superimposed shooting pains.

    On examination, there was no obvious muscle wasting of the left arm or hand. Power was graded 4/5 (on the Medical Research Council scale) in left elbow extension, wrist flexion and finger extension. The left triceps reflex was depressed. Numbness to pinprick was detected over the left middle finger. Spurling's test was positive.

What is the most likely diagnosis?

A   Left C6 radiculopathy
B   Left C7 radiculopathy
C   Left C8 radiculopathy
D   Left Erb's palsy
E   Left radial nerve palsy

3. A 25-year-old man was brought to the emergency department after suffering a traumatic head injury. He underwent a CT of the head (see **Figure 7.1**):

Figure 7.1

What does the CT of the head show?

A   Left subdural haematoma
B   Left extradural haematoma
C   Right subdural haematoma
D   Right extradural haematoma
E   Subarachnoid haemorrhage

4. A 73-year-old man presented to the emergency department after awaking with loss of vision in his left eye (see **Figure 7.2**).

What is the most likely diagnosis?

A   Central retinal artery occlusion
B   Central retinal vein occlusion
C   Cytomegalovirus retinitis
D   Preretinal haemorrhage
E   Retinal detachment

Figure 7.2 *See colour plate section.*

5. A 71-year-old man was brought to the emergency department with fever, tremor and agitation. His past medical history was of type 2 diabetes with peripheral neuropathy for which he was taking regular metformin and duloxetine. One day earlier, he had also started taking citalopram for treatment of depression.

    On examination, temperature was 38.8°C, pulse 106 beats per minute and blood pressure 142/91 mmHg.

    He was profusely sweaty, tremulous and confused with a Glasgow Coma Scale score of 12 (eyes 3, speech 4, motor 5). There was some neck stiffness, but no rash or photophobia. Cranial nerve examination revealed marked opsoclonus. Limb examination revealed increased tone and hyperreflexia throughout. Sustained clonus was elicited at the ankles.

    Investigations:

    > MRI of the brain: normal

    What is the most likely diagnosis?

    A Dopamine dysregulation syndrome
    B Malignant hyperthermia
    C Meningoencephalitis
    D Neuroleptic malignant syndrome
    E Serotonin syndrome

6. A 78-year-old diabetic man was admitted with an abrupt onset of predominantly right-sided weakness.

    On examination, he had right-sided facial weakness with frontal sparing. However, he also had a new left ptosis, with a depressed and abducted eye. The left pupil was dilated and unresponsive to light. Peripheral examination revealed a dense right hemiparesis.

    What is the most likely brainstem stroke syndrome?

    A Benedikt's syndrome (paramedian midbrain syndrome)
    B Millard–Gubler syndrome (ventral pontine syndrome)
    C Parinaud's syndrome (dorsal midbrain syndrome)
    D Wallenberg's syndrome (lateral medullary syndrome)
    E Weber's syndrome (superior alternating hemiplegia)

7. A 79-year-old man presented to the emergency department with a transient ischaemic attack (TIA) that manifested as left facial droop, dysarthria and left-sided hemiparesis. Clinical signs resolved completely within 2 hours of onset. The patient was diabetic and hypertensive, with no past medical history of TIA or stroke. His current medications include metformin, ramipril and simvastatin. He was a lifelong non-smoker.

    On examination, blood pressure is 135/85 mmHg, pulse rate 70 beats per minute and rhythm regular. There are no carotid bruits and no neurological signs.

His HbA1c was 8.1% (3.8–6.4)

Using the ABCD$_2$ assessment tool, what does the patient score?

A   3
B   4
C   5
D   6
E   7

8.   A 38-year-old woman presented with fever, back pain, paraparesis and urinary retention. An MRI of the whole spine was performed (see **Figure 7.3**).

Figure 7.3

What is the most likely diagnosis?

A   Intervertebral disc prolapse
B   Paraspinal abscess
C   Syringomyelia
D   Transverse myelitis
E   Vertebral metastases

9.   A 59-year-old woman presented with a 4-month history of continuous unilateral headache. She described a persistent, left, frontotemporal, throbbing pain with ocular involvement. Additionally, there were daily paroxysms of severe pain with associated excessive lacrimation, eyelid oedema and rhinorrhoea lasting anywhere from a few minutes to half an hour. They had been occurring approximately five times per day but did not wake her from sleep. She had no past medical history, and was taking paracetamol daily with little or no symptomatic relief. She worked as a supermarket cashier, did not smoke and did not drink alcohol.
        Physical examination was normal and fundoscopy was unremarkable.

Investigations:

MRI of the head: normal

MRA of the intracranial vessels: normal

What is the most likely diagnosis?

A   Analgesic overuse headache
B   Cluster headache
C   Hemicrania continua
D   Tension-type headache
E   Migraine without aura

10. Routine fundoscopy was performed on a 71-year-old man (see **Figure 7.4**).

Figure 7.4 *See colour plate section.*

What is the most likely diagnosis?

A   Cholesterol embolus
B   Diabetic retinopathy
C   Glaucoma
D   Macular hole
E   Normal

11. A 73-year-old man presented with a 1-year history of left hand tremor, falls and depression. He stated that he experienced a lot of difficulty using his left hand and did not feel that it was under his control. His wife also added that he is no longer able to do crossword puzzles.
    On examination, speech was non-fluent but easily intelligible. His Abbreviated Mental Test score was 8/10. He had a mild resting tremor of the left hand with abnormal flexion at the wrist. There were occasional jerking movements of the limbs. Tone was increased in the left arm, with cogwheeling at the wrist. Mild weakness was present throughout. Coordination was poor, and ideomotor apraxia was evident. Reflexes and sensation were normal. Gait was slow and unsteady. Cranial nerve examination revealed limited upgaze with diplopia. Fundoscopy was also normal.

Investigations:

> MRI of the brain: moderate frontoparietal atrophy and some evidence of small vessel ischaemic disease

A trial of dopamine conferred minimal symptomatic relief.

What is the most likely diagnosis?

A   Corticobasal degeneration
B   Frontotemporal dementia
C   Parkinson's disease
D   Progressive supranuclear palsy
E   Vascular dementia

12. A 23-year-old woman with a history of idiopathic, generalised, tonic–clonic seizures attended the outpatient clinic for her annual review. She was diagnosed, aged 18 years, following two seizures in the same year.

    She underwent MRI of the head and a sleep-deprived electroencephalogram (EEG), both of which were normal. Sodium valproate was commenced following the second seizure, and she had remained seizure free on a dose of 500 mg twice daily ever since.

    However, she is now insisting that her medication be stopped as she doesn't want to take anything that may be harmful during pregnancy.

    What is the most appropriate management?

    A   Agree to gradual cessation of treatment
    B   Discuss the matter privately with her fiancé
    C   Insist that she continue valproate in view of the risk of seizure recurrence
    D   Repeat the sleep-deprived EEG before making any decision
    E   Suggest switching to an alternative, less teratogenic antiepileptic drug

13. A 72-year-old man was brought to hospital following a fall in which he sustained a head injury. He was taking warfarin for atrial fibrillation.

    A CT of the head was performed (see **Figure 7.5**).

Figure 7.5

What is the diagnosis?

A   Bilateral acute subdural haematoma
B   Bilateral acute-on-chronic subdural haematoma

C   Bilateral chronic subdural haematoma
D   Bilateral extradural haematoma
E   Subarachnoid haemorrhage

14. A 62-year-old woman was referred by her optician, following a routine eye test (see **Figure 7.6**).

Figure 7.6 *See colour plate section.*

What is the most likely diagnosis?

A   Branch retinal vein occlusion
B   Cholesterol emboli
C   Diabetic retinopathy
D   Hypertensive retinopathy
E   Macular degeneration

15. A 45-year-old Indian man was seen in the clinic with a 1-month history of bilateral wrist weakness. For the past 4 months he had been taking an Ayurvedic medicine for chronic fatigue symptoms but now he felt worse and had also developed insomnia, abdominal discomfort and constipation. He was on no other medications and did not smoke or drink alcohol.

On examination, the patient did not appear in distress. A line of bluish-black discoloration was noted along the gingival margin. Muscle bulk was normal with no wasting or fasciculations. Tone was normal throughout. There was bilateral weakness in wrist extension. Coordination and reflexes were normal. There was no sensory involvement.

What is the most likely cause?

A   Arsenic
B   Beryllium
C   Lead
D   Mercury
E   Thallium

16. A 32-year-old woman with no past medical history presented with a generalised tonic–clonic seizure after becoming acutely confused in the third trimester of her first pregnancy.

An MRI of the brain was performed (see **Figure 7.7**).
What is the most likely diagnosis?

A   Herpes encephalitis
B   Intracerebral haemorrhage
C   Multiple sclerosis
D   Posterior reversible encephalopathy syndrome
E   Progressive multifocal leukoencephalopathy

Figure 7.7

17. A 30-year-old man was brought into the emergency department unconscious (see **Figure 7.8**).

Figure 7.8 *See colour plate section.*

What is the most likely cause of the fundoscopic appearance?

A   Branch retinal artery occlusion
B   Choroidal haemangioma
C   Cytomegalovirus retinitis
D   Myelinated fibres
E   Traction retinal detachment

18. A 38-year-old woman presented to the emergency department after awaking with complete blindness. There was no past medical history. Indeed, her only visits to the doctor had been for routine women's health checks and minor ailments. None the less, she did report feeling 'very depressed' after having been recently made redundant from her high-powered job as an executive at a city investment bank. She was single, had no financial concerns and did not use recreational drugs.

On examination, the patient was unable to differentiate between light and dark. Pupillary responses to light were normal. Visual threat response was intact. Eye movements were full and conjugate. Fundoscopy was normal. Formal assessment in the ophthalmology clinic failed to identify any organic pathology.

Investigations:

MRI of the brain: normal
Visual-evoked potentials: normal

What is the most likely diagnosis?

A   Conversion disorder
B   Factitious disorder
C   Malingering
D   Somatisation disorder
E   Undifferentiated somatoform disorder

19. A 25-year-old woman presented with severe headache, nausea and confusion. It came on abruptly while out shopping. There was no past medical history. Her only regular medication was the combined oral contraceptive pill.

On examination, her Glasgow Coma Scale score was 14. There was a receptive aphasia.

A contrast-enhanced CT was performed (see **Figure 7.9**).

Figure 7.9

What is the most likely diagnosis?

A   Dural sinus thrombosis
B   Intracerebral haemorrhage

    C   Cerebral infarction
    D   Subarachnoid haemorrhage with communicating hydrocephalus
    E   Subarachnoid haemorrhage with non-communicating hydrocephalus

20. A 55-year-old woman was referred with several months' history of increasing fatigue, weakness and intermittent double vision. Her symptoms were always worse towards the end of the day. There were no problems with her speech or swallow. She had a past medical history of hypothyroidism for which she was being treated with levothyroxine.

    On examination, muscle bulk was normal with no fasciculations. Tone, coordination, reflexes and sensation were normal. Power was initially graded as normal but there was bilateral fatigable weakness in the upper and lower limbs.

    Cranial nerve examination revealed bilateral ptosis which was worse on upgaze.

Investigations:

thyroxine 15.4 pmol/L (10–25)	thyroid-stimulating hormone 2.8 mU/L (0.4–5.0)
Antiacetylcholine receptor antibody: negative	

What is the most appropriate diagnostic serological test?

    A   Anti-Jo1 antibody
    B   Anti-muscle-specific kinase antibody
    C   Anti-smooth muscle antibody
    D   Anti-thyroid peroxidase antibody
    E   Anti-voltage-gated potassium channel antibody

21. A 61-year-old man presented to the clinic with a 5-month history of progressive weakness of his limbs, most markedly his left arm. He also reported mild difficulty in swallowing of recent onset but no cough or problems with speech. He had no significant past medical history and was on no regular medications.

    On examination, there was muscle wasting and weakness of both upper and lower limbs, with prominent 'guttering' of the dorsum of the left hand. There were numerous diffuse fasciculations. Tone and coordination were normal. Reflexes were brisk, and plantar responses were upgoing bilaterally. There was no sensory involvement. Gait was normal.

    Cranial nerve examination revealed a brisk jaw jerk, and slight wasting of the tongue with infrequent fasciculations.

Investigations:

MRI of the head and whole spine: normal
Nerve conduction studies: normal sensory study normal motor conduction velocities with no evidence of block reduced amplitude of compound muscle action potentials
Electromyography: active denervation with partial reinnervation

What is the most appropriate management?

    A   Baclofen
    B   Diazepam
    C   Galantamine
    D   Intravenous immunoglobulin
    E   Riluzole

22. An 18-year-old woman was referred by her general practitioner, following routine fundoscopy. She reported no visual disturbance (see **Figure 7.10**).

Figure 7.10 *See colour plate section.*

What is the most likely diagnosis?

A   Choroidal melanoma
B   Chorioretinitis
C   Macular degeneration
D   Macular hole
E   Photocoagulation scarring

23. A 25-year-old man was referred with a 6-month history of increasing back pain and stiffness affecting his trunk and limbs. He had also been experiencing painful spasms in his arms and legs.
     On examination, he was noted to have a bolt upright posture. There was increased tone and stiffness in the upper and lower limbs. Power and reflexes were normal.

Investigations:

> Electromyography: continuous motor unit activity in the paraspinal muscles

What is the most appropriate next investigation?

A   Anti-glutamic acid decarboxylase (GAD) antibody
B   Anti-myelin-associated glycoprotein antibody
C   Anti-*N*-methyl-D-aspartate receptor antibody
D   Anti-striated muscle antibody
E   Anti-Yo antibody

24. A 49-year-old man presented with severe headache, nausea and confusion. No other history was available.
     On examination, his Glasgow Coma Scale score was 14 and there were no focal neurological signs.
     A CT of the head was performed (see **Figure 7.11**).

What is the most likely diagnosis?

A   Dural sinus thrombosis
B   Extradural haematoma
C   Intracerebral haemorrhage
D   Subarachnoid haemorrhage with communicating hydrocephalus
E   Subdural haematoma

Figure 7.11

25. A 22-year-old man presented with blurred central vision following blunt trauma to his left eye. He commented that straight lines appeared wavy (see **Figure 7.12**).

Figure 7.12 *See colour plate section.*

What is the most likely diagnosis?

A   Drusen
B   Macular hole
C   Normal appearance
D   Optic atrophy
E   Retinal detachment

26. A 19-year-old man presented to the emergency department having been assaulted. He has superficial knife wounds to his thigh and hand. He describes the incident as his wounds are dressed and managed. Although he is in a cubicle, the police arrive after the incident was reported to them by a bystander. They talk to the receptionist and establish that a patient with knife wounds is in the department but the receptionist refers them to you for further information. He is medically fit to be interviewed but the patient does not wish to talk to the police. They are insisting on interviewing him.

What is the most appropriate course of action?

A   Take the police to the patient
B   Tell the police what you know of the patient and the incident but deny them access to him
C   Give the police the name and address of the patient only
D   Tell the police you cannot give them any information
E   Tell the police what you know of the incident only but do not give them the patient's details

27. A 55-year-old man was referred to the neurology clinic with a 6-month history of dizziness and falls. On direct questioning he also reported erectile dysfunction and episodes of urinary incontinence during this period.
     On examination, his pulse was 74 beats per minute, blood pressure 128/72 mmHg on lying which dropped to 104/58 mmHg on standing and was associated with symptoms of dizziness. He was generally slow with a marked torticollis and mildly increased tone throughout all limbs. Myoclonic jerks were noticed in the fingers of the outstretched hands. There was a generalised weakness throughout the limbs. Deep tendon reflexes were brisk throughout and plantars were upgoing bilaterally. Gait was mildly ataxic. Cranial nerve examination was normal except for slow pupillary responses to light.

Investigations:

serum ceruloplasmin 310 mg/L (200–350)	urinary copper 25 µg in 24 hours (<50)
MRI of the brain: atrophy of the putamen	

The patient's symptoms do not improve with levodopa.

What is the most likely diagnosis?

A   Corticobasal degeneration
B   Multiple system atrophy
C   Parkinson's disease
D   Progressive supranuclear palsy
E   Wilson's disease

28. A 38-year-old woman presented with rapidly progressive, bilateral, central visual field loss, as well as bilateral arm and leg weakness several weeks after a flu-like illness. She also reported a short history of bladder and bowel dysfunction. There was no past medical history.
     On examination, there was a quadriparesis, with brisk deep tendon reflexes. The patient was able to stand only with assistance. Cranial nerve examination revealed bilateral central visual field loss, with fundoscopic evidence of bilateral optic neuritis.

Investigations:

MRI of the brain: normal
MRI of the cervical spine: hyperintense cord lesion consistent with transverse myelitis (spanning C3–6)
Visual-evoked potentials: delayed
Cerebrospinal fluid: white blood cell 100/mm³ (<5)   protein 0.7 g/L (0.15–0.45)
negative for oligoclonal bands

What is the most useful diagnostic test?

A   Anti-aquaporin-4 antibody
B   Anti-GAD antibody
C   Anti-GQ1b antibody
D   Anti-*N*-methyl-D-aspartate receptor antibody
E   Anti-voltage-gated potassium channel antibody

29. A 27-year-old woman presented with several months' history of severe daily headache which was worse in the morning and associated with nausea. She also experienced episodes of pulsatile tinnitus. On a few occasions, she had experienced very brief bilateral visual loss when bending over to pick things up. Past medical history included polycystic ovarian syndrome. Her only medication was metformin.

On examination, she had some hirsutism and her body mass index was 28 kg/m². Visual acuity was 6/9 in both eyes and her visual fields were not obviously constricted. Fundoscopy revealed bilateral papilloedema. The rest of her neurological examination was normal.

Investigations:

MRI of the brain: empty sella turcica
MR venogram: normal
Lumbar puncture (cerebrospinal fluid analysis): opening pressure 30 cmH₂O (10–20) white cell count 0/mm³ (<5) protein 0.3 g/L (0.15–0.45) glucose (cerebrospinal fluid:blood ratio) 0.65 (0.5–0.8)

What is the most appropriate management?

A   Commence acetazolamide
B   Refer for insertion of a ventriculoperitoneal shunt
C   Refer for optic nerve sheath fenestration
D   Refer to a neuro-ophthalmologist for formal visual assessment
E   Serial lumbar punctures with drainage of cerebrospinal fluid to normal pressure range

30. An 82-year-old man presented with a 6-month history of progressive central visual loss (see **Figure 7.13**).

What is the most likely diagnosis?

A   Age-related macular degeneration
B   Choroidal melanoma
C   Epiretinal membrane
D   Preretinal haemorrhage
E   Retinal detachment

Figure 7.13 *See colour plate section.*

31. A 75-year-old man presented with hemiplegia.
Diffusion-weighted MRI of the brain was performed (see **Figure 7.14**).

Figure 7.14

Which of the following is the most likely diagnosis?

A   Left anterior cerebral artery territory infarct
B   Left middle cerebral artery territory infarct
C   Left posterior cerebral artery territory infarct
D   Right middle cerebral artery territory infarct
E   Right posterior cerebral artery territory infarct

32. An 18-year-old schoolgirl presented with headache. Since adolescence, she had experienced
simple headaches responsive to over-the-counter analgesia. However, these had transformed
over the past 2 years. She was now suffering from unilateral throbbing headaches, associated

with nausea and photophobia, lasting from several hours to a whole day at a time. There were no obvious triggers for the headache, and it did not wake her from sleep. She had not enjoyed a headache-free day for more than 2 months and was very anxious that the headaches would affect her performance in upcoming exams.

She wore reading glasses, and last had her sight checked by an optician 4 months ago. There was no past medical history of note. She was on the combined oral contraceptive pill and took analgesic medications such as co-codamol and ibuprofen in variable doses on a daily basis. She had no family history of migraine.

She lived with her parents, consumed five to six cups of coffee per day, smoked five cigarettes per day and drank 10 units of alcohol at weekends. She had a healthy diet but took no regular exercise.

Physical examination was completely normal and fundoscopy was unremarkable.

What is the most appropriate next step in this patient's management?

A   Avoid combined oral contraceptive
B   Commence propranolol prophylaxis
C   Lifestyle changes (reduce caffeine and alcohol intake, stop smoking, take regular exercise)
D   MRI of the head
E   Stop all analgesics

33. A 45-year-old man presented with deterioration of vision in his right eye (see **Figure 7.15**).

Figure 7.15 *See colour plate section.*

What is the most likely diagnosis?

A   Branch retinal artery occlusion
B   Branch retinal vein occlusion
C   Cholesterol embolus
D   Cytomegalovirus retinitis
E   Hypertensive retinopathy

34. A 28-year-old man with epilepsy, who had been completely seizure free for the past 3 years on treatment with sodium valproate, wished to discontinue drug therapy.

He had a clean driving licence and driving was not essential for his job. He knew that he was required to inform the Driver and Vehicle Licensing Authority, and would need to stop driving from commencement of withdrawal, but was unsure of how long he had to stop driving for.

For how long after cessation of treatment will the patient need to refrain from driving?

A   1 month
B   3 months
C   6 months
D   12 months
E   18 months

35. A CT of the head was performed on a 78-year-old man with clinical features of acute stroke. CT of the head (see **Figure 7.16**):

Figure 7.16

What is the most likely diagnosis?

A   Acute left frontal infarct and old right frontal infarct
B   Acute left parietal infarct and old left frontal infarct
C   Acute left occipital infarct
D   Acute right frontal infarct and old left frontal infarct
E   Acute right parietal infarct and old right frontal infarct

36. A 70-year-old woman presented with acute deterioration in vision in her right eye (see **Figure 7.17**).

Figure 7.17 *See colour plate section.*

What is the most likely underlying cause?

A   Diabetic retinopathy
B   Disseminated intravascular coagulation
C   Malignant hypertension
D   Retinal tear
E   Valsalva's retinopathy

37. A 32-year-old woman presented to the emergency department after awaking with diplopia
and problems with balance. She had no past medical history and was not taking any regular
medications.
     On examination, she was oriented and alert. Cranial nerve examination revealed a complex
ophthalmoplegia and reduced pupillary response to light. Fundoscopy was normal. Peripheral
nervous system examination revealed normal tone and power. However, deep tendon reflexes were
markedly depressed throughout. Plantar responses were downgoing. Moderate gait and truncal
ataxia were apparent.

Investigations:

MRI of the brain: normal	
Cerebrospinal fluid (CSF) analysis:	protein 0.6 g/L (0.15-0.45)
white blood cell 8 cells/mm^3 (<5)	CSF culture and Gram stain: no organisms seen
glucose (CSF:blood ratio) 0.6 (0.5–0.8)	CSF viral polymerase chain reaction: negative
QG1b antibody: positive	

What is the most likely diagnosis?

A   Bickerstaff's brain-stem encephalitis
B   Guillain–Barré syndrome
C   Lambert–Eaton syndrome
D   Miller Fisher syndrome
E   Wernicke's encephalopathy

38. A 36-year-old woman presented with several years' history of headache, neck pain and restricted
neck movements.
     Examination revealed a dissociated sensory loss.
     An MRI of the spine was performed (see **Figure 7.18**):

Figure 7.18

What does the MRI show?

A   Cervical spondylosis with syringomyelia
B   Cervical spondylosis and Chiari I malformation with syringomyelia
C   Cervical spondylosis and Chiari II malformation with syringomyelia
D   Chiari I malformation with syringomyelia
E   Chiari II malformation with syringomyelia

39. A 42-year-old man receiving monthly infusions of natalizumab for severe relapsing–remitting multiple sclerosis presented with a single generalised tonic–clonic seizure.

Which of the following is associated with natalizumab?

A   Acute disseminated encephalomyelitis
B   Lathyrism
C   Neuromyelitis optica
D   Progressive multifocal leukoencephalopathy
E   Transverse myelitis

40. A 57-year-old man presented with left upper limb weakness. As part of the examination, fundoscopy was performed (see **Figure 7.19**).

What is evident on fundoscopy?

A   Central retinal artery occlusion
B   Diabetic retinopathy
C   Glaucoma
D   Hypertensive retinopathy
E   Optic atrophy

Figure 7.19 *See colour plate section.*

41. A 38-year-old man was referred with a 1-year history of progressive weakness of his arms and hands. He complained of increasing difficulty in typing and troublesome cramps affecting his left arm in particular.

 On examination, there was no obvious muscle wasting. No fasciculations were observed. Tone was mildly reduced in the upper limbs. There was accompanying moderate weakness, which was most prominent in the extensors of the left arm. Lower limb tone and power were normal. Coordination was normal throughout. Reflexes were depressed. Sensory examination and gait were normal.

Investigations:

Antig-anglioside antibodies: anti-GM1 positive
MRI of the cervical spine: normal
Cerebrospinal fluid (CSF) analysis: glucose (CSF:blood ratio) 0.6 protein 0.7 (0.15–0.45) white blood cell count 1 cell/mm^3 (<5)

What is the most likely diagnosis?

A   Amyotrophic lateral sclerosis
B   Chronic inflammatory demyelinating polyneuropathy
C   Charcot–Marie–Tooth disease type 1
D   Mononeuritis multiplex
E   Multifocal motor neuropathy with conduction block

42. A 72-year-old woman was referred with a 3-year history of troublesome tremor which caused her to frequently spill drinks. She had noticed that her symptoms were worse with stress. There was a family history of an older half-sister who had recently been diagnosed with Parkinson's disease.

 On examination, the patient appeared anxious. There was prominent titubation (head tremor) as well as staggering gait and symmetrical tremor of the outstretched hands. No resting tremor was observed. Tone, power and deep tendon reflexes were normal. Tests of coordination revealed a moderate kinetic tremor. Gait was normal.

Investigations:

MRI of the brain: normal

What is the most appropriate next step in management?

A   Apomorphine challenge
B   [^{123}I] FP-CIT single photon emission computed tomography (SPECT) (DaT scan)
C   Levodopa challenge
D   Propranolol
E   Reassurance and discharge

43. A 32-year-old woman presented with reduced vision in her right eye, and pain on eye movement. There was no previous medical history. However, on direct questioning, she reported that 5 months ago she experienced an episode of numbness of her right arm lasting several days.
     On examination, there was reduced visual acuity, impaired colour vision and a relative afferent pupillary defect in the right eye. Fundoscopy revealed corresponding optic atrophy.

Investigations:

> Visual-evoked potentials: delay on the right

An MRI of the brain was performed (see **Figure 7.20**).

Figure 7.20

What is the most likely diagnosis?

A   Clinically isolated syndrome
B   Isolated cerebral angiitis
C   Limbic encephalitis
D   Multiple sclerosis
E   Small vessel ischaemic disease

44. A 45-year-old homeless man presented with confusion and unsteadiness.

On examination, the patient was unkempt and smelled strongly of alcohol. He was apathetic and restless. His Glasgow Coma Scale score was 14 (eyes 4, speech 4, motor 6), temperature 36.1°C, pulse 73 beats per minute, blood pressure 104/64 mmHg, respiratory rate 16 breaths per minute, and oxygen saturation 96% on air. Capillary blood glucose was measured as 2.9 mmol/L. Neurological examination revealed nystagmus, truncal ataxia, broad-based gait, sensorimotor peripheral neuropathy and positive Romberg's test. The Abbreviated Mental Test score was 6/10.

What is the most appropriate next step in management?

A   Intramuscular lorazepam
B   Intravenous dextrose
C   Intravenous thiamine
D   Oral aciclovir
E   Oral olanzapine

45. A 61-year-old man presented to his optician for a routine assessment (see **Figure 7.21**).

Figure 7.21 *See colour plate section.*

What is the most likely diagnosis?

A   Choroidal haemangioma
B   Chorioretinitis
C   Onchocerciasis
D   Photocoagulation scarring
E   Retinitis pigmentosa

46. A 57-year-old man presented with a 6-month history of persistent burning pains in both feet. This has been particularly troubling at night, and has been affecting his sleep. There was no past medical history and he was not taking any regular medications.

Motor examination of the lower limbs was normal. Sensory examination revealed reduced sensation to pinprick, and thermal hypoaesthesia, to low-shin level bilaterally. Proprioception and vibration sense were normal. Romberg's test was normal, as was gait.

Investigations:

oral glucose tolerance test 9.9 mmol/L at 2 hours (<7.8)
Nerve conduction studies: normal

What is the most likely diagnosis?

A   Conversion disorder
B   Diabetic amyotrophy

C Mononeuritis multiplex
D Restless legs syndrome
E Small fibre neuropathy

47. A 19-year-old woman gave a long history of infrequent headaches. There was severe, unilateral, throbbing pain, made worse on movement, with associated nausea and photophobia. The headaches used to last no longer than a day. However, recently she has been experiencing headaches on a monthly basis and they have been lasting for up to 2 days at a time. During the last attack, she experienced fortification spectra and tinnitus. The patient was otherwise well. Her only regular medication was the combined oral contraceptive pill. She took paracetamol, codeine or ibuprofen during the acute attacks but reported little symptomatic relief. Her mother had suffered from a similar problem since her mid-teens, but had noticed a dramatic improvement since starting pizotifen.

What is the most appropriate management?

A Aspirin and domperidone during acute attacks
B Regular pizotifen
C Regular propranolol
D Stop combined oral contraceptive pill (COCP)
E Sumatriptan during acute attacks

48. A 55-year-old man presented with an acute-onset severe headache.
A CT of the head was performed (see **Figure 7.22**).

Figure 7.22

What is the most likely diagnosis?

A   Arteriovenous malformation
B   Clinically isolated syndrome
C   Fahr's syndrome
D   Glioma
E   Intracerebral haemorrhage

Answers

1. D Sporadic Creutzfeldt–Jakob disease

This is a prion protein disease characterised by rapid-onset dementia, myoclonus and ataxia. Extrapyramidal features are not uncommon. Akinetic mutism rapidly ensues, and the condition typically proceeds to death within 6 months of onset. Routine blood tests are often unremarkable. MRI often reveals symmetrical hyperintensity in the striatum and/or cerebral cortex. Cerebrospinal fluid is usually normal, except for elevated 14-3-3 protein (this is a useful marker of prion protein disease; however, it may sometimes be elevated in stroke or rapidly progressive dementias). An electroencephalogram (EEG) reveals generalised periodic sharp waves in the majority of patients. Brain biopsy may be necessary for definitive diagnosis. There is no effective treatment.

There are three forms of Creutzfeldt–Jakob disease (CJD): familial, sporadic and variant. The familial form is due to heritable mutation within the prion protein (PrP) gene. It accounts for 10–15% of cases. Average onset is in the sixth decade. Sporadic CJD is due to spontaneous misfolding of the prion protein, or somatic mutation within the gene. Its incidence is 1 per million per year, and it accounts for 85–90% of cases. Peak age of onset is the seventh decade of life. Variant CJD is the human form of bovine spongiform encephalopathy (BSE) and is due to ingestion of contaminated meat products. Sporadic CJD is very difficult to distinguish phenotypically from familial CJD. Ultimately, genetic analysis may be necessary. Variant CJD, however, tends to present at a younger age (average age of onset is reported as about 27 years), has a different MRI appearance (with more prominent involvement of the pulvinar and medial thalamic nuclei), and the EEG is normal or non-specifically abnormal. Iatrogenic CJD has resulted from the use of contaminated surgical equipment, pituitary products and blood transfusion.

Corticobasal degeneration typically occurs in the seventh decade. It is a cause of dementia and myoclonus. Its progression is slower than sporadic CJD. However, there is usually akinetic rigidity with 'alien limb' phenomenon. The latter refers to the feeling that the affected limb is not under the patient's control. Protein 14-3-3 is not typically detected. Corticobasal degeneration is discussed elsewhere.

Isolated cerebral angiitis is rare. It is a granulomatous small and medium vessel vasculitis of the brain, resulting in multiple infarcts. It can present with headache, encephalopathic features and focal neurological signs.

Limbic encephalitis almost always occurs as a paraneoplastic syndrome. Paraneoplastic antibodies associated with this condition include anti-voltage-gated potassium channel, anti-Hu, anti-Ta/ma2, ANNA 3 and anti-CRMP5/CV2. Limbic encephalitis is often linked to cancers of the lung (particularly small cell lung cancer), testis, breast and thymus. It presents with anterograde and retrograde amnesia. Often, there is an acute confusional state, with personality and behavioural change. MRI typically reveals symmetrical hyperintensity within the mesial temporal lobes. Cerebrospinal fluid analysis tends to reveal a mild pleocytosis with positive oligoclonal bands. Diagnosis of this condition warrants investigation for an underlying cancer if it is not overt (typically by positron emission tomography). Initial treatment may include steroids, plasma exchange or intravenous immunoglobulin. However, definitive treatment requires identification and elimination of any underlying cancer, if possible.

Clarke C, et al (eds). Cognitive Impairment and Dementia (Chapter 7). In: Neurology: A Queen Square Textbook. Oxford: Blackwell Publishing, 2009.
Manji H, et al. Neurological Disorders (Chapter 4). In: Oxford Handbook of Neurology. Oxford: University Press, 2007.

2. B Left C7 radiculopathy

This causes pain, myotomal weakness and numbness in the pattern described. C7 is the principal root underlying the triceps jerk. C6 radiculopathy causes weakness of elbow flexion and wrist extension, depressed biceps and supinator jerks, and numbness in the lateral forearm extending to the thumb and index finger. C8 radiculopathy causes weakness in finger flexors and extensors, abductor digiti minimi and first dorsal interosseous; it causes numbness in the medial forearm extending to the ring and little fingers. Spurling's test is a manoeuvre to test for vertebral foraminal compression of the cervical nerve roots. The neck is extended and rotated towards the affected side, and downward pressure is applied on the head; the test is positive if symptoms are elicited in the affected dermatomal distribution. The test is of high specificity, but low sensitivity. Muscle wasting commonly occurs in association with longstanding or severe radiculopathies.

Erb's palsy is due to C5 and C6 root injury, which is often caused by shoulder dystocia at birth. It is characterised by the 'waiter's tip' appearance (weakness being in shoulder abduction, external rotation of the arm, elbow flexion and wrist extension).

The radial nerve and its branches are responsible for extension throughout the upper limb (elbow, wrist, fingers and thumb). The only flexion that it supports is at the elbow with the wrist semi-pronated which is achieved through its innervation of brachioradialis. The radial nerve subserves triceps and supinator jerks. It innervates skin directly in the dorsum of the hand (thumb, forefinger, middle finger and lateral half of the ring finger), and indirectly in the arm and forearm through several cutaneous branches (posterior cutaneous nerve of the arm, inferolateral cutaneous nerve of the arm and posterior cutaneous nerve of the forearm). The extent of motor and sensory involvement will depend on the point at which the nerve is injured in its anatomical course.

Snell, RS. Clinical Neuroanatomy, 7th edn. Philadelphia, PA: Lippincott, Williams & Wilkins, 2010.

3. D Right extradural haematoma

This is a typical appearance of an extradural haematoma. It is usually due to laceration of the middle meningeal artery following blunt trauma. The dura mater, which lines the cranium, peels away to the suture lines as blood collects in the extradural space; this gives rise to the convex appearance. Urgent neurosurgical referral for evacuation of the haematoma should be sought.

Perron AD. How to read a head CT scan (Chapter 69). In: Adams JG (ed.) Emergency Medicine. Philadelphia, PA: Saunders, 2008.

4. B Central retinal vein occlusion

This is a typical fundoscopic appearance of central retinal vein occlusion (CRVO); there are widespread flame-shaped intraretinal haemorrhages in all four quadrants and marked oedema of the optic disc. The condition is more common with increasing age, and can be ischaemic or non-ischaemic in aetiology. Risk factors include hypertension, dyslipidaemia, diabetes mellitus, smoking, thrombophilia and raised intraocular pressure, among others. Typically it presents with severe painless reduction of vision. Ischaemic CRVO is more severe, whereas non-ischaemic CRVO may present with fewer symptoms and signs.

Central retinal artery occlusion usually presents as acute onset of unilateral severe reduction of vision. The typical appearance is of a pale fundus with a cherry-red spot at the macula.

Cytomegalovirus retinitis is slowly progressive; fundoscopy usually reveals perivascular infiltration and haemorrhage (so-called 'pizza' appearance).

Preretinal haemorrhage usually presents as a boat-shaped haemorrhage, and is due to bleeding into the potential space between the retina and vitreous (e.g. from a posterior vitreous detachment/macroaneurysm/proliferative diabetic retinopathy). This is shown elsewhere.

In retinal detachment there is usually a well-defined border between attached and detached retina, with the latter typically being greyer in colour and out of focus. Normally, the detachment starts peripherally and progresses centrally. It presents with a curtain-like defect in the visual field, associated with sudden onset of floaters and flashing lights.

Wong T, et al. Retinal-vein occlusion. N Engl J Med 2010; 363:2135–2144.

5. E Serotonin syndrome

This patient is most likely to be suffering from serotonin (5HT) syndrome, a potentially fatal drug reaction characterised by neuromuscular excitation, autonomic stimulation and changes in mental state. It may be precipitated by the use of drugs associated with an increase in serotoninergic activity. Onset is usually within 24 hours of commencing the offending agent(s). Classes of drug that have been implicated include monoamine oxidase inhibitors (MAOIs), selective serotonin reuptake inhibitors (SSRIs), serotonin–noradrenaline reuptake inhibitors (SNRIs), tricyclic antidepressants, lithium, opiates and triptans, to name but a few.

Clinical features are variable but may include hyperthermia, tachycardia, hypertension, mydriasis, profuse sweating, hyperactive bowel sounds, increased tone, hyperreflexia, tremor, opsoclonus (uncontrolled eye movements), and spontaneous or sustained clonus. The Hunter serotonin toxicity criteria can be used to make the diagnosis. Management is by withdrawal of the suspected causative agent and basic supportive measures (airway protection, muscle relaxants, cooling, etc.). There is some anecdotal evidence supporting the use of the $5HT_2$ antagonist cyproheptadine. Similarly, some evidence exists to support the use of chlorpromazine in severe cases. Rarely, sedation, endotracheal intubation and neuromuscular paralysis are necessary. Most cases resolve within 24 hours.

Neuroleptic malignant syndrome (NMS) is characterised by hyperthermia, severe muscular rigidity and autonomic dysfunction. The syndrome may complicate the use of neuroleptic or atypical antipsychotic medications. Clinical features may include severe lead-pipe rigidity, tremor, dystonia, fever, tachycardia, labile blood pressure, tachypnoea, profuse sweating and acute confusion. Investigations may reveal leukocytosis and raised muscle enzymes. Treatment is supportive with cessation of the antipsychotic. The history of antipsychotic drug usage and clinical finding of severe rigidity can usually differentiate NMS from serotonin syndrome. Also, hyperreflexia and clonus are not prominent features of NMS.

Meningoencephalitis is not the most likely diagnosis in view of the history and clinical examination findings, which are in keeping with serotonin syndrome. The MRI of the brain is also reassuring in this regard. None the less, cerebrospinal fluid sampling would be prudent.

Dopamine dysregulation syndrome has been described in patients with Parkinson's disease who develop an addiction to their dopamine replacement therapy. Use of dopaminergic medications escalates far beyond clinical need and is associated with the development of impulse control disorders (such as pathological gambling, excessive shopping, hypersexuality).

Malignant hyperthermia occurs in patients with an autosomal dominant mutation in the ryanodine receptor. It brings about massive release of calcium from skeletal muscle sarcoplasmic reticulum which triggers severe muscle contractions and rapid-onset hyperthermia. Acidosis subsequently develops as the body's oxygen demands cannot be met. Exposure to halogenated anaesthetic gases, such as halothane, or depolarising muscular relaxants, such as suxamethonium, may precipitate the condition. There is an extremely high mortality rate in untreated patients. Standard treatment is with dantrolene sodium and general supportive measures including airway management, fluid resuscitation and cooling. Naturally, once diagnosed, future exposure to precipitants should be avoided.

Dunkley EJ, et al. The Hunter serotonin toxicity criteria: simple and accurate diagnostic decision rules for serotonin toxicity. Q J Med 2003; 96:635–642.
Boyer EW, Shannon M. The serotonin syndrome. N Eng J Med 2005; 352:1112–1120.

6. E Weber's syndrome (superior alternating hemiplegia)

This results from occlusion of the perforating branches of the proximal posterior cerebral artery which supply midbrain and cerebral peduncle. Characteristic features are ipsilateral oculomotor nerve palsy (with pupillary mydriasis and loss of response to light and accommodation) and contralateral hemiparesis.

Benedikt's syndrome is similar to Weber's syndrome. However, the red nucleus and medial lemniscus are also involved, resulting in the additional features of contralateral tremor and limb ataxia with dissociated hemisensory loss (light touch, proprioception and vibration sense).

Millard–Gubler syndrome is due to occlusion of a paramedian branch of the basilar artery at the pontine level. It comprises ipsilateral abducens and facial nerve palsy with contralateral hemiparesis.

Parinaud's syndrome is caused by a lesion of the dorsorostral midbrain. It is characterised by supranuclear gaze palsy, with convergence–retraction nystagmus on attempted upgaze. Lid retraction and dissociated pupillary responses are also common (impaired response to light, preserved response to accommodation). Causes include hydrocephalus, direct compression by tumour (e.g. pinealoma) and cerebrovascular infarction.

Wallenberg's syndrome (lateral medullary syndrome) arises variously from occlusion of the posterior inferior cerebellar artery or perforators of the distal vertebral artery. Affected territories include cerebellum and lateral medulla. Cerebellar involvement results in dysarthria, vertigo, nystagmus and ipsilateral limb ataxia. Lateral medullary involvement results in ipsilateral Horner's syndrome, ipsilateral sensory impairment of the face, ipsilateral pharyngeal and vocal cord paralysis, and contralateral sensory loss of the limbs and trunk.

Brainin M, Heiss WD (eds). Textbook of Stroke Medicine. Cambridge: Cambridge University Press, 2010.

7. D 6

The $ABCD_2$ score can be used to categorise patients presenting with TIA into low, moderate and high risk for subsequent stroke. Patients are assigned scores from 0 to 7 using the following criteria:

Age	>60 years (1 point)
Blood pressure	systolic >140 mmHg or diastolic >90 mmHg (1 point)
Clinical presentation	speech impairment without focal weakness (1 point)
	focal weakness (2 points)
Duration	10–59 minutes (1 point)
	>59 minutes (2 points)
Diabetes	yes (1 point)

The patient in question has an $ABCD_2$ score of 6 at presentation. Therefore, he is at high risk of stroke. Indeed, the risk is estimated to be 8% over the ensuing 2 days, as shown in **Table 7.1**.

Johnston SC, et al. Validation and refinement of scores to predict very early stroke risk after transient ischaemic attack. Lancet 2007; 369:283–292.

Table 7.1 Risk stratification for stroke using the $ABCD_2$ score

$ABCD_2$ score	Within 2 days	Within 7 days	Within 90 days
Low risk (<4)	1.0%	1.2%	3.1%
Moderate risk (4–5)	4.1%	5.9%	9.8%
High risk (>5)	8.1%	11.7%	17.8%

8. B Paraspinal abscess

The axial MRI reveals a large paraspinal abscess. The prevertebral collection contains septations, and there appears to be extension into the left paravertebral musculature.

Mechanical intervertebral disc prolapse is not typically associated with fever. Syringomyelia is associated with dissociated sensory loss, and is identified as a fluid-filled cavity within the central cord, usually at the level of the cervical spine. Transverse myelitis has many potential causes, and may present with back pain, fever, paraparesis and sphincter dysfunction but its appearance on MRI is, of course, different. Almost always there will be central cord enhancement on T2 weighting. Vertebral metastases again have a different appearance on MRI and may cause neurological symptoms due to cord compression, possibly as a result of pathological vertebral fracture, and may rarely be associated with fever.

Hong SH, et al. Imaging assessment of the spine: Infection or an imitation. Radiographics 2009; 29:599–612.

9. C Hemicrania continua

Hemicrania continua is a rare but distinctive headache characterised by persistent unilateral pain, with frequent superimposed episodes of severe pain and associated autonomic features such as excessive lacrimation, conjunctival injection, mild miosis, eyelid oedema, nasal congestion and rhinorrhoea. It is expected to respond completely to treatment with indometacin. Potentially worrying causes of persistent headache should still be excluded.

According to the International Classification of Headache Disorders, analgesic overuse headache is present >15 days per month. It must have at least one of the following features: bilateral distribution, pressing or tightening quality, mild/moderate intensity. There should be a clear history of worsening headache during the period of analgesic use, and it should revert to the underlying type and frequency of headache within 2 months of cessation of analgesic use.

Attacks of migraine without aura may occur at variable frequency, but usually last for between 4 hours and 3 days. At least two of the following features should be present: unilateral distribution, pulsating quality, moderate or severe intensity, aggravation by routine physical activity. In addition, nausea/vomiting and/or photophobia/phonophobia should be present.

Cluster headache is the term given to bouts of severe unilateral headache, centred on the orbital, supraorbital or temporal regions. There is usually marked parasympathetic autonomic involvement, with at least one of the following being present: ipsilateral conjunctival injection, excess tearing, nasal congestion, rhinorrhoea, eyelid oedema, facial/forehead sweating, ptosis, miosis or general restlessness. During the cluster period, the frequency of attacks is variable, ranging from one every other day up to as many as eight per day, with each lasting from 15 minutes to 180 minutes. Typically, they occur in the early morning. The frequency of attacks is, of course, less frequent outside the cluster period. Cluster headaches are more common in men.

Tension-type headache is the most common primary headache. It is broadly divided into infrequent episodic, frequent episodic and chronic forms. These, in turn, are further classified according to the presence or absence of pericranial tenderness. Two of the following need to be present: bilateral distribution, pressing/tightening quality, mild/moderate intensity, no aggravation by routine physical activity. Nausea and vomiting should not be present (mild nausea is permitted in the chronic subtype). Not more than one of photophobia or phonophobia should be present. The frequency varies by subtype, as does the duration (episodic lasts from 30 minutes to 7 days, whereas chronic may be continuous).

Refer to the International Classification of Headache Disorders for the full diagnostic criteria.
Clarke C, et al (eds). Headache (Chapter 11). In: Neurology: A Queen Square Textbook. Oxford: Blackwell Publishing, 2009.
International Headache Society. The International Classification of Headache Disorders, 2nd edn. Oxford: Blackwell Publishing, 2003.

10. A Cholesterol embolus

This is the classic appearance of a cholesterol embolus (also known as a Hollenhorst plaque). It is present in a branch of the inferotemporal retinal artery. The blood flow in this branch distal to the embolus is surprisingly good – this is due to the presence of collateral circulation from an unoccluded branch (seen just on the right of the embolus). Studies of patients with asymptomatic retinal cholesterol emboli reveal an association with hypertension and smoking. Not surprisingly, it is a marker of reduced long-term survival.

Glaucoma typically causes pallor and cupping of the optic disc. Diabetic retinopathy and macular holes are discussed elsewhere.

Hollenhorst RW. The significance of bright plaques in the retinal arterioles. JAMA 1961;178:23–29.
Bruno A, et al. Concomitants of asymptomatic retinal cholesterol emboli. Stroke 1992;23:900–902.

11. A Corticobasal degeneration

Although this patient does have parkinsonian features it is always important to be aware that atypical Parkinson's disease may be a manifestation of a different condition. In this case, the apraxia is the red flag.

Indeed, this patient most likely suffers from corticobasal degeneration, a rare neurodegenerative disorder associated with the aggregation of tau proteins. Apraxia, 'alien limb' phenomenon, and cognitive decline with prominent diminishment of executive function set against the extrapyramidal features of akinesia, rigidity and tremor, are highly suggestive of the disease. Progression is insidious with eventual involvement of all four limbs; a supranuclear gaze paresis may also develop. The clinical response to dopamine is often poor.

Parkinson's disease and progressive supranuclear palsy are discussed elsewhere.

Frontotemporal lobe dementia encompasses different clinical subtypes, all of which develop insidiously. Onset is usually in middle age. Histopathologically, there are variable degrees of cortical neuronal loss, gliosis and inclusion body formation within the frontotemporal lobes (which may appear atrophied on MRI). A strong underlying genetic basis has been described, with there being an autosomal dominant pattern of inheritance and variable penetrance in up to 50% of affected patients. Personality and behavioural change are common in the frontal variant, with blunted affect, disinhibition and perseveration being prominent findings. Episodic memory is typically unaffected. The progressive non-fluent aphasia variant presents with effortful, non-fluent speech, loss of intonation and rhythm, and word-finding difficulty. Comprehension of individual words is not usually affected, but there is often difficulty in understanding full sentences. The temporal variant presents with marked impairment of semantic memory. Patients exhibit difficulty in using and understanding both spoken and written language. Vocabulary is limited, speech is impoverished, and word-finding difficulties and paraphasias (incorrect use of words, e.g. pencil instead of pen) are common. Patients often experience difficulty in identifying familiar people as well as common objects. Parkinsonian features are relatively uncommon in the frontotemporal lobe dementias.

Vascular dementia is associated with the usual risk factors for ischaemic disease (smoking, hypertension, dyslipidaemia, diabetes and positive family history). There is often a history of stepwise deterioration. Clinical features may include dementia, pseudobulbar palsy, parkinsonian signs, pyramidal weakness with brisk deep tendon reflexes, upgoing plantars, positive primitive reflexes and the 'marche a petit pas' gait. MRI typically reveals multiple bilateral cortical and subcortical foci of high signal on T2 weighting. Leukoaraiosis may also be evident within the periventricular white matter.

Clarke C, et al (eds). Movement Disorders (Chapter 5). In: Neurology: A Queen Square Textbook. Oxford: Blackwell Publishing, 2009.

Brooks D. Diagnosis and management of atypical parkinsonian syndromes. J Neurol Neurosurg Psychiatry 2002; 72:i10–16.

12. A Agree to gradual cessation of treatment

This patient has a right to make an informed choice about her treatment and, in fact, although there is a risk of seizure recurrence on cessation of treatment, this might be expected to be relatively low in this patient who has exhibited an exemplary record of seizure control on low-dose antiepileptics (studies indicate a recurrence risk of ~40% within 2 years of commencing withdrawal in patients who have remained seizure free on medication for 2 or more years). However, the patient needs to be fully aware of the potential risks to herself and her future pregnancy should she have further generalised tonic–clonic attacks; these include potential hypoxic brain injury and sudden unexplained death in epilepsy (SUDEP). The incidence of SUDEP may be as high as 1 death per 100 patients per year, in severe epilepsy.

Sleep deprivation can decrease the seizure threshold; therefore, a repeat sleep deprivation EEG would not be unreasonable. If it were negative, as was the case previously, it would be reassuring but would not guarantee the absence of further seizures. If it were positive, however, it might help you to convince the patient that continuing antiepileptic drugs is worthwhile.

All antiepileptic drugs are associated with an increase in birth defects. Sodium valproate probably has the poorest record, with an incidence of up to 8–10% in some studies. It is most commonly associated with neural tube defects; other associations include hypospadias, heart defects, craniofacial abnormalities and developmental delay. Approaching the patient's fiancé, without her consent, would be completely inappropriate and a breach of her right to confidentiality.

Clarke C, et al (eds). Epilepsy and Related Disorders (Chapter 6). In: Neurology: A Queen Square Textbook. Oxford: Blackwell Publishing, 2009.

13. B Bilateral acute-on-chronic subdural haematoma

This CT of the head shows bilateral acute-on-chronic subdural haematoma, as evidenced by the pooling of fresh blood (hyperdense) within the existing old subdural haematomas (hypodense).

This patient requires immediate treatment with a four-factor prothrombin complex concentrate (such as Octaplex) to reverse the effects of warfarin, if it has not already been given. Note that the British Committee for Standards in Haematology has issued guidelines that recommend that such treatment be given prior to imaging in any patient on warfarin with a clear history of head injury in whom there is a strong suspicion of an intracerebral bleed. Urgent neurosurgical referral is necessary.

Perron AD. How to read a head CT scan (Chapter 69). In: Adams JG (ed.) Emergency Medicine. Philadelphia, PA: Saunders; 2008.
Keeling et al. British Society for Haematology guidelines on oral anticoagulation with warfarin, 4th edn. Br J Haematol 2011; 154:311–324.

14. C Diabetic retinopathy

The digital retinal photograph demonstrates features of mild background diabetic retinopathy. Changes include microaneurysms (dot haemorrhages) and blot haemorrhages. Preproliferative diabetic retinopathy includes background changes plus flame haemorrhages and 'cotton-wool' spots. Features of diabetic maculopathy, such as hard exudates, may also arise. Other features of preproliferative disease include intraretinal microvascular abnormalities (IRMAs – seen as small patches of fine, flat, tortuous vessels), venous beading and venous tortuosity. This condition may progress to proliferative diabetic retinopathy, which is characterised by neovascularisation (new vessel formation) on the retina or optic disc.

Branch retinal vein occlusion is more localised. Hypertensive retinopathy usually presents with fewer hard exudates. Cholesterol emboli and macular degeneration are briefly described elsewhere.

Frank, R. Diabetic retinopathy. N Engl J Med 2004; 350:48–58.

15. C Lead

In adults, lead poisoning typically manifests in non-specific symptoms such as fatigue, insomnia and irritability but can be associated with abdominal pain, constipation and peripheral motor neuropathies (especially wrist-drop and foot-drop). A bluish-black line of discoloration along the gingival margin is highly suspicious for lead poisoning. In children, lead toxicity has a significant effect on the brain and the level of exposure is said to correlate with intellectual impairment. Anaemia may also result from lead poisoning, with characteristic basophilic stippling evident on the blood film.

Acute arsenic poisoning may present with confusion, diarrhoea and vomiting, and hypovolaemic shock. Cardiac arrhythmias are a recognised feature. Chronic poisoning may present with painful peripheral sensory neuropathy, dermatitis, and hepatic and renal impairment. Mees' lines may be detected in the fingernails (these appear as transverse lines, which are usually white, and may be single or multiple).

Beryllium, if inhaled, may cause acute chemical pneumonitis or chronic granulomatous disease of the lungs (chronic beryllium disease). It may also cause contact dermatitis.

The effects of mercury poisoning vary depending on whether exposure is to inorganic elemental mercury or its organic form, methylmercury. The latter is more toxic and may result in a wide range of features including paraesthesia, tremors, ataxia, visual and auditory impairment, and cognitive decline. In severe poisoning, it may progress to coma and death. Chronic inorganic mercury poisoning is associated with an erythematous papular rash, proteinuria and anaemia. Neurological signs include tremor, ataxia and myopathy. Cognitive decline and behavioural change are common. Signs of encephalopathy may ensure.

Features of thallium poisoning include diarrhoea and vomiting, acute confusion, alopecia and Mees' lines. Chronic poisoning may cause a painful peripheral neuropathy.

Clarke C, et al (eds). Toxic, metabolic and physical insults (Chapter 18). In: Neurology: A Queen Square Textbook. Oxford: Blackwell Publishing, 2009.
Ernst E. Heavy metals in traditional Indian remedies. Eur J Clin Pharmacol 2002; 57(12):891–896.
Saper RB, et al. Heavy metal content of ayurvedic herbal medicine products. JAMA 2004; 292(23):2868–2873.

16. D Posterior reversible encephalopathy syndrome

The history and imaging findings are consistent with a diagnosis of posterior reversible encephalopathy syndrome. This form of encephalopathy is associated with acute hypertensive episodes (e.g. in eclampsia or renal disease), and the use of immunosuppressant medication (especially, following organ transplantation). It is thought that the condition results from the blood–brain barrier being overcome either by the mechanical effect of a rise in hydrostatic pressure or by a toxic effect of circulating immunosuppressant drugs.

Clinical presentation may be with confusion, depressed conscious level, headache, cortical blindness or seizures. A timely MRI of the brain may reveal evidence of vasogenic oedema within the white matter of the occipital or parietal lobes. The condition is often completely reversible if the underlying cause is promptly addressed.

Herpes encephalitis is usually caused by HSV-1 (herpes simplex virus 1) and may present with fever, headache, depressed conscious level, personality/behavioural change, dysphasia or generalised tonic–clonic seizures with olfactory or gustatory aura. The MRI of the brain usually reveals vasogenic oedema within the inferior and medial temporal lobe which may extend into the insular cortex or frontal lobe. There may be bilateral involvement.

Intracerebral haemorrhage, multiple sclerosis and progressive multifocal leukoencephalopathy are discussed elsewhere.

Clarke C, et al (eds). Disorders of consciousness and sleep (Chapter 19). In: Neurology: A Queen Square Textbook. Oxford: Blackwell Publishing, 2009.
Hinchey, J et al. A reversible posterior leukoencephalopathy syndrome. N Engl J Med 1996; 334:494–500.

17. D Myelinated fibres

This is typical of the appearance of myelinated fibres. It is a fairly common finding resulting from anomalous myelination of nerve fibres anterior to the lamina cribrosa. It is usually asymptomatic. It usually appears feather like at its edges and can obscure the retinal vessels. It follows the path of the nerve fibre layer, which sweeps in an arch from the optic disc.

Branch retinal artery occlusion, choroidal haemangioma, cytomegalovirus retinitis and traction retinal detachment have different appearances and are described elsewhere.

Golnik, K. Congenital optic nerve anomalies. Curr Opin Ophthalmol. 1998; 9(6):18–26.

18. A Conversion disorder

Of the options given, the patient is most likely to be suffering from conversion disorder. This is a condition in which there is a neurological deficit that cannot be accounted for by an underlying organic disorder. It precipitates subconsciously as a reaction to psychological stresses or conflicts, and causes significant functional impairment. In a significant number of cases, the patient exhibits what Charcot first referred to as 'la belle indifference' (i.e. a surprising lack of concern about the physical condition), although it should be noted that this is an unreliable sign. For the full diagnostic criteria, please refer to the DSM-IV (Diagnostic and Statistical Manual of Mental Disorders, 4th edn).

Factitious disorder and malingering are possibilities, but are less likely. Both are conditions in which symptoms or signs of physical or psychological disease are intentionally produced or feigned for the purpose of achieving some type of external gain. In factitious disorder, the primary motivation is to assume 'the sick role'. In contrast, the external gain in malingering is typically through financial compensation, work avoidance or access to narcotic drugs. Our patient does not fit the typical profile for either of these conditions.

Somatisation disorder can be discounted because of the fact that it is defined by the presence of many physical complaints before the age of 30 years, spanning at least several years, which have prompted treatment-seeking behaviour or have resulted in significant functional disturbance at social, occupational or other important levels. Additionally, to make the diagnosis, all of the following should have occurred at some point throughout the illness: (a) four pain symptoms, (b) two gastrointestinal symptoms, (c) one sexual symptom and (d) one pseudoneurological symptom.

Investigations should not reveal evidence of an underlying condition that can fully account for the patient's symptoms. The symptoms are not intentionally produced.

Undifferentiated somatoform disorder can also be excluded on the basis that symptoms must have been present for 6 months or longer. It is a condition in which there are one or more physical complaints that cannot be fully accounted for by any underlying medical condition, following adequate investigation. The condition causes distress to the patient or results in impaired functioning at social, occupational or other important levels. The symptoms are not intentionally produced, and they are not better accounted for by another mental health disorder

For full diagnostic criteria of the above listed conditions, please refer to the DSM-IV.

American Psychiatric Association. DSM-IV-TR: Diagnostic and Statistical Manual of Mental Disorders, 4th edn. Washington DC: American Psychiatric Association, 2000.
Stone J, et al. La belle indifférence in conversion symptoms and hysteria. Br J Psychiatry 2006; 188:204–209.

19. A Dural sinus thrombosis

The contrast-enhanced CT reveals a filling defect in the left sigmoid sinus ('empty delta' sign), consistent with dural sinus thrombosis. Furthermore, this is complicated by venous infarction of the left temporal lobe, which would account for the receptive aphasia. Onset of headache is usually gradual, but can be of the sudden 'thunderclap' type as in this case. Subarachnoid haemorrhage is an important differential, but is clearly excluded by the CT, as is an intracerebral haemorrhage. Note that the 'empty delta' sign, which is most often found in superior sagittal sinus thrombosis, is due to contrast enhancement at the margins of a non-enhancing thrombus.

Perron AD. How to read a head CT scan (Chapter 69). In: Adams JG (ed). Emergency Medicine. Oxford: Saunders, 2008.

20. B Anti-muscle-specific kinase antibody

This patient is suffering from myasthenia gravis (MG), an autoimmune disorder affecting the neuromuscular junction. It has two peaks of incidence, the first being in the second and third decades and the second in the sixth and seventh decades. It can occur as ocular or generalised forms. Clinical features may include diplopia, blurred vision, ptosis, weakness of facial muscles, speech/swallowing difficulties, respiratory compromise and proximal limb weakness.

The diagnosis is usually suggested by the history, as in this case, and can be confirmed with serological and electromyographic (EMG) tests. Three quarters of MG patients are seropositive for anti-acetylcholine receptor antibodies. Over half of the remaining ~25% of MG patients are seropositive for anti-muscle-specific kinase (MuSK) antibodies. The Tensilon test (administration of intravenous edrophonium to observe for transient alleviation of symptoms) is rarely necessary to make the diagnosis; it is contraindicated in heart disease.

EMG studies are very useful in confirming the clinical diagnosis. Jitter is a measure of variation in the interpotential interval on a single-fibre EMG (SFEMG); increased jitter is highly sensitive for MG (93% in ocular MG, 99% in generalised MG), but not highly specific as it generally signifies problems in transmission at the neuromuscular junction. Normal SFEMG in a weak muscle practically excludes the diagnosis. Decrements in compound muscle action potentials on repetitive nerve stimulation are probably the most specific finding for MG, but not the most sensitive.

Following diagnosis, CT/MRI should be performed to exclude thymoma. Approximately 15% of MG patients have a thymoma, a small minority of which have malignant features. Thymectomy is indicated for all MG patients, from late childhood to age 60 years, who are seropositive for antiacetylcholine receptor antibodies.

Medical treatment options include anticholinesterases, steroids, steroid-sparing immunosuppressants, intravenous immunoglobulin and plasma exchange.

Most patients with autoimmune hypothyroidism will be positive for antithyroid peroxidase (anti-TPO) antibodies. In this case, the patient is known to be hypothyroid and gives a history suggestive of myasthenia. Therefore, of the options given, testing for anti-TPO antibodies is not the most appropriate course of action. The remaining antibodies are associated with different conditions: anti-Jo1 with dermatomyositis, anti-smooth muscle with autoimmune hepatitis, and anti-voltage-gated potassium channel with peripheral nerve hyperexcitability (neuromyotonia) and limbic encephalitis.

Clarke C, et al (eds). Nerve and muscle disease (Chapter 9). In: Neurology: A Queen Square Textbook. Oxford: Blackwell Publishing, 2009.
Witoonpanich R, et al. Electrophysiological and immunological study in myasthenia gravis: diagnostic sensitivity and correlation. Clin Neurophysiol 2011; 122:1873–1877.

21. E Riluzole

This patient has characteristic features of amyotrophic lateral sclerosis (ALS), a subtype of motor neuron disease. The presence of mixed upper and lower motor neuron signs in both upper and lower limbs is strongly suggestive of motor neuron disease (MND). Unfortunately, this is an incurable condition. The only licensed pharmacological treatment for ALS in the UK is riluzole, which is thought to act by blocking glutamate activity. It is believed that it does so by increasing glutamate uptake by spinal neurons rather than by directly antagonising glutamate receptors. Studies show that treatment with riluzole has a small but significant effect in slowing disease progression; on average, the time to tracheostomy is prolonged by 2–4 months.

All MND patients should be referred to a specialist clinic for regular monitoring and timely supportive management.

National Institute for Health and Clinical Excellence. NICE Guidelines. TA20: Motor neuron disease: riluzole–guidance. London: NICE, 2001.

22. B Chorioretinitis

This is a typical appearance of chorioretinitis, a condition that may arise secondary to infection with *Toxoplasma gondii*, cytomegalovirus or numerous other pathogens. Infective causes may be congenital or acquired. Non-infectious causes include sarcoidosis and Behçet's disease.

Choroidal melanoma is often asymptomatic and discovered incidentally. It has a fairly characteristic appearance on fundoscopy; however, the tumour can be variably pigmented or, indeed, amelanotic.

Macular degeneration, macular holes and photocoagulation scarring are described elsewhere.

Leitman M. Manual for Eye Examination and Diagnosis, 8th edn. Chichester: Wiley-Blackwell, 2012.

23. A Anti-glutamic acid decarboxylase (GAD) antibody

This patient has features of stiff-person syndrome, a presumed autoimmune disease. It is sometimes associated with diabetes mellitus, and anti-GAD antibodies are frequently detected at high titre. Electromyography usually reveals continuous motor unit activity in affected axial and proximal limb muscles. A good response is usually achieved with high-dose baclofen or diazepam. Plasmapheresis and intravenous immunoglobulin (IVIg) have also been used successfully in these patients.

Anti-myelin-associated glycoprotein antibody is associated with demyelinating polyneuropathies. Anti-*N*-methyl-ᴅ-aspartate receptor antibody is associated with encephalitis and is found predominantly in women; a significant proportion of these cases are paraneoplastic, usually arising secondary to ovarian teratoma. Anti-striated muscle antibody is detected in a high percentage of young myasthenia gravis patients with thymoma, anti-Yo antibody is associated with paraneoplastic cerebellar degeneration. Screening for an underlying cancer should be undertaken (the antibody is linked to gynaecological and breast cancers in women).

Clarke C, et al (eds). Movement disorders (Chapter 5). In: Neurology: A Queen Square Textbook. Oxford: Blackwell Publishing, 2009.
Levy LM, et al. The stiff-person syndrome: An autoimmune disorder affecting neurotransmission of γ-aminobutyric acid. Ann Intern Med 1999; 131:522–530.

24. D Subarachnoid haemorrhage with communicating hydrocephalus

This man's CT of the head scan reveals a subarachnoid haemorrhage with communicating hydrocephalus. There is blood in the basal cisterns and in both Sylvian fissures. The dilated 4th ventricle is suggestive of a communicating hydrocephalus.

Extradural haematoma, dural sinus thrombosis, intracerebral haemorrhage and subdural haematoma are discussed elsewhere.

Perron AD. How to read a head CT scan (Chapter 69). In: Adams JG (ed). Emergency Medicine, 1st edition. Saunders; 2008.

25. B Macular hole

The appearance of a yellow ring with a central defect at the fovea is characteristic of a macular hole. The diagnosis can be confirmed with optical coherence tomography. A macular hole usually presents in the elderly female spontaneously, but can develop following blunt trauma to the eye.

Drusen are deposits of lipid and protein in Bruch's membrane, and appear as small yellowish deposits. They are the cardinal sign of early age-related macular degeneration. Optic atrophy is observed as a very pale optic disc with sharply defined margins.

Leitman M. Manual for Eye Examination and Diagnosis, 8th edn. Chichester: Wiley-Blackwell, 2012.

26. D Tell the police you cannot give them any information

Confidentiality is one of the cornerstones on which the doctor–patient relationship is based. Breach of confidentiality should occur only in exceptional circumstances and only when failure to disclose information may put the patient, or another, at risk of death or serious harm, or when it is likely to help in the prevention or prosecution of a serious crime. The General Medical Council (GMC) provides guidance on this in *Good Medical Practice* and their associated documents.

This guidance relating to gun and knife wounds outlines a two-stage strategy:
1. The police must be quickly informed when a person arrives with a gunshot or knife injury. This will enable the police to make a risk assessment of the situation. They have a responsibility of assessing further risk to the patient, hospital and staff, and other members of the public.
2. Patients should be asked if they wish to speak to the police. If they agree then a medical assessment of their fitness should be made and the timing of the interview dictated accordingly. If they are adamant that they do not wish to talk to the police the clinician responsible must make a professional judgement about whether disclosure of patient details is justified in the public interest. Where possible patients should be informed of the decision to disclose their details and the justification for this. This should also be documented in patients' notes.

General Medical Council. Good Medical Practice. London: GMC, 2006.

27. B Multiple system atrophy

Multiple system atrophy (MSA; previously known as Shy–Drager syndrome) is a sporadic, progressive, adult-onset neurodegenerative disease that may present with a combination of parkinsonian signs, autonomic dysfunction, cerebellar ataxia and pyramidal effects. It typically presents in the sixth decade. It is characterised by autonomic dysfunction with parkinsonism (MSA-P) or cerebellar ataxia (MSA-C). Clinical features may include orthostatic hypotension, urinary incontinence, erectile dysfunction, cold dusky peripheries, bradykinesia, rigidity, marked antecollis, action tremor, postural instability, dysarthria, dysphonia, dysphagia, cerebellar ataxia, emotional lability, daytime stridor/worsening snoring/sleep apnoea, etc. Resting tremor is uncommon. Cognitive decline is not considered to be in keeping with the diagnosis. MRI of the brain may be completely normal; however, putaminal, cerebellar or brainstem atrophy is not uncommon. Occasionally, the 'hot cross bun' sign (a radiological sign) may be detected in the pons on T2-weighted MRI. Treatment is supportive. Mean survival is 7 years.

Progressive supranuclear palsy (previously known as Steele–Richardson–Olszewski syndrome) is a sporadic neurodegenerative disease, defined by the presence of tau-positive neurofibrillary tangles in the substantia nigra, dentate nucleus, globus pallidus and subthalamic nucleus. Cortical involvement is variable. The defining clinical feature is a supranuclear gaze palsy affecting voluntary upgaze and/or downgaze; however, a full range of reflex eye movements is preserved (as can be demonstrated with the oculocephalic reflex). Other features include akinetic rigidity (predominantly axial), a propensity to fall backwards from early on in the disease, dysarthria, dysphagia, frontalis overactivity, impaired frontal executive function and personality change. MRI may reveal midbrain atrophy, with T2-weighted signal hyperintensity in the periaqueductal grey matter and globus pallidus. There may also be frontotemporal atrophy. As for MSA, response to levodopa is poor, management is supportive and mean survival is 7 years.

Corticobasal degeneration and Parkinson's disease do not explain this presentation and are described elsewhere. Similarly, Wilson's disease would not be expected to present in this way, and would be unlikely in a patient of this age; it is excluded by the normal copper studies.

Clarke C, et al (eds). Movement disorders (Chapter 5). In: Neurology: A Queen Square Textbook. Oxford: Blackwell Publishing, 2009.
Manji H, et al. Neurological disorders (Chapter 4). In: Oxford Handbook of Neurology. Oxford: Oxford University Press, 2007.

28. A Anti-aquaporin-4 antibody

This patient most likely has neuromyelitis optica (also known as Devic's disease), an antibody-mediated demyelinating disease. Typical presentation is with transverse myelitis and/or optic neuritis, following a prodromal flu-like illness. Optic neuritis is often painful and may be unilateral or bilateral, and can present with complete visual loss. It may follow a monophasic or relapsing and remitting course. Mean age of onset is 40 years, and it is more common in women than men (4:1). There is an association with connective tissue diseases and autoimmune endocrinopathies.

Neuroimaging usually reveals a hyperintense intrinsic cord lesion extending over at least three vertebral segments (with complete cross-sectional involvement of the cord, and evidence of enhancement with gadolinium). Brain imaging will usually be of normal appearance. Investigations should be performed to exclude other causes of transverse myelitis. Visual-evoked potentials would be expected to be delayed if there is optic nerve involvement. Anti-aquaporin-4 IgG is frequently detected in neuromyelitis optica, but is rarely detected in multiple sclerosis. Lumbar puncture usually reveals normal opening pressure, cerebrospinal fluid pleocytosis and raised protein. Oligoclonal bands are present in up to a third of patients.

Anti-GAD antibody is associated with type 1 diabetes mellitus and stiff-person syndrome; anti-GQ1b antibody is associated with Miller Fischer syndrome; anti-N-methyl-D-aspartate receptor antibody is associated with a form of encephalitis; anti-voltage-gated potassium channel antibody is associated with limbic encephalitis.

Wingerchuk DM, et al. Revised diagnostic criteria for neuromyelitis optica. Neurology 2006; 66:1485–1489.

29. A Commence acetazolamide

This woman has idiopathic intracranial hypertension (also known as pseudotumor cerebri), which can be diagnosed using these criteria:
1. Symptoms and signs of generalised intracranial hypertension in an alert and oriented patient
2. No localising signs (except nerve VI palsy)
3. Normal neuroimaging (apart from signs of raised intracranial pressure)
4. Lumbar puncture with raised opening pressure

5. Normal cerebrospinal fluid analysis
6. No other cause for intracranial hypertension.

Most patients present with severe daily headache which may be associated with nausea and vomiting or synchronous pulsatile tinnitus. There may also be retro-orbital pain associated with eye movements, transient visual obscurations associated with posture, horizontal diplopia-associated abducens nerve palsy, reduced visual acuity, relative afferent pupillary defect, constricted visual fields and an enlarged blind spot. MRI is often of normal appearance, except for signs of raised intracranial pressure (including the appearance of an empty sella turcica). It is, of course, important to exclude more significant pathology such as intracranial mass lesions and dural sinus thrombosis before making the diagnosis of idiopathic intracranial hypertension.

Patients should be reassured and advised to lose weight and restrict salt intake in the first instance. The importance of lifestyle changes should not be underestimated. In addition, pharmacological treatment is often commenced at diagnosis; first-line therapy is with the carbonic anhydrase inhibitor, acetazolamide. However, furosemide and topiramate may also be used. A referral to a neuro-ophthalmologist should be made for formal visual assessment, but surgical interventions such as optic nerve sheath fenestration or ventriculoperitoneal shunts are not usually necessary unless the patient's sight is threatened. Repeat lumbar punctures with cerebrospinal fluid drainage may provide temporary symptomatic relief, but these are rarely used in isolation.

Clarke C, et al (eds). Neuro-ophthalmology (Chapter 13). In: Neurology: A Queen Square Textbook. Oxford: Blackwell Publishing, 2009.
Friedman DI, Jacobson DM. Diagnostic criteria for idiopathic intracranial hypertension. Neurology 2002; 59(10):1492.

30. A Age-related macular degeneration

Age-related macular degeneration (ARMD) is the most common cause of irreversible visual loss in the western world. It occurs as exudative (wet) and non-exudative (dry) forms. The pathophysiology of the two related conditions is not clearly understood.

This patient has exudative ARMD, as evidenced by the characteristic appearance of subretinal blood and fluid at the macula. This leakage occurs secondary to underlying choroidal neovascularisation (CNV). The condition typically presents with blurred central vision, or central visual loss (scotoma) in severe cases. Onset is usually insidious but, in some instances, may be acute.

The non-exudative form is characterised by the presence of multiple small perimacular deposits of white/yellow extracellular material within Bruch's membrane. In a significant minority, the condition may progress to the exudative form.

Fluorescein angiography and optical coherence tomography are useful in assessing the severity of the condition. Although treatment of exudative ARMD was previously centred on the use of laser photocoagulation to destroy areas of CNV, attention is now turning to the use of anti-vascular endothelial growth factor agents to prevent CNV. Many such agents are currently being trialled.

Retinal detachment, choroidal melanoma and preretinal haemorrhage are addressed elsewhere. An epiretinal membrane (sometimes known as a macular pucker) is a transparent layer of scar tissue which forms over the surface of the retina, often in response to ageing and detachment of the posterior vitreous. As the scar tissue contracts it exerts traction on the retina and may cause distortion of vision. It can be treated surgically, by vitrectomy.

de Jong, PT. Age-related macular degeneration. N Engl J Med 2006; 355:1474–1485.

31. E Right posterior cerebral artery territory infarct

High signal is detected within the right cerebral peduncle. This is consistent with a right posterior cerebral artery territory infarct.

Caplan, LR. Caplan's Stroke: A Clinical Approach, 4th edn. Philadelphia, PA: Saunders Elsevier, 2009.
Wardlaw J. Diagnosis of stroke on neuroimaging. BMJ 2004; 328:655.
Clarke C, et al (eds). Stroke and cerebrovascular diseases (Chapter 4). In: Neurology: A Queen Square Textbook. Oxford: Blackwell Publishing, 2009.

32. E Stop all analgesics

This young woman is suffering from chronic daily headache. In the first instance, all analgesics should be stopped. It would then be reasonable to make a fuller assessment of headache type and frequency; a headache diary is useful for this purpose. Once the analgesics have been stopped, a preventive such as propranolol or amitriptyline can be introduced. It is said that preventives are often unsuccessful whereas analgesics are being overused. Clearly, lifestyle changes can be beneficial for headache, but the analgesic overuse is a more pressing issue as it is likely to be significantly contributing to her daily headache. The combined oral contraceptive does not have to be stopped as this patient is not suffering from migraine with aura (in which its use is absolutely contraindicated according to the World Health Organization); however, it can be associated with worsening headache so it may be helpful for the patient to contemplate switching to an alternative form of contraception anyway. There is no indication for MRI of the head at present.

Clarke C, et al (eds). Headache (Chapter 11). In: Neurology: A Queen Square Textbook. Oxfrod: Blackwell Publishing, 2009.
World Health Organization. Medical Eligibility Criteria for Contraceptive Use, 4th edn. Geneva: WHO, 2009.

33. B Branch retinal vein occlusion

The fundoscopic appearance of a single well-confined region of intraretinal haemorrhage within one quadrant is characteristic of branch retinal vein occlusion. Most cases are thought to be due to compression of a branch retinal vein by the corresponding artery which shares the same adventitious sheath. There is a possibility that some people are anatomically predisposed to the condition, but it has been linked to hypertension, hypercholesterolaemia and thrombophilia. It presents clinically as painless deterioration in the vision of one eye, but may be asymptomatic especially if the vein occlusion is away from the macula (i.e. nasal).

The fundoscopic appearance of an acute branch retinal artery occlusion is usually of focal retinal pallor within the affected territory. There may also be evidence of oedema, and the embolus itself may be visible within the occluded vessel. The vessel distal to the embolus may be attenuated and eventually may become thread-like in appearance.

Cholesterol embolus, cytomegalovirus retinitis and hypertensive retinopathy are discussed elsewhere.

Wong T, et al. Retinal-vein occlusion. N Engl J Med 2010; 363:2135–2144.

34. C 6 months

This is in accordance with the current Driver and Vehicle Licensing Authority guidelines. Although these guidelines are specific to the UK, other countries most likely have similar recommendations regarding driving while on antiepileptic medication.

Drivers Medical Group. For Medical Practitioners: At a glance. Guide to the current Medical Standards of Fitness to Drive. Swansea: DVLA, 2012. www.dft.gov.uk/dvla/medical/~/media/pdf/medical/at_a_glance.ashx (last accessed May 2012).

35. E Acute right parietal infarct and old right frontal infarct

The CT of the head reveals an isodense lesion within the right parietal lobe, with loss of grey–white differentiation, and sulcal effacement representing a relatively recent stroke. In addition, there is a large hypodense region in the right frontal lobe, with associated atrophy, consistent with an older established infarct.

Wardlaw J. Diagnosis of stroke on neuroimaging. BMJ 2004; 328:655.
Clarke C, et al (eds). Stroke and cerebrovascular diseases (Chapter 4). In: Neurology: A Queen Square Textbook. Oxford: Blackwell Publishing, 2009.

36. A Diabetic retinopathy

This digital retinal photograph reveals proliferative diabetic retinopathy complicated by preretinal haemorrhage. Signs of proliferative change include neovascularisation of the retina and optic disc, and retinal fibrosis. Features of background and preproliferative diabetic retinopathy such as microaneurysms, blot haemorrhages, hard exudates and 'cotton-wool' spots are also observed.

Unfortunately, neovascularisation can lead to preretinal and vitreous haemorrhage (since the new vessels are fragile and prone to bleeding), and eventually tractional retinal detachment. Panretinal laser photocoagulation is the treatment of choice, and it dramatically reduces the risk of such sight-threatening complications.

This patient should be referred urgently for ophthalmology review.

Macroaneurysm, posterior vitreous detachment, retinal tears and Valsalva's manoeuvres may all cause preretinal haemorrhage.

Frank R. Diabetic retinopathy. N Engl J Med 2004; 350:48–58.

37. D Miller Fisher syndrome

This patient is most likely to be suffering from Miller Fisher syndrome, a condition characterised by ophthalmoplegia, ataxia and areflexia. It is widely considered to be a variant of Guillain–Barré syndrome (GBS). Preceding recent infection, especially with *Campylobacter jejuni* or *Haemophilus influenzae*, predisposes to the condition. GQ1b antibody is detectable in ~95% of cases of Miller Fisher syndrome, and is thought to be pathogenic. Cerebrospinal fluid protein is elevated in ~60% of cases. The condition is usually self-limiting, and rarely requires any specific supportive care or therapeutic intervention, the exception being when it occurs as a GBS overlap syndrome, in which it may rarely progress to generalised severe weakness, requiring close monitoring and support. In such cases, treatment may entail plasma exchange or the administration of intravenous immunoglobulin.

GBS causes acute neuromuscular weakness. It develops in the wake of a predisposing infection (*Campylobacter jejuni*, cytomegalovirus, *Mycoplasma pneumoniae*, Epstein–Barr virus, HIV, *Haemophilus influenzae*). Characteristic features include acute ascending sensorimotor neuropathy and areflexia. Cranial nerve involvement and autonomic dysfunction may also be present. Arrhythmias and labile blood pressure are not uncommon. Potentially sight-threatening papilloedema may sometimes arise. Diagnosis is usually clinical, but nerve conduction studies may show patchy proximal and distal demyelination. Rarely, an axonal neuropathy may be present. Denervation may be detected on electromyography later in the course of severe disease. Anti-GM1 antibody is associated with severe GBS. However, anti-GQ1b antibody is detectable in a significant proportion of cases with ophthalmoplegia. Serological tests may also yield evidence of recent seroconversion, and add further support to the diagnosis.

Bickerstaff's brain-stem encephalitis is also associated with GQ1b antibody. The clinical features may also be similar to those of Miller Fisher syndrome; however, altered consciousness, hyperreflexia and extensor plantar responses are likely to be evident. In about one-third of cases, the MRI of the brain is also abnormal.

Wernicke's encephalopathy is associated with thiamine deficiency, often in the context of chronic alcoholism. The classic clinical triad is of confusion, ophthalmoplegia and ataxia. Signs of the condition may also be apparent on MRI of the brain. In this instance, Wernicke's encephalopathy can be excluded as the patient is oriented and alert, we are not aware of any history of alcohol abuse, the MRI of the brain is pristine and there is another more likely diagnosis. Wernicke's encephalopathy is discussed further elsewhere.

Lambert–Eaton syndrome is similar to myasthenia gravis in that it is associated with impaired acetylcholine activity at the neuromuscular junction. It is an autoimmune disorder, in which anti-voltage-gated calcium channel antibodies are usually present. If diagnosed, underlying malignancy, such as small cell lung cancer, needs to be excluded. In contrast to myasthenia gravis, strength transiently improves with repetitive activity.

Clarke C, et al (eds). Nerve and muscle disease (Chapter 9). In: Neurology: A Queen Square Textbook. Oxford: Blackwell Publishing, 2009.
Overell JR, et al. Recent developments in Miller Fisher syndrome and related disorders. Curr Opin Neurol 2005; 18(5):562–566.

38. B Cervical spondylosis and Chiari I malformation with syringomyelia

This patient's T2-weighted MRI of the cervical spine shows a small syrinx within the cervical spinal cord. In addition, there is evidence of cervical spondylosis at the C5–7 level. Inspection of the cerebellum reveals mild tonsillar descent through the foramen magnum, consistent with a Chiari I malformation.

Syringomyelia is a condition in which an abnormal cerebrospinal fluid-filled cavity forms within the central spinal cord secondary to abnormal cerebrospinal fluid dynamics. It may arise secondary to a number of other conditions, including Chiari malformations, spinal cord tumours, trauma, arachnoiditis, spinal infection and cervical spondylosis. Clinical features include a dissociated sensory loss in the upper limbs (the so-called 'cape distribution' of impaired pain and temperature sensation, with preserved proprioception and vibration sensation). This is due to disruption of the spinothalamic tracts as they cross centrally through the cord at the level of the syrinx. The dorsal columns are normally preserved. In addition, there may be muscle wasting and lower motor neuron weakness in the upper limbs. In severe cases, there may also be a spastic paraparesis below the level of the syrinx.

The Chiari I malformation is defined by descent of the cerebellar tonsils through the foramen magnum. The condition is strongly associated with syringomyelia. This is because the descended cerebellar tonsils, combined with arachnoid adhesions, can prevent normal cerebrospinal fluid pressure transmission through the foramen magnum, causing raised intracranial pressure and increased cerbrospinal fluid flow through the spinal cord aqueduct. Presentation is usually in early to mid adulthood. Clinical features may include headache, which is exacerbated by any action that increases intracranial pressure (coughing, Valsalva's manoeuvre, bending over, etc.), nystagmus and quadriparesis.

The Chiari II malformation is congenital and is associated with myelomeningocele and hydrocephalus. It is defined by downward displacement of the medulla and the cerebellar vermis and tonsils. The fourth ventricle sometimes partially herniates through the foramen magnum. Presentation is usually in the neonatal period. Clinical features may include hydrocephalus, dysphagia, respiratory distress and quadriparesis.

Clarke C, et al (eds). Spinal cord disorders (Chapter 15). In: Neurology: A Queen Square Textbook. Oxford: Blackwell Publishing, 2009.
Butteriss D, Birchall D. A case of syringomyelia associated with cervical spondylosis. Br J Radiol 2006; 79: e123–125.

39. D Progressive multifocal leukoencephalopathy

Natalizumab is a monoclonal antibody that acts to prevent immune cell migration across the blood–brain barrier. It binds to a_4-integrin, primarily at the surface of T cells, and inhibits its interaction with VCAM-1 (vascular cell adhesion molecule 1). In the UK, it is currently licensed for the treatment of rapidly evolving severe relapsing–remitting multiple sclerosis (MS) (defined as two or more disabling relapses within a 1-year period and either one or more gadolinium-enhancing lesions on MRI of the brain or a significant increase in the number of lesions evident on T2 weighting compared with the previous scan).

Clinical trials show that the drug is effective in reducing relapse frequency, delaying disease progression and reducing the number of gadolinium-enhancing lesions on MRI. Unfortunately, however, one of its most serious potential side effects is the development of progressive multifocal leukoencephalopathy (PML), a potentially fatal condition that results from reactivation of John Cunningham papovavirus. Presentation is usually with focal neurological signs, cognitive decline and sometimes seizures. MRI of the brain typically reveals single or multiple high-signal lesions on T2 weighting at the interface of the grey and white matter.

PML is usually diagnosed on account of the clinical history, characteristic appearance on MRI brain and positive cerebrospinal fluid (CSF) polymerase chain reaction result for the virus.

Lathyrism results from ingestion of *Lathyrus sativus* (grass pea). It is thought to contain a neurotoxin that damages the Betz cells of the motor cortex, causing a spastic paraparesis. Acute disseminated encephalomyelitis usually occurs in childhood following an infectious febrile illness or vaccination. It may initially present with fever, meningism, headache and focal neurological signs. The condition can progress rapidly, and seizures, coma and death may ensue. MRI reveals multifocal high-signal lesions on T2 weighting, affecting both grey and white matter, which may become confluent as the disease progresses. Transverse myelitis describes a pattern of inflammation of the spinal cord and has many potential causes, including systemic inflammatory disorders, infection, demyelination, nutrient deficiency and toxins. Neuromyelitis optica is discussed elsewhere.

Clarke C, et al (eds). Multiple sclerosis and demyelinating diseases (Chapter 10). In: Neurology: A Queen Square Textbook. Oxford: Blackwell Publishing, 2009.
Clifford D, et al. Natalizumab-associated progressive multifocal leukoencephalopathy in patients with multiple sclerosis: lessons from 28 cases. Lancet Neurol 2010;9:438–446.

40. D Hypertensive retinopathy

The fundoscopic findings of 'silver-wiring' and arteriovenous nipping are indicative of mild hypertensive retinopathy. The full grading scale is shown in **Table 7.2**.

Table 7.2 Classification of hypertensive retinopathy	
Grade	**Retinal signs**
Mild	• Generalised or focal arteriolar narrowing • Arteriovenous nipping • 'Silver-wiring'
Moderate	• Haemorrhage (dot, blot or flame) • Microaneurysms • Cotton-wool spots • Hard exudates
Malignant	• Signs of moderate retinopathy AND optic disc swelling
Adapted from Wong and Mitchell (2004).	

Central retinal artery occlusion and diabetic retinopathy are discussed elsewhere. Glaucoma causes pallor and cupping of the optic disc. Optic atrophy is recognisable as a pale optic disc with sharply defined borders.

Wong T, Mitchell P. Hypertensive retinopathy. N Engl J Med 2004; 351:2310–2317.

41. E Multifocal motor neuropathy with conduction block

This patient is most probably suffering from multifocal motor neuropathy with conduction block (MMN-CB), an autoimmune demyelinating motor neuropathy. Classically it presents lower motor neuron signs. Onset is usually in the fourth or fifth decade with asymmetrical weakness and cramping within the upper limbs. Weakness is in the distribution of specific nerves (in this case, most notably the left radial nerve) and is disproportionate to the degree of muscle wasting, which is often mild early in the condition. Indeed, muscle wasting and fasciculations tend to be late features. Cranial nerves are rarely involved. The sensory examination is usually completely normal.

Anti-GM1 antibody is detectable in a significant proportion of these patients. MRI of the cervical spine should be normal but is important in excluding other potential causes, such as radiculopathy. Cerebrospinal fluid (CSF) analysis is typically normal, except for slightly elevated protein (rarely exceeding 1 g/L). Ultimately, however, nerve conduction studies are critical in confirming the diagnosis: these are expected to show multifocal conduction block at sites other than those normally associated with extrinsic nerve compression. There may also be reduced compound muscle action potentials. The sensory study should be normal. Additionally, localised denervation may be detected on electromyography.

Chronic inflammatory demyelinating polyneuropathy (CIDP) is the main differential. However, although pure motor and sensory forms of CIDP can occur, it is characteristically a disease of mixed motor and sensory features. It has a similar age of onset with a progressive or relapsing course. Clinical features include proximal and distal weakness with areflexia and tremor. Again, weakness is disproportional to wasting, which is a late feature. Cramping is not as prominent as in MMN-CB. Distal sensory involvement, however, is common. In terms of investigations, the CSF should normally reveal raised protein and the nerve conduction studies should reveal demyelination in at least two nerves. There may be evidence of enlarged or gadolinium-enhancing nerve roots on the MRI. Anti-GM1 antibodies would not classically be expected.

Amyotrophic lateral sclerosis (ALS) would be expected to present with mixed upper and lower motor neuron signs. Fasciculations and muscle wasting are characteristically prominent features. Corticobulbar involvement is also common. Anti-GM1 would not be expected to be positive. ALS is discussed elsewhere.

Charcot–Marie–Tooth disease type 1 (CMT1) is a heritable demyelinating neuropathy. It is genetically heterogeneous, with variable patterns of inheritance. Typically it presents in the first two decades of life with predominant lower limb involvement. There is usually marked symmetrical distal wasting, weakness, depressed deep tendon reflexes and deformity of the feet. Distal sensory impairment is common.

Mononeuritis multiplex describes a pattern of disease in which at least two separate nerves have been affected. There will usually be sensory and motor impairment within the distribution of the affected nerves. It arises secondary to a large number of diseases including diabetes, vasculitis, sarcoidosis, amyloidosis and Lyme disease.

Clarke C, et al (eds). Nerve and muscle disease (Chapter 9). In: Neurology: A Queen Square Textbook. Oxford: Blackwell Publishing, 2009.
Van Schaik IN, et al. Multifocal motor neuropathy (Chapter 21). EFNS guidelines 2011. In: Gilhus NE, et al (eds), European Handbook of Neurological Management, Volume 1, 2nd edn. Oxford: Blackwell, 2011.

42. D Propranolol

This patient has essential tremor, a condition that is far more common than Parkinson's disease. Most cases are thought to have a genetic basis, and there is a positive family history in more than half of all cases. Typically, it presents with a slowly progressive, bilateral, symmetrical tremor that is predominantly kinetic or postural in nature. There may also be titubation or voice tremor. Sometimes resting tremor is also present, but it is not of the 'pill-rolling' type. Interestingly, essential tremor frequently responds well to ethanol; however, although this observation may help point towards the diagnosis, regular alcohol clearly should not be recommended as treatment. In mild cases, reassurance may be all that is necessary. In this case, however, the patient is experiencing functional difficulty and medical treatment should be offered. Propranolol or primidone is most commonly used to treat essential tremor. Rarely, in very severe intractable cases, causing significant functional impairment, deep brain stimulation or surgical ablation of the thalamic ventral intermediate nucleus may be considered.

In contrast, Parkinson's disease is usually idiopathic. Relatively rare genetic forms with variable modes of inheritance and drug-induced forms are also recognised. It is a progressive degenerative disease that typically presents with unilateral resting tremor (characteristically 'pill rolling'). Asymmetrical bilateral involvement, with more severe symptoms on the side of initial onset, is common. Patients exhibit rigidity ('cogwheeling' and 'clasp-knife'), bradykinesia and expressionless facies. The patient's voice may become hypophonic and monotonous. The gait is usually noted to be 'festinant' with increased turning time. Other features may include micrographia (small handwriting), anosmia (loss of sense of smell), drooling, depression, psychosis (with visual hallucinations), dementia, postural instability with falls, 'freezing' and sleep disturbance. Diagnosis is clinical. Response to levodopa is very good, which remains the mainstay of treatment, but motor symptoms and the 'on–off' phenomenon complicate long-term use. Dopamine agonists are, therefore, the preferred treatment in younger patients and are used to delay the time to treatment with levodopa. Diagnosis is clinical.

The National Institute for Health and Clinical Excellence guidelines advise against the use of acute levodopa or apomorphine challenges in the diagnosis of Parkinson's disease. [123I] FP-CIT SPECT (DaT scan) can be diagnostically valuable in cases where it is clinically impossible to differentiate between essential tremor and Parkinson's disease (it measures dopamine reuptake in the presynaptic terminals of striatonigral neurons). However, in this particular patient, the history and clinical findings are characteristic of a diagnosis of essential tremor.

Clarke C, et al (eds). Movement disorders (Chapter 5). In: Neurology: A Queen Square Textbook. Oxford: Blackwell Publishing, 2009.
NICE Clinical Guidelines. Parkinson's disease: diagnosis and management in primary and secondary care (CG35). London: NICE, 2012. http://publications.nice.org.uk/parkinsons-disease-cg35 (last accessed May 2012).

43. D Multiple sclerosis

This patient has multiple sclerosis (MS), an inflammatory demyelinating disease of the central nervous system. The aetiology remains unknown but it predominantly affects white people. There is also an association with some human leukocyte antigen subtypes, suggesting a genetic susceptibility. The condition is more common in women than men, and has a peak incidence in the fourth decade.

In the vast majority of patients, the disease occurs as a relapsing–remitting form. Later, it may enter a secondary progressive phase. Approximately 10% of patients have primary progressive disease. Clinical features are highly variable, depending on the location of plaque formation, but commonly include optic neuritis, cerebellar features, transverse myelitis, hemiparesis, and focal motor or sensory deficit.

The diagnosis of MS is made on the basis of the McDonald criteria. The principle is to demonstrate evidence of central nervous system inflammatory events disseminated in time and space, with other possible causes excluded. Evidence of two clinical episodes typical of MS, such as optic neuritis and a partial transverse myelitis, is sufficient to make a clinical diagnosis. MRI is increasingly used to diagnose MS. Indeed, in some cases, MS can now be diagnosed with a single MRI on presentation.

T2-weighted MRI usually reveals foci of high signal within the periventricular white matter, corpus callosum, brain stem, cerebellum or spinal cord. Visual-evoked potentials or somatosensory-evoked potentials may be delayed, supporting a process of demyelination. Additionally, in nearly all patients with MS, oligoclonal bands are found in the cerebrospinal fluid, but not in the serum. However, this finding is indicative of a local inflammatory process and, therefore, is not specific to MS. Ultimately, the diagnosis requires the demonstration of dissemination of demyelinating plaques in time and space. The MacDonald criteria, which have been revised, are frequently used to guide diagnosis.

The diagnosis of a clinically isolated syndrome is usually a forerunner to the diagnosis of MS. It is made when there is a single clinical episode of demyelination and, therefore, insufficient evidence to demonstrate dissemination of disease in time (and possibly also space, depending on MRI findings). Significant small vessel ischaemic disease would not be expected in a person of this age. Vascular dementia is discussed in more detail elsewhere. Isolated cerebral angiitis usually presents with prominent headache and focal neurological deficit secondary to small/medium vessel infarction. There may also be evidence of haemorrhage. Cerebrospinal fluid is typically positive for oligoclonal bands, but reveals a pleocytosis. Diagnosis usually rests on meningeal or brain biopsy. Limbic encephalitis is discussed elsewhere.

Clarke C, et al (eds). Multiple sclerosis and demyelinating diseases (Chapter 10). In: Neurology: A Queen Square Textbook. Oxford: Blackwell Publishing, 2009.
Polman CH, et al. Diagnostic criteria for multiple sclerosis: 2010 revisions to the McDonald criteria. Ann Neurol 2011; 69(2):292–302.

44. C Intravenous thiamine

This patient is exhibiting features of Wernicke's encephalopathy, a potentially fatal condition of thiamine deficiency. The triad of acute confusion, ataxia and ophthalmoplegia classically defines the condition. However, the clinical presentation is variable, e.g. eye signs may range from nystagmus to complete ophthalmoplegia.

The condition may develop acutely or subacutely and is most commonly reported in those who chronically abuse alcohol. However, it may occur in a wide range of conditions that cause malnutrition (such as gastrointestinal surgery, eating disorders, malignancy). The mainstay of immediate management is parenteral thiamine replacement. Timely treatment usually results in rapid resolution of the clinical signs, and avoids the significant mortality associated with the untreated condition. In practice, intravenous Pabrinex – a cocktail of B vitamins and vitamin C – is usually administered; this helps to prevent the complications of the broader spectrum of vitamin deficiency.

Thiamine has an important role as a coenzyme in a number of metabolic pathways (including the oxidation of glucose, the catabolism of amino acids and the biosynthesis of neurotransmitters). As such, the administration of dextrose to the thiamine-deficient patient potentially accelerates neurological damage by consuming the little remaining thiamine in the oxidation of glucose. Therefore, thiamine stores should be replaced before dextrose is administered (note that, in patients with low magnesium stores, the parental thiamine may be ineffective until magnesium has been restored to a normal level).

This patient is not violently agitated and does not warrant treatment with intramuscular lorazepam. Nor is there any evidence that he is psychotic and in need of treatment with antipsychotic medication. Aciclovir is an antiviral agent and is not indicated.

Clarke C, et al (eds). Toxic, metabolic and physical insults (Chapter 18). In: Neurology: A Queen Square Textbook. Oxford: Blackwell Publishing, 2009.

45. D Photocoagulation scarring

This patient has undergone extensive laser photocoagulation of the retina to treat proliferative diabetic retinopathy. In this case, a single large blot haemorrhage is also evident inferior to the disc. Panretinal photocoagulation (PRP) is typified by multiple, well-circumscribed, punched-out areas of retinal atrophy with some reactive hyperpigmentation. This is usually applied to the entire peripheral retina but avoiding the macula.

A choroidal haemangioma is a benign tumour which, as its name suggests, is located in the choroid and appears as a well-circumscribed orange–red region on fundoscopy. They are often asymptomatic and discovered incidentally. They can, however, present with visual disturbance and there is a risk of retinal detachment due to cystic degeneration. Management is usually conservative, but photodynamic therapy may have a role in some cases.

Chorioretinitis is addressed elsewhere.

Onchocerciasis is a filarial disease (also known as river blindness) which may cause choroiditis, glaucoma and optic atrophy. It also causes punctate keratitis and, in severe cases, may result in corneal fibrosis and opacification.

Retinitis pigmentosa is characterised by a 'bone-spicule' pattern of perivascular retinal hyperpigmentation in the mid-peripheries, associated with, retinal pigment epithelium atrophy. Typically the macula is spared. The retinal arteries eventually become attenuated and thread like, and the optic disc may become pale and waxy in appearance.

Bressler N, et al. Panretinal photocoagulation for proliferative diabetic retinopathy. N Engl J Med 2011; 365:1520–1526.

46. E Small fibre neuropathy

This patient is most likely suffering from a small fibre peripheral neuropathy, which may be secondary to impaired glucose tolerance. Typically, patients complain of burning, tingling or numbness in a glove-and-stocking distribution. Symptoms are often most problematic at night, and can have a significant impact on sleep. Clinical examination reveals normal motor function, normal proprioception and vibration sense. There is usually reduced sensation to pinprick and thermal hypoaesthesia, due to involvement of small unmyelinated C-fibres and lightly myelinated Aδ-fibres. The effect is usually length dependent, so the deficit tends to affect the feet first and progresses fairly symmetrically. Concurrent involvement of the small fibres of the autonomic nervous system is not uncommon; clinical features may include orthostatic hypotension and impotence, for example. Nerve conduction studies are almost always normal. However, if necessary, a skin biopsy may be performed to help make the diagnosis; this may demonstrate a reduced density of intraepithelial C-fibres. There are numerous causes of small fibre neuropathy, including 'prediabetic' states, but a large proportion of cases are idiopathic.

Psychosomatic disorders warrant consideration in the differential list of causes, but conversion disorder is clearly not the best explanation for this patient's condition. Conversion disorder is discussed elsewhere.

Diabetic amyotrophy describes a pattern of proximal muscle weakness that may complicate diabetes. It can be discounted based on the history and clinical findings.

Mononeuritis multiplex describes a pattern of nerve damage, in which there is discrete damage to at least two separate peripheral nerves, as a result of an underlying disease (e.g. diabetes mellitus, systemic lupus erythematosus, amyloidosis, sarcoidosis, Lyme disease and many more). This condition can be discounted as the patient exhibits a 'stocking' distribution of sensory involvement, rather than a 'nerve' distribution of motor and sensory deficit.

Restless legs syndrome may occur secondary to small fibre neuropathy. However, in this patient's case, the principal problem is neuropathic pain. The diagnostic criteria for restless legs syndrome are discussed elsewhere.

Clarke C, et al (eds). Nerve and muscle disease (Chapter 9). In: Neurology: A Queen Square Textbook. Oxford: Blackwell Publishing, 2009.
Devigili G, et al. The diagnostic criteria for small fibre neuropathy: from symptoms to neuropathology. Brain 2008; 131(7):1912–1925.
Papanas YN, et al. Neuropathy in prediabetes: does the clock start ticking early? Nat Rev Endocrinol 2011; 7:682–690.

47. D Stop combined oral contraceptive pill (COCP)

The COCP is contraindicated in migraine with aura, owing to the fact that it increases the risk of ischaemic stroke (approximately eightfold). Therefore, in the first instance, this patient should stop the COCP in favour of an alternative method of contraception. As far as migraine management goes, she should be reassessed after stopping the COCP. If the attacks are infrequent, it would be reasonable to attempt to manage these with aspirin and domperidone, or a similar combination, to begin with. Should these fail, a triptan would be appropriate. If, of course, the attacks are occurring frequently, typically three times per month or more, then preventive treatment should be implemented; there are many such treatments, e.g. propranolol, amitriptyline, pizotifen, topiramate, each with their own merits, limitations and side-effect profiles.

World Health Organization Press. Medical Eligibility Criteria for Contraceptive Use, 4th edn. Geneva: WHO, 2009.
Curtis KM, et al. Use of combined oral contraceptives amongst women with migraine and nonmigrainous headaches: a systematic review. Contraception 2006; 73:189–194.
Etminan M, et al. Risk of ischaemic stroke in people with migraine: systematic review and meta-analysis of observational studies. BMJ 2005; 330:63.

48. E Intracerebral haemorrhage

This CT of the brain reveals a small hyperdense lesion within the left basal ganglia, consistent with an intracerebral haemorrhage.

Arteriovenous malformations may be apparent on non-enhanced CT; foci of calcification are not uncommon within the abnormal vessels. A clinically isolated syndrome refers to a first episode of neurological symptoms resulting from neuroinflammation and lasting more than 24 hours. It is often the forerunner to a diagnosis of multiple sclerosis. However, it is not typically associated with headache and foci of demyelination are not usually evident on non-enhanced CT. Fahr's syndrome is a rare genetic disorder that results in calcification predominantly within the basal ganglia, but also within the cerebral cortex. Glioma is described elsewhere.

Wardlaw J. Diagnosis of stroke on neuroimaging. BMJ 2004; 328:655.
Clarke C, et al (eds). Stroke and cerebrovascular diseases (Chapter 4). In: Neurology: A Queen Square Textbook. Oxford: Blackwell Publishing, 2009.

Chapter 8

Oncology and palliative medicine

Questions

1. A 66-year-old man presented with symptoms of facial swelling and a feeling of fullness in the head. This had started 2 weeks ago. He had no past medical history of note and took no medication.

    On examination, he had facial plethora and swelling, raised internal and external jugular veins, and dilated veins across his superior anterior chest wall.

    Which one of the following is the least likely underlying cause of his condition?

    A   Germ cell cancer
    B   Lymphoma
    C   Myxoma
    D   Non-small cell lung cancer
    E   Small cell lung cancer

2. A 35-year-old woman was referred to the gastroenterology clinic for consideration of colorectal cancer (CRC) screening, after her brother was diagnosed with colorectal cancer at the age of 48 years.

    What is the most appropriate CRC screening programme?

    A   Colonoscopy age 45 years and then every 5 years until age 75 years
    B   Colonoscopy age 35 years, and if normal no further colonoscopies
    C   Colonoscopy age 50 years and then 10 yearly until age 70 years
    D   Colonoscopy age 55 years, and if normal no further colonoscopies
    E   Colonoscopy age 65 years and then 5 yearly until the age of 75 years

3. A 54-year-old man underwent a chest X-ray because of shortness of breath on exertion. He was a smoker of 20 cigarettes per day (35 pack-years). This demonstrated a left upper lobe mass. Further investigations are arranged.

    Investigations:

CT: 3-cm mass lesion left upper lobe ipsilateral lymphadenopathy 1.4 cm CT staging T2aN1M0 (stage IIa)
Bronchoscopy: tumour emerging from the left upper lobe bronchus
Bronchial biopsy: squamous cell carcinoma
Spirometry: forced expiratory volume$_1$ 2.4 L (83% predicted)

His case was discussed by the lung cancer multi-disciplinary team

What is the most appropriate next step in management?

A   Best supportive care
B   Chemotherapy
C   Endobronchial ultrasound
D   Lobectomy
E   Position emission tomography (PET) scan

4.   A 65-year-old woman was seen in the oncology clinic to discuss treatment of her ovarian cancer. Previously she had undergone platinum-based chemotherapy but the disease had recurred.
        Further therapy with doxorubicin chemotherapy was discussed.

Which one of the following is not a recognised side effect of anthracycline-based chemotherapy?

A   Cardiotoxicity
B   Colonic ulceration
C   Conjunctivitis
D   Peripheral neuropathy
E   Thrombocytopenia

5.   A 77-year-old man presented with a history of weight loss, fatigue and generalised aching for the preceding 6 months. He had recently developed abdominal pain and constipation. Systemic enquiry revealed no other symptoms. He had a past medical history of hypertension and angina, and his current medications were bendrofluazide, aspirin, simvastatin and nifedipine.
        On examination, he was thin; respiratory, cardiovascular and abdominal examinations were unremarkable.

Investigations:

corrected calcium 2.94 mmol/L (2.2–2.6)	alanine transaminase 32 U/L (5–35)
phosphate 1.3 mmol/L (0.8–1.4)	albumin 34 g/L (37)
parathyroid hormone 6 pmol/L (0.9–5.4)	IgG 8.0 g/L (6.0–13.0)
parathyroid hormone-related protein (PTHrP) 0.3 pmol/L (<1.8)	IgA 2.1 g/L (0.8–3.0)
	IgM 2.5 g/L (0.4–2.5)
bilirubin 18 mmol/L (1–22)	25-hydroxycholecalciferol 50 nmol/L (45–90)
alkaline phosphatase 389 U/L (45–105)	

What is the most likely diagnosis?

A   Bony metastases
B   Myeloma
C   Primary hyperparathyroidism
D   Paraneoplastic PTHrP production
E   Vitamin D deficiency

6.   A 74-year-old retired male builder presented with a 3-month history of dull right-sided chest discomfort, shortness of breath on exertion and sweating. He had no past medical history of note. He remained active and there was no limitation to his normal activities of daily living.
        A chest X-ray was performed (see **Figure 8.1**).
        Following this he had a CT of the chest and then he was referred to the thoracic surgeons for a video-assisted thoracoscopic surgical (VATS) biopsy to confirm the diagnosis.

What is the most appropriate management?

A   Cisplatin and pemetrexed

Figure 8.1

B Insertion of indwelling chest drain
C Pneumonectomy
D Radical radiotherapy
E Radiotherapy to surgical port sites

7. A 72-year-old man presented with weight loss and anaemia and was found to have a gastric carcinoma on endoscopy. He had been previously fit and well.

Investigations:

CT of the chest/abdomen/pelvis:

mass in distal gastric region

no metastases

no lymphadenopathy

Histology: gastric adenocarcinoma with HER-2-positive receptors

What is the most appropriate management?

A Chemoradiotherapy
B Chemotherapy with 5-fluorouracil
C Gastrectomy and irinotecan
D Gastrectomy and radiotherapy
E Gastrectomy, chemotherapy and trastuzumab

8. A 46-year-old Chinese man was found to have a 2.5-cm liver lesion on ultrasound. He was known to have chronic hepatitis B virus cirrhosis but was not on treatment. He was fit and well and employed as a carpenter. He had no evidence of portal hypertension and had no other past medical history.
    Physical examination was normal.

Investigations:

Triple phase CT of the liver:
liver looked cirrhotic with irregular border but normal portal vein flow and no ascites
single 2.5-cm nodule in segment 5 with arterial hypervascularity and delayed phase wash-out

bilirubin 18 mmol/L (1–22)	albumin 34 g/L (37–49)
alkaline phosphatase 196 U/L (45–105)	international normalised ratio 1.1 (<1.4)
alanine transaminase 24 U/L (5–35)	

What is the most appropriate management?

A   Liver resection
B   Liver transplantation
C   Radiofrequency ablation
D   Sorafenib
E   Transarterial chemoembolisation (TACE)

9. A 68-year-old man presented to the emergency department. He had no significant medical history and had been well until 3 weeks previously when he had started to experience increasingly severe back pain over his mid-spine. He had noticed over the last 2 days that he had had some difficulty in walking.
    On examination of his lower limbs he had increased tone bilaterally, reduced power, 3/5 proximally and 2/5 distally, brisk reflexes and up-going plantars. He had impaired sensation to a level just below his umbilicus.
    An urgent MRI of his spine confirmed a single lesion suspicious of a metastasis at T10.

Investigations:

prostate-specific antigen 90 ng/mL (<3)

What is the most appropriate next step in management?

A   Bone biopsy
B   Chemotherapy
C   High-dose steroids and discuss with spinal surgeons
D   Non-steroidal anti-inflammatory drugs, pamidronate and discuss with spinal surgeons
E   Radiotherapy

10. A 75-year-old man presented with flank pain and macroscopic haematuria.
    On examination, there was a palpable mass in the right side of his abdomen. He had a CT of the abdomen performed (see **Figure 8.2**).

Which one of the following is correct regarding the diagnosis?

A   He requires a bilateral nephrectomy
B   He requires a bone scan to assess for metastases
C   He requires a unilateral nephrectomy
D. He requires an urgent biopsy of his right kidney
E   He requires no further imaging as metastasis is rare

Figure 8.2

11. A 64-year-old man presented with a 2-week history of progressive shortness of breath at rest. He had advanced non-small cell lung cancer and severe chronic obstructive pulmonary disease. Six months ago, he completed four cycles of palliative chemotherapy, but his cancer had progressed and he was referred to the palliative care team. He was taking maximal inhaled bronchodilator and inhaled corticosteroids therapy and oral morphine 5 mg every 4 hours.

On examination, he was apyrexial, respiratory rate 14 breaths per minute and oxygen saturation 95% on air. There was a small right pleural effusion.

Investigations:

haemoglobin 10.7 g/dL (13.0–18.0)   white cell count 6.9 × 10⁹/L (4–11)

What is the best management step to improve the dyspnoea?

A   Antibiotics
B   Aspiration of effusion
C   Blood transfusion
D   Lorazepam
E   Oxygen

12. A local research and ethics committee is considering an application to investigate whether mobile phone use is associated with multiple myeloma. A hospital review is planned of mobile phone usage in hours per week of all patients diagnosed with multiple myeloma in the last 5 years. The aim is to question age-and sex-matched patients (at a ratio of 3:1 to those with multiple myeloma) from the hospital who have not been diagnosed with multiple myeloma and review their mobile phone use.

What type of clinical study is this project?

A   Case–control study
B   Cohort study

C Ecological study
D Point prevalence study
E Randomised controlled trial

13. A 74-year-old man with a history of chronic obstructive pulmonary disease and hypertension was referred to the chest clinic with worsening shortness of breath, intermittent haemoptysis and left-sided back pain. He was an ex-smoker of 50 pack-years after quitting 5 years ago. His current medications include a combination steroid and long-acting β_2-agonist inhaler, amlodipine, aspirin and he has recently commenced co-codamol.

An urgent CT of the thorax was performed (see **Figure 8.3**).

Figure 8.3

What is the most likely diagnosis?

A Aspergilloma
B Lung abscess
C Small cell carcinoma
D Squamous cell carcinoma
E Tuberculosis

14. A 64-year-old man presented with a history of dysphagia for solids and weight loss. He had no other medical problems, and took no medication.

Investigations:

Upper gastrointestinal endoscopy: 2 × 1.5 cm neoplastic appearing lesion at 15 cm from incisor teeth

CT of the chest/abdomen/pelvis:

2-cm soft tissue mass confined to the upper oesophagus

no metastases in liver or lungs

no localised lymphadenopathy

Histology: squamous cell carcinoma

What is the most appropriate therapy?

A Chemoradiotherapy

B Oesophagectomy alone
C Oesophagectomy and radiotherapy
D Oesophagectomy with neoadjuvant chemotherapy
E Radiotherapy

15. An 88-year-old woman was being treated palliatively for metastatic ovarian carcinoma. She presented with increasing abdominal pain and nausea. She had not opened her bowels for 5 days. She had been taking increasing doses of Oramorph for pain relief. She was known to have a nut allergy. On examination, she was frail and clinically dehydrated.

Which one of the following is most suitable regarding her on-going symptom management?

A Arachis oil can be given
B Co-danthramer should be avoided if the patient is incontinent
C Fybogel mebeverine should be used as a first-line agent
D Liquid paraffin can be used
E Laxatives can be withdrawn when opiate dose is stabilised

16. A 56-year-old woman with a history of ischaemic heart disease was diagnosed with human epidermal growth factor receptor-2 (HER-2)-positive early invasive breast cancer. A mastectomy with adjuvant chemotherapy and trastuzumab was planned.

Which of the following is a contraindication to treatment with trastuzumab?

A Atrial fibrillation
B Congestive cardiac failure
C Hypertension
D Mitral valve prolapse
E Previous cerebrovascular accident

17. A 57-year-old man presented with a 6-month history of intermittent abdominal pain and loose stools. He had been opening his bowel five times per day, with no associated rectal bleeding or mucus. He reported occasional episodes of facial and neck flushing. He had recently been diagnosed with asthma, for which he was taking salbutamol and beclometasone inhalers.

On examination, he looked thin. Cardiovascular, respiratory and abdominal examinations were normal.

What is the most useful diagnostic investigation?

A Adrenocorticotrophic hormone levels
B C-peptide level
C Fasting gastrin level
D Serum 5-hydroxytryptamine levels
E Urinary 5-HIAA (5-hydroxyindoleacetic acid) levels

18. An 84-year-old man with metastatic lung carcinoma was referred to hospital with a 3-day history of worsening shortness of breath. He was frail and largely housebound.

On examination, his respiratory rate was 34 breaths per minute and oxygen saturations 84% on air and 92% on 10 L oxygen. Clinically he had a large right pleural effusion confirmed on chest X-ray. He had 1000 mL aspirated with a cannula and felt better. Cytology revealed malignant cells. Three days later, the patient complained of worsening shortness of breath and a repeat chest X-ray demonstrated increased size of the pleural effusion.

What is the most appropriate next step in management?

A Chest drain insertion and talc pleurodesis
B Commence Oramorph
C Commence lorazepam
D Repeat therapeutic aspiration of 1000 mL with cannula
E Refer for video-assisted thoracoscopic surgical (VATS) drainage and talc pleurodesis

19. A 52-year-old woman was seen in the clinic after a total thyroidectomy for medullary thyroid carcinoma. She was on levothyroxine replacement but not on any other medication. She did not have any other past medical history. She complained of episodes of sweating, flushing and palpitations associated with anxiety and headaches.

    On examination, her temperature was 36.8°C, pulse 88 beats per minute, blood pressure 170/110 mmHg and respiratory rate 18 breaths per minute. There was no tremor of the outstretched hands and she was clinically euthyroid.

    What is the most useful diagnostic investigation?

    A   Serum corrected calcium
    B   Serum parathyroid hormone level
    C   Serum thyroid-stimulating hormone concentration
    D   Transthoracic echocardiogram
    E   Urine 24-hour metanephrines

20. A 58-year-old man presented with a single generalised tonic–clonic seizure on a background of several months' history of daily headache.

    An MRI of the brain was performed (see **Figure 8.4**):

Figure 8.4

    What is the most likely diagnosis?

    A   Arteriovenous malformation
    B   Cerebral toxoplasmosis
    C   Glioma
    D   Meningioma
    E   Neurocysticercosis

21. A 74-year-old woman with Alzheimer's disease (Mini Mental State Examination 17/30) has been admitted with 2 days of bilious vomiting and a diagnosis of intussusception has been made. After anaesthetic review it is thought she would survive a laparotomy and surgical resolution of the intussusception. However, she is declining the operation and in two previous clinic letters over the last 3 years note is made of her wish not to have any invasive procedures or surgery to prolong her life because of her diagnosis of Alzheimer's disease. Her daughter and her son wish for her to have the operation and are arguing strongly for it to occur without further delay.

What is the most appropriate next step in management?

A   Involve the palliative care team in the decision-making process
B   Not proceed with the operation
C   Proceed with the operation
D   Talk to the family and obtain the written permission of the next of kin for the operation to proceed
E   Try to relieve the intussusception with flexible sigmoidoscopy

22. A 67-year-old woman with was diagnosed with early oestrogen-positive invasive breast cancer. After surgery it was decided that she should have adjuvant chemotherapy.

What is the most appropriate management?

A   5-Fluorouracil
B   Anastrozole
C   Exemestane
D   Tamoxifen
E   Trastuzumab

23. A 62-year-old woman was referred to the chest clinic with right-sided chest pain, breathlessness, haemoptysis, weight loss and an abnormal chest X-ray. She was a lifelong heavy smoker (>80 pack-years).

Investigations:

CT of the chest and abdomen: large mass in the right lower lobe invading into the mediastinum and pericardium, extensive mediastinal lymphadenopathy and bone metastasis (T4N3M1b)
Bronchoscopic biopsies: squamous cell carcinoma
Mutation analysis: epidermal growth factor receptor negative

What is the most appropriate first-line therapy?

A   Cetuximab
B   Docetaxel
C   Gemcitabine and cisplatin
D   Pemetrexed
E   Vinorelbine

24. A 74-year-old man underwent Hartmann's procedure for a sigmoid tumour. He underwent a preoperative staging CT which showed tumour invading into the sigmoid wall and two enlarged mesenteric lymph nodes suggestive of metastasis. No distant metastases were seen.
     Histology of the mass showed a 5.4-cm adenocarcinoma, with complete resection margins. The tumour had invaded the muscularis propria but no adjacent structures.

What is his TNM staging classification?

A   T1N0M1
B   T2N1M0
C   T2N0M1
D   T3N1M0
E   T4N1M0

Answers

1. C Myxoma

This man has superior vena cava obstruction (SVCO) as evidenced by his facial plethora and swelling and dilated neck and chest veins. SVCO can have malignant or non-malignant aetiology, and the latter now accounts for 35% of cases of SVCO. The most common non-malignant causes are thrombosis secondary to implanted devices such as pacemakers or catheters, fibrosing mediastinitis and aortic aneurysm. The most common malignant cause is non-small cell lung cancer accounting for 50% of malignant cases, followed by small cell lung cancer (22%), lymphoma (12%), metastatic cancer (most commonly breast – 9%), germ cell tumours (3%) and thymoma (2%). Myxomas are cardiac tumours predominantly found in the atria and are most likely to present as heart failure.

Wilson LD, Detterbeck FC, Yahalom J. Superior vena cava syndrome with malignant causes. N Engl J Med 2007; 356:1862–1869.

2. D Colonoscopy aged 55 years, and if normal no further colonoscopies

The British Society of Gastroenterology colorectal cancer (CRC) screening guidelines categorise people with a family history of CRC into high, high-moderate, low-moderate or low-risk groups, based on the presence or absence of hereditary polyposis syndromes and the age and number of affected first-degree relatives. Colorectal cancer is common, and the incidence of an affected first-degree relative (FDR) among the general population is 4–10%. In the scenario given the patient has one affected FDR aged less than 50 years which equates to a low-moderate risk, and a colonoscopy at the age of 55 years is the appropriate screening test. If this is normal then no further colonoscopies need to be done.

To be high risk the patient would need to have a personal or family history suggestive of, or germline mutations indicating, Lynch's syndrome, familial adenomatous polyposis, MUTYH [mutY homologue (E. coli)]-associated polyposis (MAP), juvenile polyposis or Peutz–Jeghers syndrome. The lifetime risk of CRC in these syndromes ranges from 10% to 100%. Screening for these syndromes is covered in detail in the British Society of Gastroenterology guidelines.

The following family history would be considered high-moderate risk:
- Three affected first-degree relatives of any age. However, IF one of the three relatives is less than 50 years old then they would be considered high risk.
- If there are two affected first-degree relatives aged less than 60 OR if there are two affected relatives who have a mean age of less than 60 years AND one of them is a first-degree relative of the patient.

These patients with high-to-moderate risk should have 5-yearly colonoscopies starting at age 55 years until they are 75 years of age.

The following family history is considered to give a low-to-moderate risk:
- A single affected first-degree relative aged less than 50 years
- Two affected relatives who are aged over 60 years, of first-degree kinship.

These patients should have one colonoscopy at age 55 years and if this is normal no further colonoscopies are required.

Cairns SR, et al. Guidelines for colorectal cancer screening and surveillance in moderate and high risk groups (update from 2002). Gut 2010; 59:666–690.

3. E Position emission tomography (PET) scan

This patient has early disease (stages I to II) and should be considered for surgical resection. PET scanning should be performed prior to attempted surgical resection because it can help determine whether there is evidence of distant metastatic disease. Malignant lesions are more likely to be 'PET avid' and demonstrate uptake of fluorodeoxyglucose (FDG). If a PET scan suggests that there is lymph node involvement which would preclude surgical resection, histological confirmation needs to be done next. This approach has been shown to reduce the number of inappropriate and/or futile operations. The combination of CT and PET scanning also improves radiotherapy planning.

Techniques for nodal sampling include: endobronchial ultrasound (EBUS), which is one of the least invasive tests; endoscopic ultrasound (EUS) via the oesophagus; mediastinoscopy; mini-thoracotomy; and video-assisted thoracoscopic surgery (VATS). The last three tests necessitate general anaesthesia with its associated risks.

Patients should be considered for surgery if they are fit enough for the procedure and if predicted lung function following resection is sufficient to maintain good function. Fitness is determined by performance status, lung function [forced expiratory volume (FEV_1) >1.5 L for lobectomy, >2 L for pneumonectomy or more than 60% predicted] and other co-morbidities need to be considered.

Palliative chemotherapy and palliative care should be considered as primary treatments for patients presenting with more advanced disease and/or if other associated co-morbidities dictate that more radial treatments are too high risk and less likely to confer survival advantage.

Scherpereel A, et al. ERS/ESTS Task Force. Guidelines of the European Respiratory Society and the European Society of Thoracic Surgeons for the management of malignant pleural mesothelioma. Eur Respir J 2010; 35:479–495.

4. D Peripheral neuropathy

Doxorubicin belongs to the anthracycline class of chemotherapeutic drugs. It is used in the treatment of breast and ovarian cancer and haematological malignancies. The most important dose-related side effects are cardiotoxicity (particularly delayed cardiomyopathy in children) and myelosuppression. It is known to cause gastrointestinal side effects such as nausea and vomiting, colonic (particularly caecal) ulceration, mucositis, alopecia and ocular side effects such as conjunctivitis. It causes myelosuppression, and although it does not usually cause thrombocytopenia it can occur. Peripheral neuropathy has not been reported in clinical trials.

Monseuz JJ, et al. Cardiac side effects of cancer chemotherapy. Int J Cardiol 2010; 11:3–15.

5. A Bony metastases

The patient has hypercalcaemia, with a normal phosphate, high alkaline phosphatase (ALP), low parathyroid hormone (PTH) and normal vitamin D levels. The most likely diagnosis is bony metastases. Investigation of hypercalcaemia can helpfully be divided into two pathways, one for those with high PTH levels and one for those with low or suppressed PTH levels. If the PTH is high then the diagnosis is either primary or tertiary hyperparathyroidism or familial hypocalciuric hypercalcaemia. If the PTH level is low or normal (i.e. appropriately suppressed for the hypercalcaemia) then the most common diagnosis is malignancy. The presence of a raised alkaline phosphatase is highly suggestive of bony metastases. If the PTHrP (PTH-related protein) level is raised then a PTHrP-secreting tumour is the likely cause, the most common of which is small cell cancer of the lung. Myeloma can cause hypercalcaemia, and in this case a raised IgG (75% of cases) or raised IgA (25% of cases) level would be expected. Urinary Bence Jones protein should also be detected. Severe vitamin D deficiency can cause hypercalcaemia due to tertiary hyperparathyroidism whereby prolonged hypocalcaemia caused by vitamin D deficiency leads to overactivity of PTH which then becomes permanent, but the low PTH level rules this out together with primary hyperparathyroidism as causes of this man's hypercalcaemia.

Carroll M. A practical approach to hypercalcaemia. Am Fam Physician 2003; 67:1959–1966.
Carrol R, et al. Review: Endocrine and metabolic emergencies: Hypercalcaemia. Ther Adv Endocrinol Metab 2010; 1:225.

6. A Cisplatin and pemetrexed

The chest X-ray demonstrates a right-sided pleural effusion with associated pleural thickening and the history is very suggestive of mesothelioma. He was a retired builder and is likely to have had occupational exposure to asbestos. Asbestos is the single major cause of mesothelioma and the mean latent interval between first exposure and death is around 40 years. There is no significant association with smoking.

Patients may present with chest pain, which is usually dull in nature; however, pleuritic pain has also been described, and breathlessness. Profuse sweating may also be a feature. Weight loss and fatigue are rare at presentation, but are common features later in the disease. Imaging may demonstrate moderate-to-large pleural effusion, with nodular pleural thickening or pleural mass, uniform encasement of the lung with resulting small hemithorax and/or invasion of chest wall or other structures. The diagnosis should be confirmed histologically by ultrasound or CT-guided biopsy. Early use of thoracoscopy may provide diagnosis and enable management of large effusions with talc pleurodesis. The median survival is 9–12 months from diagnosis.

Patients with good performance status should be considered for palliative chemotherapy. The combination of cisplatin and pemetrexed has been demonstrated to have a response rate (tumour shrinkage >50%) of 41%.

Palliative radiotherapy may be useful, in selected patients, to help reduce chest wall pain, breathlessness and superior vena cava obstruction. Currently, there is no role for radical radiotherapy. Prophylactic radiotherapy to biopsy or surgical port sites may reduce chest wall invasion by tumour; however, a randomised study failed to demonstrate a benefit. Surgical resection remains controversial and currently there are no randomised controlled trials demonstrating survival advantage following pneumonectomy.

In patients with recurrent pleural effusion, who have failed talc pleurodesis or have trapped lung, an indwelling chest drain may be considered as a palliative option.

7. E Gastrectomy, chemotherapy and trastuzumab

A gastrectomy is required for this patient. Perioperative chemotherapy in gastric adenocarcinoma confers a survival benefit and is the additional treatment of choice in the UK. In those patients who are HER-2 receptor positive then addition of trastuzumab gives an overall survival benefit and improves disease-free survival, so this should be considered in all HER-2-positive patients. Chemotherapy alone is not standard practice, and there is no role for chemoradiotherapy in gastric carcinoma. Irinotecan is a second-line therapy and confers a small survival benefit over best supportive care but it is not currently recommended by the NICE.

Allum WH. BSG guidelines. Guidelines for the management of oesophageal and gastric cancer. Gut 2011; 60:1449–1472.

8. A Liver resection

This man has hepatocellular carcinoma (HCC) on a background of hepatitis B virus cirrhosis. He has early stage cirrhosis and limited stage disease, having a single lesion which is less than 3 cm in size. He has a good performance status. The American Association for the Study of Liver Diseases (AASLD) guidelines on therapy for HCC indicate that he should have a liver resection to remove the lesion. A liver transplantation would be the treatment of choice if he had up to three nodules of less than 3 cm in diameter, and no other co-morbidities, or a single lesion less than 3 cm with evidence of a raised bilirubin or portal hypertension. Radiofrequency ablation is used for patients with three nodules of less than 3 cm who have co-morbidities that preclude liver transplantation. These are all curative treatments. Patients with multinodular HCC and a performance status of 0 should have transarterial chemoembolisation, and those with multinodular HCC or portal invasion with a performance status of 1 or 2 should be offered sorafenib. Sorafenib is a multikinase inhibitor that has been proven to give a clinically relevant improvement in time to progression and in survival.

AASLD practice guideline: Update on the management of hepatocellular carcinoma. Hepatology 2011; 53(3):1020–1022.

9. C High-dose steroids and discuss with spinal surgeons

This patient has presented with signs and symptoms of spinal cord compression (SCC). It is a common oncological emergency, particularly affecting patients with prostate, lung and breast malignancy. Symptoms of weakness are commonly preceded by back pain. The majority of lesions (around 60%) are found in the thoracic spine. As well as pain, motor and gait disturbance, patients may present with bowel and bladder disturbance. Patients presenting with such symptoms should have urgent imaging of their entire spine. MRI is the modality of choice and this should include the entire spine to look for any other evidence of metastases.

If SCC is diagnosed then high-dose steroids (dexamethasone 16 mg once daily in two divided doses with proton pump inhibitor cover) should be started immediately. This relieves the inflammation around the cord and can improve neurological symptoms and long-term neurological outcome. The case should then be discussed with the on-call spinal surgeons. Although radiotherapy is a good treatment option, there is evidence that this combined with surgery rather than as an isolated treatment results in a better outcome. This is particularly true in an otherwise well patient with a good performance status, as in this case, with a single bony metastasis who would be a good surgical operative candidate. In patients who are not suitable for surgery, radiotherapy would be the best treatment after steroids are started.

Non-steroidal anti-inflammatory drugs and pamidronate are both commonly used in the treatment of bone pain caused by metastatic disease but will not improve SCC. Although bone biopsy may be of use to establish the diagnosis, it is fairly clear that this patient has metastatic prostate cancer and it is not going to alter the immediate management of his SCC. Chemotherapy is not routinely used in the treatment of SCC as most tumours causing compression will not be particularly chemoresponsive.

Patchell RA, et al. Direct decompressive surgical resection in the treatment of spinal cord compression caused by metastatic cancer: a randomised trial. Lancet 2005; 366:643–648.

10. B He should have a bone scan to assess for metastases

This patient has a diagnosis of a renal cell carcinoma (RCC). RCCs constitute 80–85% of primary renal neoplasms. They are adenocarcinomas which originate from within the renal cortex. They are more common in men and there are often bilateral lesions.

RCC can present with a variety of symptoms but the classic triad is pain, haematuria and an abdominal mass. Increasingly, asymptomatic cases are being diagnosed upon finding an incidental mass on radiographic examination. They are also associated with a paraneoplastic syndrome which includes fever, weight loss, anaemia, hepatic dysfunction and hormonal effects. Hypercalcaemia is relatively common and can be as a result of parathyroid hormone-related peptide production or bone metastasis.

Often the tumours are slow growing and patients remain asymptomatic, so metastasis at the time of diagnosis is common; therefore, it is important to assess for local and metastatic spread with CT, MRI and bone scan. A renogram may help determine split function of the kidneys which may be important in planning treatment. Needle biopsy of the mass should be avoided as it is not reliable for diagnosis and there is a risk of seeding.

Surgery is curative in the majority of patients without metastases. Treatment options include radical nephrectomy or there are a variety of nephron-sparing treatments involving partial nephrectomy or radioablative techniques.

Cohen HT, et al. Renal-cell carcinoma. N Engl J Med 2005; 353:2477–2490.

11. D Lorazepam

Dyspnoea can be defined as difficult, uncomfortable or laboured breathing, or when an individual feels the need for more air. Breathlessness is common and can be very distressing for patients with lung cancer and other severe respiratory disorders, and their care-givers. The mechanism of dyspnoea has been described as a mismatch between central motor activity and incoming afferent information form chemo- and mechanoreceptors. A patient's emotional state, personality and cognitive function can also alter its perception. It is important to give clear explanations of what is happening and to ensure that if possible the patient is sitting upright; opening windows and using a fan may also help. Regular doses of short-acting oral morphine every 2–4 hours may decrease the sensation of breathlessness. Panic and anxiety are frequently associated with breathlessness and a low dose of an anxiolytic such as lorazepam may be helpful.

Reversible causes should be treated where appropriate. For example, patients may benefit from antibiotics to treat superadded infections, blood transfusion in severe anaemia or from drainage of a moderate–large pleural effusion. A blood transfusion is not indicated in this situation; however, opinion varies as to the target haemoglobin level, some groups advising transfusion if haemoglobin <8. Similarly, this patient is unlikely to benefit from drainage of a small effusion that is not causing respiratory compromise – normal respiratory rate and oxygen saturation breathing air. Repeat pleural tap and/or drainage also increase the risk of further complications and potential for increasing distress. Oxygen therapy may help to resolve hypoxia but there is no evidence that supplemental oxygen will improve shortness of breath. Oxygen therapy should be prescribed to maintain target saturations of 94–98% or modified target of 88–92% if there is a history or significant risk of hypercapnic respiratory failure.

Kvale PA, Selecky PA, Prakash UB. Palliative care in lung cancer: ACCP evidence-based clinical practice guidelines. Chest 2007; 132(3):368S-403S

12. A Case–control study

Case–control studies review individuals based on their disease status. A group of individuals who have a given disease (are 'cases') is compared with a group of individuals who do not have the disease (the 'controls'). As in this case the control group should where possible come from the same population that gave rise to the cases. There is then a retrospective look at factors affecting both groups (cases and controls) in an attempt to find associations.

In a cohort study participants should usually be disease free when the cohort study starts, and be at risk (i.e. mobile phone user whose mobile phone use can be quantified) of developing the outcome under investigation (multiple myeloma). The cohort is followed through time to assess their later outcome status.

An ecological study is an epidemiological design that looks at populations rather than individuals. To investigate any association between mobile phones and myeloma as in this case one possible ecological study would be to obtain mobile phone use data by area (e.g. by county from mobile phone companies) and correlate this with multiple myeloma diagnoses in the same areas (e.g. from disease registries).

A point prevalence study looks at the proportion of people in a population who have a disease or condition at a particular time, and would be useful for telling you how many of the population use a mobile phone, or how many of the population are diagnosed with multiple myeloma. This information in itself is unlikely to allow an association to be shown but multiple point prevalence studies over a period of time may begin to provide more useful information.

A randomised controlled trial is useful for treatment options where there is genuine clinical uncertainty about superiority of treatment options, but ethically cannot be used to assess risk factors for disease. For example, in this case a group of individuals would have to be randomised to using mobile phones and another group to not using mobile phones, and then both groups followed up to monitor who was diagnosed with multiple myeloma.

All epidemiological study designs have benefits and disadvantages, and it is recognition of these as well as ethical considerations and financial and time constraints that dictate design choice.

Bradford-Hill A. The environment and disease: Association or causation? Proc R Soc Med 1965; 58(5):295–300.

13. D Squamous cell carcinoma

The CT scan demonstrates changes in keeping with extensive emphysema and a cavitating lung mass in the left lower lobe. The most likely diagnosis in the described clinical presentation is squamous cell lung cancer. Non-small cell lung cancer (NSCLC) accounts for 75–80% of all lung cancers. Types of NSCLC include adenocarcinoma and squamous cell carcinoma.

Squamous cell lung cancer usually presents as a mass on chest X-ray, but may cavitate and look radiologically like a lung abscess. Rarely there may be multiple cavitating lesions. Squamous cell lung cancer may also be associated with hypercalcaemia (due to bony metastases or direct tumour production of parathyroid hormone-related peptide) or finger clubbing and hypertrophic pulmonary osteoarthropathy (paraneoplastic syndromes).

Aspergilloma, lung abscess and tuberculosis may also cause areas of cavitation and, although these are potential differential diagnoses, in a man of this age group with a history of chronic lung disease the likelihood of these diagnoses is lower. The patient should be referred for urgent investigations to gain a tissue diagnosis. The lesion is relatively peripheral so direct visualisation of the tumour for biopsies may be difficult at bronchoscopy. However, the presence of cavitation increases the diagnostic yield for cytology samples in bronchial washings. In patients not fit for invasive investigation, sputum should be sent for cytological testing as this may yield a diagnosis, which although it may not dictate further active treatment may help with determining prognosis and guiding further palliative approaches. The best diagnostic approach for a peripheral lesion may be via CT-guided lung biopsy. This procedure carries a risk of pneumothorax (approximately 10% risk). This patient will need to be assessed for suitability of this procedure in view of the significant emphysematous changes.

Tuberculosis (TB) more frequently appears with cavitatory change in the upper lobes; however, other appearances are well recognised and TB is recognised as a great mimic of lung cancer and should be considered as a differential diagnosis, particularly in high-risk groups. Similarly, aspergillomas typically occur in the apices: the term is used to describe a ball of fungal hyphae within a pre-existing cavity in the lung, e.g. following previous TB infection. Small cell lung cancer is not typically associated with cavitation on chest X-ray or CT.

Pentheroudakis G, et al. Cavitating squamous cell lung carcinoma-distinct entity or not? Lung Cancer 2004; 45(3): 349–355.
Soubani A, et al. The clinical spectrum of pulmonary aspergillosis. Chest 2002; 121: 1988–1999.

14. A Chemoradiotherapy

The treatment of choice for proximal localised squamous cell carcinoma of the oesophagus is chemoradiotherapy. Middle and distal squamous cell carcinoma of the oesophagus can be treated with chemoradiotherapy alone or chemoradiotherapy in conjunction with surgery. Surgery alone would cause significant disability by removing the whole of the oesophagus and there is equally good survival with chemotherapy. There is no evidence to support the use of preoperative radiotherapy or adjuvant chemotherapy in squamous cell carcinoma of the oesophagus.

Allum WH. BSG guidelines. Guidelines for the management of oesophageal and gastric cancer. Gut 2011; 60:1449–1472.

15. B Co-danthramer should be avoided if the patient is incontinent

Constipation is a common and distressing problem in palliative care patients and its aetiology is often multifactorial. Medications including opiates (and to a lesser extent anticholinergics) are often implicated, as well as the effects of the underlying disease itself – dehydration, immobility, hypercalcaemia, poor oral intake, gastrointestinal tumours, spinal cord involvement.

There are several factors that should be addressed in the general management of a constipated patient including encouraging, where possible, a good oral fluid intake and minimising any other contributing factors. Oral laxatives should be prescribed regularly and prophylactically to all patients receiving opiate-based analgesia. The combination of a softener and a stimulant is usually recommended, but each choice should be based on the individual patient.

Dantron-containing laxatives such as co-danthramer have various side effects, including turning the urine red and causing severe perianal irritation, particularly in those with faecal incontinence. Arachis oil contains peanut oil and is thus contraindicated in patients with known nut allergies.

Bulk-forming laxatives such as fybogel mebeverine are not usually recommended as palliative care patients often struggle to maintain an adequate fluid intake and this may then result in faecal impaction and intestinal obstruction.

The use of the faecal softener liquid paraffin is not recommended because of the potential risk of lipoid pneumonia (particularly in drowsy patients where the oral route may be compromised) and anal irritation.

Laxative treatment should be regularly reassessed, even when the patient is on an unchanged analgesic regimen. Laxative treatment should also be reviewed each time an opioid medication or dose is changed.

16. B Congestive cardiac failure

Trastuzumab, more commonly known as Herceptin, should be given as an adjuvant treatment in HER-2-positive breast cancer. Cardiac function should be assessed prior to treatment and women with any of the following should not be treated with trastuzumab:

- A left ventricular fraction of 55% or less
- A history of documented congestive cardiac failure
- High-risk uncontrolled arrhythmias
- Angina pectoris requiring medication
- Clinically significant valvular disease
- Evidence of transmural infarction on electrocardiograph
- Poorly controlled hypertension.

National Institute for Health and Clinical Excellence. NICE guideline 80. Early and locally advanced breast cancer, Diagnosis and Treatment. London: NICE, 2009.

17. E Urinary 5-HIAA (5-hydroyindoleacetic acid) levels

The patient has the classic symptoms of carcinoid syndrome. This is a syndrome that occurs when neuroendocrine tumours (NETs) metastasise to the liver, causing a direct release of serotonin, tachykinins and other vasoactive compounds into the systemic circulation. Carcinoid syndrome classically presents with flushing and diarrhoea. Seventy per cent of patients report intermittent abdominal pain, 50% report diarrhoea and 30% report flushing. Patients may also complain of rhinorrhoea, episodic palpitations and lacrimation during flushing. Pellagra, wheezing and carcinoid heart disease can occur. Urinary 5-HIAA levels are a baseline investigation for patients with symptoms suspicious of an NET, and are raised in foregut and midgut carcinoid tumours. They do not confirm the diagnosis, and radiological and histological confirmation will be required. The other baseline test that should be performed in suspected NET is chromogranin A levels, which are raised in many NETs. Serum 5-hydroxytryptamine levels vary throughout the day and thus are not used clinically. Adrenocorticotrophic hormone (ACTH) levels are useful if an ectopic ACTH-producing tumour is suspected, but this patient has no symptoms to suggest Cushing's syndrome. C-peptide levels should be measured when there is a clinical suspicion of an insulinoma, but there are no symptoms of hypoglycaemia so this is unlikely. Fasting gastrin levels are raised in Zollinger–Ellison syndrome which presents with severe and recurrent duodenal ulceration.

Ramage JK, et al. BSG Guidelines for the management of gastroenteropancreatic (including carcinoid) tumours. Gut 2005; 54; 1–16.

18. A Chest drain insertion and talc pleurodesis

Malignant pleural effusions have a high risk of recurring and unless the patient has a very limited life expectancy (less than 1 month) pleurodesis should be adopted as soon as possible. Available agents include talc, bleomycin and tetracycline. Pleural aspiration should not exceed 1.5 L in a single procedure because it can be associated with the development of re-expansion pulmonary oedema.

Selected patients with malignant pleural effusions and good performance status may gain advantage from other techniques including thoracoscopy (medical or surgical video-assisted thoracoscopic surgery). Longer-term indwelling pleural catheters may also have a role in selected patients with recurrent malignant effusions, e.g. in some patients with mesothelioma.

Oramorph and lorazepam are useful agents in the palliative management of dyspnoea and may be appropriate if the patient is not a candidate for a chest drain or the effusion is not amenable to drainage.

British Thoracic Society. Pleural Disease Guideline 2010. Thorax 2010; 65(2).

19. E Urine 24-hour metanephrines

Medullary thyroid cancer (MTC) is often associated with multiple endocrine neoplasia (MEN) type 2A. The major lesion in MEN2A are medullary thyroid carcinoma, phaeochromocytoma and hyperparathyroidism.

The symptoms of episodic palpitations, anxiety and hypertension should arouse the suspicion of phaeochromocytoma in a patient with previous MTC. Hence the appropriate test in this situation would be urine 24-hour metanephrines.

Prevalence of MTC increases with age in cases of MEN2A and can reach up to 70% by the age of 70 years. After the age of 10 years the prevalence of phaeochromocytoma is up to 10–50% in this situation.

The diagnosis of clinically significant adrenal medullary disease usually follows the diagnosis of MTC. Almost all phaeochromocytomas are located in the adrenal glands. Phaeochromocytoma is almost always benign in this situation and can be bilateral in up to 50% of cases, especially after a few years.

Pacini F, et al. Medullary thyroid carcinoma. Clin Oncol (R Coll Radiol) 2010; 22(6):475–485.

20. C Glioma

All of these conditions may present with seizures. However, the appearance on the contrast-enhanced MRI of the brain is consistent with a malignant glioma. There is a large contrast-enhancing lesion in the right parietal lobe with extensive surrounding oedema. Some cystic degenerative changes are noted within the lesion.

In contrast, meningiomas are well-circumscribed extra-axial lesions. Cerebral toxoplasmosis is most common in immunocompromised individuals and usually appears as multiple ring-enhancing lesions with contrast enhancement. Arteriovenous malformations appear as an abnormal collection of entwined vessels; these may exhibit flow voids on MRI due to rapid blood flow. Cysticercosis is a parasitic disease caused by ingestion of the eggs of the pork tapeworm (*Taenia solium*). Larvae may form in the brain (neurocysticercosis). These are often very numerous and less than <1 cm diameter. They typically appear cystic and may have a visible central scolex on CT; on MRI degenerating cysts may appear as ring-enhancing lesions. Leptomeningeal enhancement is common.

Rees J, Zrinzo L. What to do with a patient who has a had a fit and the scan shows a 'glioma'? Pract Neurol 2005; 5:84–91.
Wen P, Kesari S. Malignant gliomas in adults. N Engl J Med 2008; 359:492–507.

21. B Not proceed with the operation

This patient has made repeated, sustained and documented assertions that she does not want invasive or surgical procedures to prolong her life. She now does not have capacity to make these decisions but this does not denigrate her previous statements. It is assumed that she had capacity when she made her original advance directive to refuse treatment and this must be respected. Only if there is doubt as to whether she had capacity at the time of her decision can a clinician challenge this directive, and get a court order if appropriate and there was enough time. In the emergency situation where there is not enough time for further investigations, the clinician should do whatever he can to prolong life. Deciding on the applicability of advance directives is complicated and the General Medical Council has issued guidance about considering these issues.

General Medical Council. Treatment and care towards the end of life: good practice in decision making. London: GMC, 2010.

22. B Anastrozole

First-line adjuvant chemotherapy for postmenopausal women with oestrogen receptor-positive early invasive breast cancer is an aromatase inhibitor, either anastrozole or letrozole. Exemestane is an aromatase inhibitor but should be offered only to women who have previously been treated with tamoxifen for 2–3 years. Tamoxifen is no longer considered first-line chemotherapy and it should be offered only if an aromatase inhibitor is not tolerated or contraindicated. 5-Fluorouracil is not used in the treatment of breast cancer. Trastuzumab, more commonly known as Herceptin, is used in human epidermal growth factor receptor-2 (HER-2)-positive breast cancer not oestrogen receptor-positive breast cancer and so would not be an appropriate treatment in this case.

National Institute for Health and Clinical Excellence. NICE guideline 80. Early and locally advanced breast cancer, Diagnosis and Treatment. London: NICE, 2009.

23. C Gemcitabine and cisplatin

This patient has advanced lung cancer (stage IV disease) because he has metastatic spread and so is not a candidate for curative treatment. The management of such patients is palliative chemotherapy. Tumours should be assessed for a mutation in the epidermal growth factor receptor (EGFR) to see if they would be susceptible to EGFR tyrosine kinase inhibitors such as erlotinib and gefitinib. This is not the case here. Instead this patient would need to be given combination treatment with a platinum-based agent (such as cisplatin or carboplatin) and another agent such as etoposide, vinorelbine, paclitaxel or gemcitabine. Combination treatment first line is more efficacious than using single agent therapy.

Cetuximab is a monoclonal antibody that targets EGFR, and bevacizumab is an antibody that targets vascular epidermal growth factor. Both are second-line agents and are used in combination with chemotherapy agents.

Lal R, Enting D, Kristeleit H. Systemic treatment of non-small-cell lung cancer. Eur J Cancer 2011; 47 (3):S375–377. Goldstraw P, et al. The IASLC Lung Cancer Staging Project: Proposals for the revision of the TNM stage groups in the forthcoming (seventh) edition of the TNM classification of malignant tumours. J Thorac Oncol 2007; 2:706.

24. B T2N1M0

The tumour node metastasis staging (TNM) system is overtaking the Duke's staging classification for colorectal carcinoma.

The classification is as follows (see **Table 8.1**):

Table 8.1 TNM staging criteria

TNM system for hypopharyngeal carcinoma

Primary tumour		Nodes		Metastasis	
TX	Not assessable	**NX**	Regional nodes not assessable	**MX**	Distant metastasis not assessable
T0	No evidence of tumour	N0	No regional node metastasis	M0	No distant metastasis
Tis	Carcinoma *in situ*	N1	Metastasis in single ipsilateral node ($\leq$3 cm)	**M1**	Distant metastasis
T1	Tumour invades submucosa	N2	Metastasis in one to three regional lymph nodes		
T2	Tumour invades muscularis propria	N3	Metastasis in four or more regional lymph nodes		
T3	Tumour invades through the muscularis propria into the subserosa, or into the non-peritonealised pericolic or perirectal tissues.				
T4	Tumour directly invades other organs or structures, and/or perforates visceral peritoneum				

Adapted from: Sobin LH, Gospodarowicz MK, Wittekind C (eds). TNM Classification of Malignant Tumours, 7th edn. Oxford: Wiley-Blackwell, 2009.

Chapter 9

Renal medicine

Questions

1. A 56-year-old woman with type 2 diabetes and chronic kidney disease (CKD) stage 3 was admitted for a coronary angiogram. She regularly took lisinopril and metformin, both of which were withheld for the procedure.

    Her pulse was 80 beats per minute, blood pressure 130/75 mmHg, jugular venous pressure visible at 3 cm and there no peripheral oedema. Cardiovascular and respiratory examinations were unremarkable.

    What is the most appropriate next management step to reduce the risk of contrast-induced nephropathy?

    A   0.9% NaCl 1 mL/kg per h for 12 hours pre- and post-procedure
    B   1.26% sodium bicarbonate 3 mL/kg per h for 1 hour pre-procedure and 1 mL/kg per h during and post-procedure
    C   Haemofiltration immediately before and after procedure
    D   N-Acetylcysteine 600 mg twice daily pre- and post-procedure
    E   No additional measure required

2. A 69-year-old man was admitted with a 7-day history of diarrhoea and vomiting. He had ischaemic heart disease, type 2 diabetes mellitus and gout for which his current medications were amlodipine, metformin, doxazosin, diclofenac and bisoprolol.

    On admission, his blood pressure was 120/70 mmHg, dropping to 100/53 mmHg on standing; jugular venous pressure was not visible and mucous membranes were dry.

    Investigations:

    > creatinine 420 µmol/L (90 3 months ago, normal range males 60–110)
    > lactate 2.4 mmol/L (0.6–1.8)

    Which one of the followings drug is most likely to be the cause of his acute kidney injury?

    A   Amlodipine
    B   Bisoprolol
    C   Diclofenac
    D   Gliclazide
    E   Metformin

3. A 68-year-old woman presented with worsening peripheral oedema over the past few weeks.

    On examination, she had pitting oedema to her thighs, and her blood pressure was 150/85 mmHg.

Investigations:

creatinine 180 µmol/L (females 45–90)	albumin 24 g/L (37–49)
Urinary protein:creatinine ratio 612 (<45)	
Renal biopsy (silver stain): see **Figure 9.1**	

Figure 9.1 *See colour plate section.*

Which one of the following is least likely to be associated with this condition?

A   Antiglomerular basement membrane disease (Goodpasture's disease)
B   Breast cancer
C   Hepatitis B
D   Hepatitis C
E   Systemic lupus erythematosus (SLE)

4.   A 41-year-old man returned to the nephrology clinic. He had type 2 diabetes with proliferative retinopathy and was on insulin treatment.
     Blood pressure was 150/90 mmHg and there was no peripheral oedema. Creatinine when checked 6 months ago was 158 µmol/L.

Current investigations:

creatinine 225 µmol/L (60–110)	albumin 38 g/L (37–49)
potassium 4.9 mmol/L (3.5–5.0)	HbA1c 7.7% (3.8–6.4)
Antinuclear antibody: negative	
Antineutrophil cytoplasmic antibody: negative	
Urine dipstick: protein +++, blood –	
Urinary protein:creatinine ratio 248 (<45)	

What is the most appropriate next step in management?

A   Amlodipine
B   Increase insulin
C   Low-potassium diet
D   Ramipril
E   Renal biopsy

5. A 54-year-old, 75-kg African–Caribbean man attended the renal clinic. He was known to have progressive chronic kidney disease (CKD) secondary to diabetic nephropathy. He felt well and reported no specific symptoms. He had previously been seen by the dietician and advised dietary restrictions of salt, potassium and phosphate.

   On examination, his blood pressure was 130/80 mmHg and he was assessed as being euvolaemic.

   Investigations:

creatinine 420 μmol/L (350 4 months ago, males 60–110)	iron 3 mmol/L (12–30)
	corrected calcium 2.1 mmol/L (2.2–2.6)
urea 26.0 mmol/L (2.5–7.5)	phosphate 1.84 mmol/L (0.87–1.49)
potassium 5.5 mmol/L (3.5–5.0)	parathyroid hormone 18 pmol/L (7.7–12.1)
haemoglobin 9.4 g/L (11.0–13.0)	
Urinary protein:creatinine ratio 339 (<45)	

   What is the most appropriate next step in management?

   A Add ramipril to reduce proteinuria
   B Admit and start haemodialysis
   C Erythropoietin-stimulating agent (ESA)
   D Renal ultrasound to exclude obstruction
   E Start a phosphate binder

6. A 64-year-old Afro–Caribbean man presented with fatigue and increasing dyspnoea. He had type 2 diabetes mellitus and had previously had a myocardial infarction. He was taking gliclazide, ramipril and furosemide. Prior to this presentation he had seen his general practitioner with the same complaints and had his furosemide increased and was started on a 5-day course of cephalexin for a presumed chest infection.

   On examination, his blood pressure was 125/82 mmHg sitting, 115/78 mmHg standing; jugular venous pressure was not elevated and there was no peripheral oedema.

   Investigations:

haemoglobin 8.2 g/dL (males 13–18)	corrected calcium 2.85 mmol/L (2.2–2.6)
white cell count 8.3 × 10⁹/L (4–11)	HbA1c 8.9% (3.8–6.4)
creatinine 220 μmol/L (80 3 months ago, males 60–110)	
Urine dipstick: trace protein	

   What is the most likely diagnosis?

   A Acute tubular necrosis secondary to increased furosemide
   B Acute tubulointerstitial nephritis secondary to antibiotics
   C Diabetic nephropathy
   D IgA nephropathy
   E Multiple myeloma

7. A 70-year-old man with a history of valve replacement presented with a 4-month history of general malaise and weight loss of 9 kg.

   On examination, his temperature was 37.5°C, there was splenomegaly and a soft pan-systolic murmur.

Investigations:

Urine dipstick: protein ++++, blood +++	
haemoglobin 8 g/dL (males 13–18)	C-reactive protein 60 mg/L (<10)
white cell count 3 × 10⁹/L (4–11)	C3 0.42 g/L (0.65–1.9)
platelets 45 × 10⁹/L (150–400)	C4 0.08 g/L (0.15–0.5)
creatinine 350 µmol/L (80 4 months ago, 150 2 months ago, males 60–110)	
Antineutrophil cytoplasmic antibody: positive myeloperoxidase <5 IU/mL (<5) proteinase 3 50 IU/mL (<5)	

What is the most appropriate next step in management?

A   0.5 g methylprednisolone intravenously
B   Bone marrow biopsy
C   Broad-spectrum antibiotics
D   Renal biopsy
E   Serial blood cultures

8. A 35-year-old man presented for routine clinic review having recieved a cadaveric renal transplant 6 months previously. He was taking ciclosporin, mycophenolate mofetil and prednisolone. His baseline creatinine postoperatively had settled to around 130 µmol/L. He was well with no specific symptoms.
    On examination blood pressure was 145/85 mmHg, jugular venous pressure was not elevated, and cardiovascular and respiratory examinations were unremarkable. Abdominal examination revealed slight tenderness over his transplanted kidney.

Investigations:

creatinine 190 µmol/L
Urine dipstick: protein ++
Ultrasound: normal size renal transplant kidney with no hydronephrosis seen

He was called back to clinic 3 days later in view of his change in renal function at which point creatinine had risen further to 205 µmol/L.

What is the most appropriate next step in management?

A   Cytomegalovirus polymerase chain reaction
B   Renal biopsy
C   Renal transplant artery angiogram
D   Renogram with furosemide
E   Urine culture and empirical antibiotics

9. A 78-year-old white woman presented with a 4-month history of weight loss, general malaise and occasional fevers. She was a smoker with a cough and at the time of admission had had two episodes of fresh haemoptysis. She had no significant past medical history and, other than a salbutamol inhaler, took no regular medication.
    Examination revealed a blood pressure of 130/75 mmHg, jugular venous pressure +2 cm, no peripheral oedema and nothing else of note.

Investigations:

creatinine 214 µmol/L (females 45–90)	albumin 33 g/L (37–49)
Antinuclear antibody: negative C3 normal C4 normal	Antineutrophil cytoplasmic antibody: positive (myeloperoxide <5 AU/mL, proteinase 3 <5 AU/mL)
Urine dipstick: protein +++, blood +++	
Chest X-ray: bilateral diffuse alveolar shadowing	

What is the most likely diagnosis?

A   Acute interstitial nephritis secondary to tuberculosis
B   Antiglomerular basement membrane disease
C   Membranous nephropathy associated with lung malignancy
D   Microscopic polyangiitis
E   Sepsis from a pneumonia causing acute tubular necrosis

10. A 30-year-old woman presented with a 2-month history of general malaise and intermittent fevers.
    She was found to have acute kidney injury with blood and protein on urine dipstick testing.

    Investigations:

creatinine 175 µmol/L (previously 85 µmol/L, females 45–90) haemoglobin 9 g/dL (females 11.5–16.5) white cell count 11×10^9/L (4–11)	platelets 90×10^9/L (150–400) C3 0.5 g/L (0.65–1.9) C4 0.1 g/L (0.15–0.5)

    Which one of the following is the least likely diagnosis?

    A   Infective endocarditis
    B   Lupus nephritis
    C   Mixed cryoglobulinaemia
    D   Poststreptococcal glomerulonephritis
    E   Wegener's granulomatosis (granulomatosis and polyangiitis)

11. A 72-year-old man presented to the emergency department after being found lying on the floor 24 hours after a fall at home.
    On examination, his blood pressure was 110/60 mmHg and his right calf was tense and swollen. Urine output was documented as 45 mL over the past 2 hours.

    Investigations:

potassium 7.9 mmol/L (3.5–5.0) urea 28.5 mmol/L (2.5–7.5)	creatinine 480 µmol/L (males 60–110) creatine kinase 10 000 U/L (males 25–195)
Electrocardiogram: 98 beats per minute, sinus rhythm tented T waves broad QRS complexes	

What is the most appropriate next step in his immediate management?

A   10 mL of 10% calcium gluconate given intravenously over 5 minutes
B   10 units Actrapid insulin in 50 mL of 50% dextrose given intravenously over 20 minutes
C   5 mg nebulised salbutamol followed by 15 g calcium polystyrene sulphate (Calcium Resonium) orally four times daily
D   Emergency fasciotomy
E   Haemodialyis

12. A 71-year-old woman was admitted for a semielective coronary artery bypass graft. She was known to have type 2 diabetes mellitus, hypertension and stage 3 chronic kidney disease with a creatinine of 135 µmol/L. She regularly took ramipril, atenolol and insulin. She was given intravenous co-amoxiclav perioperatively. She had a period intraoperatively where her mean arterial pressure was 60 mmHg.

   On examination postoperatively there was some slight erythema around her wound site. She was apyrexial, with pulse 84 beats per minute and blood pressure 130/75 mmHg.

Investigations:

creatinine 480 µmol/L (45–90)	C-reactive protein 18 mg/L (<10)
white cell count 9.4 × 10⁹/L (4–11)	
Urine dipstick: protein +	
Ultrasound:	
right kidney 9.4 cm	
left kidney 10.5 cm	

What is the most likely cause of her acute kidney injury?

A   Acute tubular necrosis secondary to hypotension
B   Acute tubular necrosis secondary to sepsis
C   Acute tubulointerstitial nephritis secondary to antibiotics
D   Contrast nephropathy
E   Renal artery occlusion

13. A 77-year-old white man underwent an elective coronary angiogram. He had a history of type 2 diabetes, hypertension, peripheral vascular disease and osteoarthritis. He smoked 20 cigarettes per day.

   Ten days post-procedure he developed some intermittent abdominal pain, for which he was given analgesia, and had a painful mottled right foot.

Investigations:

creatinine 463 µmol/L (pre-procedure 105, males 60–110)	eosinophils 1.1 × 10⁹/L (0.04–0.4)
	C3 0.14 g/L (0.65–1.90)
white cell count 7.8 × 10⁹/L (4–11)	
Urine dipstick: protein +	
Ultrasound:	
right kidney 9.1 cm	
left kidney 9.9 cm	

What is the most likely cause for his acute kidney injury?

A   Analgesic nephropathy
B   Cholesterol emboli

C   Contrast-induced nephropathy
D   Lupus nephritis
E   Renal artery stenosis

14. A 24-year-old woman presented with a week-long history of diarrhoea and malaise. She had seen some blood in her stool and had noticed that she was bruising easily. Her bilirubin was found to be elevated and she was referred to the gastroenterologists for investigation. She had no significant past medical history and was taking no medications.

   On examination, she had icteric sclerae and she had some areas of bruising. Urine output was 40 mL/h.

Investigations:

haemoglobin 6.1 g/dL (females 11.5–16.5)	creatinine 196 µmol/L (females 45–90)
white cell count 12 × 10⁹/L (4–11)	bilirubin 70 mmol/L (1–22)
platelets 40 × 10⁹/L (150–400)	lactate dehydrogenase 1900 U/L (10–250)
urea 13 mmol/L (2.5–7.5)	
Blood film: some fragmented red cells	

What is the most appropriate next step in her management?

A   Flexible sigmoidoscopy
B   Haemofiltration
C   Intravenous fresh frozen plasma
D   Intravenous vitamin K
E   Platelet transfusion

15. A 45-year-old peritoneal dialysis (PD) patient presented with diffuse abdominal pain and vomiting. His PD bags were draining cloudy fluid. The white cell count in the fluid was 400/mm³ (<100) with 65% neutrophils. He had been given intraperitoneal antibiotics by the PD nurses in the community.

   He was seen again on day 5 of his treatment and the effluent was still cloudy with a white cell count of 350/mm³. Gram stain was negative on both occasions.

What is the most appropriate next step in his management?

A   Admit for intravenous antibiotics in addition to intraperitoneal antibiotics
B   Assume that this is tuberculous peritonitis and start antituberculous therapy
C   Observe and follow up in outpatient clinic
D   Removal of PD on the ward under local anaesthetic
E   Surgical removal of PD catheter, minilaparotomy and wash-out

16. A 46-year-old woman came for review having recently been diagnosed with adult polycystic kidney disease. She mentioned that she had a strong family history of renal failure and haemorrhagic stroke. She was well with no symptoms of note.

   On examination, her blood pressure was 150/80 mmHg and there were bilateral masses palpable in her abdomen.

Investigations:

Urine dipstick: protein +, blood +

Which one of the following would be the next most appropriate step in her management?

A   She should be advised to arrange for her 15-year-old son to have an ultrasound screening test
B   She should be counselled that she will definitely require renal replacement therapy in the future

C   She should be counselled that there is a 25% chance that her daughter will inherit the disease
D   She should have her blood pressure repeated in 6 months to assess need for treatment
E   She should have an MR angiogram of her brain

17. A 48-year-old man from Ghana was referred by his general practitioner with unexplained renal impairment. He had no known past medical history and took no regular medications.
    His blood pressure was 135/95 mmHg with mild peripheral oedema.

Investigations from the clinic revealed:

creatinine 210 µmol/L (males 60–110)	albumin 21 g/L (37–49)
Antineutrophil cytoplasmic antibody: negative	Antinuclear antibody: negative
C3 0.7 g/L (0.65–1.9)	C4 25 g/L (0.15–0.5)
Hepatitis B and C: negative	IgG 8.4 g/L (6.0–13.0)
IgA 1.5 g/L (0.8–3.0)	IgM 1.0 g/L (0.4–2.5)
Serum electrophoresis: diffuse increase in gamma-globulins CD4 100×10^6/L (500–1200) HIV viral load 3500	
Urine dipstick: protein ++++, blood ++	

What is the renal biopsy most likely to show?

A   Cast nephropathy
B   Collapsing focal segmental glomerulosclerosis
C   Hyaline arteriosclerosis
D   Kimmelstiel–Wilson nodules
E   Minimal change

18. A 67-year-old patient presented to the transplant review clinic. He had received a cadaveric renal transplant 10 years previously. His early course had been complicated by rejection and he had been heavily immunosuppressed. At presentation he had good graft function with a baseline creatinine of 105 µmol/L and negligible proteinuria. He described symptoms of weight loss over the last 2 months and general malaise. There was no history of abdominal symptoms or fever.
    On examination, he had a large inguinal lymph node and a palpable mass in his left iliac fossa.

Investigations:

haemoglobin 8.9 g/dL (11–13)

Which one of the following is the most useful virology test?

A   BK virus
B   Cytomegalovirus
C   Epstein–Barr virus
D   Hepatitis B
E   HIV

19. A 40-year-old man underwent renal biopsy. He had been seen in the renal clinic when his general practitioner referred him having found a raised creatinine at his first attendance there. He had no old results to compare and had never seen a general practitioner before. He took no regular medications.

Investigations:

> creatinine 315 µmol/L (males 60–110)

Renal biopsy (see **Figure 9.2**):

Figure 9.2 *See colour plate section.*

Which one of the following statements regarding his condition is most likely?

A He has high blood pressure
B He needs to start renal replacement therapy (RRT) immediately
C He should be started on prednisolone and cyclophosphamide
D He will definitely have nephrotic range proteinuria
E His serum IgA will be high

20. A 50-year-old man presented with a short history of lethargy and nausea and some intermittent back lower pain. He had seen his general practitioner for the back pain and was taking diclofenac as required. He had no past medical history of note. He had noticed a reduction in urine output over the past 2 days.

His blood pressure at presentation was 190/100 mmHg and urine dipstick testing was unremarkable.

Investigations:

> haemoglobin 11 g/dL (males 13–18)
> white cell count 9 × 10⁹/L (4–11)
> erythrocyte sedimentation rate 90 mm/1st h (males 0–20)
>
> potassium 6.3 mmol/L (3.5–5.0)
> urea 42.7 mmol/L (2.5–7.5)
> creatinine 1024 µmol/L (males 60–110)
> corrected calcium 2.7 mmol/L (2.2–2.6)

He was admitted urgently to hospital and a CT was performed subsequently.
CT (see **Figure 9.3**):

Which one of the following is not a recognised cause of his condition?

A Beta-blocker
B Lymphoma
C Prostate carcinoma
D Radiotherapy
E Tuberculosis

Figure 9.3

21. A 40-year-old man presented to the emergency department feeling generally weak and tired. He complained of nausea and loss of appetite. He had previously been investigated for renal impairment and a diagnosis of diabetic nephropathy had been made, but he had defaulted clinic appointments for the past 3 years. He had no other symptoms.

On examination, his pulse was 90 beats per minute, blood pressure 160/90 mmHg and oxygen saturation 96% on air.

Investigations:

haemoglobin 5.2 g/dL (males 13–18)	bicarbonate 15 mmol/L (22–30)
mean corpuscular volume 80 fL (80–96)	urea 41.6 mmol/l (2.5–7.5)
potassium 6.4 mmol/l (3.5–5.0)	creatinine 1740 µmol/L (males 60–110)

What is the most appropriate next step in his management?

A   Initiate dialysis because serum bicarbonate is less than 17 mmol/L
B   Initiate dialysis because urea is more than 40 mmol/L
C   Initiate dialysis to facilitate packed red cell transfusion
D   Insert a central venous catheter for fluid balance
E   Urgent gastroscopy to investigate anaemia

22. A 37-year-old African man was referred because his blood pressure was found to be 230/150 mmHg. He had been diagnosed with hypertension by his general practitioner several years ago but had been non-compliant with antihypertensive medications. He was asymptomatic.

On examination, there were no focal neurological signs. Blood pressure in the left arm was 235/152 mmHg and in the right arm 245/155 mmHg. His peripheral pulses were present and there were no audible bruits; there was no evidence of papilloedema.

Investigations:

Electrocardiogram:
voltage criteria for left ventricular hypertrophy (LVH)

creatinine 190 µmol/L (males 60–110)

Urine dipstick: blood +++, protein +++

What is the most appropriate next step in management?

A Admit for intravenous antihypertensives as this is a hypertensive emergency
B Blood pressure and creatinine – re-check next week before initiating treatment
C Start on a single oral antihypertensive agent
D Urgent CT of the chest and abdomen to exclude dissection
E Urgent renal biopsy to investigate renal impairment

23. A 44-year-old female haemodialysis patient presented with increased tiredness and lethargy. The cause of her end-stage renal failure was reflux nephropathy and she had been established on regular three times a week haemodialysis for 5 years. Her haemoglobin had been noted to have been dropping recently and her erythropoietin (Epo) dose, which was given on dialysis, had been increased accordingly.

Investigations:

haemoglobin 5.9 g/dL (aim 11–12 CKD stage 5)	haematocrit 30% (36–48)
white cell count 9.2 × 10⁹/L (4–11)	reticulocytes 0% (0.5–2.5)
platelets 194 × 10⁹/L (150–400)	ferritin 620 g/L (15–300)
mean corpuscular volume 82 fL (80–96)	transferrin saturation 50%*

Gastroscopy: normal

*Transferrin saturation = ratio of serum iron and total iron-binding capacity × 100 (12–45% in females)

What is the most likely diagnosis?

A Anaemia of chronic disease
B Chronic lymphocytic leukaemia (CLL)
C Myelodysplasia
D Pure red cell aplasia (PRCA)
E Subclinical gastrointestinal blood loss

24. A 45-year-old woman was referred by her general practitioner with hypertension and abnormal renal function. She had no significant medical history and took no regular medications.
Her blood pressure was 160/95 mmHg.

creatinine 250 µmol/L (females 45–90)	albumin 29 g/L (37–49)

Urine dipstick: protein:creatinine ratio 745 (<45)
protein ++++
blood ++

Renal biopsy (see **Figure 9.4**):

Figure 9.4 *See colour plate section.*

What does the biopsy show?

A   Collapsing glomerulopathy
B   Focal necrotising crescentic glomerulonephritis
C   Membranous nephropathy
D   Mesangiocapillary glomerulonephritis (MCGN)
E   Tubulointerstitial nephritis

25. A 69-year-old man presented with a severe community-acquired pneumonia. He was known to have ischaemic heart disease and poor left ventricular function. His blood pressure was 80/40 mmHg on admission.

    He was given intravenous antibiotics and fluid resuscitated. Although his blood pressure rose to 100/70 mmHg he remained oligoanuric with a urine output of 10 mL for the next 4 hours. His jugular venous pressure was elevated to the angle of his jaw, he had fine bibasal crackles and there was bronchial breathing in the right mid-zone. There was some pedal oedema. His respiratory rate was 30 breaths per minute and oxygen saturation 92% on 28% FiO_2 (fraction of inspired oxygen).

Investigations:

haemoglobin 7.6 g/dL (males 13–18)	potassium 6.5 mmol/L (3.5–5)
white cell count 15.6 × 10⁹/L (4–11)	creatinine 250 µmol/L (baseline 100, males 60–110)

What is the most appropriate next step in management?

A   Cross-match and transfuse 2 units of packed red cells
B   Continuous venovenous haemofiltration (CVVHF)
C   Further fluid challenge (1000 mL) and monitor urine output
D   Haemodialysis
E   Inotropes, dobutamine and furosemide infusion

26. A 36-year-old man with end-stage renal failure secondary to hypertensive nephrosclerosis presented with facial pain and deformity. He had been on renal replacement via intermittent haemodialysis three times a week for 10 years. He was non-compliant with his medications which included alfacalcidol (vitamin D analogue), Calcichew (phosphate binder), ramipril, lansoprazole, sevelamer (non-calcium-containing phosphate binder) and cinacalcet (calcimimetic agent).

Investigations:

corrected calcium 2.8 mmol/L (aim 2.1–2.37 on dialysis)	parathyroid hormone >263 pmol/L (16.5–33.0)
phosphate 1.7 mmol/L (aim 1.13–1.78 on dialysis)	

CT of the head (see **Figure 9.5**):

What is the most appropriate next step in management?

A   Bone biopsy
B   Change from Calcichew to Alu-Cap
C   CT of the chest, abdomen and pelvis to exclude malignancy
D   Increase alfacalcidol
E   Parathyroidectomy

27. A 73-year-old white man was referred via his general practitioner with acute kidney injury. He had a purpuric rash over his lower limbs. He complained of generalised lethargy and weight loss. He had no significant past medical history, took no regular medication and denied any herbal remedies.

Figure 9.5

Investigations:

creatinine 450 µmol/L (previously 100, males 60–110)	C3 0.8 g/L (0.65–1.9) C4 0.04 g/L (0.15–0.5)
rheumatoid factor 390 IU/mL (<20)	
Urine: blood ++, protein +++	

Which test would be most helpful in making the diagnosis?

A   Antineutrophil cytoplasmic antibody
B   Cryoglobulins
C   Double-stranded DNA
D   Extractable nuclear antigen (ENA)
E   Erythrocyte sedimentation rate

28. A 60-year-old woman presented with acute kidney injury. She was oliguric despite fluid resuscitation.
      Initial blood results revealed:

Investigations:

white cell count 9.6 × 10⁹/L (4–11)	urea 52 mmol/L (2.5–7.5)
C-reactive protein 18 mg/L (<10)	creatinine 920 µmol/L (females 45–90)
potassium 6.0 mmol/L (3.5–5.0)	

It was decided that she should start renal replacement therapy. A dialysis catheter was inserted and she commenced dialysis heparin free. After 3 hours of haemodialysis she complained of headache and nausea. After a further half hour she became confused and had a seizure.
      On examination, she had no lateralising neurological signs and plantars were equivocal.

Investigations:

potassium 4.0 mmol/L (3.5–5.0)	creatinine 680 µmol/L (females 45–90)
urea 21 mmol/L (2.5–7.5)	

What is the most likely cause of her symptoms?

A   Cardiac arrhythmia
B   Dialyser reaction
C   Disequilibrium syndrome
D   Intracerebral bleed
E   Sepsis

29. A 42-year-old man with acute lymphoblastic leukaemia was started on chemotherapy. Over the next 48 hours his urine output was noted to decrease.

Investigations:

potassium 6.9 mmol/L (3.5–5.0)	uric acid 840 µmol/L (males 110–420)
creatinine 300 µmol/L (males 60–110)	lactate dehydrogenase 600 U/L (10–250)
phosphate 3.1 mmol/L (0.8–1.4)	

Which one of the following is the least useful treatment for this condition?

A   Allopurinol
B   Calcium gluconate intravenous
C   Mesna
D   Rasburicase
E   Sodium bicarbonate intravenously

30. A 42-year-old woman presented with lethargy, fatigue and intermittent fevers. She had a history of asthma and had had recurrent chest infections requiring several courses of oral antibiotics over the last 6 months. She had had to increase her inhaler use. She had also had intermittent abdominal pain and diarrhoea over the last month.
     On examination, her blood pressure was 140/80 mmHg and she had an isolated wheeze in her right mid-zone. Her abdomen was soft and minimally tender.

Investigations:

haemoglobin 9.5 g/dL (females 11.5–16.5)	urea 23 mmol/L (2.5–7.5)
white cell count 11.5 × 10⁹/L (4–11)	creatinine 351 µmol/L (females 45–90)
platelets 505 × 10⁹/L (150–400)	C3 1.0 g/L (0.65–1.9)
eosinophils 1.4 × 10⁹/L (0.04–0.4)	C4 0.4 g/L (0.15–0.5)

Antineutrophil cytoplasmic antibody: positive
myeloperoxide (MPO) 80 AU/mL (<5)
proteinase 3 (PR 3) <5 AU/mL (<5)

Urine dipstick: blood +++, protein +++

Blood tests repeated the following day showed that her creatinine had increased to 443 µmol/L.

Renal biopsy: focal and necrotising crescentic glomerulonephritis with one granuloma seen in the interstitium.

What is the most likely cause of her symptoms?

A   Allergic granulomatosis and angiitis (Churg–Strauss syndrome)
B   Granulomatosis and polyangiitis (Wegener's granulomatosis)
C   Post-infectious glomerulonephritis
D   Strongyloides infection
E   Tubulointerstitial nephritis secondary to antibiotics

31. A 36-year-old male haemodialysis patient was admitted for a live-related renal transplantation. Tissue typing for major antibody incompatibility was negative and blood groups were matched. He received standard immunosuppression at induction and was prescribed standard maintenance doses.

    Initially he produced good volumes of urine (>200 mL/h), but after 24 hours his urine output suddenly decreased (10 mL/h) despite adequate fluid administration and he became acutely tender over the graft.

    What is the most likely cause for these symptoms?

    A   Acute tubular necrosis
    B   Graft pyelonephritis
    C   Hyperacute rejection
    D   Obstruction
    E   Renal vein thrombosis

32. A 78-year-old man was admitted with acute kidney injury of uncertain cause. He had a background of type 2 diabetes mellitus and hypercholesterolaemia. Recently he had been suffering with diarrhoea and vomiting.

    On admission his blood pressure was 100/80 mmHg, jugular venous pressure was not visible and there was no peripheral oedema.

    Investigations:

creatinine 460 µmol/L (baseline 105, males 60–110)	urea 25.3 mmol/L (2.5–7.5)
	HbA1c 8.4% (3.8–6.4)
Urine dipstick: blood +, protein +++	

    Renal biopsy (see **Figure 9.6**):

    Figure 9.6 *See colour plate section.*

    Which one of the following is the most likely cause of his kidney injury?

    A   Acute tubular necrosis
    B   Diabetic nephropathy
    C   Hypertensive nephrosclerosis
    D   IgA nephropathy
    E   Membranous nephropathy

33. A 35-year-old woman underwent renal biopsy to investigate progressive renal impairment with proteinuria.

    Renal biopsy (Congo red staining): see **Figure 9.7**:

Figure 9.7 *See colour plate section.*

Which one of the following least applies to her diagnosis?

A   If renal biopsy is insufficient rectal biopsy can aid diagnosis
B   It is seen with familial Mediterranean fever
C   It is seen with rheumatoid arthritis
D   Prognosis is good with steroids
E   The patient should be screened for plasma cell dyscrasias

34. A 74-year-old woman presented with lethargy and back pain. A new finding was of abnormal kidney function. She had no significant past medical history and took no regular medications.

Investigations:

haemoglobin 8.8 g/dL (females 11.5–16.5)	creatinine 407 µmol/L (females 45–90)
white cell count 9.6 × 10⁹/L (4–11)	protein 96 g/L (60–76)
urea 26.4 mmol/L (2.5–7.5)	albumin 34 g/L (37–49)

Renal biopsy (see **Figure 9.8**):

Figure 9.8 *See colour plate section.*

What is the most likely underlying diagnosis?

A   AA amyloid
B   Cast nephropathy
C   Cryoglobulinaemia
D   Renal sarcoid
E   Tubulointerstitial nephritis

35. A 75-year-old woman presented feeling weak. She had had diarrhoea and vomiting for 3 days. She was initially taking bendroflumethiazide but had stopped this in the past day.

On examination, she was alert and oriented. Her pulse was 100 beats per minute and blood pressure 100/60 mmHg (standing) and 80/51 mmHg (lying).

Investigations:

sodium 120 mmol/L (135–145)	thyroid-stimulating hormone 2.0 mU/L (0.4–5.0)
urea 12.2 mmol/L (2.5–7.5)	free thyroxine 20 pmol/L (10–25)
creatinine 94 µmol/L (females 45–90)	urine osmolality 410 mosmol/kg (500–800)

What is the most appropriate management?

A   0.9% NaCl intravenously
B   2.7% NaCl intravenously
C   Demeclocycline
D   Fluid restriction <1 L/24 h
E   Tolvaptan

36. A 45-year-old woman with a history of a renal transplantation 15 years ago presented with shingles and was started on aciclovir. She had previously been heavily immunosuppressed for rejection. She had also had a recent admission for *Pneumocystis jiroveci* pneumonia and was treated with co-trimoxazole, which she was still taking at a prophylactic dose. She took ciclosporin, mycophenolate mofetil and prednisolone as her maintenance immunosuppression. In addition she had recently been started on allopurinol following an attack of gout.

She returned to the clinic 2 weeks later and had routine blood tests done.

Investigations:

haemoglobin 11.5 g/dL (aim 11–13 CKD)	urate 500 mmol/L (females 110–360)
white cell count 7.4 × 10⁹ (4–11)	corrected calcium 2.5 mmol/L (2.2–2.6)
platelets 320 × 10⁹ (150–400)	phosphate 1.1 mmol/L (0.8–1.4)
creatinine 500 µmol/L (baseline 130)	
Urine: crystals	

Which drug is the most likely cause of her acute kidney injury?

A   Aciclovir
B   Allopurinol
C   Ciclosporin
D   Co-trimoxazole
E   Mycophenolate mofetil

37. A 42-year-old woman presented with headaches and grade 3 hypertensive retinopathy. She had no significant past medical history and was otherwise well.

Her blood pressure was 190/105 mmHg in both arms, and heart sounds and peripheral pulses were normal with no delay. She had bilateral oedematous ankles.

Investigations:

sodium 140 mmol/L (135–145)	fasting glucose 4.2 mmol/L (3–6)
potassium 3.1 mmol/L (3.5–5.0)	
Urine dipstick: negative for blood and protein	
Chest X-ray: normal	

What is the most likely cause of her hypertension?

A   Acute glomerulonephritis
B   Bartter's syndrome
C   Coarctation of the aorta
D   Cushing's syndrome
E   Renal artery stenosis

38. A 51-year-old man was referred to the renal clinic for investigation of his abnormal blood results. He had a history of autoimmune thrombocytopenia and was being treated with ciclosporin. He had no other significant past medical history and, other than low-dose steroids, took no other medications. He had the following blood results:

Investigations:

sodium 136 mmol/L (135–145)	bicarbonate 17 mmol/L (22–30)
potassium 5.7 mmol/L (3.5–5.0)	chloride 115 mmol/L (95–107)
creatinine 89 µmol/L (males 60–110)	urine pH 5.1
Urinary anion gap: positive	

What is the most likely diagnosis?

A   Fanconi's syndrome
B   Type 1 renal tubular acidosis
C   Type 2 renal tubular acidosis
D   Type 3 renal tubular acidosis
E   Type 4 renal tubular acidosis

39. A 70-year-old man was referred from the diabetic clinic. He had a history of type 2 diabetes for around 20 years with no retinopathy and no neuropathy. His most recent HbA1c was 7.2% (3.8–6.4) and creatinine 6 months ago was 135 µmol/L. He was well with no recent procedures or change in his medications. He was on amlodipine and ramipril for hypertension and gliclazide for diabetes.

On examination, he had pitting oedema of his ankles and his chest was clear. His blood pressure was 115/70 mmHg.

Investigations:

potassium 4.1 mmol/L (3.5–5.0)	creatinine 535 µmol/L (males 60–90)
Urine dipstick: protein ++, blood +	
Urinary protein:creatinine ratio 120 (<45)	
Ultrasound: bilateral 10-cm kidneys	

What is the most appropriate next step in management?

A   Add an angiotensin receptor blocker for dual blockade of proteinuria
B   Add a diuretic to improve his oedema
C   Change diabetic medication to insulin
D   Renal biopsy
E   Repeat results in 1 month to monitor the trend

40. A 32-year-old man with a history of bipolar disorder was admitted felling generally unwell. He took regular lithium. He complained of increased thirst and weakness. His urine output was 4 L/24 h.

Investigations:

sodium 152 mmol/L (135–145)	glucose 7.1 mmol/L (3–6)
potassium 3.9 mmol/L (3.5–5.0)	urine osmolality 250 mosmol/kg (500–800)
corrected calcium 2.46 mmol/L (2.2–2.6)	

What is the most appropriate next step in management?

A   5% dextrose
B   0.45% saline
C   Desmopressin (DDAVP)
D   Fluid restriction
E   Thiazide diuretic

41. A 28-year-old pregnant woman at 20 weeks' gestation was referred to the joint renal-obstetric clinic by the antenatal team as she was found to persistently have 1+ protein on urine dipstick testing. She was sent for further investigations.

When interpreting these further tests, which one of the following is definitely abnormal in pregnancy?

A   Creatinine changing from 73 μmol/L in the 1st trimester to 47 μmol/L in the 3rd trimester
B   Creatinine clearance changing from 125 mL/min in the 1st trimester to 90 mL/min in the 2nd trimester
C   Glycosuria on urine dipstick
D   Sodium 132 mmol/L
E   Proteinuria 100 mg/24 hours

42. A 48-year-old woman presented to the renal transplant clinic. She recieved a deceased donor transplant 2 years ago and had had good graft function with a baseline creatinine around 100 μmol/L. Repeat blood tests, however, showed that this had increased over 6 months to 155 μmol/L with proteinuria +++ on urine dipstick testing.
    She was admitted for a biopsy which showed no rejection but did show some features consistent with her original renal disease.

Which one of the following conditions is not recognised as recurring postrenal transplantation?

A   Diabetic nephropathy
B   IgA nephropathy
C   Mesangiocapillary glomerulonephritis type II
D   Primary focal segmental glomerulosclerosis
E   Tubulointerstitial nephritis

43. A 32-year-old man presented with a short history of feeling generally unwell and weak. He had been found collapsed a home.
    On examination, he was drowsy and confused with a Glasgow Coma Scale score of 14/15. His blood pressure was 170/90 mmHg and jugular venous pressure was visible at 4 cm. There were bibasal crepitations on respiratory examination and heart sounds revealed a gallop rhythm. Neurological examination revealed an ataxic gait and bilateral nerve VII palsies.
    Biopsy showed acute tubular necrosis and deposition of calcium oxalate crystals.

Investigations:

sodium 139 mmol/L (135–145)	creatinine 460 μmol/L (males 60–110)
potassium 6 mmol/L (3.5–5.0)	chloride 104 mmol/L (95–107)
urea 32 mmol/L	bicarbonate 15 mmol/L (22–30)
Urine dipstick: protein +++, blood ++	

What is the most likely cause?

A   Ethylene glycol ingestion
B   Rhabdomyolysis
C   Severe community-acquired pneumonia
D   Salicylate overdose
E   Vasculitis with a rapidly progressive glomerulonephritis

Answers

1. A 0.9% NaCl 1 mL/kg per h for 12 hours pre- and post-procedure

Contrast-induced nephropathy is common. It is defined as a rise in serum creatinine by >25% or by 44 µmol following the use of radiocontrast. It is often undetected as renal function may not be checked post-procedure. It usually occurs 24–48 hours after exposure, with creatinine levels peaking 5–7 days later. Although renal function often returns to normal about 7–10 days later, contrast-induced nephropathy is still an important cause of iatrogenic renal failure, morbidity and mortality. Those most at risk are patients with pre-existing renal impairment, and particularly those with diabetes. Although it is correct to stop nephrotoxins for 48 hours pre- and post-procedure there is also evidence that good hydration helps to prevent contrast nephropathy. Intravenous fluids will increase renal blood flow and minimise the prerenal effects of a post-contrast diuresis. Sodium bicarbonate may also be of benefit, but not over 0.9% NaCl. It is important to examine the patient first – with signs of volume depletion, larger fluid volumes than suggested here may be required. Likewise if there are signs of volume overload, further fluids would be contraindicated. This patient seems to be clinically euvolaemic and 0.9% NaCl 1 mL/kg per h for 12 hours pre- and post-procedure would suffice. Large meta-analyses suggest that N-acetylcysteine confers no significant benefit, although it causes no harm. Continuous venovenous haemofiltration does remove circulating contrast but there have been no large-scale trials to prove its benefit and it is clearly invasive, expensive, time-consuming and not without risk.

European Society of Urogenital Radiology Guidelines. Contrast Media. ESUR, 2008. http://www.esur.org/Contrast-media.51.0.html (last accessed May 2012).
Solomon R, Dauerman HL. Contrast-induced acute kidney injury. Circulation 2010; 122(23):2451–2455.

2. C Diclofenac

Amlodipine and bisoprolol both lower blood pressure and thus can contribute to the progression to acute tubular necrosis, but they are not directly toxic to the kidneys. Gliclazide is a sulfonamide that has no association with acute kidney injury. Metformin is known to cause lactic acidosis in the presence of renal impairment and the general consensus is that it should be withdrawn when creatinine is >150 µmol/L, but it does not cause acute kidney injury. Non-steroidal anti-inflammatory drugs (NSAIDs; such as diclofenac) and cyclo-oxygenase (COX) inhibitors are inhibitors of prostaglandin synthesis. In situations of normal renal blood flow (RBF) prostaglandins, (namely prostacyclin and prostaglandin E_2) have little haemodynamic effect on the kidney; in situations of reduced renal blood flow (e.g. hypovolaemia, as present here, any type of shock, congestive cardiac failure or cirrhosis) they cause significant change in renal haemodynamics. In the presence of a reduced RBF there are normally two actions of prostaglandins: compensatory afferent arteriolar dilatation to maintain glomerular perfusion, and blockade of the diuretic effect of antidiuretic hormone. These effects are attenuated by NSAID/COX inhibitors use, leading to dramatic reduction in renal blood flow and resulting in acute kidney injury.

Murray MD, Brater DC. Renal toxicity of the nonsteroidal anti-inflammatory drugs. Annu Rev Pharmacol Toxicol 1993; 33:435.

3. A Antiglomerular basement membrane disease (Goodpasture's disease)

This patient has presented with nephrotic syndrome with the triad of proteinuria (6 g in 24 hours), hypoalbuminaemia and peripheral oedema. The biopsy is classic for membranous nephropathy with numerous small 'spikes' seen on the glomerular basement membrane (seen best on silver stain). Light microscopy may be normal or there may be glomerular basement membrane (GBM) thickening. On electron microscopy there will be subepithelial immune deposits. Membranous nephropathy has many associations – most importantly infections and malignancy. Detection of malignancies may be preceded by membranous nephropathy by several years.

Associations include:

Infections
Hepatitis B and C
Malaria
Streptococcal infection
Syphilis
Schistosomiasis

Neoplasms
Solid tumours – carcinoma of breast, lung, kidney, gastrointestinal tract
Haematological malignancy – Hodgkin's disease, non-Hodgkin's disease

Systemic disease
Systemic lupus erythematosus
Sarcoidosis
Autoimmune thyroiditis

Toxins
Captopril
Non-steroidal anti-inflammatory drugs
D-Penicillamine
Gold

Anti-GBM disease is a rare pulmonary–renal syndrome which presents with a rapidly progressive glomerulonephritis showing a focal and segmental necrotising crescentic glomerulonephritis on renal biopsy and is not associated with nephrotic syndrome.

Protein:creatinine ratio (PCR) is more reproducible and generally more useful than 24-hour collections. A PCR of 100 mg/mmol is approximately equal to 1 g protein per 24 hours, and a PCR of >300 mg/mmol suggests 'nephrotic range' proteinuria (see Renal Association guidelines).

4. D Ramipril

Diabetic nephropathy is the most common cause of end-stage renal failure in Europe and the USA with an increased incidence in males. Renal biopsy is seldom required to establish the diagnosis, particularly in the presence of advanced retinopathy, negative immunology testing and no microscopic haematuria.

Good blood pressure control has been shown to slow down progression of all renal disease, particularly diabetic nephropathy which typically progresses quickly with glomerular filteration rate (GFR) declining by up to 12 mL/min per 1.73 m^2 each year. This can be reduced to 5 mL/min per 1.73 m^2 each year with tight blood pressure control. Amlodipine is a reasonable choice of antihypertensive; however, use of a long-acting, tissue-bound, angiotensin-converting enzyme (ACE) inhibitor (such as ramipril) or an angiotensin receptor blocker may slow decline further to as little as a loss of 0.3 mL/min per 1.73 m^2 each year and should be tried as first-line antihypertensive therapy (the RENAAL trial – see below). Tight diabetic control is also important but with hypertension and heavy proteinuria the most appropriate first step is to control blood pressure. A low-salt diet would be indicated but in the absence of hyperkalaemia a low-potassium diet is less important; none the less potassium should be monitored closely after the addition of an ACE inhibitor. Renal artery stenosis is common, particularly in type 2 diabetes, and should be considered if creatinine increases by >20% after initiation of an ACE inhibitor or if fluid retention becomes problematic.

MacGregor MS, Taal MW. Renal Association Guidelines – Detection, monitoring and care of patients with CKD. The Renal Association, 2011. http://www.renal.org/ClinicalGuidelinesSection/Detection-Monitoring-and-Care-of-Patients-with-CKD.aspx (last accessed May 2012).
KDOQI Guidelines. Diabetes and Chronic Kidney Disease. National Kidney Foundation. USA, 2007. http://www.kidney.org/professionals/KDOQI/guideline_diabetes (last accessed May 2012).

Brenner BM. Effects of losartan on renal and cardiovascular outcomes in patients with type 2 diabetes and nephropathy. N Engl J Med 2001; 345(12):861–869.

5. E Start a phosphate binder

This patient has blood results consistent with progressive chronic kidney disease (CKD) stage 4. Although he has a declining glomerular filtration rate (GFR) corrected for race (16 mL/min per 1.73 m^2 by the MDRD equation*) he is well and has no uraemic symptoms. He should be counselled that the need for renal replacement therapy is inevitable in the near future, and ideally he should be assessed for either elective formation of arteriovenous fistula for haemodialysis or insertion of a Moncrieff or Tenckhoff catheter for peritoneal dialysis. Younger patients should also be assessed for their suitability for transplantation, have any appropriate cardiological investigations, have possibility of live donors looked into or, failing that, be placed on the deceased donor transplantation list. The gold standard is that all of this should be done before the need to start dialysis.

Here the patient is anaemic but needs adequate iron replacement before starting erythropoietin. An angiotensin-converting enzyme (ACE) inhibitor to reduce proteinuria would be appropriate in a less advanced state of CKD; potassium of 5.5 mmol/L (3.5–5.0) would also be a contraindication.

Although his creatinine has risen by 70 µmol/L this actually corresponds only to a drop in GFR of 3 mL/min per 1.73 m^2 (19–16**) and is very unlikely to be caused by obstruction.

The calcium is low and phosphate is high, with evidence of secondary hyperparathyroidism from a raised parathyroid hormone (PTH). Starting a phosphate binder would be appropriate here to keep bone turnover as normal as possible and to stabilise PTH. Hyperphosphataemia is known to exert a direct calcifying effect on vascular smooth muscle cells; when prolonged it can cause calcification of coronary arteries, cardiac valves and pulmonary tissues, all seen in CKD, contributing to increased cardiovascular morbidity and mortality.

Kidney Disease: Improving Global Outcomes (KDIGO) issues guidelines regarding calcium and phosphate control, and management of secondary hyperparathyroidism. These recommend that serum phosphate should be maintained between 0.87 and 1.49 mmol/L (2.7 and 4.6 mg/dL) in patients with CKD stages 3 and 4 (as in this case), and between 1.13 and 1.78 mmol/L (3.5 and 5.5 mg/dL) in patients with CKD stage 5. They also publish guidelines for PTH, as well as the recommended frequency of measurement for PTH, calcium and phosphate.

NKF KDOQI guidelines – K/DOQI Clinical Practice Guidelines for Bone Metabolism and Disease in Chronic Kidney Disease. *Am J Kidney Dis* 2003; 42(4):suppl 3.
*The Modification of Diet in Renal Disease (MDRD) equation has been widely accepted as a formula to calculate estimated GFR (eGFR). It takes into account serum creatinine, age, race and gender.
**eGFR can be easily calculated using the above equation which can be found on the Renal Association website: http://www.renal.org/eGFRcalc (last accessed May 2012).

6. E Multiple myeloma

Acute tubulointersitial nephritis does occur with antibiotic use but is relatively rare; there might be a blood eosinophilia, and protein and leukocytes in the urine. Diabetic nephropathy is a possibility but it would be unusual for renal impairment to progress this quickly, particularly in the absence of significant proteinuria. There is no suggestion that the patient is hypovolaemic, making acute tubular necrosis less likely. The rate of decline of renal function, relatively bland urine and normal blood pressure also go against IgA nephropathy.

Acute kidney injury with anaemia and hypercalcaemia should always raise the suspicion of multiple myeloma. Serum electrophoresis, immunoglobulins, Bence Jones proteins, a bone marrow biopsy and a renal biopsy are all indicated here. Note that Bence Jones proteins (urinary light chains) are not detectable by urine dipstick testing.

Goldschmidt H, et al. Multiple myeloma and renal failure. Nephrol Dial Transplant 2000; 15(3):301–304.

7. E Serial blood cultures

The two broad differential diagnoses here are a small vessel vasculitis (SVV) with a rapidly progressive glomerulonephritis (RPGN) or infective endocarditis (IE). There are features that would suggest either diagnosis. The patient clearly has rapidly progressing renal impairment with blood and protein on dipstick testing, and the positive antineutrophil cytoplasmic antibody (ANCA) suggests the diagnosis of an SVV. The complements are, however, consumed which is not in keeping with a vasculitis but rather IE, supported by the pancytopenia, splenomegaly and valvular history. A renal biopsy would be helpful (showing a focal and segmental necrotising crescentic glomerulonephritis with vasculitis and a proliferative glomerulonephritis with infection) but is unsafe here because of thrombocytopenia. Pulse methylprednisolone can be given empirically if the suspicion of RPGN is high (particularly in the context of a strongly positive ANCA), but there are too many factors pointing towards infection in this case. Broad-spectrum antibiotics would be important but not until after serial blood cultures. Echocardiogram (transthoracic or transoesophageal) should be done urgently. Bone marrow biopsy is unlikely to aid in distinguishing between SVV and IE.

It is well recognised that ANCA can be positive in conditions other than vasculitis. Infection, particularly endocarditis, and occult malignancy should be looked for where the diagnosis is not clear.

Csernok E, et al. Clinical and immunological features of drug-induced and infection-induced proteinase 3-antineutrophil cytoplasmic antibodies and myeloperoxidase–antineutrophil cytoplasmic antibodies and vasculitis. Curr Opin Rheumatol 2010; 22(1):43–48.

8. B Renal biopsy

The key thing to exclude here is rejection. The patient has recieved a fairly recent cadaveric transplant with good baseline function which has deteriorated suddenly and is continuing to worsen. An ultrasound scan has already been performed and is normal with no suggestion of hydronephrosis, thus there is little value in doing a renogram at this point to look for obstruction. His blood pressure is on the high side but there is no suggestion of salt and water retention, making a renal artery stenosis less likely. There is nothing to suggest infection in his urine or systemically so, although urine culture should be sent, there is no indication to commence empirical antibiotics. Although cytomegalovirus polymerase chain reaction should be monitored regularly post-transplantation, it is not indicated urgently here. Renal biopsy is the definitive way to diagnose rejection and should be performed under ultrasound guidance urgently to assess for signs of rejection and to allow prompt treatment, which has been shown to improve long-term graft outcome. Kidney Disease: Improving Global Outcomes (KDIGO) guidelines suggest that renal allograft biopsy should be performed before treating acute rejection, unless facilitating the biopsy will substantially delay potential treatment. They also recommend that kidney biopsy be performed when there is a persistent, unexplained increase in serum creatinine, or when there is new onset of proteinuria or unexplained proteinuria ≥3 g/24 h.

KDIGO. Guidelines for Care of the Kidney Transplant Recipient. Am J Transplant 2009; 9 (3):S1–S157.

9. B Antiglomerular basement membrane disease

This patient presents with acute kidney injury and evidence of pulmonary haemorrhage. Antiglomerular basement membrane (anti-GBM) disease (Goodpasture's disease) is a rare pulmonary–renal syndrome. It may present acutely with fulminant pulmonary haemorrhage and renal failure or more gradually, as in this case, with generalised symptoms of fatigue and weight loss, and symptoms of subclinical pulmonary haemorrhage. Pulmonary haemorrhage is more common and severe in smokers and cigarette smoking has been proposed as a possible trigger, exposing antigenic epitopes on the basement membrane that are normally 'hidden'. Wegener's granulomatosis (granulomatosis with polyangiitis) is another cause of pulmonary–renal syndrome which may present in a similar way but cANCA (cytoplasmic antineutrophil cytoplasmic antibody) proteinase 3 is positive in the majority of patients (>95%) making it a less likely diagnosis in this case. Microscopic polyangiitis is also a small vessel vasculitis, usually pANCA (perineural ANCA) myeloperoxide positive, and does not typically cause respiratory involvement. Given her age and race tuberculosis would be unusual, and with an acute nephritis there might be leukocytes in urine. There is nothing to suggest a membranous nephropathy (she is not nephrotic) and the chest X-ray description is more suggestive of pulmonary haemorrhage than malignancy. She is not haemodynamically compromised or obviously septic so acute tubular necrosis (ATN) is less likely and, again, the chest X-ray is more suggestive of pulmonary haemorrhage (with bilateral changes) than pneumonia.

Anti-GBM disease is caused by IgG anti-GBM antibodies against the α_3 chain of type IV collagen (found in the glomerular and alveolar basement membranes) which bind and fix complement and cause local injury. Renal biopsy will show a focal and segmental, necrotising crescentic glomerulonephritis. Bowman's capsule may be ruptured. Immunofluorescence shows linear capillary wall staining for anti-GBM (IgG) and C3 deposition.

Treatment is immunosuppression with methylprednisolone and cyclophosphamide, haemodialysis if oligoanuric (often with no renal recovery) and plasma exchange to attempt to remove circulating antibodies. Patients can be dual ANCA and anti-GBM positive and this group tends to have a better outcome.

10. E Wegener's granulomatosis (granulomatosis and polyangiitis)

In a patient presenting with acute kidney injury in the context of systemic symptoms there are several important differential diagnoses. Often a renal biopsy is required in order to confirm the diagnosis but it is vital to first undertake a full nephritic screen. Here the main pointer is the complements which are low (see **Table 9.1**). Complement may be low in all of these conditions except Wegener's granulomatosis which is an ANCA-associated small vessel vasculitis where complement is normal. In infective states (such as post-streptococcal glomerulonephritis and infective endocarditis) there will be consumption of complement. In lupus nephritis there are immune deposits seen in the kidney on histology.

Table 9.1 Hypocomplementaemia

Disease	C3	C4
Infective endocarditis	↓	↓
Postinfectious glomerulonephritis	↓	↓/↔
Systemic lupus erythematosus	↓	↓
Essential mixed cryoglobulinaemia	↔	↓
Mesangiocapillary glomerulonephritis (MCGN) type II	↓	↔
Cholesterol emboli	↓	↔

11. A 10 mL of 10% calcium gluconate given intravenously over 5 minutes

This patient presents with acute kidney injury in the context of rhabdomyolysis. Because of widespread cell death there is accumulation of intracellular elements, particularly creatine kinase (CK), myoglobin and potassium.

In this case there is evidence of myocardial irritation on his ECG caused by hyperkalaemia, and the first and most important step is to stabilise this using 10 mL of 10% calcium gluconate given intravenously over 2–5 minutes (or 5 mL of 10% calcium chloride). If there is no improvement in ECG changes, this can be repeated after 5 minutes, up to a total of 40 mL calcium gluconate. It is important to remember that this calcium gluconate (or chloride) is cardioprotective only and does not actually lower serum potassium. In addition, its protective effects will last for under an hour and so other measures must be taken to identify the cause of hyperkalaemia and to lower the potassium concentration. The first measure to lower potassium would be an insulin/dextrose infusion (using 10 units of fast-acting insulin in 50 mL of 50% dextrose which can be given over 10–20 minutes through a large-bore peripheral cannula). This can lower potassium by 0.5–1.5 µmol/L and the effects will last between 2 and 4 hours. It can be repeated after 2–4 hours, but beware of hypoglycaemia developing. It works by insulin increasing $Na^+/K^+/ATPase$ activity which moves potassium into cells. If this fails to adequately control potassium then the next step is haemodialysis or haemofiltration. This will bring potassium quickly under control within 30 minutes and results in extracorporeal removal of potassium.

Compartment syndrome occurs either if there is compromise to the blood supply of a limb because of immobility, or from generalised muscle injury in the case of toxic or virally induced rhabdomyolysis. An urgent fasciotomy is required here, as is careful fluid balance and replacement, because it will ultimately help treat the cause of the hyperkalaemia and may save the limb. First, however, the patient must be stabilised cardiovascularly. Nebulised salbutamol and Calcium Resonium have little to add to the management of hyperkalaemia that insulin dextrose doesn't achieve. Salbutamol (10–20 mg) will lower serum potassium by around 1 µmol/L but acts on the same Na^+/K^+-ATPase pump that insulin/dextrose does and has a slower onset of action, so it therefore confers no additional benefit. In acutely unwell patients with underlying cardiac disease it may also precipitate tachyarrhythmias. Calcium Resonium is a cation exchange resin which exchanges sodium for potassium in the gastrointestinal tract. It can be given orally or rectally (more effective) and its effect will be maximal at 24–48 hours.

Steddon S, et al. Oxford Handbook of Nephrology and Hypertension. Oxford: Oxford University Press, 2006.

12. A Acute tubular necrosis secondary to hypotension

The causes of postoperative acute kidney injury are many and should always be considered, particularly looking for sepsis. The obvious period of low blood pressure here makes acute tubular injury secondary to hypotension the most likely cause of her rising creatinine, especially in the context of her risk factors and pre-existing kidney disease. A mean arterial pressure of less than 70 mmHg is the limit below which renal autoregulation is impaired and the glomerular filtration rate falls. Sepsis is another common cause of postoperative acute kidney injury but unlikely here. Although her wounds look a little red she is systemically well and her inflammatory markers are not elevated. Acute tubulointerstitial nephritis is less likely. It is less frequently seen with co-amoxiclav than some other antibiotics, although there are reported cases. The relatively bland urine and lack of raised white cell count (eosinophilia is often seen) make this diagnosis unlikely here. Contrast is not given for coronary bypass grafting. Renal artery occlusion is also unlikely because, although there is a slight variation in kidney size, this is within acceptable limits and they are essentially normal sized. In addition there is no evidence of salt and water overload or hypertension which you might expect with renal artery stenosis or occlusion, and there are no symptoms of an acute arterial occlusion.

13. B Cholesterol emboli

Cholesterol emboli are the most obvious diagnosis in view of age, risk factors and atherosclerotic history. White men over the age of 50 years are the most susceptible group. It most frequently occurs in them after vascular instrumentation or surgery, most commonly angiography. It also occurs in the context of thrombolysis or anticoagulation. Showers of cholesterol crystals from destabilised plaques cause partial occlusion of small arteries which results in infarcts in the endarterial territories, typically the digits and the gut. Damage in the kidneys can either be acute (1–4 weeks post-procedure) from similar downstream ischaemia in the small renal vessels or more chronic (can be months after the initial insult) and progressive from a secondary fibrotic response. Urine is often bland although patients can present with heavy proteinuria. A blood eosinophilia is common and hypocomplementaemia is often seen. Treatment is limited and may comprise use of statins, despite paucity of evidence. Mortality and morbidity are high from cardiovascular causes, and renal function often fails to recover, requiring long-term renal replacement therapy.

Contrast-induced nephropathy would also be a possible cause of acute kidney injury here but the systemic signs and the patient's symptoms point more towards cholesterol emboli. Also the timing of the presentation is a little late for contrast-induced nephropathy which typically causes a creatinine rise 24–48 hours post-exposure to contrast.

Although this patient is at risk of having renal artery stenosis given his vascular risk factors, again the acute presentation, signs and ultrasound findings go against this.

Lupus nephritis is associated with hypocomplementaemia but it would be a very unlikely presentation in an elderly white man.

Analgesic nephropathy would not present in such an acute way, although pain killers can be associated with acute tubulointerstitial nephritis.

Dupont PJ, et al. Lesson of the week: Cholesterol emboli syndrome. BMJ 2000; 321:1065–1067.

14. C Intravenous fresh frozen plasma

This patient has haemolytic uraemic syndrome (HUS) associated with a diarrhoeal illness. HUS is the triad of microangiopathic haemolytic anaemia, red cell fragmentation on blood film and acute kidney injury. It may be typical, associated with a diarrhoeal illness (D+), or atypical which includes genetic mutations (of complement or von Willebrand's factor), pregnancy induced and secondary to drugs (D–).

In D+ HUS pathogenic bacteria produce toxins which translocate across the inflamed mucosa of the bowel into the blood, causing endothelial damage. This is particularly damaging to the glomerular endothelium which is involved in the pathogenesis of the acute kidney injury. More generally the endothelial damage leads to platelet activation, increased prothrombotic factors and release of ultra-large von Willebrand's factor. There is resultant thrombocytopenia and thrombotic microangiopathic anaemia. HUS and thrombotic thrombocytopenic purpura (TTP), in which there is less kidney involvement and more neurological involvement, are part of the same clinical spectrum. Presentation with HUS may quickly progress to multiorgan failure.

Treatment is supportive and the first line is infusion of fresh frozen plasma, but not platelets which may worsen the outcome. Plasma exchange is indicated if there is neurological involvement, or if TTP is expected. There is no indication for haemofiltration or haemodialysis in this case as the patient is still passing urine, although renal impairment may progress and dialysis may be still required. There is no role for vitamin K in the treatment of HUS. Flexible sigmoidoscopy is not indicated and would be unsafe with this patient's degree of anaemia and thrombocytopenia, but stool culture should be performed.

Clark WF. HUS/TTP Update. Kidney Int 2008 (75):S1–S3.

15. E Surgical removal of PD catheter, minilaparotomy and wash-out

This patient has a diagnosis of culture-negative peritoneal dialysis (PD) peritonitis. An elevated dialysate white cell count of >100 /mm^3 of which at least 50% are polymorphonuclear neutrophils is supportive of the diagnosis. Patients with cloudy fluid and either abdominal pain and/or fever should have prompt initiation of empirical intraperitoneal antibiotic therapy. He has had appropriate treatment in the community for 5 days with intraperitoneal antibiotics and his peritoneal infection has not resolved. This constitutes refractory peritonitis and the recommended approach would be to admit him, arrange for a surgical removal of his peritoneal dialysis (PD) catheter and a wash-out, and convert him, at least temporarily, to haemodialysis. PD catheters can be removed medically on the wards without an operation but in the case of peritonitis this is not recommended as there would obviously be no option for wash-out. In addition the subcutaneous 'cuffs', which secure the catheter in place where it is tunnelled under the skin, are often retained, serving as a further source of infection.

Although there is no growth in the PD fluid there is nothing else in the history to suggest tuberculosis and the white cells are predominantly neutrophils, not lymphocytes. At laparotomy it is standard to send further fluid and peritoneal biopsies for culture and histology, particularly looking for granulomas or presence of acid-fast bacilli.

Adding intravenous antibiotics will not add anything to the treatment of the infection as the patient will already be therapeutically covered with intraperitoneal dosing. The watch-and-wait strategy has already been in place for 5 days and there has been little improvement and it is clear that this now a non-resolving infection which requires further intervention.

ISPD Guidelines/Recommendations. Peritoneal Dialysis-Related Infections Recommendations: 2010 update. Perit Dial Int 2010; 30:393–423.

16. E She should have an MR angiogram of her brain

Adult polycystic kidney disease (APKD) is a common inherited disease. It is inherited as an autosomal dominant disease, so there is a 50% chance of offspring being affected. There are two mutations, found on chromosome 16 and chromosome 4, which are responsible for the phenotype seen. These mutations code for polycystin-1 (PKD-1) and polycystin-2 (PKD-2) respectively. PKD-1 is more common than PKD-2. Both polycystin-1 and polycystin-2 are involved in the regulation of cell proliferation and differentiation in the tubular epithelium and in the maturation of these cells. When this mechanism fails in APKD there is dysregulated cell turnover and uncontrolled growth which results in the formation of multiple cysts. These cysts enlarge over time and there is ongoing ischaemic and fibrotic damage which culminates in renal impairment.

Patients often present with a positive family history, flank or loin pain, haematuria, nocturia or hypertension. Ultrasound is the imaging of choice for diagnosis. For the best negative predictive value this should be done only after the age of 20 years.

The Ravine criteria are used to interpret the scan and confirm the diagnosis (only valid for PKD-1) as shown in **Table 9.2**.

Table 9.2 Ravine criteria		
Age	**Positive family history**	**Negative family history**
<30 years	2 cysts in either kidney	5 cysts in either kidney
30–60 years	4 cysts in either kidney	5 cysts in either kidney
>60 years	8 cysts in either kidney	8 cysts in either kidney

PKD-2 often presents later than PKD-1. Hypertension is often the first sign of APKD and may be present even when renal function is normal. Not all patients with APKD will progress to renal failure. A worse renal prognosis is associated with patients who are diagnosed earlier or have early hypertension, and those with PKD-1 mutations.

Polycystic kidneys are associated with both extrarenal cysts (particularly polycystic livers) and an increased risk of intracranial aneurysms. Around 5–10% of patients with APKD will have an intracranial aneurysm and this tends also to be familial. Patients with a strong family history of intracerebral bleeds should have screening with an MR angiogram. Most commonly the aneurysms rupture in younger patients with poor blood pressure control and confer high mortality and morbidity.

Her blood pressure at present is too high and she should be promptly started on antihypertensives to help preserve renal function.

Belibi F, Edelstein C. Unified ultrasonographic diagnositic criteria for polycystic kidney disease. J Am Soc Nephrol 2009; 20(1):6–8.

17. B Collapsing focal segmental glomerulosclerosis

This patient has significant renal impairment with a negative nephritic screen except for positive HIV virology. A low CD4 count and a high viral load indicate untreated, or undertreated, disease. HIV infection is associated with many different types of renal lesion but the most common one described is HIV-associated nephropathy (HIVAN), followed by HIV immune-complex kidney (HIVICK) disease. In HIVAN, which is predominantly seen in patients of African descent, there is typically a collapsing variant of focal segmental glomerulosclerosis (FSGS) caused by HIV infection of the renal proximal tubular cells and podocytes. HIVICK refers to a collection of immunoglobulin-related glomerulonephritides which are more commonly seen in non-African patients. HIVAN is characterised by heavy proteinuria (often nephrotic range, i.e. >3 g/24 h), microscopic haematuria, albuminuria and high rates of progression to end-stage renal disease. It occurs when HIV infection is advanced (CD4 <200) and often in the context of an AIDS-defining illness.

Hyaline arteriosclerosis is caused by uncontrolled hypertension; this patient's blood pressure is only marginally elevated and he is not on antihypertensive agents. Kimmelstiel–Wilson nodules are typically associated with diabetic nephropathy and there is no suggestion of diabetes in this case. Minimal change, although a common cause of nephrotic syndrome, is not as a rule associated with abnormal creatinine or dipstick haematuria. There would also be a greater degree of peripheral oedema with such proteinuria and hypoalbuminaemia. Typically HIVAN will present with massive proteinuria and hypoalbuminaemia, but relatively little peripheral oedema. Cast nephropathy is seen in association with multiple myeloma. The normal full blood count, immunoglobulins and serum electrophoresis exclude multiple myeloma, and in cast nephropathy there would not be such a degree of proteinuria and hypoalbuminaemia.

Kaufman L, et al. The pathogenesis of HIV-associated nephropathy. Adv Chronic Kidney Dis 2010; 17(1):36–43.

18. C Epstein–Barr virus

This patient has a 10-year history of immunosuppression with a history of rejection earlier in his transplant history which would have necessitated stronger immunosuppression at the time for treatment of this. All the viruses listed are important and can cause problems throughout the post-transplantaton course. The key here is in interpreting the clinical picture and the time frame.

The weight loss, anaemia, lymphadenopathy and a palpable abdominal mass are clear pointers towards malignancy. Patients who have received long-term immunosuppression are at increased risk of malignancy. In transplant recipients this is known as post-transplantation lymphoproliferative disease/disorder (PTLD) and is often driven by Epstein–Barr virus which can cause uncontrolled B cell proliferation. It occurs in 1–5% of renal transplant recipients, often in those who have been most heavily immunosuppressed. Patients often respond to a reduction in their immunosuppression, but may require chemotherapy.

Cytomegalovirus (CMV) is important to remember as a major complication of transplantation. CMV polymerase chain reaction should be performed regularly post-transplantation. Patients can be asymptomatic but can present with systemic symptoms, colitis, pneumonitis and graft dysfunction. Although it should be checked, in this case CMV infection would not account for all the features.

BK virus (named after the initials of the first renal transplant recipient in whom the virus was isolated) is a polyoma virus that can cause graft dysfunction and ureteric stenosis but there is nothing to suggest BK nephropathy here. Equally there is nothing to suggest HBV infection in this case. HIV should be considered but again there is nothing else in the history that points towards it.

Steddon S, et al. Oxford Handbook of Nephrology and Hypertension. Oxford: Oxford University Press, 2006.

19. A He has high blood pressure

The biopsy picture is consistent with malignant hypertension. The picture shows hyaline arteriosclerosis, and the vessel seen in the centre of the biopsy has a typical 'onion skin' appearance of the media, with complete occlusion of the lumen. Vascular changes in the renal vessels from uncontrolled hypertension are as a result of endothelial injury and intimal thickening. There are sub-endothelial lipid deposits and hyaline thrombi. Fibrinoid necrosis is seen in the small renal arteries.

Although this section of the biopsy looks to be severely damaged by hypertensive changes, it is impossible to comment on his prognosis based on one small segment. So, despite the fact that his renal function is already significantly impaired, it would be impossible to say that he needs immediate dialysis, although it is highly likely that renal function will continue to deteriorate over time, particularly if his blood pressure remains poorly controlled.

Starting immunosuppression would suggest that there is clear evidence of an inflammatory or autoimmune lesion seen which is not the case, either in this small section of biopsy or in the history.

It is possible that this patient could have IgA nephropathy as well as malignant hypertension, but again a larger biopsy sample including glomeruli is required to consider this diagnosis, as well as specific staining for IgA deposition. Even if this were the diagnosis, serum IgA would not always be raised in IgA nephropathy.

Finally it is not possible to comment on the extent of proteinuria just by looking at vessels on a renal biopsy. Protein leak suggests intrinsic renal disease, in particular glomerular lesions, and again there is insufficient biopsy material here to assess. Even then it is difficult to predict quantities of proteinuria from biopsy alone.

20. C Prostate carcinoma

This patient has a diagnosis of retroperitoneal fibrosis (RPF) as seen by the inflammatory mass on the CT surrounding the aorta. He has presented with acute kidney injury secondary to obstruction from ureteric involvement (which may be as a result of reduced contractility as opposed to simply mechanical obstruction) and the kidneys can be seen as dilated on the imaging. There is also evidence on the CT of a nephrostomy tube in the left kidney to decompress the system.

RPF is a relatively uncommon condition and typically presents in men between the ages of 40 years and 60 years. It is characterised by extensive fibrosis throughout the retroperitoneum and causes obstruction of the mid- to lower-third of the ureters. Renal impairment develops as a result of obstructive uropathy. In many cases it is idiopathic and in these cases the pathogenesis is thought to involve an immunological response to antigens within atherosclerotic plaques and leakage of proinflammatory material across the wall of an atheromatous aorta. It is also associated with aortic aneurysms.

In other cases RPF is associated with a variety of causes including drug induced (classically beta-blockers but also methysergide), lymphoma or other lymphoproliferative disorders, tuberculosis and metastatic malignancy. The patient should have a full CT to assess any further evidence of malignancy or lymphadenopathy, and the inflammatory mass should be biopsied to aid diagnosis. The aim should be to preserve renal function by relieving the obstruction promptly, and ureteric stenting is often required, sometimes preceded by nephrostomy as in this case. Immunosuppression in the form of corticosteroids may reduce the inflammation and thus improve renal function, but there is an absence of evidence base for long-term immunosuppression. Definitive surgery would include ureterolysis and omental wrapping.

Prostatic malignancy and hypertrophy can also present with bilateral hydronephrosis but the level of obstruction is lower (bladder outflow obstruction) and it would not be expected to see the para-aortic inflammatory mass on CT. The treatment of prostate cancer with radiotherapy could, however, cause RPF.

21. C Initiate dialysis to facilitate packed red cell transfusion

This patient has presented with end-stage renal failure and symptoms of uraemia, particularly lethargy, nausea and loss of appetite. He has a diagnosis of diabetic nephropathy and has not been followed up for several years. His blood pressure is uncontrolled. This probably represents the natural progression of his underlying kidney disease.

There is no reason to insert a central venous catheter here, as there is nothing to suggest volume depletion or overload. Central lines are not routinely required to monitor patients with kidney injury and are not without risk. Volume status as far as possible should be assessed clinically, using primarily lying and standing blood pressures, heart rate, jugular venous pressure measurement, fluid balance charts and daily weights.

Acidosis itself is not an indication to start dialysis, except in cases of acute kidney injury with pH <7.1 and myocardial depression. There is no absolute cut-off urea value when dialysis should be started. Patients have variable tolerance of uraemia. This patient is beginning to display some uraemic symptoms but the more pressing indication to start dialysis is his anaemia and hyperkalaemia. He clearly requires blood transfusion and with potassium of 6.4 mmol/L it would be unsafe to do this without simultaneously dialysing him.

His anaemia is most likely secondary to his end-stage renal failure. There is nothing to suggest active bleeding and he is not haemodynamically unstable. He requires urgent transfusion and thereafter to be established on iron replacement and an erythropoietin-stimulating agent. In patients with an eGFR (estimated glomerular filtration rate) of >30 mL/min per 1.73 m^2 it cannot be assumed that anaemia is due to renal impairment and in these cases further investigations should be considered. This patient, however, has an eGFR of <5 mL/min per 1.73 m^2.

22. C Start on a single oral antihypertensive agent

Hypertensive crises can be defined as urgencies or emergencies. Emergencies would include severe hypertension with encephalopathy, stroke, pulmonary oedema and cardiac ischaemia. This patient presents as a hypertensive urgency, not emergency. He does have evidence of target organ damage (left ventricular hypertrophy, renal impairment) but this is probably not acute as he has a long-standing history of hypertension and no symptoms. There is nothing to suggest a dissection, but if he had presented with chest pain or back pain or had a discrepancy between blood pressure in different arms then this would require urgent investigation.

He does have evidence of renal impairment with blood and protein in his urine and this should be monitored. A renal biopsy is probably required prognostically as much as diagnostically and should be performed when his blood pressure is safe to do so. His renal function may in fact improve with better blood pressure control, and the blood and protein in his urine may improve.

A hypertensive emergency (encephalopathy, dissection, acute left ventricular failure) should be treated with an intravenous infusion of antihypertensives, aiming for a blood pressure of 160/100 mmHg in the first day, and even lower if there is aortic dissection. Labetalol or glyceryl trinitrate is commonly used.

In this case a single oral agent can be used, e.g. amlodipine 5 mg, and titrated. Aim to bring the blood pressure down relatively slowly with a diastolic of 100 mmHg initially and then reassess every 2 days. It would not be reasonable to simply wait for a week and repeat as, in the face of obvious target organ damage, this will not represent so-called 'white-coat hypertension' and should be treated straight away.

If hypertension is left untreated there is a 1-year mortality rate of >90%. This falls to <10% with appropriate treatment.

Cherney D, et al. Management of patients with hypertensive urgencies and emergencies: A systematic review of the literature. J Gen Intern Med 2002; 17(12):937–945.
Steddon S, et al. Oxford Handbook of Nephrology and Hypertension. Oxford: Oxford University Press, 2006.

23. D Pure red cell aplasia (PRCA)

This patient presents with worsening anaemia despite adequate treatment with erythropoietin. It is not sufficient to attribute this to anaemia of chronic disease as she should be able to maintain her haemoglobin with appropriate iron replacement and erythropoietin. The normal white cell count makes chronic lymphocytic leukaemia unlikely. The normal mean corpuscular volume and normal gastroscopy with the elevated ferritin and transferrin make blood loss unlikely. Myelodysplasia is also unlikely with normal white cell and platelet count, and absence of reticulocytes.

Acquired pure red cell aplasia is a rare condition. It can be idiopathic, associated with underlying haematological/autoimmune disorders and viral infections, or secondary to neutralising autoantibodies against erythropoietin. The latter is the most likely cause in this case. Typically patients have been on erythropoietin for 6–18 months. PRCA is characterised by profound anaemia, very low/absent reticulocytes and the virtual absence of erythroblasts in the bone marrow. Serum transferrin saturations and ferritin rise as iron cannot be incorporated into new erythrocytes. Bone marrow aspirate should be performed and the anti-erythropoietin antibodies be measured. Treatment includes withdrawal of erythropoietin and transfusions for symptoms. Immunosuppressive treatment should be considered.

Casadeval N, et al. Epoetin-induced autoimmune pure red cell aplasia. J Am Soc Nephrol 2005; 16:S67–S69.

24. A Collapsing glomerulopathy

This biopsy shows a classic collapsed glomerulus in the left upper quadrant of the picture which would be most likely expected in HIV-associated nephropathy (HIVAN). There is also extensive acute tubular injury (ATN) with large dilated tubules (especially in the lower central part of the picture). A collapsing glomerulopathy is typically associated with nephrotic range proteinuria often with hypoalbuminaemia. This patient should be tested for HIV urgently and started on HAART (highly reactive antiretroviral therapy) as appropriate. Rarely, collapsing glomerulopathy can be caused by other causes, including HTLV, pamidronate and hepatitis C infection.

The small vessel ANCA-positive vasculitides [granulomatosis with polyangiitis (Wegener's granulomatosis) and microscopic polyangiitis] would be associated with a focal necrotising crescentic glomerulonephritis. This diagnosis should be considered in anyone presenting with acute kidney injury with blood and protein in the urine, but this is not the typical biopsy picture.

In membranous nephropathy the glomeruli have typically thick basement membranes with a 'spiky' appearance on silver stain. In tubulointerstitial nephritis the glomeruli are normal, which is clearly not the case here, and the interstitium shows an inflammatory cell infiltrate. Mesangiocapillary glomerulonephritis (MCGN) (or membranoproliferative glomerulonephritis – MPGN), of which there are three types, refers to a pattern of glomerulopathy including mesangial proliferation, thick capillary walls and so-called double contours.

Davison Y, et al. Oxford Textbook of Nephrology, 3rd edn. Oxford: Oxford University Press, 2006.

25. B Continuous venovenous haemofiltration (CVVHF)

This patient has presented with severe sepsis and acute kidney injury, most likely due to acute tubular necrosis (ATN). The associated mortality is high.

Although he is anaemic and would benefit from transfusion, it is not safe to do at present – he is showing signs of volume overload and is already hyperkalaemic. Equally, although he is oliguric it would not be safe to give him any more fluid, especially up to 1 L, as he already has an elevated jugular venous pressure, peripheral oedema and bibasal crepitations in the context of known left ventricular dysfunction. He most likely will require inotropic support but there is little evidence to support the use of dobutamine or furosemide infusions in the context of ATN.

He is oliguric with rising potassium and not responding to simple fluid resuscitation and thus needs renal replacement. The choice is between intermittent haemodialysis (IHD) and haemofiltration (CVVHF) – see **Table 9.3**. In this situation haemofiltration is preferable as it is associated with greater haemodynamic stability and, in a patient who is hypotensive with known left ventricular impairment, is more likely to be tolerated than haemodialysis. Haemofiltration is the most common method of renal replacement therapy in the intensive care unit, where this patient should be managed.

Ronco C, Bellomo R. Dialysis in intensive care unit patients with acute kidney injury: Continuous therapy is superior. Clin J Am Soc Nephrol 2007; 2(3):597–600.

Table 9.3 Intermittent haemodialysis versus continuous venovenous haemofiltration

	Intermittent haemodialysis	Continuous venovenous haemofiltration
Location	Outpatient, inpatient, home	Mainly high-dependency/intensive care unit setting
Patients	Haemodynamically stable	Haemodynamically compromised
Principles	Intermittent No fluid replacement required Dialysate required Solute clearance by diffusion	Slow and continuous Fluid replacement required No dialysate required Solute clearance by convection
Benefits	Independence for the well patient Form of long-term treatment	Slower more controlled fluid shifts
Disadvantages	Large fluid shifts Rapid correction of electrolytes	High intensity care required Temporary treatment

26. E Parathyroidectomy

This patient has biochemical evidence of tertiary hyperparathyroidism. Secondary hyperparathyroidism develops in renal failure secondary to phosphate accumulation. In addition there are low levels of

1,25(OH)$_2$-vitamin D and associated hypocalcaemia. Parathyroid hormone (PTH) rises in response to these. If this is uncontrolled then prolonged stimulation of the parathyroid glands will result in hyperplasia and autonomous secretion of PTH. This is tertiary hyperparathyroidism and the overactive parathyroid glands will not respond to medical therapy. Cinacalcet is a calcimimetic agent that acts essentially as a 'medical parathyroidectomy' but some patients will be intolerant or non-compliant. Parathyroidectomy should be considered in this case as he is not responsive to medical treatment and has clear radiological evidence of resultant bony deformity and brown tumours (osteitis fibrosa cystica). These changes may slowly recover postoperatively.

A bone biopsy is not always required and imaging and biochemistry are often sufficient to diagnose. There is little benefit in changing phosphate binder from Calcichew to Alu-Cap (another non-calcium-containing, aluminium-based phosphate binder) here and more definitive treatment is required. The CT and biochemistry are not suggestive of metastatic disease so a full body CT is not justified. Increasing his alfacalcidol would further increase his calcium and phosphate so would not help.

KDOQI. Clinical Practice Guidelines for Bone Metabolism and Disease in Chronic Kidney Disease. http://www.kidney.org. (Last accessed May 2012)

27. B Cryoglobulins

This man has acute kidney injury with active urinary sediment and a rash. This makes some form of vasculitis the most likely diagnosis. The low complement level limits what this is likely be due to there being only a few conditions associated with hypocomplementaemia. Small vessel (i.e. ANCA positive) vasculitis is, therefore, less likely. Systemic lupus erythematosus (SLE) would be a possibility, but this patient's age, race and sex make lupus an extremely unlikely diagnosis, so double-stranded DNA (dsDNA) is not going to help. Extractable nuclear antigen (ENA) is useful if antinuclear antibody (ANA) is positive and in distinguishing between various connective tissue/autoimmune disorders, but in this case we are not told that he is ANA positive thus ENA is unlikely to aid in the diagnosis. Erythrocyte sedimentation ratio is a non-specific marker of several autoimmune and inflammatory conditions and does not help distinguish between them.

The strongly positive rheumatoid factor, low complements (C4 > C3) with rash and acute kidney injury (AKI) all point to cryoglobulinaemia. Cryoglobulins are a heterogeneous group of immunoglobulins which precipitate from plasma/serum at temperatures <37°C. There are several types of cryoglobulins and different ways to classify them but essentially there are three categories: type I (simple, monoclonal) accounts for around 10% of cryoglobulinaemias and is associated with lymphoproliferative disorders; type II (mixed, monoclonal–polyclonal immune complex); type III (mixed polyclonal–polyclonal immune complex) contains rheumatoid factors (usually IgM) which form complexes with the Fc portion of polyclonal IgG. They account for 90% of cryoglobulinaemias and are almost always associated with hepatitis C infection.

Other important investigations would include hepatitis C (and B) serology, C3 nephritic factor, immunoglobulins and serum electrophoresis (warm), and a renal biopsy.

Ramos-Casals M, et al. The cryoglobulinaemias. Lancet 2012; 379:348–60.

28. C Disequilibrium syndrome

This patient has typical signs of disequilibrium syndrome. Disequilibrium is a central nervous system disorder that can affect haemodialysis patients, causing acute symptoms that develop during or immediately after haemodialysis. Early symptoms include headache, nausea, disorientation, restlessness and blurring of vision. More severely affected patients progress to confusion, seizures and coma. The symptoms are mainly thought to be due to cerebral oedema. It occurs when there is insufficient time for urea equilibration and haemodialysis rapidly reduces the blood urea nitrogen. There is resultant water movement into the brain. New dialysis patients are at highest risk, particularly those who are elderly and with a high urea (>60 mmol/L). First dialysis sessions are usually for a maximum of 2 hours, with slow blood flow rates and minimal fluid removal to minimise this complication. Treatment involves stopping the dialysis session and treating the seizure. Improvement should occur.

There is no indication here that the patient has had an arrhythmia and her potassium has been lowered effectively. There is nothing to suggest sepsis in the blood tests or history. A dialyser reaction would typically occur shortly after (minutes to half an hour) starting dialysis and not after 2 or 3 hours as in this case. It would present with an anaphylactoid reaction. Intracerebral bleed is also a possibility, but she has had heparin-free dialysis and the lack of focal neurological signs would go against it. She should, however, have a CT to formally exclude this diagnosis.

Levy J, et al. The Oxford Handbook of Dialysis, 3rd edn. Oxford: Oxford University Press, 2009.

29. C Mesna

This patient has tumour lysis syndrome (TLS). TLS occurs at initiation of treatment of malignancies, most commonly haematological. It may also occur spontaneously if the tumour burden is large. Uric acid is primarily responsible for renal injury following necrosis of large numbers of malignant cells. Acute kidney injury results, associated with hyperkalaemia, hyperphosphataemia and high uric acid levels. Lactate dehydrogenase will also be high.

Ideally at-risk patients should be identified, prehydrated with 0.9% NaCl and given allopurinol.

In patients with established TLS the treatment includes aggressive fluid resuscitation to maintain a high urine output and allopurinol to prevent metabolism of xanthine and thus uric acid. Sodium bicarbonate to alkalinise the urine may help prevent precipitation of uric acid into crystalline casts, although maintaining a good urine output with NaCl may suffice. Rasburicase is recombinant urate oxidase which rapidly reduces uric acid levels. Treatment of hyperkalaemia, which would include calcium gluconate to stabilize the myocardium, may be required. If the patient is oliguric and potassium is not controllable, haemodialysis is indicated.

Mesna provides bladder protection from haemorrhagic cystitis in patients treated with ifosfamide or cyclophosphamide.

Howard SC, et al. The tumour lysis syndrome. N Engl J Med 2011; 364:1844–1854.

30. A Allergic granulomatosis and angiitis (Churg–Strauss syndrome)

This patient presents with classic features of Churg–Strauss syndrome (allergic granulomatosis and angiitis) which is a small and medium vessel vasculitis presenting as allergic rhinitis, asthma and eosinophilia, usually in the third to fifth decades. There are typically three stages: initially the allergic phase in which asthma begins, then the eosinophilic stage characterised by eosinophilic infiltration of various organs, and finally the vasculitic phase in which patients present with symptoms of a systemic vasculitis. Around 30% of patients have renal involvement, many of whom will have a rapidly progressive glomerulonephritis (RPGN), and antineutrophil cytoplasmic antibody (ANCA) is often positive in those who do. The patient displays the classic picture of increasingly difficult to control asthma, eosinophilia, abdominal pain and diarrhoea, which could be as a result of gut infiltration, and constitutional symptoms.

Granulomatosis and polyangiitis (Wegener's granulomatosis) is a possibility but is not associated with the asthmatic symptoms or raised eosinophil count. It is associated with a positive ANCA but typically proteinase 3 (PR 3) rather than myeloperoxide.

A post-infectious glomerulonephritis (GN) would often be associated with hypocomplementaemia and would not show a necrotising GN on biopsy. Furthermore ANCA would not be positive. Similarly tubulointerstitial nephritis would most likely be ANCA negative and would not cause a necrotising GN.

Although strongyloides could be responsible for some of the gastrointestinal and even respiratory symptoms, with an eosinophilia, it would not be associated with an ANCA-positive, rapidly progressive glomerulonephritis.

Lanham JG, et al. Systemic vasculitis with asthma and eosinophilia: a clinical approach to the Churg–Strauss syndrome. Medicine (Baltimore) 1984; 63:65–81.
Katzenstein AL. Diagnostic features and differential diagnosis of Churg–Strauss syndrome in the lung. Am J Clin Pathol 2000; 114:767–772.

31. E Renal vein thrombosis

There are many causes for graft dysfunction postrenal transplantation and distinguishing between them depends in part on the history and timings of the deterioration, and in part on the findings on renal biopsy.

Acute tubular necrosis (ATN) is a common cause of delayed graft function and is often because of the type of transplant and the length of cold ischaemic time (e.g. kidneys from non-heart-beating deceased donors would be expected to initially have ATN whereas kidneys from uncomplicated living donors would not). In this case also there is an initial good urine output which suddenly drops; this, in the absence of any other insult, would not be typical of ATN. It would also be very unusual to develop graft pyelonephritis 24 hours postoperatively, although in the longer term infections are common. Hyperacute rejection (i.e. within minutes, often seen on the operating table where the kidney is initially pink and turns mottled and blue) is virtually never seen now as a result of more sophisticated cross-match testing and the use of ABO-compatible donors (although increasingly ABO-incompatible living transplants are being performed but with preoperative immunosuppression/plasma exchange/immunoabsorption to remove anti-blood group antibodies). Obstruction would also be uncommon at this early stage as the patient will still be catheterised. It is possible to have a degree of obstruction due to external compression from a haematoma or lymphocele but the acute graft tenderness is not typical of obstruction.

The most likely diagnosis is, therefore, renal vein thrombosis. This is a relatively rare (up to 3% of transplants) postoperative transplantation complication but will usually result in graft loss. It may be related to technical problems or thrombophilic tendencies, but often there is no cause found. In any patient where renal vein thrombosis is suspected an urgent ultrasound should be requested which may show increased resistive indices in the transplant renal arteries and no flow in the transplant renal vein. The patient will then most likely be taken back to theatre for re-exploration and attempted thrombectomy but nephrectomy is common.

32. A Acute tubular necrosis

The history is suggestive of acute tubular necrosis (ATN) with an acute deterioration from a relatively normal baseline. There is clear documentation of a hypotensive episode and his history of diarrhoea and vomiting may suggest that he has been volume deplete prior to his admission. Furthermore he has a background of diabetes and is elderly, so his kidneys will be much more susceptible to such insults. The biopsy confirms the diagnosis with widespread tubular atrophy, widely spread dilated tubules with flattened epithelium and debris within the lumina.

Although he has poorly controlled diabetes and proteinuria there is nothing on the biopsy to suggest diabetic nephropathy. The main changes seen would be in the glomerulus and there are only tubules shown on this section. The same applies for IgA nephropathy, which can be associated with a rapidly progressive glomerulonephritis but usually with high blood pressure, and membranous nephropathy, which is associated with nephrotic syndrome but there is no evidence of this here. In hypertensive nephrosclerosis you would expect to see changes within the vessels or the glomerulus (glomerulosclerosis), neither of which is seen here.

33. D Prognosis is good with steroids

The diagnosis is renal amyloid as shown by the dense deposition of amorphous hyaline material in the glomerulus, with positive staining on Congo red. There are two main forms of amyloid that affect the kidney: AA and AL. AA amyloid is a reactive amyloid associated with chronic inflammatory conditions, such as rheumatoid arthritis, bronchiectasis, chronic abscesses and inflammatory bowel disease. It is also associated with familial Mediterranean fever, an autosomal recessive disorder affecting predominantly Jews, Armenians and Turks. AL amyloid, also known as primary amyloid, is caused by monoclonal light chains produced by a plasma cell dyscrasia.

Renal involvement typically presents with heavy proteinuria ± nephrotic syndrome and progressive renal impairment. Deposits of pale hyaline material are seen in the mesangium and the capillary loops on renal biopsy and electron microscopy will show amyloid fibrils.

If the diagnosis of amyloidosis is suspected, biopsy is the definitive investigation. In the absence of renal involvement or if renal biopsy is not possible, fine-needle fat-pad biopsy and rectal biopsy have both been described as the investigation of choice, giving positive results in 80–90% of cases.

The prognosis depends on the type of amyloid (AL worse than AA) and the extent of involvement. Steroids alone will not suffice as a treatment. Treatment includes removing the cause, i.e. treating the plasma cell dyscrasia in AL and the underlying inflammation in AA. Chemotherapy with melphalan and steroids is used in AL, as is haematopoietic cell transplantation. Prognosis is very poor. In those with AA amyloid there may be some role for cytotoxic, immunosuppressive and anti-cytokine drugs, and newer agents that interfere with fibril development are under investigation.

Dember M. Amyloidosis-associated kidney disease. J Am Soc Nephrol 2006; 17:3458–3471.

34. B Cast nephropathy

The patient has presented with multiple myeloma. The clues in the history are lethargy and back pain with otherwise unexplained acute kidney injury. In addition there is a high total protein count with a low normal albumin, thus suggesting a high globulin level. The biopsy shows cast nephropathy with large fractured casts within the tubules. There is tubular atrophy and some inflammatory cells are seen.

Myeloma may cause kidney impairment in several ways. Cast nephropathy (myeloma kidney) is the most common. Light chains, or fractures of them, cause obstruction of the tubules and are directly toxic to them. In addition myeloma can affect the kidney secondary to deposits of paraproteins, causing either amyloidosis or light chain deposition disease. This biopsy does not have any clear features of amyloid, and it would be AL amyloid that would be associated with a plasma cell dyscrasia. Other factors such as hypercalcaemia (which is common), analgesic use (particularly non-steroidal anti-inflammatory drugs) and hypovolaemia may also contribute.

Renal involvement in myeloma is associated with poorer outcome and increased mortality. Those with findings suggestive of cast nephropathy should be treated and considered for chemotherapy (bortezomib or thalidomide with dexamethasone). Trials are ongoing into the use of haemodialysis with a high-flux membrane.

There is little in the history to suggest a cryoglobulinaemia and on the biopsy you would expect to see glomerular abnormalities with either a membranoproliferative glomerulonephritis or glomerular deposits, whereas the glomerulus seen in the top right-hand corner of this picture is relatively normal. With both a tubulointerstitial nephritis (TIN) and sarcoid (which causes a TIN) you would expect a much denser inflammatory cell infiltrate in the interstitium than seen here, with granulomas in the case of sarcoid. Neither of these diagnoses would explain the presence of the large casts in the tubules.

35. A 0.9% NaCl intravenously

When considering hyponatraemia and its appropriate treatment it is vital to consider the underlying cause and, in particular, identify the patient's fluid balance status (see **Figure 9.9**). Hyponatraemia can occur with volume depletion, volume overload or euvolaemia, and there are different causes for each group.

Symptomatic hyponatraemia occurs when the sodium level drops quickly or at levels below around 125 mmol/L. Treatment depends on identifying the underlying cause. In this case the patient is clearly volume deplete with a postural drop and a resting tachycardia, and a history of diarrhoea. She is also on a thiazide diuretic. The urinary osmolality is difficult to interpret in the context of diuretic use but in general a high urine osmolality is associated with diuretic use, adrenal insufficiency, cerebral salt wasting, salt-wasting nephropathy and the syndrome of inappropriate antidiuretic hormone (ADH) secretion (SIADH).

In the absence of encephalopathy, as in this patient, the treatment involves trying to slowly restore euvolaemia and treat/remove any underlying causes. It is important to assess whether the hyponatraemia is acute or chronic and to aim to correct slowly to avoid neurological complications such as central pontine myelinolysis. When the patient is volume deplete it is sufficient to resuscitate with 0.9% saline. Hypertonic saline in general should be considered only in the context of encephalopathy and should be given cautiously in a high dependency setting via a central line.

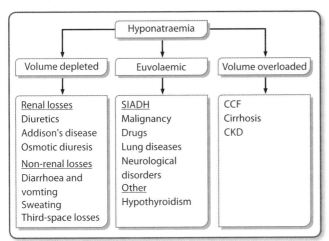

Figure 9.9 Approach to diagnosing hyponatraemia. CCF, congestive cardiac failure; CKD, chronic kidney disease; SIADH, syndrome of inappropriate antidiuretic hormone secretion.

It is not necessary in this case. When the patient is overloaded or euvolaemic they should be fluid restricted to <1 L/24 hours. If SIADH is diagnosed (hyponatraemia not on diuretics, euvolaemic, normal renal/adrenal/thyroid function, ↑urine sodium, ↑urine osmolality) demeclocycline may be used to reverse the effects of ADH by inducing a nephrogenic diabetes insipidus. Tolvaptan is a new V_2-receptor (ADH receptor) blocker which is shown to effectively raise sodium levels in patients with euvolaemic or hypervolaemic hyponatraemia. Neither of these measures is, therefore, appropriate in this case.

Sterns RH, et al. The treatment of hyponatraemia. Semin Nephrol 2009; 29(3):282–299.
Schrier RW, et al. Tolvaptan, a selective oral vasopressin V2-receptor antagonist, for hyponatraemia. N Engl J Med 2006; 355:2099–2112.

36. A Aciclovir

This patient has an acute kidney injury and is on many potentially toxic drugs. The distinguishing finding is crystalluria which can be caused by several drugs that precipitate in the urine. This in turn can lead to acute kidney injury. Drugs in particular that cause crystalluria include antivirals (aciclovir and indinavir), methotrexate and some antibiotics (sulfadiazine, amoxicillin).

Allopurinol itself is not nephrotoxic but the dose should be adjusted in renal impairment. It should not be given with azathioprine as this can cause severe pancytopenia.

Ciclosporin is a commonly used immunosuppressant in renal transplantation which must be monitored closely using trough levels because it can also be nephrotoxic at higher levels. Nephrotoxicity is manifested in various histopathological ways but may include acute tubular necrosis, ischaemia secondary to changes in renal blood flow/vasoconstriction, fibrosis and a thrombotic microangiopathy.

Co-trimoxazole again is not nephrotoxic itself but must be dose adjusted in renal impairment. It can cause leukopenia.

The main side effects of mycophenolate mofetil are gastrointestinal in nature and it may also cause a low white cell count.

37. E Renal artery stenosis

This woman presents with uncontrolled hypertension which is not acute – she has evidence of target organ damage with established retinopathy. This is not likely to be due to an acute glomerulonephritis as she is otherwise well and there is no blood or protein in her urine. Although her potassium is low, patients with Bartter's syndrome are usually normotensive. Hypertension is common in Cushing's syndrome, affecting over 80% of patients, and blood tests often show low potassium. However, a high serum glucose level, often in the diabetic range, would be expected.

Coarctation of the aorta causes hypertension in children and young adults, more commonly in males. Clinically there would be higher blood pressure in the upper limbs, radiofemoral delay and a mid-systolic murmur. Abnormalities in the chest X-ray may be seen with rib notching and a 'figure-3' sign in the upper mediastinum from pre- and poststenotic dilatation of the aorta.

Renal artery stenosis (RAS) refers to atherosclerotic narrowing of the larger renal vessels. It typically presents with hypertension which is difficult to control, and evidence of salt and water overload. Renal function is often impaired and potassium is often low because of secondary hyperaldosteronism. Urine dipstick is bland. Ultrasound should be performed and a difference in size between the kidneys of >1.5 cm is suggestive. Thereafter further imaging using an isotope test (captopril MAG-3), CT angiogram or MR angiogram may be useful in making the diagnosis. Treatment of RAS is controversial with only some nephrologists favouring angioplasty. The ASTRAL trial suggested no significant clinical benefit with intervention.

The ASTRAL investigators. Revascularization versus medical therapy for renal-artery stenosis. N Engl J Med 2009; 361:1953–1962.

38. E Type 4 renal tubular acidosis

This patient has evidence of a renal tubular acidosis shown by low serum bicarbonate and a low urinary pH. Broadly speaking the renal tubular acidoses (RTAs) are divided into proximal and distal, and differentiating between them involves interpreting the clinical context as well as the results of blood and urine. They all cause a normal (hyperchloraemic) anion gap acidosis as in this case.

Type 1 RTA (distal) is due to impaired secretion of H^+ in the collecting duct. It manifests as a hyperchloraemic hypokalaemic metabolic acidosis. It is associated with renal stones and hypophosphataemic metabolic bone disease. It can be secondary to Sjögren's syndrome, systemic lupus erythematosus, rheumatoid arthritis, amyloidosis, analgesic nephropathy and lithium. Typically serum potassium is low, serum bicarbonate is very low (<10 mmol/L) and the urine pH is >5.3. The urinary anion gap (u-AG = u-[$Na^+ + K^+$] – u-[Cl^-]) is positive.

Type 2 RTA (proximal) is due to impaired retention of bicarbonate in the proximal tubule, causing bicarbonate wasting and systemic acidosis; it also presents as a hyperchloraemic hypokalaemic metabolic acidosis. It is caused by myeloma, amyloidosis, Wilson's disease, heavy metal toxicity and drugs (aminoglycosides, acetazolamide and antiretrovirals). Typically serum potassium is low, serum bicarbonate is low (12–20 mmol/L) and the u-AG is positive. Patients often present with other features of proximal tubular dysfunction known as Fanconi's syndrome. Fanconi's syndrome is marked by failure to absorb many substances by the proximal tubules, including amino acids and phosphate, and often presents with bone pain and osteomalacia. Serum phosphate is low and there is glucose and protein on urine dipstick.

Type 4 RTA is also distal and is associated with hypoaldosteronism. There is resultant hyperkalaemia and associated acidosis. It is caused by diabetes mellitus, drugs (particularly ciclosporin and non-steroidal anti-inflammatory drugs), obstructive uropathy and Addison's disease. Serum potassium is high and bicarbonate is low, although not usually below 16 mmol/L. Urinary pH is typically <5.3 and the u-AG is positive.

Confusingly, there is no type 3 RTA!.

Steddon S, et al. Oxford Handbook of Nephrology and Hypertension. Oxford: Oxford University Press, 2006.

39. D Renal biopsy

Although there is a longstanding history of diabetes the patient has no evidence of microvascular complications (no retinopathy) and has a well-controlled HbA1c. This makes the diagnosis of diabetic nephropathy less likely. He does have a degree of proteinuria but with a well-controlled blood pressure. Even if the diagnosis were diabetic nephropathy, it would be unlikely to progress at this rapid rate when these parameters are well controlled.

Although dual blockade of the renin–angiotensin–aldosterone system may be beneficial in the context of heavy proteinuria, his blood pressure is already well controlled, and the addition of another agent is unlikely to help or solve the problem of why his function has deteriorated so quickly. Equally furosemide may give a little symptomatic relief but will not help his renal function. The peripheral oedema may well be a side effect of amlodipine.

It is inappropriate to leave this patient another month as he clearly has a rapid jump in his creatinine which cannot be attributed to diabetes alone. He also has blood as well as protein in his urine which may indicate another glomerular lesion. He should have an urgent nephritic screen and an urgent renal biopsy to determine the cause in his drop in function and to allow treatment to be initiated as appropriate.

40. E Thiazide diuretic

Hypernatraemia is relatively rare and should not generally be seen where there is free access to water. Groups of patient who are more susceptible are very young and elderly people and those who are otherwise unwell.

Broadly speaking hypernatraemia is caused by an excess of hypertonic fluids (intravenous infusions, enteral or parenteral nutrition), excess water loss and decreased thirst (in the risk groups mentioned above). In terms of excess water loss, this may be renal (diabetes insipidus, diuretics, osmotic diuresis), gut (diarrhoea and vomiting, nasogastric losses) or skin (sweating and burns).

Treatment involves identifying and treating the underlying cause and aiming to restore normal sodium values. If the hypernatraemia is acute then it may be reversed quickly. If chronic (>24 hours) is should be corrected slowly at a rate of no more than 0.5 mmol/L per h. The most appropriate fluid resuscitation is normal water orally or nasogastrically. If it must be given intravenously then either 0.45% saline or 5% dextrose may be used.

The diagnosis of diabetes insipidus (DI) can be made here partly based on clinical information – he is polyuric suggesting an increased loss renal, there is no history of diuretic use and he does not have diabetes mellitus, making an osmotic diuresis unlikely. The diagnosis is supported by lab results which show inappropriately dilute urine. DI can be either cranial in origin or nephrogenic. Cranial causes would include infections, vasculitis, tumour, tuberculosis or trauma, and the treatment of cranial DI is with desmopressin (DDAVP). Nephrogenic DI, on the other hand, is often drug induced (particularly with lithium which makes the distal tubules resistant to the actions of vasopressin) but may be congenital, secondary to hypercalcaemia or medullary cystic disease. The treatment is with a thiazide diuretic which causes reduced water delivery to the collecting duct, or with non-steroidal anti-inflammatory drugs which can antagonise the effect of antidiuretic hormone.

Waise A, Fisken RA. Unsuspected Nephrogenic Diabetes Insipidus. BMJ 2001;323:96–97.

41. B Creatinine clearance changing from 125 mL/min in the 1st trimester to 90 mL/min in the 3rd trimester

There are many physiological changes that affect the mother's kidneys during pregnancy, reflecting the increased renal blood flow and glomerular filtration rate (GFR). These begin to take place from as early as 6 weeks' gestation. The effective renal blood flow increases from around 480 mL/min pre-pregnancy to a peak of around 890 mL/min in the second trimester. With this the GFR and creatinine clearance rise, peaking in the 2nd trimester, and thus it is worryingly abnormal to drop creatinine clearance from the 1st to 2nd trimester which represents acute kidney injury that must be investigated urgently. A fall in creatinine, conversely, simply reflects the increased GFR.

Secondary to changes in renal haemodynamics and tubular function, it can be normal to see a degree of proteinuria. This should be no more than 260 mg/24 h. Changes in tubular function can also cause glycosuria which does not necessarily indicate impaired glucose tolerance. If glycosuria is seen persistently or heavily then further investigations for diabetes are warranted.

Finally the changes in fluid status, including up to 8 L increase in total body water, can cause hyponatraemia and normal sodium for a pregnant woman is probably 132–140 µmol/L.

Williams D, Davison J. Chronic kidney disease in pregnancy. BMJ 2008; 336:211–215.

42. E Tubulointerstitial nephritis

After a renal transplantation it is possible that the same disease affecting the kidneys originally will recur and this will be identified on renal biopsy. Recurrence of original disease affects up to 10–20% of patients and accounts for around 5% of graft failures at 10 years.

Primary focal segmental glomerulosclerosis is known to have a recurrence rate of around 20–30% and can occur within days of transplantation. It is thought to lead to graft loss in around 50% of cases. IgA nephropathy also commonly recurs with rates quoted between 20% and 60%. Progression of disease is usually slow but can result in graft loss in the long term.

Mesangiocapillary glomerulonephritis (MCGN), particularly type II although to a lesser extent type I, has also been seen to recur in allografts. Rates of between 50% and 100% are quoted for MCGN type II.

Other primary diseases that may recur include membranous nephropathy and haemolytic uraemic syndrome/thrombocytic thrombocytopenic purpura.

Various systemic diseases also recur in the transplanted kidney, the most common of which are lupus nephritis and diabetic nephropathy.

Tubulointerstitial nephritis is commonly secondary to drugs, or less commonly tuberculosis and sarcoid, and is not reported to recur in renal transplantation.

Golgert WA, et al. Recurrent glomerulonephritis after renal transplantation: An unsolved problem. Clin J Am Soc Nephrol 2008; 3(3):800–807.

43. A Ethylene glycol ingestion

Oxalate crystals can be ovoid or pyramidal in shape and are present in hyperoxaluria or hypercalciuria. They are also a diagnostic clue in ethylene glycol poisoning. Another clue in his investigations is the raised anion gap (AG) acidosis (AG = 26 here, normal 8–16, calculate by $[Na^+ + K^+] - [Cl^- + HCO_3^-]$).

Ethylene glycol itself causes inebriation but, more harmfully, is metabolised in the liver by successive oxidations to toxic metabolites responsible for the symptoms seen. One of these is glycolic acid which is then metabolised to oxalic acid. Classically there are three clinical stages of presentation. Stage 1 is the central nervous system stage where patients display depression, ataxia, speech slurring, hallucination, convulsions, coma and vomiting. Stage 2 is the cardiorespiratory stage with tachycardia, tachypnoea, hypertension, pulmonary oedema, pneumonitis and shock. Finally stage 3 is the renal stage with proteinuria, haematuria, flank pain, crystalluria and acute kidney injury.

Although rhabdomyolysis is also a cause of a raised AG acidosis there are no other clues pointing to rhabdomyolysis in the history, apart from the collapse, and it would not explain the patient's cardiovascular, respiratory or neurological symptoms or the crystals on the biopsy, although it would cause acute tubular necrosis.

Equally severe sepsis, often with raised lactate, can cause an increased AG acidosis but again pneumonia would not account for all of the other symptoms in this patient. Salicylate poisoning causes neurological signs and pulmonary oedema, as well as an increased AG acidosis but does not cause acute kidney injury. Haemodialysis can be used to effectively remove salicylate.

Although a small vessel vasculitis might account for some of the patient's constitutional and neurological symptoms (vasculitis is most commonly associated with mononeuritis multiplex or peripheral neuropathy), a focal and segmental necrotising crescentic glomerulonephritis would be expected on the biopsy.

Chapter 10

Respiratory medicine

Questions

1. A 74-year-old man was referred to the chest clinic from the emergency department. He presented following a fall on ice and was treated with simple analgesia for a minor soft tissue injury. No other injuries were sustained. He was otherwise fit and well with no history of cough, shortness of breath, chest pain or weight loss. He stopped smoking 20 years ago. He was a retired dock-yard ship-builder.

   Clinical examination was normal.

   Chest X-ray (see **Figure 10.1**):

Figure 10.1

Which one of the following statements is least likely regarding the diagnosis?

A Benign asbestos-related pleural effusions usually occur within 10 years of exposure
B Diffuse pleural thickening may be seen in patients with a history of heavy asbestos exposure
C High-resolution CT is more sensitive than chest X-ray in detecting pleural plaques
D Pleural plaques are a premalignant finding
E Pleural plaques are usually asymptomatic

2.   A 21-year-old female student nurse was referred to the chest clinic for further advice following pre-employment screening. She had been previously well with no past medical history of note. She was born in London; her parents immigrated to the UK from Bangladesh 40 years ago. She lived with her parents and her three siblings and had had frequent holidays to visit relatives in Bangladesh. She received a BCG vaccine at school aged 13 years as confirmed by a scar on her left deltoid.

   Physical examination was normal.

Investigations:

Mantoux test: 18 mm (<5 mm negative, 5–14 mm positive, >15 mm strongly positive)

Chest X-ray: lungs are clear
normal mediastinal contours

Interferon release assay: positive

What is the most appropriate next step in management?

A   Bronchoscopy
B   Chest physiotherapy for induced sputum sampling with hypertonic saline
C   CT of the chest
D   Start quadruple therapy with rifampicin, isoniazid, pyrazinamide and ethambutol
E   Treat with rifampicin and isoniazid

3.   A 84-year-old man, presented to the emergency department with a 5-day history of increased breathlessness and a cough productive of green sputum. He felt tired and lethargic and had lost his appetite. His exercise tolerance had decreased such that he was short of breath on minimal exertion (baseline exercise tolerance 10 metres). He had a history of severe chronic obstructive pulmonary disease (COPD), diabetes and osteoarthritis.

   On examination, he was alert, but appeared tired. He had a low-grade fever 37.8°C and was haemodynamically stable. He was able to speak in short sentences with a respiratory rate of 34 breaths per minute. He was centrally cyanosed. Pulse oximetry showed oxygen saturation of 87% on air and 91% on 2 L/min O_2 via nasal cannulae. On auscultation, there was widespread mild wheeze.

Investigations:

| white cell count 14.3×10^9/L (4–11) | C-reactive protein 76 mg/L (<10) |
| neutrophils 10.8×10^9/L (1.5–7.0) | |

Chest X-ray:
emphysematous change in keeping with COPD
no focal consolidation or mass lesion seen

Arterial blood gases on arrival (on 2 L/min O_2 via nasal cannulae):	PaO_2 7.3 kPa (11.3–12.6)
	base excess 4 mmol/L ($\pm$2)
pH 7.35 (7.35–7.45)	
$PaCO_2$ 7.6 kPa (4.7–6.0)	

He was commenced on antibiotics, steroids, and nebulised salbutamol and ipratropium.

What is the most appropriate next step in management?

A   Aminophylline infusion
B   Continue present treatment and re-assess within 1 hour
C   Doxapram infusion
D   Non-invasive ventilation
E   Reduce oxygen to 1 L/min via nasal cannulae and re-assess within 1 hour

4. A 68-year-old woman presented with a 12-hour history of left-sided pleuritic chest pain and shortness of breath. She had a past medical history of hypertension and a right mastectomy for breast cancer 6 months ago. Her current medications included amlodipine and tamoxifen.

   On examination, she appeared to be in moderate discomfort, but was alert and oriented and with good peripheral perfusion. Her pulse was 118 beats per minute, blood pressure 130/80 mmHg, respiratory rate 22 breaths per minute and oxygen saturation 91% on room air. Heart sounds were normal and chest was clear on auscultation. There was some swelling and tenderness of the left calf.

   Investigations:

   > Chest X-ray: blunting of the left costophrenic angle

   What is the most useful diagnostic investigation?

   A   CT pulmonary angiogram (CTPA)
   B   D-dimer
   C   Echocardiogram
   D   Isotope lung scan
   E   Doppler ultrasound of the left leg

5. A 23-year-old female nursing student attended the chest clinic for routine review. She had had asthma since age 5 years and had needed multiple hospital admissions, including one admission to an intensive therapy unit for mechanical ventilation and four admissions over the past 12 months for this condition. She was a non-smoker. She had good compliance with her medications, which included: budesonide 200 µg/formoterol fumarate 6 µg two inhalations twice daily, salbutamol 100 µg two inhalations as required – used about eight times per day, montelukast 10 mg daily and, for the last year, a maintenance dose of prednisolone 20 mg daily. She was intolerant of oral theophyllines.

   Investigations:

   > Skin-prick tests:
   > strong positive reaction to house-dust mite
   > negative for other common aeroallergens
   >
   > total IgE 308 IU/mL (<30)

   What is the most appropriate next step in management?

   A   Adrenaline by intramuscular injection for self-administration in case of emergencies
   B   Aminophylline modified-release tablets
   C   Home nebuliser with salbutamol and ipratropium nebulised solutions
   D   Maintenance dose of prednisolone should be increased to 40 mg daily
   E   Trial of omalizumab

6. A 74-year-old woman presented with a 2-year history of increasing shortness of breath on exertion and a cough productive of white sputum. Her symptoms had not responded to three courses of antibiotics. There was no history of any fevers, night sweats or weight loss. She was born in Bangladesh and migrated to the UK 40 years ago. Her exercise tolerance was limited to 50 metres at a gentle pace. She had type 2 diabetes mellitus and hypertension. She had no previous history of respiratory illness and had never smoked. She had no known tuberculosis contacts. She was a housewife and lived with her extended family. Her current medications included gliclazide, amlodipine, aspirin and salbutamol.

   On examination, her oxygen saturation was 93% breathing room air and respiratory rate 24 breaths per minute. Chest auscultation revealed mild scattered wheeze. She also had mild ankle swelling. There was no BCG scar.

Investigations:

Spirometry:	FVC 1.20 L (normal range 1.60–1.72)
FEV$_1$ 0.60 L (normal range 1.18–1.26)	FVC post-BD 1.18 L
FEV$_1$ post-BD 0.62 L	

(FEV$_1$ = forced expiratory volume in 1 second; FVC = forced vital capacity; BD = bronchodilator)

What is the most likely diagnosis?

A   Adult onset asthma
B α_1-Antitrypsin deficiency
C   Congestive cardiac failure
D   Chronic obstructive pulmonary disease (COPD) secondary to biomass fuel exposure
E   Tuberculosis

7.   A 78-year-old man with chronic obstructive pulmonary disease (COPD) presented to his general practitioner. He had a chronic cough and produced approximately two egg-cupfuls of white/cream-coloured sputum each morning. His exercise tolerance was limited to 5 metres; he was largely house bound and was dependent on carers for daily activities.

He had recently lost 3 kg in weight and had a poor appetite. His general practitioner noted that he also suffered from night sweats. During the last 12 months he had suffered two infective exacerbations requiring oral antibiotics and steroids. He was an ex-smoker and had no known tuberculosis (TB) contact.

His general practitioner recently sent sputum samples for microscopy, culture and sensitivities (MC&S), and alcohol acid-fast bacilli (AFB) and TB culture.

Investigations:

MC&S: purulent sputum, no organisms seen, cultures negative
AFB: smear negative
TB culture: scanty growth, probable *Mycobacterium* species identified
Chest X-ray: loss of volume in right upper lobe with consolidation and cavitation emphysematous changes noted

What is the most appropriate next step in management?

A   Commence azithromycin
B   Commence ethambutol and rifampicin for 9 months
C   Commence ethambutol and rifampicin for 24 months
D   Commence standard antituberculous therapy to include ethambutol, isoniazid, pyrazinamide and rifampicin
E   Send two more sputum samples for AFB and TB culture

8.   A 28-year-old woman was referred to the medical admissions unit after consulting her obstetrician. She was 26 weeks' pregnant with her first child. Six hours ago, she had sudden-onset, left-sided pleuritic chest pain and shortness of breath. The obstetrician examined her and reassured her that there were no concerns with the progression of the pregnancy, but requested a medical review. She had no past medical history of note.

On examination, she appeared anxious, but was comfortable at rest. Her pulse was 98 beats per minute and regular, blood pressure 110/84 mmHg, respiratory rate 24 breaths per minute and oxygen saturation 95% on air. Auscultation of the chest revealed a pleural rub at the left base. She had mild swelling of the ankles bilaterally.

Investigations:

Chest X-ray: no abnormality detected
Electrocardiogram: rate 102 per minute, sinus rhythm

What is the most appropriate next investigation?

A CT pulmonary angiogram
B D-dimer
C Doppler ultrasound of the legs
D Echocardiogram
E Perfusion scan

9. A 23-year-old man presented to the emergency department complaining of sudden-onset, right-sided chest pain and shortness of breath. He had no past medical history of note.

On examination, he appeared distressed with pain, respiratory rate was 30 breaths per minute, oxygen saturation 97% breathing FiO_2 (inspired oxygen fraction) 0.6 via a facemask, blood pressure 110/74 mmHg and heart rate 98 beats per minute. There were reduced breath sounds on the right.

An urgent chest X-ray was performed (see **Figure 10.2**).

Figure 10.2

What is the most appropriate next step in management?

A Continue high-flow oxygen and observe
B Needle aspiration in right second intercostal space in the mid-clavicular line
C Insertion of large-bore surgical chest drain

D   Ultrasound-guided chest drain insertion using small-bore tube in right mid-axillary line in fifth intercostal space

E   Ultrasound-guided needle aspiration anterior to right mid-axillary line in fifth intercostal space

10. A 23-year-old woman presented to her general practitioner complaining of a cough, night sweats, shortness of breath and weight loss. She was born in China and had lived in the UK for 5 years.

Investigations:

haemoglobin 10.2 g/dL (11.5–16.5)	lymphocytes 2.5 × 10⁹/L (1.5–4.0)
white cell count 24.6 × 10⁹/L (4–11)	neutrophils 20.8 × 10⁹/L (1.5–7.0)
platelets 463 × 10⁹/L (150–400)	monocytes 1.2 × 10⁹/L (0–0.8)

Chest X-ray (see **Figure 10.3**)

Figure 10.3

What is the most likely diagnosis?

A   Bronchogenic cyst
B   Germ cell tumour
C   Lymphoma
D   Retrosternal goitre
E   Thymoma

11. A 74-year-old woman was referred by her general practitioner to the chest clinic with a 3-year history of cough and progressive shortness of breath. Her general practitioner had prescribed her four courses of antibiotics and two short courses of steroids with little benefit. She was a non-smoker and was not taking any regular medication. She described cough productive of purulent sputum and had noticed a few episodes of blood streaking in the sputum. There was no weight loss or night sweats, but she did complain of lethargy. She had no known tuberculosis contact, but she had been admitted to hospital with a pneumonic illness in childhood.

What is the most appropriate diagnostic test?

A   Bronchoscopy
B   Chest X-ray
C   High-resolution CT of the chest
D   Serum α_1-antitrypsin level
E   Tuberculin skin test

12. A 24-year-old man with a history of asthma presented to the emergency department with a 2-day history of worsening wheeze and shortness of breath. His regular medication included budesonide/formoterol combination inhaler one puff twice daily and as required, plus montelukast. He was under outpatient follow-up with the respiratory clinic and a clinic letter stated that his best peak flow was 620 L/min.

   On arrival he was alert but appeared tired and was unable to complete sentences, his oxygen saturation was 95% breathing 40% oxygen, respiratory rate 30 breaths per minute, pulse 130 beats per minute and on auscultation there was widespread wheeze. His peak flow was 180 L/min.

   He was commenced on prednisolone, salbutamol nebulisers and continuous oxygen therapy (40%).

Investigations:

Chest X-ray: hyperexpanded lungs no acute lung pathology detected
Electrocardiogram: rate 102 per minute, sinus rhythm
Arterial blood gases on 40% oxygen: $PaCO_2$ 4.2 kPa (4.7–6.0) pH 7.37 (7.35–7.45) PaO_2 14.3 kPa (11.3–12.6)

What is the most appropriate next step in management?

A   Increase oxygen therapy to 60%
B   Intravenous ketamine
C   Intravenous magnesium
D   Intravenous salbutamol
E   Intubation and mechanical ventilation

13. A 34-year-old man presented to the chest clinic with a 6-month history of increasing shortness of breath and a non-productive cough. He smoked 10 cigarettes per day. He had no past medical history of note and did not take any regular medication. He worked in an office with no exposure to dust or fumes. He did not keep any pets and had not recently travelled abroad.

   On examination, he had finger clubbing and coarse crackles on auscultation of the lower zones. Oxygen saturation was 93% on air.

Investigations:

Chest X-ray: bilateral consolidation with thickened interlobular septa
CT of the chest: 'crazy paving pattern' of patchy airspace shadowing, with areas of normal lung
Bronchoalveolar lavage (BAL): profuse milky washings
BAL microscopy culture and sensitivity (MC&S): no organisms seen, culture negative
BAL acid-fast bacilli (AFB) / tuberculosis (TB) culture: AFB not seen, TB cultures negative
BAL cytology: granular, acellular, eosinophilic, PAS (periodic acid–Schiff)-positive deposits and foamy macrophages

What is the most appropriate treatment?

A   Antituberculous therapy
B   Co-trimoxazole
C   High-dose oral prednisolone
D   Pulsed intravenous methylprednisolone
E   Whole lung lavage

14. A 32-year-old woman was referred to the chest clinic following a third spontaneous left-sided pneumothorax. She reported shortness of breath on exertion and had previously suffered an episode of self-limiting haemoptysis. She also complained of abdominal bloating.
    Physical examination was normal.

Investigations:

Pulmonary function tests: no abnormality detected
Chest X-ray: hyperinflated lungs with reticular shadowing   no mass lesion or pneumothorax seen
CT of the thorax: multiple small (<1 cm) thin-walled cysts   small left-sided effusion

What is the most likely diagnosis?

A α_1-Antitrypsin deficiency
B   Catamenial pneumothorax
C   Cystic fibrosis
D   Lymphangioleiomyomatosis
E   Pulmonary Langerhans' cell histiocytosis

15. A 72-year-old man was referred to the medical admissions unit by his general practitioner. He had a 5-day history of cough with green sputum and left-sided chest pain. He was feverish and confused and had lost his appetite. He had type 2 diabetes mellitus, hypertension and hypercholesterolaemia. His medications included metformin, ramipril, simvastatin and aspirin. He was a non-smoker and lived with his wife.
    On examination, he was mildly confused, but oriented in time, place and person. He appeared flushed and was pyrexial at 38.4°C, but had cool peripheries with a systemic blood pressure of 108/58 mmHg. He had a respiratory rate of 24 breaths per minutes and oxygen saturation on air of 95%. There were coarse crackles audible in the left lower zone with dullness to percussion.

Investigations:

haemoglobin 15.4 g/dL (13.0–18.0)	potassium 5.8 mmol/L (3.5–5.0)
white cell count 18.4 × 10⁹/L (4–11)	urea 13.4 mmol/L (2.5–7.5)
neutrophils 14.7 × 10⁹/L (1.5–7.0)	creatinine 178 µmol/L (60–110)
sodium 124 mmol/L (135–145)	

What is the most appropriate next step in management?

A   Admission to the high dependency unit for intensive monitoring
B   High-flow oxygen
C   Intravenous co-amoxiclav and clarithromycin

D   Intravenous hydrocortisone

E   Stop current medications, prescribe intravenous fluids, and oral amoxicillin and clarithromycin

16. A 16-year-old girl presented to the emergency department with a 3-day history of increasing shortness of breath, lethargy, fevers and right-sided neck discomfort. She had consulted her general practitioner 10 days previously complaining of a sore throat and was prescribed a 5-day course of erythromycin. She had no past medical history of note and did not take any regular medications. She was allergic to penicillin.

On examination, she appeared unwell with temperature 38.6°C and pulse 110 beats per minute. There was tenderness of the right side of the neck. Examination of the oropharynx revealed mild erythema and bilateral tonsillar enlargement; no exudate seen. Examination of respiratory, abdominal and nervous systems was normal.

Investigations:

Chest X-ray: thin-walled cavitating lesions in left mid-zone and right lower zone
HIV negative

What is the most likely causative pathogen?

A   *Cryptococcus neoformans*
B   *Fusobacterium necrophorum*
C   *Mycobacterium tuberculosis*
D   *Pneumocystis jiroveci*
E   *Staphylococcus aureus*

17. A 22-year-old male student attended a routine asthma clinic follow-up appointment. He was planning a trip to the Everest Base Camp. He suffered from mild asthma in early childhood, but had not needed to take any regular or reliever medications for more than 10 years. He had never smoked and was athletic, regularly competing in running events for his university.

He was concerned about the potential risk of developing high-altitude pulmonary oedema.

What is the most appropriate advice?

A   Keep ascent to ≤300 m/day and rest every third day
B   Keep ascent to ≤800 m/day and rest every fifth day
C   Prophylactic dexamethasone
D   Prophylactic nifedipine
E   The trip should not be contemplated in view of his past medical history of asthma

18. A 36-year-old man was referred to the chest clinic following a routine medical examination as part of the visa application process for a 2-year secondment to America. He worked for a bank and had never smoked tobacco or other substances. He had no past medical history of note other than mild viral illnesses during early childhood, for which he did not require any specific treatment, and there was no family history of respiratory disease. He was fit and well.

Investigations:

Chest X-ray: right lung appeared hyperlucent with reduced vascular marking and small pulmonary artery

What is the most likely diagnosis?

A α_1-Antitrypsin deficiency
B   Congenital lobar emphysema
C   MacLeod's syndrome

D   Pneumothorax
E   Pulmonary sequestration

19. A 29-year-old woman presented to the emergency department with a 3-day history of increased shortness of breath and wheeze. She had a history of minor coryzal symptoms and was coughing up yellow sputum. There was no history of chest pain, haemoptysis or leg swelling. She had a history of asthma, but had stopped her regular inhalers 6 weeks ago, after she discovered that she was pregnant and was concerned about the risk of steroid inhalers to the baby. Her prescribed medication consisted of a combination inhaled corticosteroid and long-acting β_2-agonist two puffs taken twice daily and as required. At presentation she was taking folic acid only and no other medication.

  On examination, she appeared stable and was able to speak in full sentences. She was afebrile. Respiratory rate was 14 breaths per minute and oxygen saturation 98% on air. There was mild wheeze throughout both lungs but no other added sounds. Peak flow rate (PEFR) was 520 L/min (patient's best previous PEFR was 540 L/min). Pulse was 80 beats per minute and blood pressure 110/76 mmHg.

  She was keen to go home. She lived with her husband and 2-year-old child. She agreed to return if her symptoms deteriorated and she was referred to the asthma clinic for further follow-up.

  What is the most appropriate next step in management?

  A   Admit for regular nebulisers and observation
  B   Advise chest physiotherapy and relaxation techniques
  C   Amoxicillin and prednisolone
  D   Montelukast
  E   Restart regular inhaler corticosteroid and long-acting β_2-agonist

20. An 84-year-old man presented with haemoptysis of approximately three teaspoonfuls over the previous 24 hours. He had a 5-day history of cough productive of yellow sputum. There was no preceding history of weight loss, but he gave a 6-month history of general malaise which he had attributed to 'old age'. He had suffered from pulmonary tuberculosis in his teens and recalled that he was in hospital for 12 months. He had not had any operations. There was no other past medical history and he did not take any regular medication. He was a retired school teacher and there was no history of foreign travel or contact with industrial dusts or fumes. He was active and independent.

  One hour after arrival in the emergency department he suffered an episode of massive haemoptysis – approximately 1.5 L of fresh red blood. His pulse was 120 beats per minute and blood pressure 80/40 mmHg. He was able to maintain his own airway and his oxygen saturation was found to be 95% breathing high-flow oxygen.

  Large-bore venous access was gained and the intensive care teams were assisting in the resuscitation.

  What is the most appropriate next step in management?

  A   Arterial embolisation
  B   Fresh frozen plasma
  C   Itraconazole
  D   Surgical resection
  E   Tranexamic acid

21. A 28-year-old woman with cystic fibrosis attended for a routine follow-up appointment. She discussed with the specialist nurse that she was planning to start a family. Her genotype was ΔF508 /ΔF508. She had been well recently and had not suffered from any pulmonary exacerbations of the disease for 4 years. She did not take any regular antibiotics, performed twice daily chest physiotherapy and took regular mucolytic nebulisers. She had pancreatic insufficiency for which she took Creon 10 000 units as directed and vitamins A, D, E and K, folic acid and calcium supplements. Her husband was not a carrier of the common cystic fibrosis genes.

On examination, her chest was clear, her oxygen saturation was 97% on breathing room air and her body mass was index 17 kg/m².

Investigations:

> Spirometry:
> FEV₁ 91% predicted
> FVC 93% predicted

What is the most appropriate advice with regard to pregnancy?

A   Ciprofloxacin is the preferred antibiotic for a pulmonary exacerbation during pregnancy
B   Colomycin is the preferred antibiotic for a pulmonary exacerbation during pregnancy
C   Pregnancy should be avoided as there is a significant risk of lung function decline
D   She is unlikely to conceive without assisted conception
E   She should commence dietary supplements

22. A 54-year-old man attended the chest clinic accompanied by his wife, who complained that he was a heavy snorer and she slept in another bedroom as the snoring was so loud. The patient said he felt tired and lethargic during the day and needed to urinate at least three times during the night. His wife said that she had observed some episodes where he seemed to stop breathing and then woke up coughing and choking, but the patient did not recall these events. He often woke with a dry mouth and had occasional morning headaches.

He had gained weight recently and wore a 46 cm (18") collar shirt. He smoked 20 cigarettes per day and drank 40 units of alcohol per week. He had hypertension and type 2 diabetes mellitus and his regular medications included metformin, ramipril and bendroflumethiazide.

On examination, his weight was 110 kg and height 1.75 m. He had no obvious craniofacial abnormality. His chest was clear.

Investigations:

> Epworth Sleepiness Score: 6/24 (<9)
>
> Sleep study: apnoea–hypopnea index 11.4/h (<5)

What is the most appropriate management?

A   Bariatric surgery
B   Continuous positive airway pressure
C   Dietary and lifestyle advice
D   Domiciliary non-invasive ventilation
E   Mandibular advancement device

23. A 76-year-old woman presented to the chest clinic complaining of a 4-month history of progressive shortness of breath, right-sided chest discomfort and a dry cough. She had weight loss of 2 kg and poor appetite. She had ischaemic heart disease, type 2 diabetes mellitus and hypertension. Two years ago, she had triple-vessel coronary artery bypass grafting (CABG) and had not experienced any further angina. She had stopped smoking 4 years ago. Her current medications included aspirin, bisoprolol, metformin, ramipril and simvastatin.

Examination of the chest revealed reduced chest expansion on the right with dull percussion note and absent breath sounds.

Thoracic ultrasound confirmed a large right pleural effusion and a diagnostic pleural tap was performed.

Blood-stained fluid 20 mL was aspirated and sent for analysis together with matched venous samples:

Investigations:

Pleural fluid microbiology: Gram stain negative, no organisms seen, no growth after 5 days

Pleural fluid cytology: atypical, reactive mesothelial cells, no malignant cells seen

Pleural fluid biochemistry:
protein 31 g/L
lactate dehydrogenase 568 U/L
glucose 4.9 mmol/L (>3.3)
pH 7.4 (>7.4)

Venous biochemistry:
total protein 54 g/L (60–76)
lactate dehydrogenase 674 U/L (10–250)
glucose 8.4 mmol/L (fasting 3.0–6.0)

What is the most likely cause of the pleural effusion?

A   Dressler's syndrome
B   Malignancy
C   Meigs' syndrome
D   Parapneumonic effusion
E   Rheumatoid arthritis

24. A 38-year-old woman presented with a 6-week history of shortness of breath and cough. She had no significant past medical history and did not take any regular medication. She smoked 20 cigarettes per day. There was no history of recent foreign travel and she did not keep any birds or pets. She worked in an office and there was no history of exposure to industrial dusts or fumes.
    On examination, there was finger clubbing and fine inspiratory crackles in the lower zones on auscultation.

Investigations:

Chest X-ray: no abnormality

High-resolution CT of the thorax: ground-glass opacity in lower zones and peripheries

What is the most likely diagnosis?

A   Acute interstitial pneumonitis
B   Cryptogenic organising pneumonia
C   Desquamative interstitial pneumonia
D   Respiratory bronchiolitis-associated lung disease
E   Usual interstitial pneumonia

25. A 23-year-old female university student presented with a 2-week history of a dry cough and left-sided chest discomfort on coughing. She had no previous history of respiratory illness and did not take any regular medication. She was a non-smoker and had recently moved into a shared rented house. She appeared tired but physical examination was normal.

What is the most likely diagnosis?

A   Adult-onset asthma
B   Allergic rhinitis
C   Gastro-oesophageal reflux
D   Inhaled foreign body
E   Self-limiting viral illness

26. A 24-year-old man was admitted to the acute medical ward with right lower lobar pneumonia. He had no past medical history and was not taking any regular medication. There was no history of recent travel, he was a non-smoker and he worked in an office.

On admission his temperature was 38.8°C, pulse 120 beats per minute, blood pressure 124/68 mmHg, respiratory rate 34 breaths per minute and oxygen saturation 92% on air. He was not confused.

Chest X-ray showed consolidation in the right lower zone and loss of clarity of right hemi-diaphragm. He was commenced on high-flow oxygen therapy, intravenous co-amoxiclav and clarithromycin, and intravenous fluids. The next day as he had improved clinically he was switched to oral antibiotics. Forty-eight hours after admission his condition deteriorated and he had spiking fevers, complaining of worsening shortness of breath, and respiratory rate was 28 breaths per minute with oxygen saturations of 94% on 40% oxygen.

What is the most likely cause of the deterioration in the clinical condition?

A   Acute respiratory distress syndrome
B   Complication of different underlying lung pathology
C   Lung abscess
D   Inappropriate antibiotic prescribing
E   Parapneumonic effusion

27. A 46-year-old male lorry driver was referred to the sleep clinic by an occupational health physician working for the haulage company. He had recently been involved in a road traffic accident and it was suggested that he may have been at fault because of lack of due care and attention when driving.

He had no past medical history of note. He rarely drank any alcohol and smoked 20 cigarettes per day. He did not have a partner and so there was no collateral history; however, he had previously been told that he was a snorer and he reported that he frequently woke gasping for breath. He confirmed that he had excessive daytime somnolence (Epworth Sleepiness Score 16/24), poor concentration and early morning headaches.

An urgent sleep study was performed (see **Figure 10.4** on page 336):

What is the most appropriate advice?

A   Commence domiciliary non-invasive ventilation
B   Commence modafinil
C   Inform the Driver and Vehicle Licensing Authority (DVLA) and stop driving until he has received adequate treatment
D   Lifestyle and dietary advice
E   Surrender his licence and do not drive again

28. A 34-year-old female Zimbabwean office worker presented with progressive shortness of breath on exertion. She was diagnosed HIV positive 4 years ago and was receiving antiretroviral therapy.

Pulse oximetry demonstrated desaturation on exercise. She had a loud second heart sound but no audible murmurs. Chest was clear to auscultation.

Investigations:

Chest X-ray:
no focal consolidation
prominent pulmonary arteries

CD4 count: 348 cells/mm³ (400–1600)

Viral load: undetectable

What is the most likely diagnosis?

A   Chronic thromboembolic disease
B   Intracardiac shunt across an atrial septal defect (ASD)
C   Physical deconditioning secondary to sedentary lifestyle
D   *Pneumocystis jirovecii* pneumonia
E   Pulmonary arterial hypertension

29. A 34-year-old Norwegian man was referred to the chest clinic because the chest X-ray that his general practitioner had ordered was reported as abnormal. He had a 6-week history of lethargy, fevers, painful wrists and ankles, and tender erythematous nodules on his shins. He had had no recent infective illnesses. He had no past medical history of note and was not taking any regular medication.

Investigations:

Chest X-ray (see **Figure 10.5**, opposite).

Respiratory events summary						
Parameter	Obstructive	Central	Mixed	All apnoeas	Hypopnoea	All events
Number	543	62	217	822	100	922
Per hour	57.6	6.6	23.0	87.1	10.6	97.7
Average duration (mm/s)	0:23	0:21	0:24	0:23	0:21	0:23
Longest duration (mm/s)	2:02	0:55	0:54	2:02	1:09	2:02
	(2:33:21)	(23:34:31)	(23:42:53)	(2:33:21)	(6:56:27)	(2:33:21)
Apnoea–hypopnoea index (AHI)	97.7					

Figure 10.4

Figure 10.5

What is the most likely prognosis?

A   30% chance of central nervous system involvement
B   30% chance of progressive pulmonary infiltration
C   50% chance of progressive renal dysfunction
D   50% chance of symptomatic hypercalcaemia
E   90% chance of resolution of disease within 2 years

30. A 34-year-old woman with a history of asthma presented to the emergency department with cough, wheeze and breathlessness. Her symptoms had been triggered by being exposed to a dusty environment while decorating her house. Her asthma was normally well controlled and she attended the nurse-led asthma clinic in the community. Her normal medications included beclomethasone and salbutamol inhalers.

On examination, she was alert and able to speak in short sentences. Oxygen saturation was 95% breathing air, respiratory rate 20 breaths per minute, pulse 120 beats per minute and peak flow rate 200 L/min (40% predicted). On auscultation there was widespread wheeze.

She was given prednisolone 40 mg and salbutamol 5 mg via an oxygen-driven nebuliser. Fifteen minutes later she remained wheezy and a second salbutamol nebuliser was given.

What is the most appropriate next step in management?

A   Amoxicillin
B   Intravenous aminophylline
C   Ipratropium bromide by oxygen-driven nebuliser
D   Montelukast
E   Salbutamol by Heliox-driven nebuliser

31. A 72-year-old woman presented to the chest clinic with a 9-month history of progressive shortness of breath and dry cough. Her exercise tolerance was limited to 10 metres. She did not notice any diurnal variation in her symptoms, but she was unable to lie flat and slept with three pillows. She had hypertension and hypercholesterolaemia. She was a non-smoker. Her current medications included ramipril, bendroflumethiazide, aspirin and simvastatin.

On examination, there was ankle oedema and fine end-inspiratory crackles. Oxygen saturation was 92% on air.

A CT of the chest was performed (see **Figure 10.6**).

Figure 10.6

What is the most likely diagnosis?

A Bronchiectasis
B Cough secondary to angiotensin-converting enzyme inhibitor
C Congestive cardiac failure
D Desquamative interstitial pneumonia
E Usual interstitial pneumonitis

32. A 56-year-old man was referred by the stroke team for an opinion regarding an abnormal chest X-ray. He presented with sudden-onset, left-sided weakness and was making a steady recovery with rehabilitation. The physiotherapists were concerned that he showed desaturation on standing and mobilising. He had no previous history of respiratory symptoms and no past medical history of note. He was a non-smoker.

On examination, there was telangiectasia and finger clubbing. Oxygen saturations were 93% on air. His chest was clear to auscultation.

Investigations:

Chest X-ray: 3-cm, smooth, round, intrapulmonary mass in right lower zone

What is the most likely diagnosis?

A Asbestos-related pleural plaque
B Lung abscess
C Previous tuberculosis infection
D Pulmonary arteriovenous malformation
E Pulmonary embolism

33. A 38-year-old white businessman presented to the chest clinic with a persistent cough, wheeze and shortness of breath on exertion. He also had ongoing lethargy, fevers and minor weight loss. He suffered a flu-like illness 6 weeks ago, when on a business trip to Malaysia. He had a past medical history of mild asthma and occasionally used a salbutamol inhaler. The inhaler had not been effective recently. He did not smoke but kept a dog.

Investigations:

haemoglobin 13.5 g/dL (13.0–18.0)	lymphocytes 3.3 × 10⁹/L (1.5–4.0)
white cell count 21.0 × 10⁹/L (4–11)	eosinophils 4.2 × 10⁹/L (0.04–0.4)
neutrophils 12.3 × 10⁹/L (1.5–7.0)	erythrocyte sedimentation rate 46 mm/1st h (0–20)

Mantoux test: 11 mm (<5 mm negative, 5–14 mm positive, >15 mm strongly positive)

Chest X-ray: bilateral reticular nodular infiltrates

What is the most likely diagnosis?

A   Churg–Strauss syndrome
B   Löffler's syndrome
C   Miliary tuberculosis
D   *Pneumocystis jirovecii* pneumonia
E   Tropical pulmonary eosinophilia

34. A 64-year-old man with bullous emphysema presented to the emergency department with sudden onset of shortness of breath and left-sided chest pain. A chest X-ray confirmed a large left-sided pneumothorax. The emergency department team inserted small bore (12 Fr) intercostal chest tube with underwater seal, and the X-ray was repeated which demonstrated that the chest tube was in a satisfactory position near the left apex and there was partial re-expansion of the left lung.

   He was prescribed regular simple analgesia and oxygen therapy to maintain oxygen saturation 94–98% and was referred to the medical team for on-going care. Forty-eight hours after admission the chest drain was still bubbling profusely. A third chest X-ray again confirmed that the chest tube remained in a satisfactory position and the lung had further expanded; however, a large left pneumothorax persisted (>2 cm rim).

   What is the most appropriate next step in management?

A   Apply low-volume high-pressure suction to chest drain
B   Clamp chest tube
C   Flush chest drain with 10 mL 5% saline solution using aseptic technique
D   Insert large-bore chest drain
E   Refer to cardiothoracic surgeons

35. A 28-year-old man presented to the emergency department with a 4-week history of cough with purulent sputum, fever, night sweats and weight loss of 3 kg. He had no past medical history. He was a smoker of 20 cigarettes per day and drank excessive alcohol (>70 units per week). He was unemployed and of no fixed abode but was living in a charity-run shelter.

   On examination, he was unkempt and malnourished. His temperature was 37.2°C, pulse 94 beats per minute, blood pressure 110/68 mmHg, respiratory rate 18 breaths per minute and oxygen saturation 94% on air. There was no palpable lymphadenopathy. He had reduced breath sounds in the right upper zone. Cardiovascular, abdominal and nervous system examinations were normal.

Investigations:

haemoglobin 11.8 g/dL (13.0–18.0)	lymphocytes 0.7 × 10⁹/L (1.5–4.0)
mean corpuscular volume 110 fL (80–96)	sodium 134 mmol/L (135–145)
white cell count 7.8 × 10⁹/L (4–11)	urea 4.5 mmol/L (2.5–7.5)
neutrophils 6.4 × 10⁹/L (1.5–7.0)	creatinine 54 μmol/L (60–110)

Chest X-ray (see **Figure 10.7**):

Figure 10.7

What is the most appropriate next step in management?

A   Admit to general respiratory ward for intravenous amoxicillin and clarithromycin
B   Admit to respiratory isolation room and send sputum samples for acid-fast bacilli and tuberculosis (TB) culture
C   Discharge with ethambutol, isoniazid, pyrazinamide and rifampicin
D   Discharge with oral amoxicillin and clarithromycin
E   Discharge with urgent follow-up in chest clinic for CT of thorax and bronchoscopy

36. A 54-year-old woman was referred by her general practitioner to the chest clinic with a 6-month history of persistent dry cough. Her symptoms occurred throughout the day but were particularly troublesome at night and when speaking on the telephone. There was no history of rhinitis or postnasal drip. She had a history of hypertension. There was no previous history of respiratory illness or atopy. Her general practitioner reviewed her medications and had stopped perindopril 8 weeks ago. Her current medications included bendroflumethiazide and candesartan; she also took over-the-counter remedies for occasional dyspepsia. She was a non-smoker and worked as a telephone receptionist. She was distressed that cough was interfering with her work.

On examination, she appeared well but had a dry cough. Body mass index was 34 kg/m², oxygen saturation 94% on room air, heart sounds normal and chest clear to auscultation.

Investigations:

> Chest X-ray: no abnormality detected
>
> ---
>
> Spirometry:
> FEV$_1$ 2.23 L (80% predicted)
> FEV$_1$ postbronchodilator 2.28 L (82% predicted)
> FVC 2.76 L (85% predicted)
> FVC postbronchodilator 2.73 L (83% predicted)
> DLCO 78% predicted
> corrected DLCO 96% predicted
>
> ---
>
> (FEV$_1$ = forced expiratory volume 1 second; FVC = forced vital capacity; DLCO = diffusion capacity of lung to carbon monoxide)

What is the most appropriate next step in management?

A   Gastric emptying studies
B   High-resolution CT of the chest
C   Oesophageal pH manometry
D   Omeprazole
E   Prednisolone

37. A 24-year-old man with cystic fibrosis presented to the emergency department with a 6-day history of worsening shortness of breath on exertion, thick dark-green sputum with streaks of haemoptysis that was difficult to expectorate, loss of appetite and lethargy. He commenced a course of oral ciprofloxacin 4 days ago with no improvement in his symptoms. He had no known drug allergies.

On examination, his temperature was 37.6°C, respiratory rate 34 breaths per minute and oxygen saturation 96% on 4 L oxygen via nasal cannulae. He had gross finger clubbing and coarse crackles audible in the upper zones bilaterally with scattered wheeze.

Investigations:

> Chest X-ray: chronic bronchiectatic changes with patchy consolidation right mid and upper zones and evidence of mucus plugging
>
> ---
>
> Sputum culture of routine sample taken at last clinic visit 8 weeks ago: *Pseudomonas aeruginosa*

What is the most appropriate antibiotic regimen of choice?

A   Intravenous ceftazidime and tobramycin
B   Intravenous meropenem
C   Intravenous piperacillin–tazobactam
D   Oral amoxicillin and clarithromycin
E   Oral ciprofloxacin

38. A 72-year-old man, with type 2 diabetes mellitus, was admitted with a 4-day history of cough, drenching sweats, chest pain and loss of diabetic control.

Investigations:

> Chest X-ray: large right-sided pleural effusion
>
> ---
>
> Ultrasound-guided diagnostic pleural tap: purulent thick green fluid

What is the most likely infecting organism?

A   *Bacteroides* species
B   Enterobacteriaceae
C   *Staphylococcus aureus*
D   *Streptococcus milleri*
E   *Streptococcus pneumoniae*

39. A 34-year-old man presented to the chest clinic with a chronic productive cough and several episodes of haemoptysis. He gave a history of recurrent chest infections since childhood. He and his partner had recently been referred for fertility treatment.

On examination, he had finger clubbing and scattered crackles throughout both lung fields.

What is the most likely diagnosis?

A   Bronchiectasis
B   Cystic fibrosis
C   Primary ciliary dyskinesia
D   Pulmonary fibrosis
E   Pulmonary tuberculosis

40. A 56-year-old man presented with a 6-month history of a dry cough and progressive shortness of breath on exertion. The symptoms first occurred following a flu-like illness. There was no history of weight loss or on-going fevers. He had a history of rheumatoid arthritis, for which he was taking methotrexate weekly. He had never smoked.

On examination, a left-sided effusion was detected. The aspirated fluid was turbid looking. Following simple bench centrifugation, the pleural fluid remained turbid and a clear supernatant did not appear.

What is the most likely nature of the effusion?

A   Chylothorax
B   Empyema
C   Malignant effusion
D   Pseudochylothorax
E   Rheumatoid effusion

41. A 75-year-old man was referred to the chest clinic by his general practitioner. Eight weeks ago he presented with a 2-week history of cough productive of yellow sputum and his general practitioner requested a chest X-ray which was found to be abnormal. By the time of outpatient consultation, he had recovered completely; the cough had resolved and he was feeling well. He had no loss of appetite or weight. He had previously worked at a granite quarry. He had never smoked.

On examination, there was no finger clubbing, his chest was clear and oxygen saturation was 94% on air.

Investigations:

Chest X-ray: multiple, small, dense nodules bilaterally, mainly in the upper zones

What is the most likely diagnosis?

A   Asbestosis
B   Kaolinosis
C   Progressive massive fibrosis
D   Silicosis
E   Stannosis

42. A 68-year-old woman was referred to the chest clinic following an infective exacerbation of chronic obstructive pulmonary disease (COPD). She had made a good recovery and her exercise tolerance was back to her baseline of 250 metres on flat ground. She planned to travel to Spain on a 3-hour flight in 6 weeks' time and her general practitioner requested an in-flight oxygen assessment.

Investigations:

Oxygen saturation at rest breathing air: 93%

PaO_2 after hypoxic challenge test using 15% FiO_2 for 20 min: 7.8 kPa

Forced expiratory volume in 1 second (FEV_1): 1.48 (48% predicted)

What is the most appropriate advice?

A   Reassess in 3 weeks
B   She can fly with in-flight oxygen at a flow rate of 2 L/min
C   She can fly with in-flight oxygen at a flow rate of 4 L/min
D   She can fly without the need for in-flight oxygen
E   She should undergo exercising testing as a prelude to flying

43. A 64-year-old man was admitted with severe pneumonia and septicaemia. He was treated with oxygen and intravenous antibiotics (co-amioxiclav and clarithromycin), and had repeated fluid challenges to a total volume of 400 mL (equivalent to 60 mL/kg) of sodium chloride 0.9%.
    On examination, his pulse was 134 beats per minute, blood pressure 86/44 mmHg, central venous pressure 12 mmHg, respiratory rate 28 breaths per minute and oxygen saturation 92% on 40% oxygen.

What is the most appropriate next step in management?

A   Adrenaline
B   Colloid
C   Furosemide
D   Further crystalloid
E   Noradrenaline

44. A 74-year-old man was admitted to hospital with severe shortness of breath. He had a history of emphysema.
    On examination, he had diminished breath sounds over the left side of the chest; the trachea was central.

Investigations:

Chest X-ray: large left pneumothorax

What is the most appropriate next step in management?

A   Insert 14 Fr drain immediately above a rib margin in the scalene triangle
B   Insert 14 Fr drain immediately below a lower rib margin in the scalene triangle
C   Insert 14 Fr drain in the second intercostal space in the mid-clavicular line
D   Insert 28 Fr drain immediately above a rib margin in the scalene triangle
E   Insert 28 Fr drain immediately below a lower rib margin in the scalene triangle

45. A 53-year-old woman presented with a 2-year history of increasing wheeze and shortness of breath on exertion. She was a current smoker (30 pack-years) and had started working at a local bakery as a cleaner 3 years previously. Her wheeze improved on holiday and was better on her days off.
    On examination, she had nasal congestion and marked expiratory wheeze.

What is the most likely diagnosis?

A   Atopic asthma
B   Chronic bronchitis
C   Emphysema
D   Hypersensitivity pneumonitis
E   Occupational asthma

46. The local research and ethics committee is considering an application to collect spirometry data from over 65 year olds presenting to a hospital with breathlessness. The aim is to collect data from 100 people who have been formally diagnosed as having chronic obstructive pulmonary disease (COPD) and from 100 people who have not had this diagnosis. Then the aim is to compare these two groups and draw conclusions as to the validity of spirometry in elderly people for making the diagnosis of COPD. The data collected are depicted below.

	Known COPD	No previous diagnosis of COPD
EV_1 (L)	2.8	3.1
FEV_1/FVC ratio (%)	68	74
PEFR	390	480

The data demonstrate gaussian distribution.

What is the most appropriate statistical test that you should use?

A χ^2 test
B   Mann–Whitney test
C   Paired one-sided t-test
D   Pearson's correlation
E   Unpaired two-sided t-test

Answers

1. D Pleural plaques are a premalignant finding

Pleural plaques are the most common manifestation of asbestos exposure and may be found in up to 50% of asbestos-exposed workers. Plaques typically develop 20–30 years after exposure and the incidence increases with prolonged exposure. Pleural plaques are usually asymptomatic and present as an incidental finding. Patients with extensive plaques may present with breathlessness. There is no evidence that plaques are premalignant. Patients with isolated pleural plaques do not necessarily need further investigations or regular follow-up; however, high-resolution CT scanning is a more sensitive test to detect pleural plaques. Other forms of benign asbestos-related pleural disease include benign asbestos-related pleural effusion, diffuse pleural thickening and rounded atelectasis. Benign pleural effusions occur relatively early within 10 years of exposure and may be asymptomatic or present with chest pain, dyspnoea and fever, and tend to resolve spontaneously. They may recur and progress to diffuse pleural thickening. There is no clear association with mesothelioma. On chest X-ray, diffuse pleural thickening may be defined as a smooth pleural opacity extending over at least a quarter of the chest wall. Symptoms are relatively common and include dyspnoea and chest pain. Pleural biopsy may be required to differentiate diffuse pleural thickening from mesothelioma.

British Thoracic Society Standards of Care Committee. Statement on malignant mesothelioma in the United Kingdom. Thorax 2001; 56:250–265

2. E Treat with rifampicin and isoniazid

As in the case above, screening may identify cases of latent tuberculosis (TB). Active TB infection should be excluded by medical history, physical examination and chest X-ray. If there is no evidence of active TB infection and the chest X-ray is normal then further investigation including bronchoscopy, induced sputa and CT scanning is not necessary and may have potential risks and side effects including significant discomfort and radiation exposure. Mantoux (with appropriate interpretation and knowledge of prior BCG vaccination) and/or interferon-γ screening tests may identify cases of latent TB infection. Certain groups with latent TB, including patients under the age of 35 years, HIV-positive patients and health-care workers should be offered TB chemoprophylaxis. The most frequently offered treatment is 3 months of isoniazid and rifampicin. Patients who decline TB chemoprophylaxis should be counselled to seek medical advice if they develop any symptoms suggestive of active disease and the chest X-ray should be repeated at 3 and 12 months.

National Institute for Health and Clinical Excellence. NICE Guidance 117: Tuberculosis: Clinical diagnosis and management of tuberculosis, and measures for its prevention and control. London: NICE, 2011.

3. B Continue present treatment and re-assess within 1 hour

Non-invasive ventilation (NIV) should be considered for all patients presenting with respiratory acidosis (pH<7.35 and $PaCO_2$>6 kPa) secondary to an exacerbation of chronic obstructive pulmonary disease (COPD), if standard medical treatment (controlled oxygen therapy, nebulised salbutamol and ipratropium, prednisolone ± antibiotic therapy if indicated) has not improved the situation within 1 hour. A clearly documented treatment plan for NIV, with ceilings of treatment and/or suitability for escalation to invasive ventilatory support, should be discussed and documented at the outset of treatment. If there is impairment of consciousness and/or pH<7.2, then there should be a lower threshold for invasive support if it is deemed appropriate. In patients with type 2 respiratory failure (PaO_2 <8 kPa, $PaCO_2$ >6 kPa) oxygen therapy should be controlled to target SaO_2 between 88% and 92% and PO_2 >7.2 kPa. It would be inappropriate to reduce the oxygen flow rate to 1 L/min as this would lead to worsening hypoxia; however, it would be appropriate to use a controlled delivery system such as a Venturi device delivering 24–28% oxygen. Nebulised treatment should continue and be delivered using air rather than high-flow oxygen to avoid over-oxygenation and possible loss of hypoxic drive.

Aminophylline may be used in reversible airway obstruction and acute severe asthma; however, there is little evidence of benefit in acute exacerbations of COPD and it may cause arrhythmias, convulsions and hypotension.

With widespread availability of NIV, respiratory stimulants, e.g. doxapram, have little role in the management of respiratory failure and are associated with a number of side effects including arrhythmias, chest pain, agitation, hallucinations and seizures.

Roberts CM, et al. Non-invasive ventilation in chronic obstructive pulmonary disorder: management of acute type 2 respiratory failure. RCP/BTS Concise guideline. London: British Thoracic Society, 2008.

4. A CT pulmonary angiogram (CPTA)

The history is suggestive of venous thromboembolic (VTE) disease with an acute pulmonary embolism (PE). The diagnosis of a PE can be difficult and involves a clinical assessment of probability. Risk factors, clinical presentation and clinical signs are taken into account and tests are performed to add weight to the clinical decision. Scoring systems such as the modified Wells score may be employed to estimate the pretest probability of a PE (see **Table 10.1**).

Table 10.1 Wells clinical prediction rule for pulmonary embolism (PE)	
Clinical feature	**Points**
Clinical symptoms of deep vein thrombosis (DVT)	3
Other diagnosis less likely than pulmonary embolism (PE)	3
Heart rate greater than 100 beats per minute	1.5
Immobilisation or surgery within past 4 weeks	1.5
Previous DVT or PE	1.5
Haemoptysis	1
Malignancy	1

Adapted from: Wells PS, et al. Derivation of a simple clinical model to categorize patient's probability of pulmonary embolism: increasing the models utility with the SimpliRED D-dimer. Thromb Haemost 2000; 83(3):416–420.

Risk score interpretation (probability of PE):
- >6 points: high risk
- 2–6 points: moderate risk
- <2 points: low risk

[In the clinical scenario described in the question there are clinical features of a DVT, PE is more likely than another diagnosis, the heart rate is greater than 100 beats per minute and there is active malignancy (total score 8.5 = high risk).]

D-dimer testing has an important role in diagnosing and excluding PE and should be used only after a pretest probability assessment. D-dimers are a sensitive test for VTE but not specific. D-dimers are generated as a result of fibrinolysis, which occurs in many clinical situations, including VTE, sepsis, pregnancy and neoplasia.

A low or intermediate pretest probability score, combined with a negative D-dimer has a 92% probability for excluding PE. If there is a high clinical suspicion of PE (i.e. Wells score >6) a D-dimer should not be performed and patients should be referred for appropriate imaging. CTPA is the recommended initial lung imaging modality for non-massive PE. Urgent bedside echocardiography may be useful for diagnosing massive PE in haemodynamically compromised patients.

Ventilation–perfusion (nuclear medicine) scans may be useful if the chest radiograph is normal and if facilities are readily available. If the patient presents with signs of a deep vein thrombosis,

Doppler ultrasound may be sufficient to confirm the diagnosis, but should not be used as a sole test to exclude the diagnosis.

The British Thoracic Society Standards of Care Committee, Pulmonary Embolism Guideline Development Group. British Thoracic Society guidelines for the management of suspected acute pulmonary embolism. Thorax 2003; 58:470–484.

5. E Trial of omalizumab

This patient with severe asthma remains poorly controlled and dependent on regular oral steroids. She may be a candidate for a trial of omalizumab. This is a humanised monoclonal antibody which binds to circulating serum IgE. It is administered by subcutaneous injection and should be initiated only in specialist centres managing patients with severe and difficult asthma. If the trial of omalizumab is successful, as indicated by improvement of symptom control, lung function and reduction in serum IgE, oral steroids may be tapered and stopped.

Patients with severe and difficult asthma should have self-management plans. With good inhaler technique and compliance with medications home nebulisers are not normally required. This patient has been intolerant of theophyllines and therefore commencing aminophylline modified-release tablets would not be appropriate. Patients may require additional oral corticosteroids to treat acute exacerbations. However, long-term high-dose steroids have a number of deleterious side effects, including osteopenia, immunosuppression, weight gain and impairment of glucose tolerance, so dose should be minimised where possible. Increasing the regular dose would not be a satisfactory long-term strategy.

It would not be appropriate to recommend adrenaline by intramuscular injection for self-administration in case of emergencies unless there was a history of anaphylaxis.

British Thoracic Society and Scottish Intercollegiate Guidelines Network. British Guideline on the Management of Asthma – a national clinical guideline. London: BTS and SIGN, 2009.

6. D Chronic obstruction pulmonary disease (COPD) secondary to biomass fuel exposure

The history and spirometry findings are suggestive of COPD. Tobacco smoking is the leading cause of COPD; however, exposure to biomass fuels is an increasingly recognised cause of respiratory disease. Wood and charcoal are used by a third of the world's population for cooking and heating, and burning of these fuels indoors results in the generation of large amounts of noxious gases including carbon monoxide, hydrocarbons, oxygenated and chlorinated organics, and free radials which have been found to increase the incidence of respiratory disease, cardiovascular disease and all-cause mortality.

α_1-antitrypsin (α_1AT) deficiency is an autosomal recessive disorder that is associated with early development of emphysema. The glycoprotein protease inhibitor α_1AT is produced by the liver and acts in the lungs to oppose neutrophil elastase, which destroys alveolar wall connective tissue. Insults such as tobacco smoke and infection stimulate pulmonary neutrophils and macrophages to produce increased levels of the elastase. If α_1AT is deficient, the elastase cannot be opposed and the lungs are subject to proteolytic attack leading to emphysema.

Adult-onset asthma is also increasing in prevalence and congestive cardiac failure may also be a differential diagnosis; however, the fixed obstructive defect seen in the spirometry would not support either of these diagnoses.

The history is not particularly suggestive of tuberculosis (TB); however, this patient may be considered at high risk of reactivation of latent disease especially considering her ethnic background and co-morbidities, including diabetes mellitus. Patients with diabetes are at increased risk of re-activation of latent TB. Patients presenting with a chronic cough – a cough of more than 8 weeks' duration – should have a chest X-ray and patients considered to be at high risk of TB should be screened by sending three early morning sputum samples for alcohol acid-fast bacilli testing and TB culture.

Salvi SS, Barnes PJ. Chronic obstructive pulmonary disease in non-smokers. Lancet 2009; 374:733–743.

7. E Send two more sputum samples for AFB and TB culture

This patient has a chronic productive cough and a background history of COPD (chronic obstructive pulmonary disease). The chest X-ray findings and positive sputum culture demonstrating a probable *Mycobacterium* species should prompt referral to the chest clinic for further review and investigation. In the first instance, two more sputum samples for acid-fast bacilli (AFB) and TB (tuberculosis) culture should be sent.

This patient does not have any obvious risk factors for *Mycobacterium tuberculosis* and the history may be more suggestive of an atypical or opportunistic organism. These organisms occur throughout the environment, including soil, water and animal hosts. The significance of isolating these organisms depends on the specific identity, number of isolates and intensity of growth. Patients with underlying chronic respiratory disease and/or immunocompromise are more at risk of significant infection with these organisms. These infections are most frequently encountered in elderly men with COPD. The risk of contagion from person to person is low and therefore identification of these organisms is not notifiable and contact tracing is not necessary.

Opportunistic mycobacteria causing pulmonary disease need prolonged treatment regimens. Regimens may include combinations of rifampicin, isoniazid, ethambutol and/or other agents for up to 2 years. Antituberculous therapy should be prescribed and monitored by a chest physician or a doctor with a special interest in the management of TB. Significant drug interactions and side effects are common problems, especially in elderly patients already receiving polypharmacy.

Subcommittee of the Joint Tuberculosis Committee of the British Thoracic Society. Management of opportunistic mycobacterial infections: Joint Tuberculosis Committee Guidelines 1999. Thorax 2000; 55:210–218.

8. E Perfusion scan

Pulmonary embolism (PE) is the leading cause of maternal death. The diagnosis of PE in the general population is sometimes difficult and this may be more complicated in pregnancy and the postpartum period as some of the symptoms of PE may be some of the normal symptoms of pregnancy. Accurate diagnosis is essential to reduce the risks of the side effects of inappropriate treatments, and morbidity and mortality risks of undetected PE for both the mother and the fetus. Serum levels of D-dimer increase in pregnancy, and therefore this test is not clinically useful in pregnancy. There is a high prevalence (70%) of deep vein thrombosis (DVT) in patients with proven PE in pregnancy and therefore Doppler ultrasound of the leg veins may be a useful test to confirm the diagnosis without the risks associated with ionising radiation. However, physiological changes associated with hormonal effects and the compressive effects of the gravid uterus increase leg swelling in pregnant women in the absence of a DVT and a negative Doppler should not be used to rule out PE.

Nuclear medicine imaging (ventilation–perfusion scan) is often the imaging modality of choice in this group as it carries a low radiation dose. If the perfusion scan is completely normal a significant PE can be excluded. This modality may not be available locally and a number of the scans (approximately 20%) are indeterminate and a further test will need to be performed.

CT pulmonary angiogram (CTPA) has a high sensitivity and specificity and is often preferred as the PE may be directly seen and/or an alternative cause for the patient's presentation may be identified. This modality carries a risk of radiation to the fetus and breast of the woman. The risks and benefits should be considered and the risk to both fetus and mother is greater if the mother has an untreated PE.

British Thoracic Society Standards of Care Committee Pulmonary Embolism Guideline Development Group. British Thoracic Society guidelines for the management of suspected acute pulmonary embolism. Thorax 2003; 58:470–484.
Matthews S. Imaging pulmonary embolism in pregnancy: what is the most appropriate imaging protocol? Br J Radiol 2006; 79:441–444.

9. B Needle aspiration in right second intercostal space in the mid-clavicular line

This patient has presented with a classic history of a primary spontaneous pneumothorax (PSP) as confirmed by the chest X-ray. He has a large pneumothorax (complete collapse of right lung) and, although distressed and in pain, is still haemodynamically stable.

The clinical situation guides the management of PSP. If a patient presenting with PSP is asymptomtaic and clinically stable, then a conservative approach may be appropriate. The administration of high-flow oxygen may treat associated hypoxia, but has also been demonstrated to increase the rate of resolution of the pneumothorax.

If the patient is distressed, tachypnoeic and/or hypoxic, the intial management of choice is attempted needle aspiration of up to 2.5 L of air followed by repeat chest X-ray to ensure that the lung has re-expanded. If this is succesful, then no further immediate treatment may be necessary, and if the lung has partially re-expanded and the overall clinical picture has improved, then the patient may be observed. Needle aspiration may be as effective as insertion of a large-bore chest drain and may reduce the length of stay. If however, needle aspiration is unsuccsesful, a small-bore chest drain may be the next best step.

Thoracic ultrasound will identify specific diagnostic features of a pneumothorax, but this practice is not necessary for routine management. Thoracic ultrasound should, however, be used for other pleural procedures including diagnostic pleural taps and chest drain insertion for pleural effusion.

MacDuff A, et al. Management of spontaneous pneumothorax: British Thoracic Society pleural disease guideline 2010. Thorax 2010; 65(2):ii18–eii31.

10. C Lymphoma

The chest X-ray demonstrates a large anterior mediastinal mass. The most likely cause of the mediastinal mass in a woman of this age group and with the blood test presented is lymphoma. The mediastinum is commonly involved in patients with Hodgkin's lymphoma. To establish the histological diagnosis of lymphoma, an adequate tissue sample is required; this should be in the form of a biopsy which may be either CT guided, via endobronchial ultrasound (EBUS), or surgical.

Common symptoms of mediastinal disease include cough, chest pain and dyspnoea, as well as symptoms relating to structural compression, e.g. dysphagia, stridor or superior vena cava obstruction. Mediastinal disorders may also be asymptomatic and found incidentally on chest X-ray. The likely nature of a mediastinal mass may be determined according to anatomical site.

Anterior mediastinal mass:
- thymoma (superior)
- thyroid (superior)
- germ cell tumour
- lymphoma
- ascending aortic aneurysm
- pleuropericardial cyst
- pericardial fat pad
- anterior diaphragmatic hernia

Superior mediastinal mass:
- bronchogenic cyst

Posterior mediastinal mass:
- neural tumour
- foregut duplication cyst
- lipoma
- descending aortic aneurysm
- posterior diaphragmatic hernia

Germ cell tumours arise from immature germ cells during development. Mature cystic teratomas represent 80% of germ cell tumours. These are benign and occur in young adults (prevalence male = female) and appear on a chest X-ray or as a well-defined mass which may contain flecks of calcification. Seminomas occur in men aged 20–40 years and are malignant.

Retrosternal goitre is usually asymptomatic unless there is tracheal compression leading to dyspnoea. Surgical resection is recommended if there is airway compromise.

Thymomas are tumours arising from the thymus and may contain functioning thymic tissue. Myasthaenia gravis (MG) occurs in 30–40% patients with thymomas; frequently this does not respond to thymectomy and may even occur after resection. Twenty per cent of patients with MG are found to have thymoma.

Duwe BV, Sterman DH, Musani AI. Tumors of the mediastinum. Chest 2005; 128(4):2893-2909

11. C High-resolution CT of the chest

The history is suggestive of bronchiectasis which may present as recurrent lower respiratory tract infections and the expectoration of purulent sputum. Symptoms may also include chest pain, dyspnoea and haemoptysis, and the condition may progress to respiratory failure.

A chest X-ray should be performed in all suspected cases and is recommended for all patients presenting with a chronic cough (>8 weeks). The imaging modality of choice for diagnosing bronchiectasis is high-resolution CT (HRCT), which will demonstrate the pathognomonic features of bronchial wall thickening and dilatation. HRCT may demonstrate certain features suggesting a cause for the condition, e.g. allergic bronchopulmonary aspergillosis (ABPA) or cystic fibrosis (CF). Some routine blood tests should be performed in the work-up of all patients presenting with bronchiectasis, including serum immunoglobulins and protein electrophoresis, plus total IgE and skin-prick testing or serum IgE testing to *Aspergillus* species. Bronchoscopy is not routinely performed, unless there is a suspected endobronchial lesion, or foreign body, with associated distal bronchiectasis. Bronchoalveolar lavage may be useful to gain a microbiological diagnosis if mycobacterial infection is suspected.

α_1-Antitrypsin levels should not be routinely requested in these patients, but may be useful if HRCT demonstrates basal emphysema. A tuberculin skin test is unlikely to be helpful in a patient of this age group and is not the test of choice. Tuberculin skin tests are useful to identify cases of latent tuberculosis infection but need to be interpreted with knowledge of previous BCG vaccination history.

M C Pasteur, D Bilton, A T Hill. British Thoracic Society guideline for non-CF bronchiectasis. Thorax 2010; 65:i1–i58.

12. C Intravenous magnesium

This patient has features of life-threatening asthma as suggested by peak flow rate (PEF) <33% of best. Other features of life-threatening asthma include the presence of: (1) silent chest, cyanosis or feeble respiratory effort; (2) arrhythmia or hypotension; (3) exhaustion, altered consciousness.

Following the administration of oxygen-driven nebulised salbutamol or terbutaline and ipratropium bromide and steroids, intravenous magnesium sulphate 1.2–2.0 g infusion over 20 minute should be considered. Intravenous magnesium has bronchodilator effects; however, the exact mechanism of action is unclear.

As the patient has features of life-threatening asthma, a senior physician should be called to review the patient and the patient should be referred to the intensive care team to consider transfer to the intensive care unit. If the patient is not improving the senior clinician may consider use of intravenous β_2-agonist (salbutamol) or intravenous aminophylline, or progression to mechanical ventilation.

Oxygen therapy should be given to maintain oxygen saturation between 94 and 98%; there is no benefit in maintaining saturation >98% with increased oxygen therapy. In cases of life-threatening asthma requiring intubation and mechanical ventilation, intravenous ketamine may sometimes be used to relieve intractable bronchospasm but requires expert anaesthetic supervision.

Scottish Intercollegiate Guidelines Network. SIGN Guidelines. Guideline 101: British Guideline on the Management of Asthma. Edinburgh: SIGN, 2011.
www.sign.ac.uk/guidelines/fulltext/101/index.htmlCached - Similar (last accessed May 2012).
Scottish Intercollegiate Guidelines Network. SIGN Guidelines. Management of acute severe asthma in adults in hospital, 2008. http://www.sign.ac.uk/pdf/sign101a42008.pdf (last accessed May 2012).

13. E Whole lung lavage

The history, radiological findings and bronchoalveolar lavage (BAL) results are suggestive of pulmonary alveolar proteinosis (PAP). PAP is a rare alveolar defect due to failure of alveolar macrophages to remove surfactant, leading to the accumulation of proteinaceous material within the alveoli. The condition presents between 30 and 50 years age and male smokers are at higher risk. Patients may present with breathlessness and a dry cough and/or with superadded infection, causing acute onset of symptoms in association with fever. Opportunistic infection is the major complication (*Nocardia* species, fungi and mycobacteria) due to the impaired host defence secondary to surfactant accumulation.

Diagnosis is usually made by typical CT appearances – 'crazy paving pattern' of patchy airspace shadowing, with areas of normal lung. The treatment of choice is repeated therapeutic whole lung lavage. This is performed at specialist centres under general anaesthetic using single lung ventilation via a double-lumen endotracheal tube. Repeated warm saline lavage is used to wash the bronchial tree and characteristic milky lavage fluid is obtained. The prognosis with whole lung lavage is generally good.

Atypical infections are common and specific antibiotics should be administered if cultures are positive. There is no role for empirical antituberculous therapy or co-trimoxazole. There is no benefit from treatment with steroids which may increase the risk of opportunistic infections.

Borie R, et al. Pulmonary alveolar proteinosis. Eur Respir Rev 2011; 20(120):98–107.

14. D Lymphangioleiomyomatosis

Lymphangioleiomyomatosis (LAM) is a disorder characterised by the abnormal proliferation of smooth muscle cells throughout the lungs, airways, blood vessels and lymph system. Progressive nodular infiltration of the lymphatics and airways leads to the formation of cysts throughout the lungs. The disease affects women of child-bearing age (and postmenopausal woman taking hormone replacement therapy). It is a rare disorder, affecting 1 in 1.1 million, and is of unknown cause. Of adult women with tuberous sclerosis 40% develop the pulmonary changes seen in LAM.

Clinical features include pneumothorax (often recurrent), dyspnoea, chest pain, cough, haemoptysis, and pulmonary haemorrhage, chylothorax and pleural effusion. Other organs may be affected by the condition. Angiomyolipoma, a benign renal tumour, occurs in 50% of LAM patients and patients should be screened for these lesions with abdominal CT. Within the pelvis, cystic masses (lymphangioleiomyomas) may occur that enlarge during the day, leading to fullness and bloating.

Patients should be referred to a specialist centre for further management. The course and prognosis of LAM are very variable. Hormonal manipulation with progesterone has been tried, but there are no large studies. Oestrogens should be avoided. Patients should be advised to use contraception as pregnancy may accelerate the disease process. Lung transplantation may be necessary; however, LAM can recur in the transplanted lung.

α_1-Antitrypsin deficiency, catamenial pneumothorax (pneumothorax occurring during menstruation probably secondary to thoracic endometriosis), cystic fibrosis and pulmonary Langerhans' cell histiocytosis (rare condition of pulmonary infiltration with histiocytes) may also present or be complicated by recurrent pneumothoraces; however, the CT appearance described is not typical of these conditions (see **Table 10.2**).

Harari S, Torre O, Moss J. Lymphangioleiomyomatosis: what do we know and what are we looking for? Eur Respir Rev 2011; 20(119):34–44.

Table 10.2 Typical CT finding of conditions associated with recurrent pneumothorax

Diagnosis	Typical CT findings/notes
α_1-Antitrypsin deficiency	Bullous emphysema
Catamenial pneumothorax	Often normal CT – diagnosis confirmed by video-assisted thoracoscopic surgery (VATS)
Cystic fibrosis	Bronchiectasis – predominantly in upper zones
Lymphangioleiomyomatosis	Multiple, small (<1 cm), thin-walled cysts
Pulmonary Langerhans' cell histiocytosis	Multiple nodules, thin and thick walled, varying sizes (reflecting different ages of nodules), may cavitate

15. C Intravenous co-amoxiclav and clarithromycin

This patient has the history, signs and investigation findings suggesting severe community-acquired pneumonia (CAP). Patients with severe pneumonia should be treated as soon as possible with intravenous antibiotics, e.g. co-amoxiclav and clarithromycin.

The severity of pneumonia may be graded according to the CURB65 score and the score should be interpreted in conjunction with clinical judgement. One point is scored for each positive finding to provide a score out of 5.

C – confusion [Abbreviated Mental Test (AMT) score <8/10]
U – urea >7.0 mmol/L (normal range 2.5–7.5 mmol/L)
R – respiratory rate >30 breaths per minute (normal range 12–18 breaths per minute)
B – blood pressure <90 mmHg systolic or <60 mmHg diastolic
65 – age >65 years

Patients with a CURB65 score >3 are at higher risk of morbidity and mortality. Patients with CURB65 scores of 4 and 5 should be considered for transfer to the critical care unit. These patients should have early senior review.

Patients with a low CURB65 score (0 or 1) are at low risk and may be treated with oral antibiotics at home if there are no concerning features and the patient has sufficient support in the community.

Oxygen saturations should be monitored and patients should be prescribed and administered appropriate oxygen therapy to maintain an oxygen saturation of 94–98% (unless there is a history or significant risk of hypercapnic respiratory failure). There is no evidence for the routine use of steroids in the management of severe pneumonia.

British Thoracic Society Standards of Care Committee. The British Thoracic Society Guidelines for the management of community acquired pneumonia in adults. Update 2009. Thorax 64 (suppl III).

16. B *Fusobacterium necrophorum*

The history of an infective illness in a previously well young person with pharyngitis, 'angina' (neck pain) and lung cavitation is suggestive of Lemierre's syndrome. This rare illness is caused by the anaerobe *Fusobacterium necrophorum*, an organism that can colonise the oral cavity, but may occasionally lead to bacteraemia. The history described is typical of the condition which, although still rare, appears to be increasing in incidence with recent efforts to reduce inappropriate antibiotic prescribing for pharyngitis-type illnesses, and the organism is not sensitive to erythromycin and other macrolides so the infection is not effectively treated.

The infection can spread to the neck and carotid sheath, leading to thrombosis of the internal jugular vein (suppurative thrombophlebitis). Septic embolisation to the lung may occur with subsequent cavitation and/or abscess formation. Other complications may also include empyema, and abscesses in bones, joints and other organs. Treatment of the condition requires a prolonged course of metronidazole (6 weeks) and a penicillin (or appropriate alternative if penicillin allergic). The role of anticoagulation is controversial.

Cryptococcus neoformans, Pneumocystis jirovecii, Rhodococcus species and fungi are causes of lung cavitation in HIV infection and other immunocompromised patients. Lung cavitation may occur secondary to community-acquired pneumonia and may complicate approximately 16% of *Staphylococcus aureus* pneumonias. *Staphylococcus aureus* is also the most common causative organism of lung abscesses secondary to septic embolisation in right heart endocarditis in intravenous drug abusers. Tuberculosis may cause lung cavitation; however, the typical presentation would be more prolonged than the case described above.

Riordan T. Human infection with *Fusobacterium necrophorum* (necrobacillosis), with a focus on Lemierre's syndrome. Clin Microbiol Rev 2007;20:622–659.

17. A Keep ascent to ≤300 m/day and rest every third day

Minor effects of altitude sickness may be due to hyperventilation provoked by hypoxia at altitude and may include light-headedness, fatigue, peripheral paraesthesia, nausea and anorexia, headaches and sleep disturbance. The major concerns of altitude sickness are high-altitude pulmonary oedema (HAPE) and high-altitude cerebral oedema (HACE). These conditions are caused by hypoxia itself, may develop rapidly and are potentially fatal.

The risk of altitude sickness increases with the rate at which altitude is attained. The risk may be reduced by keeping the ascent to ≤300 m/day and resting every third day. Minor symptoms resolve with rest, analgesia and adequate hydration but descent may be necessary to control the symptoms. Acetazolamide may be useful as prophylaxis and to treat minor symptoms, by provoking a mild metabolic acidosis and allowing greater hyperventilation in response to hypoxia without the usual alkalosis. It is recommended when rapid ascent is unavoidable.

Such a trip should be planned and expert medical advice may be needed, but many patients who suffer from mild asthma in childhood are not affected later in adult life and so this should not be an absolute contraindication to the trip.

Nifedipine may be used in the treatment of HAPE to reduce pulmonary artery pressure although its use for prophylaxis is controversial. Dexamethasone is used in the management of HACE to reduce cerebral oedema.

Imray C, et al. Acute altitude illnesses. BMJ 2011; 343:d4943.

18. C MacLeod's syndrome

MacLeod's syndrome is due to parenchymal and vascular maldevelopment, following childhood bronchitis or bronchiolitis. The condition is usually asymptomatic and may be diagnosed on routine chest X-rays, which may demonstrate a hyperlucent lung, with reduced vascular markings and a small pulmonary artery.

α_1-Antitrypsin deficiency is an autosomal recessive condition associated with early onset emphysema. Emphysematous change is accelerated in smokers and causes bilateral disease.

Congenital lobar emphysema is a congenital abnormality that causes the overinflation of a lobe due to localised bronchomalacia or bronchial obstruction. It may cause wheeze and/or chest wall deformity. The condition may resolve spontaneously during development through childhood.

In cases of pneumothorax there would be absent rather than reduced pulmonary markings if complete or a visible lung edge in partial collapse; there is more likely to be a typical history of either trauma or sudden-onset pleuritic pain and shortness of breath.

Pulmonary sequestration is a congenital abnormality resulting from a segment of lung without a bronchial connection and therefore reduced ventilation. The segment of lung may be supplied by an aberrant artery. Most are left sided (most common in left lower lobe). This condition is often associated with other congenital abnormalities, but may be detected on routine chest X-rays. Surgical resection may be necessary if there is repeated infection.

19. E Restart regular inhaler corticosteroid and long-acting β_2-agonist

The presentation suggests a mild exacerbation of asthma which may be as a result of a viral illness and is probably exacerbated by stopping the regular prescribed medications. The patient is well and lives with her husband and so may be safely discharged home with advice.

Pregnancy can affect asthma and asthma can affect the outcome of pregnancy. Generally, a third will improve during pregnancy, a third will notice no change in their symptoms and a third will deteriorate. The course of asthma is likely to be similar in successive pregnancies.

Pregnant women with asthma should be counselled to continue their normal asthma medications and should be monitored closely throughout pregnancy and provided with a written asthma management plan. Smoking cessation advice should be given if indicated.

The risk to the fetus of uncontrolled asthma outweighs any small risk of asthma medication and steroid should be continued. With this history provided above there is no clear indication for admission for nebuliser or for oral antibiotics or steroids. Relaxation techniques may be of use but only in addition to the recommended medication.

There are limited data for the safety of leukotriene receptor antagonists, e.g. montelukast, and manufacturers recommend that these drugs are not commenced in pregnancy but should be continued if this is already an established medication as the risk of deterioration of symptoms outweighs the potential for side effects.

Scottish Intercollegiate Guidelines Network (SIGN). Guideline 101: British Guideline on the Management of Asthma. Edinburgh: SIGN, 2011.
www.sign.ac.uk/guidelines/fulltext/101/index.htmlCached – Similar (last accessed May 2012).

20. A Arterial embolisation

Massive haemoptysis (>500 mL in 24 hours) is a life-threatening emergency, with a mortality of up to 80%. Priorities need to include: airway protection and ventilation, cardiovascular support with large-bore ± central access, fluid resuscitation with blood and clotting factors ± inotropes. Tranexamic acid may be useful. Cross-sectional imaging if the patient is stable and early bronchoscopy are indicated. The management of choice, if available locally, is interventional radiology and arterial embolisation. Surgical resection may be necessary if other measures fail. In some cases, active treatment may be inappropriate and palliative treatment with oxygen and opiates may be necessary.

The history suggests that an aspergilloma may be the cause of the haemoptysis. An aspergilloma is a ball of fungal hyphae occurring within a cavity in the lung. Aspergillomas are often asymptomatic; however, up to 75% will present with haemoptysis. Superadded infections may provoke exacerbations. Sometimes there are systemic symptoms such as malaise and fever, and treatment with itraconazole may be considered. Itraconazole will not eradicate the fungus, but may reduce the cavity size and reduce the chance of haemoptysis.

Lordan J L, Gascoigne A, Corris PA. The pulmonary physician in critical care. Illustrative case 7: Assessment and management of massive haemoptysis. Thorax 2003; 58:814–819.

21. E She should commence dietary supplements

Women with cystic fibrosis (CF) are often subfertile; however, some patients may conceive naturally and if possible pregnancy should be planned to optimise the mother's physical and nutritional status. The outcome of a pregnancy is improved by optimising and maintaining pulmonary function and weight gain throughout the pregnancy. She has a body mass index (BMI) of 17 and should be advised to optimise her nutritional status before becoming pregnant. It is likely that dietary supplementation will be necessary. Close monitoring with regular dietician, chest physiotherapy and support from the other members of the multi-disciplinary CF team is essential throughout pregnancy. Pregnancy does not affect survival when compared with the entire female CF population, but impaired pulmonary function with forced expiratory volume$_1$ <60% predicted is the main predictor of worse maternal and fetal outcome.

Most antibiotics used to treat pulmonary exacerbations of CF are safe in pregnancy; however, ciprofloxacin, chloramphenicol, metronidazole and intravenous colimycin should be avoided. Aminoglycosides should be used with caution and close level monitoring carried out as there is a risk of fetal ototoxicity.

Genetic counselling and screening should be offered to CF patients and their partners. CF is an autosomal recessive disorder. The *CFTR* gene is located on the long arm of chromosome 7. Carrier frequency in the white population is 1:25. ΔF508 is the most common mutation. More than 1000 different mutations of the *CFTR* gene are recognised and the 30 commonest abnormalities (>99.5% of the abnormalities) are screened for by a screening blood test, so if the partner is not a carrier of these mutations, there is a minimal chance that the child will have CF; however, the child will be a carrier of the CF gene.

McArdle JR. Pregnancy in cystic fibrosis. Clin Chest Med 2011; 32(1):111–120.
Davies J, et al. Clinical review. Cystic fibrosis. BMJ 2007; 335:1255–1259.

22. C Dietary and lifestyle advice

This middle-aged man has a history suggestive of sleep-disordered breathing. He is obese (body mass index 35 kg/m^2) and has hypertension and diabetes. Obesity, especially upper body obesity (and collar size >43 cm [17"]), is a risk factor for obstructive sleep apnoea (OSA). OSA is part of a spectrum, ranging from snoring at one end and complete obstruction of the upper airway with frequent nocturnal awakenings at the other, with significant sleep fragmentation and excessive daytime somnolence. The combination of OSA identified by a sleep study together with symptoms of excessive daytime somnolence leads to the diagnosis of obstructive sleep apnoea syndrome. OSA is increasingly recognised as a risk factor for hypertension, cardiovascular and cerebrovascular disease, and complications of the metabolic syndrome, and is a major contributing factor to a large proportion of road traffic accidents.

It is important to differentiate sleepiness – tendency to fall asleep due to inadequate sleep from tiredness – feelings of exhaustion that may be multifactorial but not associated with a tendency to fall asleep. The severity of sleepiness may be assessed using the Epworth Sleepiness Score (ESS). This is scored out of 24; 0–9 is considered normal and >9 excessively sleepy.

Sleep studies are performed to confirm the diagnosis. These studies may vary from simple overnight oximetry, to oximetry with some other modalities of monitoring, e.g. chest and abdominal wall movements and oronasal flow (limited sleep study), to full polysomnography with EEG, electro-oculography (EOG) and electromyography (EMG), to stage sleep physiology. This will depend on local availability and protocols.

The sleep study is used to determine the severity of OSA; however, the values may vary according to each sleep centre. Expertise is needed to grade the sleep studies according to the apnoea–hypopnoea index (AHI), i.e. the number of events per hour.

As a guide:
  AHI <5 = normal
  AHI 5–15 = evidence of mild OSA – does not normally require treatment, advise conservative measures if symptomatic
  AHI 10–15 = mild OSA may require CPAP if very symptomatic
  AHI 15–30 = moderate OSA – advise trial of CPAP
  AHI > 30 = severe OSA – advise referral for urgent CPAP
  (CPAP = continuous positive airway pressure)

Not all patients need treatment. The evidence for significant treatment benefit rests on symptoms, which drive treatment, rather than the degree of OSA on a sleep study.

This patient is not excessively sleepy – ESS <9 and the sleep study demonstrates an AHI of 11.4, i.e. mild OSA. Conservative approaches such as weight loss, reduction in alcohol consumption, smoking cessation and trying to sleep in the decubitus rather than the supine position should be recommended.

Mandibular advancement devices may be of benefit to snorers with mild OSA, assuming adequate dentition. Severe OSA with evidence of CO_2 retention may require non-invasive ventilation. Bariatric surgery may be needed for significant weight loss in morbidly obese patients.

Johns MW. A new method for measuring daytime sleepiness: The Epworth Sleepiness Scale. Sleep 1991; 14:540–545.
Scottish Intercollegiate Guidelines Network. SIGN Guideline No. 73: Management of obstructive sleep apnoea/ hypopnoea syndrome in adults. Edinburgh: SIGN, 2003.

23. B Malignancy

Initial pleural fluid analysis should include the assessment of:
- Pleural fluid appearance
- Biochemistry (protein and lactate dehydrogenase)
- Cytology (for malignant cells and differential cell count)
- Microbiology (Gram stain and microscopy, culture, acid-fast bacilli (AFB) and tuberculosis (TB) culture)
- pH.

Determining whether an effusion is a transudate or an exudate is helpful to narrow the differential diagnosis. The pleural effusion described is an exudate. In patients with a normal serum protein, pleural fluid protein <30 g/L = transudate and protein >30 g/L = exudates. Additional pleural fluid investigations include cholesterol, triglycerides, haematocrit, glucose and amylase in certain clinical circumstances.

Common causes of exudative effusions include: empyema, TB and other infections, oesophageal rupture, pancreatitis, other connective tissue diseases and autoimmune conditions, and post-cardiac injury (Dressler's syndrome). An exudative effusion in a patient in this age group is most likely to be malignant. The sensitivity for pleural fluid cytology is about 60%. In a young patient; parapneumonic effusion is a more likely cause.

Table 10.3 Common causes of exudative effusions	
Parapneumonic effusion	May complicate 40% of bacterial pneumonias – most common cause of exudates in young patients
Malignancy	Most common exudative effusion in patients >60 years
Mesothelioma	Pleural fluid cytology – low sensitivity
Pulmonary embolism	Haemorrhagic effusion
Rheumatoid arthritis	Low glucose in pleural fluid (often <1.6 mmol/L)

Pleural effusions are common after coronary artery bypass grafting or post-cardiac injury syndrome (Dressler's syndrome), and typically occur as small, left-sided effusions with most resolving spontaneously. It would be unusual for this effusion to recur after 1 year and an alternative diagnosis should be sought.

Meigs' syndrome is a unilateral (often right sided) or bilateral benign transudative pleural effusion which may occur in women with ascites and ovarian tumours.

Pulmonary changes, including pleural effusions, may be the first manifestation of rheumatoid arthritis; however, rheumatoid pleurisy is more common in men (70% male). The pleural fluid glucose is typically low (<1.6 mmol/L) and pH is typically reduced (<7.3). These effusions can persist for months to years, although duration may be several weeks.

Pleural Disease Guidelines 2010. British Thoracic Society Pleural Disease Guideline 2010. Thorax 2010; 65(2). Light RW. Pleural effusion. N Engl J Med 2002; 346:1971–1977.

24. C Desquamative interstitial pneumonia

Desquamative interstitial pneumonia (DIP) is rare and the majority of patients are smokers, although it may occur with passive smoking. It typically occurs in patients aged 30–50 and presents with gradual inset of breathlessness and cough over weeks to months. Finger clubbing is common. High-resolution CT (HRCT) of the thorax may show ground-glass opacities in the lower zones and peripheries, with mild reticulation and honey-combing. Bronchoalveolar lavage may reveal an increase in pigmented macrophages; however, surgical biopsy is necessary for diagnosis. Smoking cessation is essential and corticosteroids are often used; however, their efficacy has not been studied. With smoking cessation, the prognosis is usually good.

Acute interstitial pneumonitis is a rapidly progressive (over days) form of interstitial lung disease (ILD) characterised by diffuse alveolar damage – formerly known as Hamman–Rich syndrome. The mean age of onset is 50 years. It is often preceded by 'viral'-type illness. It rapidly leads to respiratory failure requiring ventilator support; immunosuppressive therapy should be considered. The overall mortality rate is at least 50%.

Cryptogenic organising pneumonia (COP) is a disease of unknown cause characterised by 'plugging' of alveolar spaces with granulation tissue which may extend into the bronchioles. It is more common in non-smokers, with a mean age of onset of 55. There is typically a short (<3 months) history of breathlessness and cough, with malaise, fever and weight loss. Chest X-ray and HRCT demonstrate patchy areas of consolidation with air bronchograms which may migrate – 'flitting changes'. Transbronchial biopsy may often confirm the diagnosis. The management is with steroids and the prognosis is generally good.

Respiratory bronchiolitis-associated interstitial lung disease (RB-ILD) may present similarly to DIP; however, HRCT may demonstrate centrilobular nodules, ground-glass changes, thick wall airways and centrilobular emphysema. Surgical biopsy is necessary for diagnosis which will demonstrate accumulation of brown pigmented macrophages. Prognosis is good with smoking cessation.

Usual interstitial pneumonitis (UIP) is an ILD of unknown cause. It typically presents in older patients, mean age 67 years; its prevalence increases with age. HRCT typically demonstrates subpleural reticulation, with minimal ground-glass changes and progressive fibrotic change with honey-combing.

Wells AU. Interstitial Lung Interstitial lung disease guideline: the British Thoracic Society in collaboration with the Irish Thoracic Society, Thoracic Society of Australia and New Zealand. Thorax 2008; 63:v1–v58.

25. E Self-limiting viral illness

This patient presents with an acute cough (<3 weeks' duration). This is the most common presentation to general practice. An acute cough is usually self-limiting and as a result of a viral illness. Ninety-three per cent of patients with flu-like illnesses may experience cough symptoms. Pneumonia and/or the inhalation of a foreign body may also cause an acute cough but there are no features to point to these diagnoses in the scenario described.

A cough lasting more than 8 weeks is defined as chronic and may be reported by 10–20% of adults and is more common in obese females. A careful history alone may identify the cause of the cough; however, a chest X-ray should be performed in all adults presenting with chronic cough. Common causes of cough with a normal chest X-ray include: smoking, gastro-oesophageal reflux, asthma, allergic rhinitis and angiotensin-converting enzyme inhibitor use.

Morice A H, McGarvey L, Pavord I. Recommendations for the management of cough in adults, on behalf of the British Thoracic Society Cough Guideline Group. Thorax 2006; 61(I):i1–i24.

26. E Parapneumonic effusion

This young man presented with the typical history and clinical features of community-acquired pneumonia (CAP) and was previously well with no past medical history of note. This patient was considered to have a low risk of mortality–CURB65 score 1/5 (respiratory rate >30 breaths per minute); however, the clinical decision was made to commence intravenous antibiotics. Some patients with CURB65 0–1 may be considered for oral antibiotics and discharged home. Patients who are initially prescribed intravenous antibiotics should be reviewed early and switched to oral antibiotics if appropriate, as indicated by clinical improvement in terms of resolution of fever for >24 hours. If patients fail to improve, then they should be reviewed and it may be necessary to seek further senior advice, review the history and examination, and/or repeat the chest X-ray, inflammatory markers and review microbiology results if available. Parapneumonic effusion may complicate 40% of cases of CAP and early thoracocentesis is recommended. Rarer complications of CAP may include lung abscess (which typically occurs later in the clinical course) or development of adult respiratory distress syndrome (may be associated with severe sepsis). An underlying lung pathology is less likely in a young, previously fit patient; however, patients with CAP should have a follow-up chest X-ray at 6 weeks to ensure that the consolidation has resolved.

British Thoracic Society Standards of Care Committee. The British Thoracic Society Guidelines for the management of community acquired pneumonia in adults. Thorax 2009; 64(III).

27. C Inform the DVLA and stop driving until he has received adequate treatment

The oximetry demonstrates repeated episodes of desaturation suggestive of sleep-disordered breathing/obstructive sleep apnoea (OSA) and the patient is subjectively very sleepy – a diagnosis of obstructive sleep apnoea/hypopnoea syndrome (OSAHS). He should be told that he must stop driving and inform the DVLA of his diagnosis. He should be referred for urgent CPAP (continuous positive airway pressure) and will need appropriate follow-up to ensure that his overnight desaturation has improved and his symptoms of excessive daytime somnolence have resolved on therapy. The DVLA medical advisors will review his case and advise when he may return to driving. As he is a heavy-goods vehicle driver specialist consideration and close follow-up will be required. However, if he has been successfully treated and demonstrated good compliance with treatment, he may be able to resume his work.

All patients with sleep-disordered breathing problems will benefit from lifestyle and dietary advice (if overweight/obese); however, as this patient has evidence of severe OSAHS he will need treatment with CPAP.

Modafinil is a central nervous system-stimulating drug that may be used to treat narcolepsy. It was previously used to treat patients with OSA who were still symptomatic despite CPAP therapy;

however, the licence for this application of the drug has been withdrawn due to concerns of addiction to the medication.

Johns MW. A new method for measuring daytime sleepiness: The Epworth Sleepiness Scale. Sleep 1991; 14:540–545.

Scottish Intercollegiate Guidelines Network. SIGN Guideline No. 73: Management of obstructive sleep apnoea/ hypopnoea syndrome in adults. Edinburgh: SIGN, 2003.

28. E Pulmonary arterial hypertension

Primary pulmonary arterial hypertension (PPH), as defined by resting mean pulmonary artery pressure >25 mmHg, in the absence of significant underlying respiratory, cardiac or connective tissue disease, may be either familial or sporadic. The chest X-ray may demonstrate enlargement of central pulmonary arteries, with 'pruning' of peripheral vessels.

Sporadic cases of PPH may be associated with certain drug exposures (including fenfluramine, cocaine and amphetamines), human immunodeficiency virus (HIV), human herpesvirus (HHV)-8 or portal hypertension.

HIV-related pulmonary arterial hypertension (HIV-PAH) is a rare complication of the disease of uncertain cause. Other causes of PPH should be excluded. HIV patients are at increased risk of thromboembolic disease. The chest X-ray may demonstrate asymmetrical pulmonary vascular markings, but an CT pulmonary angiogram is the gold standard for diagnosis. An atrial septal defect may give subtle clinical features of a fixed split second heart sound. *Pneumocystis jiroveci* pneumonia is an opportunistic infection with insidious onset of dyspnoea and dry cough, with perihilar shadowing progressing to diffuse interstitial infiltration on the chest X-ray associated with significant desaturation on exercise.

Cicalini S, Chinello P, Petrosillo N. HIV infection and pulmonary arterial hypertension. Expert Rev Respir Med 2011; 5(2):257–266.

29. E 90% chance of resolution of disease within 2 years

The chest X-ray demonstrates bilateral hilar lymphadenopathy (BHL). The history of fevers, arthralgia and erythema nodosum together with the chest X-ray finding of BHL in a white person is most likely to be due to a diagnosis of Löfgren's syndrome (acute sarcoidosis). Löfgren's syndrome typically occurs as a mild acute disease, which is usually non-progressive. It is common in Irish, Scandinavian and African women. The diagnosis may be found by taking a detailed clinical history alone; however it is important to exclude other causes of BHL (see **Table 10.4**). High-resolution CT of the chest and lymph node aspiration and/or biopsy may be needed. Histology will demonstrate non-caseating granulomas.

Table 10.4 Differential diagnosis of bilateral hilar lymphadenopathy on chest X-ray
Sarcoidosis
Tuberculosis
Lymphoma
Coccidioidomycosis and histoplasmosis
Berylliosis
Hypogammaglobulinaemia and recurrent infections

It is important to assess the extent and severity of the disease and to look for extrapulmonary involvement. Baseline biochemistry (urea and electrolytes, liver function tests and bone profile), full blood count and serum angiotensin-converting enzyme should be measured in all patients, and patients should have pulmonary function testing and an ECG.

Löfgren's syndrome has a good prognosis and 90% experience complete disease resolution within 2 years. Löfgren's syndrome does not need any specific treatment; however, conservative approaches such as simple analgesia/non-steroidal anti-inflammatory drugs and rest may be needed for some patients. The average time for BHL to resolve is 8 months. Fifteen per cent of patients will suffer progressive lung infiltration.

Neurological involvement occurs in up to 20% of patients and can affect any part of the central or peripheral nervous system. Most common is facial nerve lower motor neuron involvement; mononeuritis multiplex is also recognised and some patients may present with less specific features and psychiatric illness. Renal involvement may occur in one-third of patients; however, progression to renal failure is rare. Hypercalcaemia may be a feature due to conversion of vitamin D_3 to active 1,25-dihydroxycholecalciferol in the granulomas and is more common in summer months.

Costabel U, Ohshimo S, Guzman J. Diagnosis of sarcoidosis. Curr Opin Pulm Med 2008; 14(5):455–461.

30. C Ipratropium bromide by oxygen-driven nebuliser

This patient has features of acute severe asthma [peak expiratory flow (PEF) 33–50% of predicted and pulse ≥110 beats per minute]. The immediate management should include oxygen therapy if necessary to maintain oxygen saturation at 94–98%, bronchodilators via oxygen-driven nebuliser (either salbutamol 5 mg or terbutaline 10 mg and ipratropium bromide 0.5 mg) and prednisolone 40–50 mg orally or intravenous hydrocortisone 100 mg if the patient is too dyspnoeic to swallow.

This patient had oxygen saturation of 95% breathing air, therefore supplemental oxygen therapy is not required, but continuous monitoring with pulse oximetry should be performed to detect deterioration and oxygen commenced if necessary.

An infective exacerbation of asthma is most likely to be viral in aetiology and routine prescription of antibiotics should be avoided unless clinically indicated. Intravenous aminophylline is unlikely to convey additional benefit over conventional initial therapy with nebulised bronchodilators and steroids. Side effects of aminophylline include arrhythmia which may further complicate the clinical picture. Current evidence does not support use of leukotriene receptor antagonists, e.g. montelukast in acute asthma. However, these medications may be a useful adjunct in the management of chronic asthma. Routine administration of Heliox to manage acute asthma is not supported in the current medical literature.

Scottish Intercollegiate Guidelines Network. British Guideline on the Management of Asthma. A national clinical guideline. Edinburgh: SIGN, 2012 http://www.sign.ac.uk/pdf/sign101a42008.pdf (last accessed May 2012).

31. E Usual interstitial pneumonitis

Usual interstitial pneumonitis (UIP) may be diagnosed with typical clinical findings and on high-resolution CT (HRCT) which demonstrates the typical features of bilateral, peripheral and subpleural reticulation with honey-combing, traction bronchiectasis and minimal or no ground-glass opacification. Lung biopsy is not normally required for diagnosis unless there are atypical features.

The cause of UIP is unknown. The mean age at presentation is 67 years. Patients typically present with progressive dyspnoea and cough with an average of 9 months' history prior to presentation. Examination will reveal fine late inspiratory ('Velcro') crackles, finger clubbing in 50%, and signs of cyanosis or cor pulmonale in severe disease. Pulmonary function tests will demonstrate a restrictive lung defect with reduced gas transfer and arterial blood gases may demonstrate type I respiratory failure.

Bronchiectasis should be suspected in cases of chronic cough with sputum production – typically purulent and daily. HRCT will confirm the diagnosis with airway dilatation and thickening and mucus plugging.

Congestive cardiac failure should be excluded by performing echocardiography and serum BNP (brain natriuretic peptide). HRCT may demonstrate bilateral pleural effusion and dependent changes of interstitial oedema.

ACE inhibitors (ACEIs) are a common cause of chronic dry cough (side effect noted in up to 10% of women taking ACEIs), because of accumulation of bradykinin in the lung. Interstitial pneumonitis and pulmonary infiltration with eosinophilia are extremely rare complications of ACEIs. The patient may benefit from switching the ACEI to an angiotension II receptor blocker.

Desquamative interstitial pneumonia (DIP) is a very rare condition that occurs in smokers, typically aged 30–50 years. The HRCT demonstrates ground-glass opacification (present in all cases); reticulation and honey-combing may also occur.

Wells AU, et al. Interstitial Lung Interstitial lung disease guideline: the British Thoracic Society in collaboration with the Irish Thoracic Society, Thoracic Society of Australia and New Zealand. Thorax 2008; 63; v1–v58.

32. D Pulmonary arteriovenous malformation

Patients with pulmonary arteriovenous malformations (PAVMs) often present with an abnormal chest X-ray, typically demonstrating a smooth, rounded, intrapulmonary mass with draining or feeding vessels. Symptoms may include dyspnoea, haemoptysis and atypical chest pain. PAVMs may present with acute stroke or cerebral abscesses; 50% of patients are asymptomatic. Clinical examination may reveal mild hypoxia (because of right-to-left shunt), orthodeoxia hypoxia on standing due to increase in blood flow to dependent lung areas (70% of PAVMs are basal), finger clubbing and bruits audible to auscultation. Eighty per cent of PAVMs occur in patients with hereditary haemorrhagic telangiectasia and patients and their families should be screened for PAVMs because of the associated potential for neurological sequelae. Patients with PAVMs should be referred to a specialist centre for further assessment and consideration of embolisation to prevent shunting, hypoxia and risk of embolic stroke.

Asbestos-related pleural plaques typically occur as calcified areas of pleural thickening or a characteristic 'holly-leaf' appearance and are asymptomatic. Lung abscesses present with symptoms of productive cough, fevers and a cavitating lesion on chest X-ray.

A patient may be at risk of developing a lung abscess following a stroke if it is complicated by dysphagia and aspiration pneumonia; however, this patient does not have symptoms suggesting an infective aetiology. Old tuberculosis may be found incidentally on a chest X-ray which may demonstrate a calcified granuloma (Ghon focus), typically in the upper zone.

Patients may be at increased risk of developing pulmonary emboli (PEs) following a period of reduced mobility and would be associated with sudden-onset pleuritic chest pain and hypoxia. Often the chest X-ray appearance will be normal or may demonstrate a small unilateral effusion. Pulmonary infarction secondary to PE may lead to a wedge-shaped opacity on a chest X-ray; a rounded opacity would not be a typical feature of PEs.

Hsu CC, et al. Embolisation therapy for pulmonary arteriovenous malformations. Cochrane Database Syst Rev 2010; (5):CD008017.

33. E Tropical pulmonary eosinophilia

Tropical pulmonary eosinophilia is caused by hypersensitivity to the migrating larvae of filarial worms, *Wucheria bancrofti* and *Brugia malayi*. It occurs in the Indian subcontinent, south-east Asia and South Pacific islands. It presents with gradual-onset (weeks to months) cough, wheeze, sputum, dyspnoea, chest pain and fever, weight loss and fatigue. Chest X-ray typically demonstrates diffuse patchy shadowing. Blood tests demonstrate significant eosinophilia and raised IgE, and filarial complement is positive. Sputum and bronchoalveolar lavage contain eosinophils.

Löffler's syndrome (simple pulmonary eosinophilia) is caused by parasitic infection, usually *Ascaris lumbricoides*, but also *Strongyloides* and *Ankylostoma* species. The passage of larvae through the lung causes an allergic reaction and may be asymptomatic or present with cough, malaise, anorexia, low-grade fevers and night sweats. The illness typically last for around 2 weeks. Chest X-ray may show transient bilateral perihilar shadowing and there is low-level blood eosinophilia.

Miliary tuberculosis (TB) is is a more common presentation of disseminated TB in immunocompromised individuals. Chest X-ray demonstrates a typical 'miliary' or 'millet-seed' pattern of diffuse nodularity. Full blood count may demonstrate lymphopenia – eosinophilia would not be a typical feature.

Pneumocystis jirovecii pneumonia is an opportunistic infection in immunocompromised individuals. Patients present with progressive dyspnoea and dry cough. Hypoxia and desaturation on exertion are common features. Chest X-ray demonstrates bilateral perihilar infiltrates that progress to alveolar shadowing. Full blood count is often normal.

Churg–Strauss syndrome is characterised by asthma, blood eosinophilia and eosinophilic granulomatous inflammation of the respiratory tract. It is often associated with sinusitis and other systemic features including vasculitic neuropathy and skin involvement.

Campos LE, Pereira LF. Pulmonary eosinophilia. J Bras Pneumol 2009; 35(6):561–573.

34. E Refer to cardiothoracic surgeons

This patient has a history of chronic lung disease and presented with a large pneumothorax – secondary spontaneous pneumothorax (SSP). Patients presenting with SSP should be admitted for further management. Supplemental oxygen should be administered in accordance with the British Thoracic Society guidelines for the use of oxygen in adults. Most patients presenting with SSP will require a small-bore chest drain attached to an underwater seal and early opinion from a respiratory physician should be sought to guide further management. Suction should not be used routinely, but high-volume, low-pressure suction may be recommended in some circumstances to aid re-expansion of the collapsed lung. Ongoing bubbling or failure of re-expansion may suggest persistent air leak and these cases should be discussed with a thoracic surgeon at 48 hours. The thoracic surgeon may employ one of the following techniques:
- Open thoracotomy and pleurectomy
- Video-assisted thoracoscopic surgery (VATS) with pleurectomy and/or pleural abrasion
- Surgical chemical pleurodesis with talc

Patients with persistent SSP who are unfit for general anaesthesia and/or surgical intervention may be considered for talc pleurodesis via the chest tube or for domiciliary management with a Heimlich valve, which is a one-way valve that prevents air from travelling back up a chest drain. There is no strong evidence that large-bore chest tubes will offer benefit over small-bore tubes.

The chest drain is still bubbling profusely, therefore flushing is not indicated and potentially risks introducing infection. A bubbling chest drain should never be clamped as it may lead to tension!

British Thoracic Society. Pleural Disease guidelines 2010. Thorax 2010; 65(2).

35. B Admit to respiratory isolation room and send sputum samples for acid-fast bacilli and TB (tuberculosis) culture

The clinical history, risk factors (homelessness and alcohol abuse) and chest X-ray demonstrating significant consolidation with loss of volume in the right upper lobe are strongly suggestive of pulmonary TB. People with TB (pulmonary or non-pulmonary) should not be admitted to hospital for diagnostic tests or for care unless there is a clear clinical or socioeconomic need, such as homelessness. If hospital admission is necessary, patients should be managed in respiratory isolation and separated from immunocompromised patients. If the clinical signs and symptoms are strongly suggestive of TB, three early morning sputum samples for acid-fast bacilli and culture should be sent and treatment should be initiated early – this may be before culture results are available. The four-drug initiation regimen is recommended (rifampicin, isoniazid, pyrazinamide and ethambutol) for 2 months and the regimen may be reduced to rifampicin and isoniazid for a further 4 months if the cultures demonstrate a fully sensitive organism. Directly observed therapy may be particularly useful to compliance in certain at-risk groups, including homeless people with active TB.

This patient is not overtly septic so it may be possible to wait for sputum acid-fast bacilli smear results and seek specialist respiratory opinion regarding commencing antituberculous therapy, rather than commencing empirical antibiotics for community-acquired pneumonia. A CT scan and bronchoscopy may not be necessary if the diagnosis is confirmed on sputum results – sputum induction with nebuliser saline and physiotherapy may increase the diagnostic rate.

National Institute for Health and Clinical Excellence. NICE Guidelines No. 117: Tuberculosis. Clinical diagnosis and management of tuberculosis, and measures for its prevention and control. London: NICE, 2011.

36. D Omeprazole

Chronic cough (cough lasting longer than 8 weeks) is more likely to occur in middle-aged women. Gastro-oesophageal disorders, including reflux (GORD) and oesophageal dysmotility, may be the cause in up to 40% of cases of chronic cough and may occur in the absence of heartburn or typical reflux symptoms. Proton pump inhibitors (e.g. omeprazole 20 mg twice daily for at least 8 weeks) may help in 75–100% of cases and an empirical trial of treatment should be considered as first-line therapy. Prokinetic agents such as metoclopramide or erythromycin may help some patients. All patients should be advised regarding conservative measures to reduce GORD including: weight loss; reducing caffeine and alcohol intake; taking main meal at lunch time; and elevating head of bed by 5 cm.

Some patients with resistant symptoms may require referral for specialist review and investigation including oesophageal ambulatory 24-hour pH measurement and/or oesophageal manometry, barium meal and gastric emptying studies. Selected patients may benefit from fundoplication.

Angiotensin-converting enzyme inhibitors cause cough in about 10% of patients (women > men) – these medications should be stopped. The cough may take up to 40 weeks to resolve.

The patient has a mild restrictive lung defect (probably related to body habitus) with normal gas transfer and normal chest X-ray. There are no features in the history to suggest an interstitial or suppurative pathology – referral for a high-resolution CT scan of the thorax would not be the first appropriate investigation. Similarly, there are no features to suggest asthma/atopic disease and prednisolone may exacerbate reflux symptoms.

Morice AH, McGarvey L, Pavord I. Recommendations for the management of cough in adults, on behalf of the British Thoracic Society Cough Guideline Group. Thorax 2006; 61(I):i1–i24.

37. A Ceftazidime and tobramycin

Pulmonary disease is the leading cause of morbidity and mortality in patients with cystic fibrosis (CF). Successful treatment of pulmonary exacerbations requires a number of coordinated approaches, including appropriate antibiotics, chest physiotherapy and inhaled medications to aid sputum clearance, plus optimisation of nutritional status and other co-morbidities. Patients with CF are particularly susceptible to *Pseudomonas aeruginosa*. The prevalence of *P. aeruginosa* increases with age and more than 70% of adult CF patients are chronically colonised.

Oral antibiotics may be appropriate for mild exacerbations (using, e.g., oral ciprofloxacin), but intravenous antibiotics are needed for the management of severe exacerbations, if there is known bacterial resistance to oral medications and/or if the patient has failed to improve after a course of oral antibiotic therapy. Generally, pulmonary exacerbations in patients with *P. aeruginosa* are managed with two agents to reduce the risk of emergence of further bacterial resistance. A typical regimen may include tobramycin plus a penicillin with antipseudomonal properties (e.g. pieracillin–tazobactam), a third-generation cephalosporin (e.g. ceftazidime) or a cabapenem (e.g. meropenem).

Oral amoxicillin and clarithromycin are the antibiotics of choice to treat community-acquired pneumonia in the general adult population. Cystic fibrosis patients are susceptible to different bacterial pathogens, as discussed above, and therefore antibiotic therapy to treat infective exacerbations should be tailored to the known sputum culture results and sensitivities.

Flume PA, Mogayzel PJ, Robinson KA, et al. Cystic fibrosis pulmonary guidelines: Treatment of pulmonary exacerbations. Am J Respir Crit Care Med 2009; 180:802–808.
Davies J, et al. Clinical review. Cystic fibrosis. BMJ 2007; 335:1255–1259.

38. D *Streptococcus milleri*

The clinical history and pleural aspirate are strongly suggestive of empyema. Immunocompromised patients, including people with diabetes, those who abuse drugs and alcohol, and patients with recurrent aspiration are at increased risk of developing empyema.

A pleural tap should be performed if empyema is suspected and may demonstrate turbid fluid or frank pus, pleural fluid pH <7.2 and/or positive Gram stain on bacterial culture. All of these features are indicators for the insertion of a chest drain. Forty per cent of pleural infections are culture negative. Bacterial causes of empyemas are shown in **Table 10.5**.

British Thoracic Society. Pleural Disease Guidelines 2010. Thorax 2010; 65(2).

Table 10.5 Bacterial causes of empyema

Community-acquired infection (% of cases)		Hospital-acquired infection (% of cases)	
Streptococcus milleri	28%	Meticillin-resistant S. aureus	27%
Anaerobes	19%	Staphylococcus aureus	22%
Streptococcus pneumoniae	14%	Enterobacteria	20%
Staphylococcus aureus	12%	Enterococci	12%
Other organisms: enterobacteria, Haemophila influenzae, Pseudomonas species, TB, Nocardia species		Other organisms: Streptococcus species, Pseudomonas species, anaerobes	

39. B Cystic fibrosis

Patients with cystic fibrosis (CF) are usually diagnosed as neonates or in childhood; however, some patients may be diagnosed in adulthood and these patients usually have milder phenotypes. Some patients may be detected following screening for male infertility. Male CF patients may be infertile due to failure of the normal development or blockage of the vas deferens, seminal vesicle, ejaculatory duct or epididymis; however, in some patients fertility may be preserved.

Primary ciliary dyskinesia (PCD) is a rare genetic disorder causing chronic respiratory disease because of abnormal cilia and reduced mucociliary clearance, microbiological colonisation and chronic infection, and the development of bronchiectasis. PCD is also associated with infertility in men because of functional abnormalities of the ductus epididymis and reduced sperm motility because the sperm tails have the same morphological defect as the cilia and do not beat correctly.

Bronchiectasis has a number of other causes including genetic (two examples described above), postinfective (tuberculosis or pertussis) and postobstructive (e.g. distal to an inhaled foreign body). Many of these conditions are not associated with infertility.

Pulmonary fibrosis would be an unusual diagnosis in a patient of this age group with a long history of recurrent infections. Tuberculosis should be considered in patients from high-risk groups presenting with a chronic productive cough; however, this would not lead to the history as outlined above.

Davies J, et al. Clinical review. Cystic fibrosis. BMJ 2007; 335:1255–1259.

40. D Pseudochylothorax

A cloudy, milky effusion is suggestive of chylothorax or pseudochylothorax. If the milky fluid is passed through a centrifuge or left to rest on the laboratory bench for 1 hour and fails to clear, it is suggestive of a pseudochylothorax. This may be confirmed on further testing with the identification of rhomboid-shaped crystals of cholesterol and the presence of raised total cholesterol, but normal triglyceride, levels. Causes of a pseudochylothorax include chronic pleural inflammation relating to persistent tuberculous effusion or rheumatoid pleuritis.

Chylothorax may occur following disruption of the thoracic duct, and pleural fluid may appear turbid, milky, serous or blood stained. The presence of pleural fluid chylomicrons or pleural fluid triglyceride level >110 mg/dL confirms the diagnosis. Causes include: malignancy (particularly lymphoma), trauma, following lobectomy and pulmonary lymphangioleiomyomatosis.

Pleuritis and pleural effusions are commonly associated with rheumatoid arthritis (up to 30% of patients). Pleural effusions are usually asymptomatic and the fluid is typically exudative and straw coloured, with a low glucose and low pH and typically lymphocytic. Malignancy should be considered in the differential diagnoses, especially in patients in this age group; however, a milky effusion, as described above, would not be typical of malignancy.

Hillerdal G. Chylothorax and pseudochylothorax. Eur Respir J 1997; 10:1157–1162.
British Thoracic Society. Pleural Disease Guidelines 2010. Thorax 2010; 65(2).

41. D Silicosis

Pneumoconioses are non-malignant respiratory disease caused by the reaction of the lung to the inhalation of mainly mineral or organic dusts. Tiny inhaled particles (<5 μm) can reach the terminal airways and alveoli where they are slowly cleared by macrophages or alveolar cells, leading to inflammatory reactions and characteristic patterns of disease and radiological features.

Silica is used in industries such as ceramics and stone masonry. Acute silicosis may occur within 1–2 months of working with the dust and presents as a dry cough and rapid-onset shortness of breath. Chest X-ray typically demonstrates patchy bilateral lower airspace shadowing. Chronic silicosis occurs with lower dust concentration and patients are often asymptomatic. The chest X-ray may demonstrate mid- and upper zone nodularity which will calcify after about 10 years and can be associated with calcified hilar lymphadenopathy.

Inhalation of asbestos may lead to asbestosis, which is a form of chronic interstitial fibrosis that is made worse with cigarette smoking. It typically presents with shortness of breath and dry cough but after a long latency period that is often decades after initial exposure. The chest X-ray may be normal in early disease but may later show bilateral reticulonodular shadowing, predominantly affecting the lower zones, which may progress to affect the mid- and upper zones.

Coal workers' pneumoconiosis is caused by the deposition of coal dust within the lung and the risk increases with the duration and amount of exposure. The disease is characterised by the formation of nodules in the alveoli. With progressive massive fibrosis these nodules can extend to the chest wall also. Symptoms typically consist of dyspnoea and blackened sputum. The chest X-ray demonstrates nodules located in the upper zones which enlarge and become increasingly radiodense.

Kaolinosis is a form of pneumoconiosis acquired by inhaling china clay dust (kaolin), which is used in the production of paper, ceramics, soaps, toothpaste and some medicines. Stannosis is another rare pneumoconiosis associated with tin oxide.

Sirajuddin A, Kanne JP. Occupational lung disease. J Thorac Imaging 2009; 24(4):310–320.

42. D She may fly without the need for in-flight oxygen

If there is concern regarding a patient's fitness to fly because of medical conditions a flight assessment should be performed. This should be done when the patient is stable and has recovered form any recent exacerbations. This patient has recovered from an infective exacerbation and is back to baseline function so the assessment may be performed now.

Flight assessments are performed by conducting a hypoxic challenge test. The patient receives 15% oxygen for 20 minutes and then arterial blood gases are performed to determine recommendations for in-flight oxygen.

If PaO_2 >6.6 kPa (>50 mmHg) or oxygen saturation 85% then in-flight oxygen not required.
If PaO_2 <6.6 kPa (<50 mmHg) or oxygen saturation <85% then in-flight oxygen required at 2 L/min via nasal cannulae.

Lung volumes (forced expiratory volume$_1$) and oxygen saturations using pulse oximetry may be useful indicators of disease severity; however, it is more difficult to predict patient outcomes during flight when the available oxygen may be reduced to 15%. A hypoxic challenge test performed for 20 minutes may not replicate the patient's experience of a long-haul flight and should be interpreted with caution.

Patients with infectious tuberculosis, pneumothorax, large-volume haemoptysis and respiratory failure requiring >4 L/min oxygen should be advised not to travel by air.

Shrikrishna D, Coker RK. Managing passengers with stable respiratory disease planning air travel: British Thoracic Society recommendations. Thorax 2011; 66:831–833.

43. E Noradrenaline

This patient has developed septic shock as a result of pneumonia. Patients with septic shock should receive intravenous fluids as soon as possible to help maintain circulating volume and recover blood pressure to perfuse vital organs. The requirement for volume replacement is not easy to determine and so patients should be managed with repeat fluid challenges with close clinical review. If fluid therapy alone fails to restore an adequate blood pressure to perfuse the organs, mean arterial pressure >65 mmHg, then a vasopressor should be commenced. However, adequate fluid resuscitation is a prerequisite for the success of vasopressor therapy in patients with septic shock. First-line vasopressor agents to manage septic shock include noradrenaline and dopamine. However, noradrenaline helps overcome hypotension more effectively than dopamine and dopamine must be administered via central access.

There is an ongoing debate over the relative advantages of crystalloids versus colloids in the management of shocked patients; however, clinical studies and a number of meta-analyses have failed to demonstrate a significant difference in outcome of response to therapy. Furosemide would not be beneficial in this situation as it would worsen hypotension.

Dellinger RP, et al. Surviving Sepsis Campaign: International guidelines for management of severe sepsis and septic shock. Intensive Care Med 2008; 34(1):17–60.

44. A Insert 14 Fr drain immediately above a rib margin in the scalene triangle

This patient presents with severe symptoms and a large pneumothorax on a background of emphysema. This is a secondary spontaneous pneumothorax (SSP). Patients with SSP may often be more symptomatic and suffer greater compromise than patients presenting with primary spontaneous pneumothoraces due to reduction in physiological reserve. SSPs are less likely to resolve spontaneously and most patients will need some form of intervention. Oxygen therapy should be used with caution in patients at risk of carbon dioxide retention. Needle aspiration may be considered in some cases to try to avoid chest drain insertion; however, most cases will require the insertion of a chest drain to adequately treat the pneumothorax. A small-bore drain (14 Fr) will generally be sufficient and there is no evidence that these drain are inferior to large-bore chest (e.g. 28 Fr) drains.

Chest drains and all other procedures should be performed immediately above a rib margin to reduce the risk of injury to the neurovascular bundle that is situated below a lower rib margin. Similarly, where possible, all procedures should be performed in the 'triangle of safety' – the scalene triangle to reduce risk of injury to other organs and reduce risk of bleeding from intercostal arteries.

MacDuff A, Arnold A, Harvey J. Management of spontaneous pneumothorax: British Thoracic Society pleural disease guideline 2010. Thorax 2010; 65(suppl 2):ii18–ii31.

45. E Occupational asthma

The history is very suggestive of occupational asthma. The symptoms have commenced since she started working in a bakery. Occupational asthma is due to specific workplace sensitisers and may account for 10% of adult-onset asthma and more than 300 work-related allergens are recognised. The diagnosis may be difficult to establish and it is important to take a careful history of exposure to all of the potentially irritant substances and to document the temporal relationship of contact with development of symptoms. Early diagnosis is important, as an earlier removal from the workplace in affected individuals leads to a better outcome. The symptoms improve away from work, but can take several days to settle. Serial peak flow measurements should be recorded every 2 hours from waking to sleep for 4 weeks, although there are no changes to treatment. Holidays and periods away from work should be documented. There may be associated rhinitis and urticaria. Smoking increases the risk of developing occupational asthma and smoking cessation should be encouraged.

Hypersensitivity pneumonitis is a group of lung diseases caused by inhalation of an organic antigen to which the patient has been previously sensitised. It may follow an 'acute' or 'chronic' course. Many different antigens have been reported, including 'farmers' lung' and 'bird-fanciers' lung'. The condition typically presents with breathlessness, dry cough and constitutional symptoms including fevers and weight loss.

British Thoracic Society and Scottish Intercollegiate Guidelines Network. British Guideline on the Management of Asthma – a national clinical guideline. London/Edinburgh: BTS/SIGN, 2009.

46. E Unpaired *t*-test

Choosing the right statistical test is dependent upon the nature of the data being analysed and three decisions must be made:

1. If the data have a gaussian, or normal, distribution a parametric test can be used. Tests that do not make assumptions about the population distribution are referred to as non-parametric tests. These tests are also called distribution-free tests.
2. Tests can either be one or two sided. The one-sided *P* value relates to the probability that two sample means would differ in the direction specified by the hypothesis. The two-sided *P* value allows for the probability that the sample means may differ in either direction.
3. A pared or unpaired test can be used. An unpaired test should be used to compare groups when the individual values are not paired or matched with each other. A paired test can be used when values represent repeated measurements on one subject (before and after an intervention) or measurements on matched subjects.

In this case the data have a gaussian (normal) distribution, a two-sided result must be allowed for (either cohort could have higher or lower recorded values, even though it is expected that those with known chronic obstructive pulmonary disease will have lower values), and the cohorts are unpaired. As such the student *t*-test allowing for these factors should be used (see **Table 10.6**).

Table 10.6 Indications for using different statistical tests			
Goal	**Normally distributed data**	**Rank, score or not-normally distributed data**	**Binomial data**
Describe one group	Mean	Median	Proportion
Compare two unpaired groups	Unpaired *t*-test	Mann–Whitney test	Fisher's test (χ^2 for large groups)
Compare two paired groups	Paired *t*-test	Wilcoxon's test	McNemar's test
Quantify association between two variables	Pearson's coefficient	Spearman's coefficient	

Chapter 11

Rheumatology

Questions

1. A 34-year-old woman presented with a deep vein thrombosis of the left femoral vein. Apart from a weekend break to Spain, she had not travelled recently. She was usually fit and active and swam at least twice a week. Apart from two miscarriages at 11 and 13 weeks' gestation, there was no past medical history of note.

   On examination she had a swollen, tender, left calf.

   What is the most useful diagnostic investigation?

   A Activated protein C
   B Anticardiolipin antibodies
   C Anti-dsDNA antibodies
   D Antithrombin III
   E Homocysteine

2. A 56-year-old man presented with a history of shortness of breath and numbness in his feet, causing difficulty in mobilising. He had also noticed a rash on his arms. He had a past medical history of asthma which was diagnosed 3 years ago. He had no other past medical history. Current medications were salbutamol and beclometasone inhalers. He did not smoke or drink alcohol.

   On examination he had a purpuric rash on both forearms. Respiratory rate was 20 breaths per minute and oxygen saturation 96% on air. Respiratory examination revealed mild bilateral wheeze. Neurological examination showed a peripheral sensory neuropathy of his lower limbs.

   Investigations:

haemoglobin 13.4 g/dL (13.0–18.0)	lymphocytes 2.3 × 10⁹/L (1.5–4.0)
white cell count 7.2 × 10⁹/L (4–11)	eosinophils 2.0 × 10⁹/L (0.04–0.4)
platelets 168 × 10⁹/L (150–400)	sodium 142 mmol/L (135–145)
erythrocyte sedimentation rate 64 mm/1st h (0–20)	potassium 3.9 mmol/L (3.5–5.0)
	urea 4.1 mmol/L (2.5–7.5)
C-reactive protein 24 mg/L (<5)	creatinine 94 µmol/L (60–110)
neutrophils 3.2 × 10⁹/L (1.5–7.0)	

   Antinuclear antibody 1:160 (<1:80)
   Anti-dsDNA: negative
   Myeloperoxidase and antineutrophil cytoplasmic antibody: positive

   Urinary protein: negative

   What is the most likely diagnosis?

   A Churg–Strauss syndrome
   B Microscopic polyangiitis

C   Polyarteritis nodosa
D   Takayasu's arteritis
E   Wegener's granulomatosis

3.   A 65-year-old man presented with new-onset headache, tenderness over both of his temporal arteries and jaw claudication.

Investigations:

haemoglobin 10.5 g/dL (males 13–18)	creatine kinase 100 U/L (25–195)
erythrocyte sedimentation rate 110 mm/1st h (males 0–20)	

Which of the following does not apply to his diagnosis?

A   Colour duplex ultrasound can aid with diagnosis
B   He must have an urgent temporal artery biopsy before starting any treatment
C   His symptoms should settle within 2 weeks of starting steroids
D   It is closely associated with polymyalgia rheumatica
E   Temporal artery biopsy may be normal

4.   A 37-year-old woman presented with symptoms of severe Raynaud's phenomenon and arthralgia of the small joints of her hands. She had recently developed indigestion. She had no other relevant past medical history and her current medication was omeprazole 20 mg once daily.
    On examination, she had digital ulceration and swelling. On respiratory examination there were fine bi-basal crackles.

Investigations:

haemoglobin 11.2 g/dL (11.5–16.5)	erythrocyte sedimentation rate 46 mm/1st h (0–30)
white cell count 4.3 × 10⁹/L (4–11)	C-reactive protein 10 mg/L (<10)
platelets 167 × 10⁹/L (150–400)	
Antinuclear antibody 1:160 (<1:80)	
Rheumatoid factor 60 (<20)	
Anti-dsDNA: negative	
Anticentromere antibody: positive	

What is the most likely diagnosis?

A   Diffuse cutaneous systemic sclerosis
B   Limited cutaneous systemic sclerosis
C   Mixed connective tissue disease
D   Rheumatoid arthritis
E   Systemic lupus erythematosus

5.   A 19-year-old woman presented with a 6-month history of fatigue. This had been associated with intermittent fevers, and migratory arthralgia in her small and large joints. She had noticed a pruritic rash on her face. She had no past medical history and took no medications.
    On examination, she had tenderness and mild swelling of her left knee and the distal interphalangeal joints of her right hand. There was an erythematous, maculopapular rash on her face affecting the forehead and cheeks.

Investigations:

haemoglobin 10.2 g/dL (11.5–16.5 g/dL)	platelets 136 × 10⁹/L (150–400)
white cell count 2.8 × 10⁹/L (4–11)	erythrocyte sedimentation rate 38 mm/1st h (0–30)

Antinuclear antibody 1:160 (<1:80)
Anti-dsDNA 1:160 (<1:80)
Anticentromere antibody: negative

What is the most likely diagnosis?

A   Mixed connective tissue disorder
B   Polymyositis
C   Rheumatoid arthritis
D   Systemic lupus erythematosus
E   Systemic sclerosis

6.   A 24-year-old man presented with a 1-week history of fever, polyarthralgia, sore throat and skin rash. The rash was salmon-pink coloured and occurred with the fever, fading as the fever resolved. He had a temperature of 38.5°C, pulse 100 beats per minute, blood pressure 130/75 mmHg and oxygen saturation 99% on air.
     On examination, he had a pericardial rub. Examination of both small and large joints was normal.

Investigations:

haemoglobin 11.9 g/dL (13.0–18.0)	alanine aminotransferase 189 U/L (5–35)
white cell count 15.9 × 10⁹/L (13.0–18.0)	alkaline phosphatase 87 U/L (45–105)
neutrophils 9.7 × 10⁹/L (1.5–7.0)	erythrocyte sedimentation rate 89 mm/1st h (0–30)
platelets 608 × 10⁹/L (150–400)	C-reactive protein 54 mg/L (<5)
bilirubin 7 mmol/L (1–22)	ferritin 6030 g/L (15–300)
albumin 31 g/L (37–49)	

Rheumatoid factor: negative
Antinuclear antibody: negative
Antineutrophil cytoplasmic antibody: negative

What is the most likely diagnosis?

A   Adult Still's disease
B   Churg-Strauss syndrome
C   Haemophagocytosis
D   Periodic fever syndrome
E   Wegener's granulomatosis

7.   A 36-year-old woman was admitted with shortness of breath. She had progressive dyspnoea for the last 2 months and now could only walk up to 200 metres on the flat. She did not have chest pain. She had a cough which produced only white sputum. Over the last month she had had occasional bouts of fever. She also had weakness and pain in her left arm and numbness in the lateral part of her right thigh. She had a past history of recurrent rhinitis, sinusitis and asthma.

On examination, her temperature was 38.4°C, pulse 102 beats per minute, blood pressure 104/70 mmHg, respiratory rate 20 breaths per minute and oxygen saturation 94% on air. There were purpuric spots and a maculopapular rash over the extensor aspect of left forearm. She had a polyphonic wheeze. There was a gallop rhythm at the apex and a pericardial rub. There was a left wrist drop as well as sensory loss over the lateral cutaneous nerve of right thigh.

Investigations:

haemoglobin 11.2 g/dL (11.5–16.5)	potassium 5 mmol/L (3.5–5.0)
mean corpuscular volume 84 fL (80–96)	urea 8 mmol/L (2.5–7.5)
white cell count 12 ×10⁹/L (4–11)	creatinine 134 µmol/L (45–90)
platelets 349 × 10⁹/L (150–400)	albumin 45 g/L (37–49)
neutrophils 6 × 10⁹/L (1.5 –7.0)	bilirubin 3 mmol/L (1–22)
lymphocytes 3 × 10⁹/L (1.5–4.0)	alanine transaminase 39 U/L (5–35)
eosinophils 3 × 10⁹/L (0.04–0.4)	alkaline phosphatase 102 U/L (45–105)
sodium 138 mmol/L (135–145)	

Urinalysis: protein 2+, blood 2+, leukocytes +, nitrites

Electrocardiogram: sinus tachycardia

Echocardiogram:
left ventricle was slightly enlarged with ejection fraction of 50%
small pericardial effusion

Chest X-ray: infiltrates in both the lower lobes of the lung

What is the most likely diagnosis?

A   Cardiac amyloidosis
B   Churg–Strauss syndrome
C   Goodpasture's syndrome
D   Löffler's syndrome
E   Sarcoidosis

8.   A 33-year-old woman presented with a 2-month history of pain and swelling in her hands and feet. She had no past medical history of note and was on no regular medication.
    General examination was normal with normal heart sounds.
    On examination of skin and joints there was obvious dactylitis in the fingers of both hands and arthropathy affecting the distal interphalangeal joints. Examination of her feet revealed tenderness over the calcaneus bilaterally with onycholysis of most of her toenails.

Investigations:

Rheumatoid factor: negative
Antinuclear antibody: negative
Extractable nuclear antigen: negative
Antineutrophil cytoplasmic antibody: negative
Antiendomysial antibodies: negative

erythrocyte sedimentation rate 78 mm/1st h (0–30)

What is the most likely diagnosis?

A   Enteropathic arthropathy
B   Jaccoud's arthropathy
C   Psoriatic arthropathy

D   Reiter's syndrome
E   Rheumatoid arthritis

9. A 41-year-old woman presented with pain and colour change in her fingers related to cold temperatures. She was a non-smoker who exercised regularly. On systems review she also reported some dysphagia to liquids.
    On examination, she had thickening of the skin in her fingers with some oedema of the digits. There were tender, white nodules over some of her interphalangeal joints. Around her mouth there were some telangiectasias.

Investigations:

> Rheumatoid factor: negative
>
> Antinuclear antibody: negative
>
> Antineutrophil cytoplasmic antibody: negative
>
> ---
>
> erythrocyte sedimentation rate 89 mm/1st h   C-reactive protein 14 mg/L (<10)
> (0–30)

What is the most appropriate treatment for her presenting complaint?

A   Clopidogrel
B   Doxazosin
C   Losartan
D   Nifedipine
E   Sildenafil

10. A 19-year-old Irish woman was referred with recurrent fever occurring five to six times a year for the last 10 years. On each occasion the fever lasted for 7–8 days and could be accompanied by abdominal pain, arthralgia and intermittent macular eruptions. Investigations during each febrile episode had always proved negative. She was adopted and had no siblings.
    She was currently apyrexial and systemic examination was normal.

Investigations:

> IgG 18.9 g/L (6.0–13.0)   IgA 2.9 g/L (0.8–3.0)
>
> IgM 4.1 g/L (0.4–2.5)   IgD 70 (range 0–80) (0.0–8.0)
>
> ---
>
> Urinary porphobilinogen not detected
>
> *MEFV* mutation not detected
>
> *TNFRSF1A* mutation detected

What is the most likely diagnosis?

A   Acute intermittent porphyria (AIP)
B   Familial hibernian fever or tumour necrosis factor (TNF) receptor-associated periodic syndrome (TRAPS)
C   Familial Mediterranean fever (FMF)
D   Hyperimmunoglobulinaemia D syndrome (HIDS)
E   Systemic lupus erythematosus (SLE)

11. A 33-year-old woman presented with arthralgia in the small joints of both hands and myalgia. She had suffered from Raynaud's phenomenon for many years, and this had recently worsened. She had no other relevant past medical history and was not on any medication.
    On examination, she looked well. There was tenderness of the distal interphalangeal joints of both hands, and swelling of her fingers bilaterally. Palpation of the muscles in her limbs revealed tenderness.

Investigations:

haemoglobin 11.3 g/dL (11.5–16.5)	lymphocytes 1.2×10^9/L (1.5–4.0)
white cell count 3.1×10^9/L (4–11)	platelets 145×10^9/L (150–400)
neutrophils 2.1×10^9/L (1.5–7.0)	

Rheumatoid factor: negative
Antinuclear antibody: 1/160
Anti-dsDNA: negative
Anti-U1-ribonucleoprotein: 1/1000
Anticentromere: negative

What is the most likely diagnosis?

A   Mixed connective tissue disease (MCTD)
B   Polymyositis
C   Rheumatoid arthritis (RA)
D   Scleroderma
E   Systemic lupus erythematosus (SLE)

12. A 36-year-old woman presented with a 2-month history of arthralgia and a recurrent itchy rash over her trunk and limbs. She had started antihistamine therapy with no benefit.
     On examination, there were urticarial lesions all over the trunk. Skin biopsy revealed leukocytoclastic vasculitis and a diagnosis of urticarial vasculitis was made.

What is the most appropriate next step in management?

A   Azathioprine
B   Dapsone
C   Hydroxychloroquine
D   Naproxen
E   Prednisolone

13. A 40-year-old woman with type 2 diabetes and a history of stage 3 chronic kidney disease presented with an acutely painful, swollen and hot left knee. There was no history of trauma and she did not have any joint prosthesis. She also complained of a swollen and painful left elbow.
     On examination, she was afebrile. Her left knee was swollen, red, hot and tender to touch. There was reduction in the range of movements. Her left elbow also seemed swollen and red with a reduced range of movements.

Which one of the following statements is most likely concerning her diagnosis?

A   Plain joint radiographs will be useful in the acute diagnosis
B   The absence of a fever makes septic arthritis unlikely
C   The most likely causative organism is group a β-haemolytic streptococcus
D   The presence of crystals in join aspirate allow differentiation between a septic arthritis and a crystal arthropathy
E   The involvement of more than one joint does not exclude septic arthritis

14. A 52-year-old man presented with painful joints. He complained of swelling and stiffness of his wrists, knees and ankles. He had also noticed a rash on his face. He felt generally weak and tired and thought that he may have lost some weight. There was a history of poorly controlled hypertension, for which he took amlodipine, doxazosin and hydralazine, and asthma, for which he had a salbutamol inhaler. He had a chest infection last month and had completed a course of amoxicillin.

Investigations:

haemoglobin 9.7 g/dL (males (13–18.0)	erythrocyte sedimentation rate 70 mm/1st h (0–20)
Antinuclear antibody 1/160 Extractable nuclear antigen: negative	
C3 0.88 g/L (0.65–1.9)	C4 0.15 g/L (0.15-0.5)
Antihistone antibodies: positive	

Which drug is most likely to have caused his symptoms?

A   Amlodipine
B   Amoxicillin
C   Doxazosin
D   Hydralazine
E   Salbutamol

15. A 33-year-old man presented with pain and swelling in his wrists and elbows. He also gave a history of red eyes with blurred vision. He had one mouth ulcer and had recently had an episode of epididymitis. He had a history of intermittent diarrhoea. There was no significant family history, he took no regular medications and denied any recent sexual activity.

What is the most likely diagnosis?

A   Behçet's disease
B   Crohn's disease
C   Reactive arthritis
D   Rheumatoid arthritis
E   Syphilis

16. A 58-year-old man presented with fever, weight loss of 6 kg over the past 2 months and generalised arthralgia.
    His blood pressure was 190/85 mmHg.

Investigations:

creatinine 285 µmol/L (males 60–110)	erythrocyte sedimentation rate 100 mm/1st h (0–20)
Urine dipstick: blood ++, protein ++	

He proceeded to have a renal biopsy. Post-biopsy he had significant macroscopic haematuria and a drop in blood pressure raising the suspicion of a post-biopsy bleed.
    To investigate this further he had a renal angiogram (see **Figure 11.1**).

Which one of the following features is least likely to be associated with the underlying diagnosis?

A   ANCA-associated vasculitis
B   Elevated creatine kinase
C   Hepatitis B viral infection
D   Medium vessel vasculitis
E   Presentation with hypertension and loin pain

Figure 11.1

17. A 64-year-old man presented with severe breathlessness and a non-productive cough. He had a past medical history of giant cell arteritis diagnosed by temporal artery biopsy 4 months previously. He smoked 20 cigarettes per day. His medication included prednisolone 20 mg daily and methotrexate 20 mg weekly.

On examination, his oxygen saturation was 92% on air, respiratory rate 18 beats per minute and there were bi-basal, fine, end-inspiratory crackles.

Investigations:

haemoglobin 14.2 g/dL (13.0–18.0)	creatinine 74 µmol/L (60–110)
white cell count 7.4 × 10⁹/L (4–11)	C-reactive protein 47 mg/L (<5)
HIV antibodies: negative	

A CT of the chest was performed (see **Figure 11.2**):

What is the most likely diagnosis?

A   Aspergillosis
B   Cardiac failure
C   Methotrexate pneumonitis
D   *Pneumocystis jiroveci* pneumonia
E   Staphylococcal pneumonia

Figure 11.2

18. A 24-year-old man presented with a 10-day history of tender lumps over the shins, painful ankles, shortness of breath and lethargy. There was a preceding history of a mild coryzal-type illness.

   On examination, there were erythematous, subcutaneous nodules over the shins and synovitis of the ankles.

   What is the most useful diagnostic investigation?

   A   Antinuclear antibodies
   B   C-reactive protein
   C   Chest X-ray
   D   Kveim's test
   E   Skin biopsy

19. A 58-year-old man was referred to the clinic. He had a 15-year history of asthma. Recently he had developed symptoms of worsening shortness of breath and wheezes, and had required three courses of prednisolone for acute exacerbations. Each course of steroids led to a significant improvement in his symptoms, but, on stopping the steroids, his symptoms worsened again. He suffered from chronic rhinitis and nasal polyps. He had recently developed a left-foot drop and complained generally of myalgia and lethargy.

   His current medication included: budesonide/formoterol combination inhaler and montelukast.

   Investigations:

white cell count 8.4×10^9/L (4–11)	eosinophils 2.8×10^9/L (0.04–0.4)
High-resolution CT of the chest: widespread patchy ground-glass opacification	
Multiple tiny (few millimetres only) pulmonary nodules	
No lymphadenopathy	

   What is the most likely diagnosis?

   A   Adult-onset asthma
   B   Churg–Strauss syndrome
   C   Giant cell arteritis
   D   Goodpasture's disease
   E   Montelukast-induced pneumonitis

20. A 61-year-old woman was referred following an atraumatic vertebral fracture. She had a past medical history of an oesophageal pouch and gastro-oesophageal reflux for which she was taking omeprazole 40 mg. Two years ago, she was diagnosed with breast carcinoma for which she had a resection and remained on tamoxifen. She had no other medical problems and had received no previous corticosteroids.

Investigations:

corrected calcium 2.35 mmol/L (2.2–2.6)
MRI: T12 crush fracture
Bone scan: no bony metastases
Dual-energy X-ray absorptiometry (DXA) scan: T-score –3.7 Z-score –1.3

What is the most appropriate treatment?

A   Alendronate
B   Risedronate
C   Raloxifene
D   Strontium
E   Teriparatide

21. A 64-year-old man presented with recurrent epistaxis and sinusitis.
On examination he had painful red eyes and a purpuric rash on his lower limbs. Urine output was 50 mL/h.

Investigations:

potassium 4.8 mmol/l (3.5–5.0) urea 25 mmol/L (2.5–7.5)	creatinine 452 µmol/L (males 60–110)
Antinuclear antibody: negative Antineutrophil cytoplasmic antibody: positive myeloperoxide <5 IU/L (<5)	proteinase 3 >100 IU/L (<5)
Anti-glomerular basement membrane (GBM): negative	
Urine dipstick: blood +++, protein ++++	
Chest X-ray: normal	

What is the most appropriate next step in management?

A   Broad-spectrum antibiotics
B   Haemodialysis
C   Plasma exchange
D   Prednisolone and cyclophosphamide
E   Prednisolone and methotrexate

22. A 29-year-old female student, originally from Korea, presented with a history of transient left arm weakness. She also gave a history of intermittent blurred vision for the last few months. She had lost 5 kg of weight over this period. She had no other significant past medical history, no relevant family history and took no regular medication. She was a non-smoker and did not drink alcohol.

On examination, there was an audible bruit over her right carotid artery and her left radial pulse was absent. Her blood pressure was 110/80 mmHg in the left arm and, although difficult to auscultate, approximately 80/60 mmHg in the right arm.

Investigations:

haemoglobin 9.8 g/dL (11.5–16)	erythrocyte sedimentation rate 90 mm/1st h (0–30)
Antinuclear antibody: negative	

What is the most likely diagnosis?

A   Atherosclerosis
B   Giant cell arteritis
C   Polyarteritis nodosa
D   Systemic lupus erythematosus (SLE)
E   Takayasu's arteritis

Answers

1. B Anticardiolipin antibodies

The diagnosis of antiphospholipid syndrome (APS) is based on the Sapporo classification criteria which uses clinical and laboratory criteria – patients need one of each:

A. Clinical:
- Evidence of vascular [deep vein (but not superficial vein), arterial or small vessel] thrombosis

  OR
- Pregnancy morbidity: unexplained fetal loss at ≥10 weeks' gestation, or one or more premature births ≤34 weeks' gestation due to pre-eclampsia, eclampsia or placental Insufficiency, or three or more embryonic losses ≤10 weeks' gestation.

B. Laboratory: persistent presence in the serum of at least one type of antiphospholipid antibody (aPL) on two or more occasions at least 12 weeks apart and no more than 5 years before the manifestation of symptoms. The types of aPL can include IgG or IgM anticardiolipin antibodies, IgG or IgM β_2-glycoprotein I antibodies, or lupus anticoagulant antibodies.

Although not part of the diagnostic criteria, APS is associated with heart valve disease, livedo reticularis, thrombocytopenia, nephropathy and neurological manifestations such as stroke.

Activated protein C deficiency and antithrombin III deficiency are associated with venous thrombosis, but are not associated with a significant increase in pregnancy loss. Homocysteinaemia is associated with cerebrovascular accidents and myocardial infarction. Raised levels of anti-dsDNA are associated with systemic lupus erythematosus. This can be associated with APS, but this patient has no other diagnostic features of lupus, and therefore the diagnosis is most likely to be APS.

Miyakis S, et al. International consensus statement on an update of the classification criteria for definite antiphospholipid syndrome (APS). J Thromb Haemost 2006; 4(2):295.

2. A Churg–Strauss syndrome

Churg–Strauss syndrome is a small vessel vasculitis that is characterised by eosinophil-rich and granulomatous inflammation involving the respiratory tract and a necrotising vasculitis involving small to medium size vessels. It predominantly affects the respiratory, cardiovascular and neurological systems. In 70% of cases it is associated with a positive MPO-ANCA (myeloperoxidase, antineutrophil cytoplasmic antibody), and nearly all affected patients have an eosinophilia. It is associated with asthma and usually manifests within 3 years of the onset of asthma. In an ANCA-positive patient the presence of asthma and eosinophilia, and the absence of renal involvement, make Churg–Strauss syndrome the most likely diagnosis. There are two other ANCA-associated small vessel vasculitides: Wegener's granulomatosis and microscopic polyangiitis. Wegener's granulomatosis characteristically affects both the upper and the lower respiratory tract, with symptoms of sinusitis as well as lower respiratory tract symptoms, and approximately 80% of patients will go on to develop glomerulonephritis. Microscopic polyangiitis has the same pattern of clinical manifestations as Wegener's granulomatosis, but it does not cause granulomatous disease. It is the most common cause of the pulmonary–renal syndrome. Polyarteritis nodosa does not give a positive ANCA result, and Takayasu's arteritis is a large vessel vasculitis that causes thickening of the involved arteries and subsequent luminal narrowing and inflammation. It typically presents in women in their 20s and 30s, with diminished pulses in their upper limbs and blood pressure discrepancies between right and left arms because of subclavian stenosis. It can present with neurological sequelae because of carotid artery involvement, aortic regurgitation because of aortic root dilatation and hypertension because of renal artery stenosis.

Jennet JC, Falk RJ. Small vessel vasculitis. N Engl J Med 1997; 335(21):1512–1523.
Weyand CM, Goronzy JJ. Medium and large vessel vasculitis. N Engl J Med 2003; 349:160–169.

3. B He should have an urgent temporal artery biopsy before starting treatment

This patient has presented with giant cell arteritis (GCA), also known as temporal arteritis. The American College of Rheumatology criteria for diagnosis include:

- Age >50 years
- New-onset headache
- Abnormality of the temporal arteries
- ESR (erythrocyte sedimentation rate) >50 mm/1st h
- Positive temporal artery biopsy.

Three or more of these criteria will give the diagnosis with 97% sensitivity and 79% specificity. This patient has four of these criteria. Of patients with GCA, 95% will have an ESR >50 mm/1st h.

It is recognised that there is a strong association between polymyalgia rheumatica (PMR) and GCA, and some consider them to be part of the same disease spectrum. Of patients with GCA, 50% will also have symptoms of PMR and up to 15% of patients with PMR will have evidence of GCA on temporal artery biopsy.

The suspicion of GCA should prompt immediate treatment with high-dose corticosteroids (prednisolone 40–60 mg) to prevent the significant risk of blindness. Treatment should not be delayed by waiting for temporal artery biopsy. It is generally accepted that a temporal artery biopsy will still be useful up to 10–14 days after starting steroids.

Upon starting steroids, symptoms should quickly settle within 1–2 weeks. For those with PMR, the PMR symptoms will settle more quickly, within 2–3 days.

Temporal artery biopsy remains the gold standard for making the diagnosis, although colour duplex ultrasound is increasingly being used to complement this and may offer an alternative in the future. It has a negative predictive value of around 95%. A negative temporal artery biopsy does not exclude GCA as there may be skip lesions. It is accepted that a unilateral biopsy of at least 1 cm, but ideally 1.5–3.0 cm, in length will be around 85–90% sensitive. In the face of strong clinical suspicion steroids should be continued.

Hunder GG, et al. The American College of Rheumatology 1990 criteria for the classification of giant cell arteritis. Arthritis Rheum 1990; 33:1122–1128.
Rahman W, et al. Giant cell (temporal) arteritis: An overview and update. Surv Ophthalmol 2005; 50(5):415–428.

4. B Limited cutaneous systemic sclerosis

Systemic sclerosis is a connective tissue disorder characterised by scleroderma (thickening and fibrosis of the skin) and a distinctive pattern of internal organ involvement. There are two recognised patterns of disease: limited cutaneous systemic sclerosis and diffuse cutaneous systemic sclerosis. In limited cutaneous systemic sclerosis fibrosis is mainly restricted to the hands, arms and face, with the onset of Raynaud's phenomenon occurring years before diagnosis and pulmonary hypertension usually present. Anticentromere antibodies are seen in 50–90% of patients. Diffuse cutaneous systemic sclerosis is usually rapidly progressive and affects a much larger area of skin, with one or more internal organs affected. It is associated with anti-topoisomerase I, anti-RNA polymerase and anti-fibrillin antibodies. Up to 99% of those with systemic sclerosis of either subclass will have Raynaud's phenomenon at some point in the disease. Common manifestations of systemic sclerosis are arthralgia, pulmonary fibrosis, sclerodermal renal crisis and gastrointestinal motility disorders. It is associated with a positive antinuclear antibody in 90% of cases and a positive rheumatoid factor in 30% of cases. Anticentromere antibodies are specific to limited cutaneous systemic sclerosis and are not associated with any of the other diagnoses. Mixed connective tissue disease is associated with a positive anti-U1-RNP.

Gabrielli A, et al. Scleroderma. N Engl J Med 2009; 360:1989–2003.

5. D Systemic lupus erythematosus

Systemic lupus erythematosus (SLE) is a multisystem, autoimmune, connective tissue disorder with a wide spectrum of clinical presentations. It has a female:male ratio of 9:1 and its peak onset in women is in their late adolescence or early 40s. Its most common manifestations are constitutional symptoms of fatigue and fever, skin manifestations of a butterfly or photosensitivity rash, and musculoskeletal symptoms of arthralgia, arthritis and myositis. It can also manifest itself in a number of other systems: renal, haematological, neuropsychiatric, reticuloendothelial, gastrointestinal, respiratory and cardiac. The American College of Rheumatology diagnostic criteria for SLE are outlined below. To be diagnosed with SLE individuals need to fulfil at least four of the following criteria.

Manifestations:
- Oral ulcers
- Photosensitivity
- Malar rash
- Discoid rash
- Seronegative arthritis
- Evidence of serositis such as pleural effusion or pericarditis
- Renal involvement
- Neurological involvement
- Haematological involvement
- Positive for anti-dsDNA, anti-Sm, IgG or IgM anticardiolipin antibodies, or lupus anticoagulant
- Positive for antinuclear antibody (ANA).

Although the other conditions could have a similar presentation, antibodies to double-stranded DNA are highly specific for SLE.

Hochberg MC. Updating the American College of Rheumatology revised criteria for the classification of systemic lupus erythematosus. Arthritis Rheum 1997; 40(9):1725.
D'Cruz DP, et al. Systemic lupus erythematosus. Lancet 2007; 369:587–596.

6. A Adult Still's disease

This man presents with a systemic inflammatory condition with markedly high ferritin and a negative autoantibody screen. This is typical of adult Still's disease, a multisystem disease of unknown aetiology. In addition to the symptoms noted in this case pleuritis, weight loss and adenopathy can feature. The pathophysiology is driven by interleukins-1 and -6, interferon-γ, and tumour necrosis factor-α. There is no single diagnostic test for adult Still's disease, with diagnosis requiring exclusion of infectious, neoplastic and other autoimmune conditions. A leukocytosis, elevated acute phase reactants, a moderate transaminitis and, in particular, extremely elevated serum ferritin levels are suggestive of the diagnosis. Rheumatoid factor and antinuclear antibodies are usually absent. Treatment includes the use of non-steroidal anti-inflammatory drugs and corticosteroids in the first instance. Steroid-sparing immunosuppressants can then be introduced including methotrexate, azathioprine and ciclosporin. In refractory cases biologic agents including anakinra (an interleukin-1 receptor agonist) and etanercept (a tumour necrosis factor antagonist) have been successfully used. Prognosis actually tends to be more favourable when systemic symptoms predominate.

　　Haemophagocytosis is a multisystem disorder characterised by fever, hepatosplenomegaly, lymphadenopathy, jaundice and rash, with lymphocytosis, anaemia, neutropenia and thrombocytopenia, markedly elevated serum ferritin levels and abnormal liver enzymes. The absence of cytopenias or hyperbilirubinaemia makes this diagnosis less likely in this case. Churg–Strauss syndrome is a medium vessel vasculitis involving the lungs, gastrointestinal system, peripheral nerves and kidneys. Wegener's granulomatosis is a small vessel vasculitis that affects the nose, lungs and kidneys. Wegener's is closely associated with cytoplasmic antineutrophil cytoplasmic antibodies (cANCAs) and Churg–Strauss with pANCA (perinuclear ANCA). Periodic fever syndrome can also present in a similar way to this case and can have an associated leukocytosis and raised inflammatory markers. It is not commonly associated with the marked transaminitis or raised ferritin evident here.

Efthimiou P, et al. Diagnosis and management of adult onset Still's disease. Ann Rheum Dis 2006; 65(5):564–572.

7. B Churg–Strauss syndrome

The history of recurrent sinusitis, rhinitis, asthma and prominent eosinophilia should raise the suspicion of Churg–Strauss syndrome (CSS). The presence of mononeuritis multiplex, purpuric spots and rash should also raise suspicions of a vasculitis process. Additional clues to the presence of CSS is the cardiac and renal involvement. Presence of blood and protein in urine should raise suspicion of a glomerulonephritic process. Thus, the total picture is in keeping with CSS. Antineutrophil cytoplasmic antibodies (ANCAs) might be absent in more than 50% of cases. However, in the presence of renal involvement pANCA (perinuclear ANCA) is usually positive.

Cardiac amyloidosis usually does not present with a history of asthma, mononeuritis multiplex and vasculitis. Goodpasture's syndrome also has pulmonary and renal involvement, but eosinophilia and cardiac involvement are not present.

Sarcoidosis does not present with a vasculitic picture with purpuric rash, glomerulonephritic renal involvement and recurrent sinusitis.

CSS is an eosinophil-rich granulomatous vasculitis affecting small-to-medium arteries with involvement of the respiratory tract and gastrointestinal tract.

In CSS, an allergic rhinitis-like picture is the usual presentation along with recurrent sinusitis. Asthma usually manifests in the fourth decade and once a full vasculitic picture develops the asthma subsides. Pulmonary infiltrates are common; however, unlike Wegener's granulomatosis epistaxis and haemoptysis are not common.

Cardiac involvement can occur with myocardial infarction, conduction abnormalities, pericardial effusion and congestive cardiac failure, as in this patient. This is the usual cause of life-threatening complications.

Renal involvement usually takes the form of focal segmental glomerulonephritis or vasculitic manifestations.

The American College of Rheumatology criteria for diagnosis:
- Eosinophilia >10%
- Extravascular eosinophils seen on blood vessel biopsy
- Neuropathy (mono- or polyneuropathy)
- Asthma
- Non-fixed pulmonary infiltrates
- Paranasal sinus abnormality.
 (Four criteria are needed for diagnosis.)

Treatment is with steroids – either oral prednisolone or intravenous methylprednisolone. Steroids can be combined with cyclophosphamide to induce remission in resistant cases. Once remission is achieved, azathioprine can be used instead of cyclophosphamide, or steroids alone can be used and then tapered.

Masi AT, et al. The American College of Rheumatology 1990 criteria for the classification of Churg–Strauss syndrome (allergic granulomatosis and angiitis). Arthritis Rheum 1990; 33(8):1094.
Sinico RA, Bottero P. Churg-Strauss angiitis. Best Pract Res Clin Rheumatol 2009; 23(3):355–366.

8. C Psoriatic arthropathy

This woman presents with a small joint arthropathy, dactylitis, a plantar fasciitis, psoriatic nail changes and a negative autoantibody screen – all consistent with a diagnosis of psoriatic arthropathy. Psoriatic arthropathy usually occurs in those with marked dermatological disease but can occur in those with any degree of psoriasis and affects 5% of those with the skin condition. Clinically five main categories of psoriatic arthritis are described:
- Asymmetrical: this category predominates representing 70% of psoriatic arthropathy and is generally mild. It usually involves fewer than three joints.
- Symmetrical: accounting for 25% of cases, joints on both sides of the body are affected and presentation is similar to rheumatoid arthritis.

- Arthritis mutilans: a severe, deforming progressive arthropathy. Arthritis mutilans has also been called chronic absorptive arthritis and a similar process can be seen in rheumatoid arthritis.
- Spondylitis: symptoms are predominated by spinal stiffness, but hand and foot involvement can occur as in the symmetrical arthritis form. May occur with or without sacroiliitis.
- Distal interphalangeal predominant: characterised by inflammation and stiffness in the distal interphalangeal joints. Nail changes are often marked.

Treatment is with non-steroidal anti-inflammatories and immunomodulatory agents. Methotrexate, leflunomide and azathioprine are often used and also improve the dermatological manifestations. Tumour necrosis factor-α inhibitors can be used in refractory cases.

Jaccoud's arthropathy is a chronic, non-erosive, rheumatoid-like deformity of the hands associated with rheumatic fever and systemic lupus erythematosus. The absence of valvular abnormalities makes rheumatic fever-associated Jaccoud's arthropathy unlikely, and the case does not fit with systemic lupus erythematosus. Enteropathic arthropathy (similar to psoriatic disease) is commonly associated with HLA-B27 but there is no history of enteric disease in this case. Reiter's disease is similarly associated with an antecedent infection, most commonly enteric or genitourinary, but in addition to the arthropathy evident in this case Reiter's disease manifests with conjunctivitis and urethritis.

Mease PJ. Psoriatic arthritis: update on pathophysiology, assessment and management. Ann Rheum Dis 2011; 70 (1):77–84.

9. D Nifedipine

This woman is presenting with scleroderma (CREST syndrome – calcinosis, Raynaud's phenomenon, oesophageal dysmotility, sclerodactyly and telangiectasia). The question relates to her presenting complaint of Raynaud's phenomenon: episodes of digital pallor, cyanosis and rubor in response to cold or emotional stress. Colour changes are often accompanied by pain and paraesthesia and symptoms can last minutes to hours, but with an absence of symptoms between episodes. The mainstay of treatment is with calcium channel blockers. Short-acting agents are effective, but frequently associated with adverse effects (headache, flushing, oedema).

Use of angiotensin-converting enzyme inhibitors such as losartan (and angiotensin II receptor blockers) has no proven benefit over calcium channel blockers, but some evidence points to their utility in decreasing severity and frequency of episodes of vasospasm. Anti-platelet agents have had varied results in Raynaud's phenomenon, ticlopidine has shown benefits in one series but was ineffective in another study. Clopidogrel's effectiveness has not yet been studied in relation to Raynaud's phenomenon.

α-Adrenergic antagonists have provided some symptomatic relief in Raynaud's phenomenon. Physiological studies have shown that digital vasoconstriction is mainly mediated by adrenoceptors of the α_2-subtype rather than the α_1-adrenoceptors antagonised by doxazosin.

Phosphodiesterase inhibitors such as sildenafil have also been shown to be effective in Raynaud's phenomenon but should be used primarily as a second-line therapy.

Pope JE. The diagnosis and treatment of Raynaud's phenomenon: a practical approach. Drugs 2007; 67(4):517–525.

10. B Familial hibernian fever or tumour necrosis factor (TNF) receptor-associated periodic syndrome (TRAPS)

This woman is presenting with a periodic fever syndrome, with the laboratory results indicating familial hibernian fever, also known as TNF receptor-associated periodic syndrome (TRAPS). There are a number periodic fever diseases described:

- TRAPS – characterised by episodes of fever, abdominal pain and painful, flitting, erythematous skin lesions. Attacks usually last for longer than 1 week and longer than in hyperimmunoglobulinaemia D syndrome and familial Mediterranean fever. It is caused by mutations in *TNFRSF1A*, detection of which is diagnostic. Suggestive laboratory results in a compatible clinical picture include polyclonal gammopathy as in this case. Treatment with non-steroidal anti-inflammatory drugs (NSAIDs) has been the mainstay of therapy but recently etanercept (an anti-TNF agent) has been shown to decrease the frequency, duration and severity of attacks.

- Familial Mediterranean fever (FMF) – caused by mutations in *MEFV*. The majority of patients have their first attack before 18 years of age, which is characterised by fever developing over 2–4 hours and lasting from 6 hours to 4 days. The metaraminol provocation test can be used prior to genetic testing. NSAIDs are used for acute attacks and colchicine reduces attack frequency.
- Hyperimmunoglobulinaemia D syndrome (HIDS) – manifests as high fever, abdominal pain, vomiting and diarrhoea, and frequently joint pain. Diagnosis is with persistently high IgD levels.
- Muckle–Wells syndrome – a rare syndrome characterised by intermittent febrile episodes, progressive sensorineural deafness and AA amyloidosis with nephropathy.
- Familial cold autoinflammatory syndrome – a rare condition whereby cold exposure can produce a systemic inflammatory response involving fever, urticaria and arthralgia.

Acute intermittent porphyria is characterised by abdominal pain, neuropathies and constipation, but, unlike most types of porphyria, rashes are not part of the presentation. Although systemic lupus erythematosus can present with symptoms similar to those presented here and can manifest with a relapsing–remitting course, the overall recurrent but non-progressive clinical picture favours a periodic fever.

Hull KM, et al. The expanding spectrum of systemic autoinflammatory disorders and their rheumatic manifestations. Curr Opin Rheumatol 2003; 15(1):61–69.

11. A Mixed connective tissue disease

Mixed connective tissue disease (MCTD) is an overlap syndrome with many features of systemic lupus erythematosus (SLE) and other connective tissue diseases. It most commonly presents with arthralgia or arthritis, with no particular pattern of distribution. Eighty-five per cent of those with MCTD suffer from Raynaud's phenomenon, and 66% have swollen fingers. MCTD had erroneously been thought to be the only cause of swollen fingers but they can occur in early scleroderma, eosinophilic fasciitis and anti-tRNA synthetase antibody overlap syndrome. The most concerning features of the disease are myositis, fibrosing alveolitis and pulmonary hypertension; patients should be routinely monitored for signs of these. Pulmonary hypertension is the most common cause of death. The presence of anti-U1-RNP antibodies in a high titre with negative antibodies to double-stranded DNA is diagnostic of MCTD. None of the other diagnoses given is associated with this antibody pattern, although SLE, scleroderma and rheumatoid arthritis could all present with similar clinical features.

Venables PJW. Mixed connective tissue disease. Lupus 2006; 15:132.

12. E Prednisolone

Urticarial vasculitis, also named hypocomplementaemic urticarial vasculitis, has a marked female predominance and may occur with other connective tissue disease including systemic lupus erythematosus, Sjögren's syndrome and cryoglobulinaemia. It presents with recurrent bouts of prolonged atypical urticaria, persisting for >24 hours and fading to leave brown pigmentation due to extravasation of red cells. Skin lesions tend to be painful and burn rather than itch.

Steroids should be used as first-line treatment to gain control of symptoms and the disease. Antimalarials, such as hydroxychloroquine, or dapsone may be used as second-line agents. Steroid-sparing agents such as azathioprine may also have a role in the long-term management but not in the acute setting. Non-steroidal anti-inflammatory drugs such as naproxen may help alleviate some discomfort, but will not resolve the lesions.

Venzor J, Lee WL, Huston DP. Urticarial vasculitis. Clin Rev Allergy Immunol 2002; 23(2):201–216.

13. E The involvement of more than one joint does not exclude septic arthritis

Any patient presenting with an acutely swollen, hot and red joint must be treated as an emergency and as having a septic arthritis until proven otherwise. The diagnosis is suspected clinically and confirmed with joint aspiration and culture. Diabetic patients, intravenous drug users and those with pre-existing joint disease or joint prosthesis are most at risk.

The most common causative organisms are Gram-positive cocci, the most common of which is *Staphylococcus aureus* [including MRSA (meticillin-resistant *S. aureus*)], followed by group A β-haemolytic streptococci. Unless specific risk factors are identified or the patient is immunocompromised there is no need to introduce empirical antibiotics against Gram-negative organisms, *Neisseria gonorrhoeae* (which has increasing prevalence in the USA and Australia) or *Haemophilus influenzae* type b, the incidence of which has dramatically reduced following introduction of vaccination.

Crystals and sepsis can coexist in a joint so the presence of crystals alone does not exclude a septic arthritis.

More than one joint is affected in up to 20% of patients with septic arthritis.

The presence or absence of a fever is not a reliable indicator as to whether a patient has a septic arthritis and 45% of patients with a septic arthritis will not present with a raised temperature.

Plain films of the affected joint may be useful as a baseline investigation in terms of assessing joint damage in the future, as well as for assessing for the presence of osteomyelitis. They may also show chondrocalcinosis, but they are not useful in the actual diagnosis of septic arthritis. Equally, a bone MRI will help distinguish between septic arthritis and osteoarthritis but will not differentiate between joint sepsis and inflammatory changes.

Coakley G, et al. BSR & BHPR, BOA, RCGP and BSAC guidelines for management of the hot swollen joint in adults. Rheumatology 2006; 45:1039–1041.

Christadoulou C, et al. Polyarticular septic arthritis. BMJ 2006; 333:1107–1108.

14. D Hydralazine

This patient has drug-induced lupus erythematosus (DILE). There is a list of around 80 drugs that have been recorded as being associated with this condition, but the five most common are hydralazine, minocycline, isoniazid, quinidine and procainamide. Others include angiotensin-converting enzyme inhibitors, anticonvulsants, antifungals and some of the biologic agents [interleukin, interferon and tumour necrosis factor (TNF)-α antagonists].

Drug-induced lupus has many similar presenting features to systemic lupus erythematosus (SLE), including presentation with arthralgia, myalgia, fever, rash, serositis and positive antinuclear antibodies. Central nervous system and renal involvement is rare in DILE. Although SLE is predominantly seen in younger women, DILE is typically seen in an older age group (aged 50–70 years) and has a roughly equal sex distribution. White people are affected more frequently than African–Caribbean patients. There are some laboratory differences that will help distinguish DILE from SLE including normal complements (which are often consumed in SLE), antihistone antibodies (which are typically positive in DILE) and anti-ssDNA (single-stranded DNA) antibodies being more common than anti-dsDNA antibodies (reverse in SLE).

Of the list of medications that this patient is on hydralazine is by far the most commonly associated with DILE. Although some antibiotics are associated, there are no reports with amoxicillin. Diltiazem has been reported as a causative agent but not amlodipine; there are no reports of salbutamol, and doxazosin has only very rarely been documented.

Anti-inflammatory drugs or steroids may have a short-term role in treating symptoms of DILE and symptoms should settle upon withdrawal of the causative drug. Autoantibodies may persist longer term.

Vedove CD, et al. Drug-induced lupus erythematosus. Arch Dermatol Res 2009; 301(1):99–105.

15. A Behçet's disease

Behçet's disease (or syndrome) is a chronic, relapsing, multi-system inflammatory disorder. It typically affects patients in their third and fourth decades and is more common in patients from the Middle East and Asia.

There are no particular clinical or lab findings specific to Behçet's disease and the International Study Group guidelines suggest that to make the diagnosis the patient must have oral aphthous ulcers (at least three times in 12 months) along with two out of the four of the following symptoms:
- Genital ulcers (including anal ulcers and swollen testicles or epididymitis)

- Ocular inflammation (including iritis and anterior or posterior uveitis)
- Cutaneous manifestations (erythema nodosum, folliculitis, acneiform lesions)
- Pathergy (papule >2 mm diameter 24–48 hours after needle prick).

Other symptoms recognised include diarrhoea, neurological involvement (rare), polyarthritis (commonly affecting the knees and ankles, elbows and wrists), superficial thrombophlebitis, cardiac involvement (coronary vasculitis, myocarditis, pericarditis) and lung involvement (pulmonary vasculitis, effusions, pulmonary hypertension).

Although this patient could have inflammatory bowel disease or rheumatoid arthritis, the spectrum of symptoms would be more clearly associated with Behçet's disease. Reactive arthritis would not explain his oral or ocular symptoms. Syphilis, which causes a primary chancre, and could account for his oral ulcers and arthralgia, is less likely based on the history.

International Study Group. Criteria for diagnosis of Behçet's disease. Lancet 1990; 335(8697):1078–1080.

16. A ANCA-associated vasculitis

This patient's angiogram, done to look for a source of bleeding post-biopsy, shows multiple medium vessel aneurysms and is typical of classic polyarteritis nodosa (PAN). PAN is a rare necrotising arteritis which affects the medium vessels in the gut (presenting with abdominal pain and bloody diarrhoea), skin (causing livedo reticularis), nerves (manifesting as mononeuritis multiplex or peripheral neuropathy) and kidneys. Renal impairment results from ischaemic change or infarction and patients may be hypertensive as a result, or present with haematuria or loin pain from segmental infarcts. Vessels show transmural fibrinoid necrosis in medium-sized vessels. The antineutrophil cytoplasmic antibody (ANCA)-associated vasculitides affect small vessels and do not typically give this picture. They are often diagnosed by renal biopsy where you would expect a focal and segmental necrotising glomerulonephritis.

PAN may be associated with hepatitis B infection. Creatine kinase is elevated as a result of muscle injury. ANCA is negative.

Treatment centres on immunosuppression. This includes prednisolone with the addition of cyclophosphamide in the so-called 'high-risk' group (older patients with renal, gut or coronary involvement). With concomitant hepatitis B infection the evidence base for treatment is sparse but current opinion is that interferon treatment plus plasma exchange may also be required.

17. C Methotrexate pneumonitis

Methotrexate pneumonitis is the most likely diagnosis in this situation. Pulmonary complications may be seen in 4–10% of patients treated with methotrexate. The chest X-ray or CT may demonstrate bilateral diffuse pulmonary infiltrates; pleural effusions may also be seen. Risk factors for developing methotrexate-induced lung disease include: diabetes; rheumatoid or other lung/pleural disease; daily rather than intermittent therapy; age >60 years; and smoking. It does not appear to be dose related and can occur at doses <20 mg per week. The condition may present acutely with interstitial pneumonitis, fever and eosinophilia, or in the more common subacute form within a year of treatment, presenting with dyspnoea, fever, cough, hypoxia and basal crackles. Treatment consists of drug withdrawal. The benefit of steroids is not proven.

Aspergillosis may be seen in patients with a history of longstanding, often poorly controlled asthma. It may present with a recurrent episodes of mucus plugging, fever and malaise, and expectoration of dark mucus plugs, sometimes as casts of the airways. The chest X-ray demonstrates flitting infiltration and the diagnosis may be supported by blood tests including positive IgG precipitins, positive IgE RAST (radioallergosorbent test) to *Aspergillus* species, raised total serum IgE and eosinophilia (may be suppressed if on steroids).

Patients receiving immunosuppressive therapy are at risk of developing opportunistic infections such as *Pneumocystis jiroveci* pneumonia (PCP – formoly *P. carinii* pneumonia). The condition may present with gradual onset breathlessness and dry cough with retrosternal tightness. Fever and tachypnoea may occur. Chest examination is typically normal. PCP may present with pneumothorax. The chest X-ray pattern demonstrates bilateral perihilar infiltrates that progress to alveolar shadowing. The chest X-ray may be normal in about 10% of cases.

The clinical presentation described above may be due to cardiac failure; however, it is a less likely cause in the absence of a previous cardiac history and, with the degree of chest X-ray changes, the patient is more likely to complain of a cough productive of frothy white sputum. A staphylococcal pneumonia is more likely to present with a lobar pneumonia and more pronounced inflammatory response. This patient may be more at risk of developing pneumonia as he is immunosuppressed; however, this is not the most likely diagnosis in this scenario.

Salliot C, van der Heijde D. Long-term safety of methotrexate monotherapy in patients with rheumatoid arthritis: a systematic literature research. Ann Rheum Dis 2009; 68(7):1100–1104.

18. C Chest X-ray

The clinical picture described is very suggestive of Löfgren's syndrome (acute sarcoidosis). This is a mild disease, which is usually non-progressive and presents with fevers, bilateral lymphadenopathy on chest X-ray, erythema nodosum (as described above) and arthralgia. It occurs particularly in white people. It has a good prognosis and resolves completely and spontaneously in 80% of patients within 1–2 years. Only a minority of patients may develop further lung disease. The typical history, as described above with a chest X-ray demonstrating bilateral hilar lymphadenopathy, is often sufficient to form the diagnosis without the need for further investigation. These patients should be advised to rest and take simple analgesia and non-steroidal anti-inflammatory drugs. The patients should be monitored and if there is diagnostic doubt further investigations may be necessary to exclude more serious causes of bilateral hilar lymphadenopathy including tuberculosis and lymphoma. Serum acetylcholinesterase levels may be raised; however, the level may also be normal in active sarcoid, following the trend of levels may be more useful in disease monitoring.

A skin biopsy may be useful to confirm the diagnosis if there is clinical doubt to confirm evidence of non-caseating granuloma. C-reactive protein may be elevated in many inflammatory conditions and has a poor specificity.

The Kveim test is no longer performed clinically because of the risks of transmissible disease. It involved injecting splenic tissue from a patient with known sarcoid to determine whether a granulomatous reaction occurred.

Costabel U, Ohshimo S, Guzman J. Diagnosis of sarcoidosis. Curr Opin Pulmon Med 2008; 14(5):455–461.

19. B Churg–Strauss syndrome

The clinical features and findings are suggestive of Churg–Strauss syndrome, a rare condition (2.4 per million) affecting middle-aged adults, male:female ratio 2:1. The cause of the condition is unknown. The disease is characterised by asthma, blood eosinophilia and eosinophilic granulomatous inflammation of the respiratory tract, with necrotising vasculitis affecting medium and small vessels. Perinuclear antineutrophil cytoplasmic antibody (pANCA) and anti myeloperoxidase (MPO) positive in two thirds of patients.

A diagnosis of Churg–Strauss syndrome can be made if four out of six of the following criteria are present:
- Asthma – often present for many years, with maturity onset and difficult to control
- Blood eosinophilia >10%
- Vasculitic neuropathy
- Pulmonary infiltrates on high-resolution CT (HRCT) of the chest
- Sinus disease
- Extravascular eosinophils on biopsy.

Although not necessary for diagnosis, a number of other systems can also be involved:
- Myocardial involvement (cardiomyopathy, coronary artery inflammation, pericardial effusion)
- Gastrointestinal symptoms (related to eosinophilic infiltration of mesenteric vessels)
- Alveolar haemorrhage
- Proteinuria (rare)

- Skin nodules and purpura
- Constitutional symptoms – myalgia, fevers and weight loss.

Montelukast was previously thought to be a cause of the syndrome; however, it is likely that the addition of montelukast to a patient with 'poorly controlled asthma' enabled dose reduction of prednisolone with subsequent 'unmasking' of the underlying disease, misdiagnosed as asthma.

Adult-onset asthma is increasingly recognised and is often relatively resistant to treatment; many patients may require long-term low-dose oral steroids to gain symptomatic control. HRCT would be normal unless there is another underlying diagnosis.

Giant cell arteritis is the most common form of systemic vasculitis affecting large and medium sized vessels. Minor pulmonary complications of cough and hoarseness occur in up to 25% cases; however chest X-ray and HRCT are normal.

Noth I, et al. Churg–Strauss syndrome. Lancet 2003; 361:587–594.

20. D Strontium

This woman has had a crush fracture and has a dual-energy X-ray absorptiometry scan consistent with osteoporosis. She therefore fits the NICE (National Institute for Health and Clinical Excellence) guidance for secondary prevention of further osteoporotic fractures in postmenopausal women. Strontium ranelate is indicated for use in those who cannot tolerate bisphosphonate therapy and has approval from NICE in these circumstances. It acts through decreasing bone resorption but also increasing new bone formation. Contraindications for use include chronic kidney disease and concomitant use of tetracycline antimicrobials, and care should be taken in those at increased risk of venous thromboembolic disease.

Alendronate is recommended for osteoporosis secondary prevention therapy when osteoporosis is confirmed (with a T-score ≥ -2.5) in postmenopausal women. As with most of the bisphosphonate class of agents, upper gastrointestinal side effects including dyspepsia are common. They should therefore be used with care in those with known oesophageal and gastric pathology. Selective oestrogen receptor modulators, such as raloxifene, aim to maximise the beneficial effects of oestrogen on bone without having a marked impact on endometrial or breast tissue. However, raloxifene is still contraindicated in those in whom there is either confirmed breast or uterine pathology or in whom there is symptomatology consistent with potential pathology (e.g. per vaginum bleeding or breast lumps). In those who are unable to take bisphosphonates, strontium or raloxifenes or in those who have had an unsatisfactory response to these agents a recombinant human parathyroid hormone, teriparatide, is available which has some effect in stimulating new bone formation.

National Institue for Health and Clinical Excellence. NICE Guidelines. TA161 Osteoporosis – secondary prevention including strontium ranelate: guidance. London: NICE, 2011.

21. D Prednisolone and cyclophosphamide

This patient presents with typical symptoms and investigations suggesting a diagnosis of granulomatosis with polyangiitis (GPA – formerly Wegener's granulomatosis). GPA is a small vessel vasculitis characterised by ANCA (antineutrophil cytoplasmic antibody) positivity, typically proteinase 3 (PR 3 or cytoplasmic ANCA – cANCA). It is a rapidly fatal disease and, without treatment, 2-year mortality rate is around 90%. Upon diagnosis treatment to achieve remission should be initiated as soon as possible. There have been increasing numbers of trials over the last few years looking at the optimum agents and their duration both to achieve remission and for long-term maintenance. The current recommendations are that cyclophosphamide (oral or intravenous, varies among various renal units) and prednisolone (3 days of intravenous methylprednisolone then high-dose oral prednisolone) are the treatment of choice to achieve remission. Thereafter prednisolone and azathioprine are the usual maintenance agents. Rituximab may also be an option for inducing remission or treating relapse.

There are no indications in this case for haemodialysis. He is still passing reasonable volumes of urine and his potassium is safe. Methotrexate should not be used in renal impairment, particularly not if glomerular filteration rate <30 mL/min per 1.73 m^2. There is nothing in the history to suggest a focal infection so there is no reason to give broad-spectrum antibiotics.

Plasma exchange has been shown in trials to be of benefit if there is pulmonary haemorrhage, dialysis-requiring, rapidly progressive glomerulonephritis, creatinine >500 μmol/L or coexisting anti-glomerular basement membrane antibodies, none of which this patient has.

Hoffman GS. Therapeutic interventions for systemic vasculitis. JAMA 2010; 304(21):2413–2414.

22. E Takayasu's arteritis

Takayasu's arteritis (TA) is a rare large vessel vasculitis most commonly affecting women under the age of 40 years, and in particular those from Asia. The term TA is used to describe a granulomatous inflammation of the aorta and its major branches, and its symptoms reflect varying sites and stages of involvement. The aetiology is unknown. Patients present with constitutional symptoms, including headache, malaise and weight loss, vascular features, including bruits and absent distal pulses, and neurological features such as transient ischaemic attacks.

The American College of Rheumatology published a classification in 1990 for TA whereby the presence of factors diagnoses the disease with a sensitivity of 90.5% and a specificity of 97.8%. These factors include age at onset (≥40 years), significant difference in systolic blood pressure in each arm (>10 mmHg), arteriographic changes suggesting aortic occlusion or branch occlusion, poor brachial pulse, subclavian/aortic bruits and distal claudication.

A diagnosis of atherosclerosis is unlikely as she is young and has no other significant risk factors. Equally she is not in the age group for giant cell arteritis which typically affects those over the age of 50 years. Although polyarteritis nodosa may present with general symptoms of malaise, headache and visual disturbance, it would not typically cause the absent pulses or discrepancy in blood pressures. Systemic lupus erythematosus should be considered in a young woman presenting with non-specific constitutional symptoms but again would not explain the vascular findings and one would expect antinuclear antibody to be positive.

Arend WP, et al. The American College of Rheumatology 1990 criteria for the classification of Takayasu arteritis. Arthritis Rheum 1990; 33(8):1129–1134.
Johnston SL, et al. Takayasu arteritis: a review. J Clin Pathol 2002; 55:481–486.

Chapter 12

Therapeutics and toxicology

Questions

1. A 25-year-old woman was brought to the emergency department in a stuporous state 3 hours after attempting suicide by ingesting around 100 mL of antifreeze.

   On examination, her Glasgow Coma Scale score was 12 (eyes 3, speech 4, motor 5). Her pulse was 72 beats per minute, blood pressure 125/89 mmHg, respiratory rate 20 breaths per minute and oxygen saturation 97% on air.

   Investigations:

Arterial blood gas on air:	sodium 140 mmol/L (135–145)
pH 7.32 (7.35–7.45)	potassium 5.1 mmol/L (3.5–5.0)
PCO_2 3.1 kPa (4.7–6.0)	urea 6.4 mmol/L (2.5–7.5)
PO_2 15.9 kPa (11.3–12.6)	creatinine 82 µmol/L (45–90)
bicarbonate 18.8 mmol/L (22–30)	glucose 5 mmol/L (3.0–6.0)
base excess –6 mmol/L (± 2)	lactate 4 mmol/L (0.6–1.8)
anion gap 17.5 mmol/L (8–16)	osmolar gap 18.1 (<10)

   What is the most appropriate management?

   A   Activated charcoal
   B   Fomepizole
   C   Gastric lavage
   D   Lorazepam
   E   Sodium bicarbonate

2. A 32-year-old woman with Crohn's disease wished to become pregnant. She had ileal Crohn's disease which was currently well controlled on budesonide 9 mg once daily and azathioprine 100 mg once daily. She had had perineal disease in the past which had been successfully treated with infliximab infusions.

   Which one of the following treatments for Crohn's disease should always be discontinued during pregnancy?

   A   Azathioprine
   B   Budesonide
   C   Infliximab
   D   Mesalazine
   E   Methotrexate

3. A 47-year-old woman was referred with continuous headache and a clinical diagnosis of hemicrania continua was subsequently made.

What is the most appropriate management?

A   Aspirin with domperidone
B   Ergotamine
C   Indometacin
D   Sumatriptan
E   Verapamil

4. A 75-year-old woman was diagnosed with Alzheimer's dementia during an inpatient admission. Mini-Mental State Examination revealed a score of 9/30. Agitation was a prominent feature.

What is the most appropriate pharmacological treatment?

A   Donepezil
B   Galantamine
C   Memantine
D   None
E   Rivastigmine

5. A 27-year-old man presented with a 1-month history of fatigue, easy bruising and frequent epistaxis. He had no past medical history of note and was not taking any medications.
   Following investigation, he was diagnosed with immune thrombocytopenia [formerly known as idiopathic thrombocytopenic purpura (ITP)].

Investigations:

His blood tests revealed:	international normalised ratio 1.1 (<1.4)
haemoglobin 11.1 g/dL (13.0–18.0)	activated partial thromboplastin time 30 s (30–40)
platelets 31 × 10^9/L (150–400)	

What is the most appropriate treatment?

A   Corticosteroids
B   Plasma exchange
C   Platelet transfusion
D   Rituximab (anti-CD20)
E   Romiplostim

6. A 27-year-old man with a history of previous substance abuse had recently been commenced on antituberculous therapy for pulmonary tuberculosis. His current medications include rifampicin, isoniazid, pyrazinamide, ethambutol, pyridoxine and methadone. He was receiving directly observed therapy and was under close supervision of the drug rehabilitation team. He had been compliant with his medications, but the patient was complaining of increasing symptoms of anxiety, insomnia and muscle aches.

What is the most appropriate next step in management?

A   Citalopram
B   Diazepam
C   Increase dose of methadone
D   Increase dose of pyridoxine
E   Stop all antituberculous therapy and check liver function tests

7. A 24-year-old man presented in the early hours of the morning with confusion, headache and jaw pain. He had been at a nightclub and had taken two ecstasy pills prior to feeling unwell. He had no past medical history and took no prescribed medications.

On examination, he was disoriented in time and place. His temperature was 38.4°C, pulse 110 beats per minute and blood pressure 156/100 mmHg. Neurological examination revealed nystagmus and ataxia. The rest of his examination was normal.

Which of the following is not a recognised complication of MDMA ingestion?

A   Cerebral venous sinus thrombosis
B   Coronary vasospasm
C   Hyperpyrexia
D   Rhabdomyolysis
E   Serotonin syndrome

8. A 64-year-old woman was referred with a high stoma output, dehydration and oedema following a jejunostomy 5 weeks ago for mesenteric infarction. She had lost 5 kg in weight and her stoma output was over 1.5 L per day. Parenteral nutrition was initiated shortly after her operation and then stopped 3 weeks ago. She had been prescribed intravenous fluids, and was tolerating an oral diet.

On examination, she weighed 43 kg, and had bilateral peripheral oedema to her mid-thigh. Abdominal examination revealed a jejunostomy and midline laparotomy scar. No abnormalities were detected on further physical examination.

Investigations:

haemoglobin 12.4 g/dL (11.5–16.5)	urea 4.6 mmol/L (2.5–7.5)
white cell count 5 × 10⁹/L (4–11)	creatinine 96 µmol/L (45–90)
platelets 167 × 10⁹/L (150–400)	magnesium 0.6 mmol/L (0.75–1.05)
sodium 138 × 10⁹/L (150–400)	C-reactive protein 3 mg/L (<5)
potassium 3.6 mmol/L (3.5–5.0)	

What is the next most appropriate step in management?

A   Loperamide
B   Octreotide
C   Omeprazole
D   Low-fat, high-carbohydrate diet
E   Reduction of oral hypotonic fluids to less than 500 mL/day

9. A 73-year-old woman was referred because of an unpleasant 'crawling' sensation in her legs. It was worse in the evenings and was relieved by movement. She was unable to sit still for more than a couple of minutes without moving her legs. There was no past medical history of note. She did not drink alcohol.

Neurological examination was normal.

What is the most appropriate treatment?

A   Amitriptyline
B   Baclofen
C   Clonazepam
D   Dihydrocodeine
E   Ropinirole

10. A 24-year-old man was diagnosed with fully sensitive pulmonary tuberculosis. He was commenced on standard quadruple therapy (rifampicin, isoniazid, pyrazinamide and ethambutol).

What is the most likely mechanism of action of rifampicin in the treatment of mycobacterial infection?

A   Increases mycobacterial cell wall permeability

    B   Inhibits mycobacterial protein synthesis
    C   Inhibits mycobacterial RNA polymerase
    D   Inhibits synthesis of mycobacterial fatty acids
    E   Inhibits synthesis of mycolic acid in mycobacterial cell wall

11. A 31-year-old man presented with a 2-day history of flushing, vertiginous dizziness, diarrhoea and restlessness. Five days ago he was prescribed linezolid for a paraspinal lumbar abscess. He had a past medical history of depression and was on a number of medications: linezolid, tramadol, amitriptyline, citalopram and paracetamol.

    On examination, he had a pulse of 120 beats per minute and blood pressure 175/105 mmHg. Physical examination was normal.

What is the most likely cause?

    A   Amitriptyline interaction with citalopram
    B   Amitriptyline interaction with linezolid
    C   Citalopram interaction with linezolid
    D   Inadvertent tramadol overdose
    E   Tramadol interaction with linezolid

12. A 36-year-old man presented to the emergency department with a 'staggered' paracetamol overdose over the course of 24 hours. He had a history of depression and deliberate self-harm. He took 32 × 500 mg paracetamol tablets in total. He had no other medical problems. He took regular venlafaxine, but no other medications.

    He was admitted, started on an *N*-acetylcysteine infusion and fluid resuscitation. Twenty-four hours after admission he became confused.

Investigations:

haemoglobin 14 g/dL (13.0–18.0)	urea 12 mmol/L (2.5–7.5)
white cell count 8 × 10⁹/L (4–11)	creatinine 346 µmol/L (60–110)
platelets 234 × 10⁹/L (150–400)	bilirubin 340 mmol/L (1–22)
prothrombin time 102 s (11.5–15.5)	alkaline phosphatase 184 U/L (45–105)
international normalised ratio 10 (< 1.4)	alanine transaminase 1342 U/L (5–35)
sodium 134 mmol/L (135–145)	albumin 32 g/L (37–49)
potassium 5 mmol/L (3.5–5.0)	

Arterial blood gases on air:	bicarbonate 12 mmol/L (22–30)
pH 7.18 (7.35–7.45)	base excess 8 mmol/L (± 2)
PO_2 18 kPa (11.3–12.6)	lactate 2.8 mmol/L (0.6–1.8)
PCO_2 2 kPa (4.7–6.0)	

What is the one criterion that determines urgent liver transplantation referral?

    A   Bilirubin
    B   Creatinine
    C   Lactate
    D   pH
    E   Prothrombin time

13. A 20-year old man was referred because of excessive daytime somnolence which was affecting his work and personal life. He had had this problem from childhood and had performed poorly academically at school. There was no previous medical or family history. He drank 15 units of alcohol per week but did not smoke or take any recreational drugs. Although his nightly sleep pattern was regular, he reported broken sleep with very vivid dreams. Occasionally, on waking he would be unable to move for a few seconds. He reported no episodes of sudden collapse.

An overnight polysomnogram with multiple sleep latency testings confirmed the diagnosis. Unfortunately, his condition did not improve with a trial of methylphenidate.

What is the most appropriate treatment?

A   Clomethiazole
B   Ephedrine
C   Mephedrone
D   Modafinil
E   Promethazine

14. A 56-year-old man from Guinea Bissau presented with fever and all-over body pain. He was diagnosed with type 2 diabetes 5 years ago and started on oral hypoglycaemics. Three years ago, he had had a non-ST segment myocardial infarction and was started on secondary preventive medications. Three months ago, after being found to have *Cryptosporidium* he had been diagnosed with HIV and commenced on antiretroviral therapy.

He was on a number of medications: aspirin, simvastatin, atenolol, ramipril, metformin, and Atripla (combination of efavirenz, emtricitabine and tenofovir).

On examination, he had tender muscle groups over his thighs and upper arms bilaterally.

Investigations:

sodium 138 mmol/L (135–145)	albumin 35 g/L (37–49)
potassium 4.0 mmol/L (3.5–5.0)	alanine transaminase 46 U/L (5–35)
urea 8.9 mmol/L (2.5–7.5)	alkaline phosphatase 103 U/L (45–105)
creatinine 136 µmol/L (60–110)	creatine kinase 13 780 U/L (25–195)
bilirubin 7 mmol/L (1–22)	lactate 1.2 mmol/L (0.6–1.8)

What is the most likely cause of his presentation?

A   Efavirenz-induced myositis
B   Metformin-induced lactic acidosis
C   Metformin-induced myositis
D   Statin-induced myositis
E   Tenofovir-induced lactic acidosis

15. A 34-year-old agricultural worker presented to the emergency department with a 2-hour history of confusion, tremor, blurred vision, diarrhoea and vomiting. He was using pesticide earlier.

On examination, he had tearing eyes with pinpoint pupils, and was drooling excessively. His Glasgow Coma Scale score was 14 (eyes 4, speech 4, motor 6), pulse 48 beats per minute, blood pressure 90/54 mmHg, respiratory rate 10 breaths per minute and oxygen saturation 92% on air. Auscultation of the lungs revealed widespread wheeze. Heart sounds were normal. The abdomen was soft, with hyperactive bowel sounds. Neurological examination revealed extensive tremor and dystonia.

Apart from oxygen and fluid resuscitation, what is the next most appropriate step in management?

A   Adrenaline
B   Atropine
C   Diazepam
D   Glycopyrrolate
E   Pralidoxime

16. A 36-year-old man underwent investigations for secondary hypertension. His results showed high urine levels of catecholamine metabolites in urine. A subsequent CT and MIBG (*meta*–iodobenzylguanidine) scan showed a 3 × 4 cm mass in the left adrenal suggestive of a phaeochromocytoma.

He was started on phenoxybenzamine 10 mg twice daily in preparation for tumour removal before being subsequently increased to 30 mg twice daily. The blood pressure was still 150/100 mmHg.

What is the most appropriate next antihypertensive agent?

A   Atenolol
B   Bendrofluazide
C   Doxazosin
D   Furosemide
E   Spironolactone

17. A 58-year-old man with a renal transplant attended for review. He had good graft function with a creatinine of around 140 μmol/L. His immunosuppression comprised tacrolimus and azathioprine with a low dose of steroids. He had recently had an episode of gout and was started on allopurinol by his general practitioner. He had also had a lower respiratory infection and been given a course of amoxicillin and clarithromycin. He complained of tiredness and lethargy at clinic.

Investigations:

haemoglobin 6.3 g/dL (aim 13.0–18.0)	platelets 129 × 10⁹/L (150–400)
white cell count 1.5 × 10⁹/L (4–11)	

What is the most likely cause if his pancytopenia?

A   Allopurinol
B   Amoxicillin
C   Clarithromycin
D   Prednisolone
E   Tacrolimus

18. A 30-year-old woman attended the emergency department with a 7-day history of worsening headache. Over the course of the past day she had developed fever, nausea, photophobia and neck stiffness. She had been quite drowsy for the past few hours.

On examination, her Glasgow Coma Scale score was 14 (eyes 3, verbal 5, motor 6). Her temperature was 39°C. There was no rash. Cardiorespiratory and abdominal examinations were unremarkable. Neurological examination revealed a positive Kernig sign.

Investigations:

MRI of the brain: mild hydrocephalus	
Cerebrospinal fluid: opening pressure 34 cmH₂O (5–18)	
white cell count 10 x 10⁹/L (<5)	protein 0.8 g/L (0.15–0.45)
90% lymphocytes, 10% neutrophils	glucose 3 mmol/L (3.3–4.4)
India ink stain of cerebrospinal fluid: encapsulated cells	

What is the most appropriate treatment?

A   Intravenous amphotericin B and flucytosine
B   Intravenous caspofungin
C   Intrathecal fluconazole
D   Oral ketoconazole
E   Oral pyrimethamine, sulfadiazine and folinic acid

19. A 78-year-old woman was referred by her general practitioner after being found to have a raised white blood cell count on two routine blood samples. The patient had a past medical history of diabetes and hypothyroidism. Her only medications were metformin and thyroxine.

   On examination, she appeared well. There were no skin changes. She had a mild non-tender lymphadenopathy affecting the cervical, axillary and inguinal regions. There was no organomegaly on abdominal examination. Cardiovascular, respiratory and neurological examinations were normal.

Investigations:

haemoglobin 11.1 g/dL (11.5–16.5)	lymphocytes 30 × 10⁹/L (1.5–4)
white cell count 34 × 10⁹/L (4–11)	platelets 167 × 10⁹/L (150–400)

haemoglobin 11.1 g/dL (11.5–16.5)   lymphocytes 30×10^9/L (1.5–4)
white cell count 34×10^9/L (4–11)   platelets 167×10^9/L (150–400)

Blood film (see **Figure 12.1**):
Immunophenotyping: CD19, CD5 and CD23 positive
Weak expression of surface immunoglobulin (IgM κ light chains)

Bone marrow aspirate:
35% lymphocytes
diffuse involvement

Figure 12.1 *See colour plate section.*

What is the most appropriate next step in management?

A   Alemtuzumab
B   Chlorambucil
C   Fludarabine
D   Observation and follow-up
E   Rituximab

20. A 58-year-old man with mild chronic obstructive pulmonary disease and epilepsy was referred to the smoking cessation clinic. He smoked 20 cigarettes per day and was keen to give up smoking. He had failed to stop smoking using will-power and nicotine replacement therapy, and was attending group counselling sessions. The counsellor had recommended that he may be a suitable candidate for another medication.

What is the most appropriate treatment?

A   Acamprosate
B   Bupropion
C   Citalopram
D   Disulfiram
E   Varenicline

21. A 22-year-old man presented with pain in his elbows, shoulders and knees, 3 weeks after commencing quadruple therapy for pulmonary tuberculosis.

Investigations:

haemoglobin 12.3 g/dL (13.0–18.0)	platelets 204 × 10⁹/L (150–400)
white cell count 7.2 × 10⁹/L (4–11)	erythrocyte sedimentation rate 32 mm/1st h (0–30)

Antinuclear antibody 1:40 (negative at 1:20 dilution)
Rheumatoid factor 38 kIU/L (<30)
Anticyclic citrullinated 15 (negative <20)
Protein antibodies (anti-CCP)

What is the most likely cause of his symptoms?

A   Ethambutol arthropathy
B   Isoniazid-induced systemic lupus erythematosus
C   Paradoxical reaction
D   Pyrazinamide-induced arthralgia
E   Rheumatoid arthritis

22. A 72-year-old man was admitted to hospital with an international normalised ratio (INR) of 9.2. He had been taking warfarin for atrial fibrillation (target INR 2–3), and his regular maintenance dose was 6 mg daily. Five days ago, he was found to have acute, severe prostatitis for which he had been started on ciprofloxacin.

On examination, the patient was well and there was no clinical evidence of bleeding.

What is the most appropriate management for this patient?

A   Halve the dose of warfarin and monitor INR daily
B   Omit warfarin for 2 days
C   Stop the ciprofloxacin and continue warfarin at 1 mg per day
D   Stop warfarin and prescribe 1 mg oral vitamin K
E   Stop warfarin and prescribe 1 unit of fresh frozen plasma

23. A 21-year-old woman with a history of complex partial seizures attended the neurology outpatient clinic for review. Despite complying with escalating doses of carbamazepine for the past 6 months, seizure control remained poor. She was now keen to try an alternative medication to achieve better seizure control.

The plan was to switch to lamotrigine; however, she was concerned about side effects.

Which one of the following is a recognised side effect of lamotrigine?

A   Alopecia
B   Blurred vision
C   Menstrual irregularities
D   Skin rash
E   Tremor

24. A 43-year-old woman presented with fever and malaise for the last month. Examination revealed a pansystolic murmur and splinter haemorrhages. Her weight was recorded as 125 kg.

Three sets of blood cultures grew an α-haemolytic streptococcus sensitive to penicillin and gentamicin. A transthoracic echocardiogram showed a mobile vegetation on her posterior mitral leaflet. She was commenced on benzylpenicillin 2.4 g intravenously 4 hourly and gentamicin 70 mg intravenously three times daily.

After 24 hours her gentamicin levels were measured:

Investigations:

peak 1.2 mg/L (target 3–5 mg/L)	trough <1 mg/L (target <1 mg/L)

What is the next most appropriate step in management?

A   Decrease in frequency of gentamicin dosing
B   Increase in frequency of gentamicin dosing
C   Use of actual body weight to dose gentamicin
D   Use of dose-determining weight to dose gentamicin
E   Use of ideal body weight to dose gentamicin

25. A 41-year-old man had started treatment for chronic hepatitis C. He was an ex-intravenous drug user but was not taking any other medications, illicit drugs or alcohol.
     He was hepatitis C virus (HCV) genotype 1a and his pretreatment RNA was 4.6 log IU/mL. Liver ultrasound showed an irregular liver with coarse echotexture.
     After 12 weeks of treatment with pegylated interferon and ribavirin he had repeat blood tests.

Investigations:

haemoglobin 13.7 g/dL (13.0–18.0)	alkaline phosphatase 184 U/L (45–105)
white cell count 5.6 × 10⁹/L (4–11)	alanine transaminase 34 U/L (5–35)
platelets 198 × 10⁹/L (150–400)	albumin 40 g/L (37–49)
bilirubin 14 mmol/L (1–22)	HCV RNA 4.5 log IU/mL

What is the next step in management?

A   Continue pegylated interferon and ribavirin until 24 weeks of treatment is completed
B   Continue pegylated interferon and ribavirin until 48 weeks of treatment is completed
C   Continue pegylated interferon and ribavirin until 24 weeks and repeat HCV RNA levels. If they have not reduced by at least 3 log IU/mL stop treatment
D   Perform a liver biopsy and if cirrhosis is present continue treatment for 48 weeks
E   Stop pegylated interferon and ribavirin treatment

26. A 68-year-old man presented after returning from Ghana with a fever. He was shown to have 2.0% *Plasmodium falciparum* malaria on his blood film and was commenced on appropriate antimalarial therapy.
     Three hours later, he had a cardiac arrest with the initial rhythm being torsades de pointes. After one cycle of defibrillation he had a return of spontaneous circulation. He had a past medical history of atrial fibrillation and heart failure, and was on a number of medications: quinine, aspirin, atorvastatin, furosemide, bisoprolol and digoxin.

What is the most likely cause of the ventricular tachycardia?

A   Digoxin interaction with quinine
B   Digoxin toxicity
C   Diuretic-induced hypomagnesaemia
D   Hypoglycaemia
E   Quinine toxicity

27. A previously fit and well 28-year-old man with a 1-week history of bleeding gums was found to have an excess of myeloid blast cells containing prominent granules and Auer rods on his blood film. Bone marrow biopsy confirmed an excess of promyelocytes. Cytogenetic studies confirmed the presence of a t(15:17) translocation.
     He had no active bleeding points at presentation, but had stopped brushing his teeth because it was making his gums bleed for several hours afterwards.

Investigations:

haemoglobin 9.2 g/dL (13.0–18.0)	international normalised ratio 1.2(<1.4)
white cell count 27 × 10⁹/L (4–11)	activated partial thromboplastin time 35 s (30–40)
platelets 63 × 10⁹/L (150–400)	fibrinogen 3.1 g/L (1.8–5.4)

The most appropriate treatment for this patient is standard induction chemotherapy for acute myeloid leukaemia (e.g. daunorubicin, cytosine arabinoside, etoposide).

What should this treatment be combined with?

A   All-*trans*-retinoic acid
B   Dexamethasone
C   Regular transfusions of fresh frozen plasma
D   Rituximab
E   Thalidomide

28. A 44-year-old woman presented to the emergency department with drowsiness, a persistent throbbing headache, nausea and vomiting. She had had difficulty concentrating at work and had noticed that she had been quite irritable recently. Her symptoms were worse in the morning, and were relieved when she was at work. She had recently moved house, and her cat had died shortly after moving home so she had initially put her symptoms down to stress.

    She had no past medical history, and took no medications.
    Physical examination was unremarkable.

Investigations:

haemoglobin 13 g/dL (11.5–16.5)	C-reactive protein 4 mg/L (<5)
white cell count 4.5 × 10⁹/L (4–11)	carboxyhaemoglobin 35%: non-smoker (<2%), smoker (3–15%)
platelets 167 × 10⁹/L (150–400)	

What is the most important management step?

A   Administration of continuous positive airway pressure ventilation
B   Charcoal administration
C   Continuous venous–venous haemofiltration
D   High-flow oxygen therapy
E   Hyperbaric oxygen therapy

29. A 53-year-old man presented to the emergency department with headache, intraoral tingling, cramping abdominal pain and diarrhoea 15 minutes after eating tuna steak at a seafood restaurant.

    On examination, he was anxious with a flushed appearance. A blanching erythematous macular rash was noted predominantly over the trunk. His temperature was 37.4°C, pulse 110 beats per minute, blood pressure 98/54 mmHg, respiratory rate 22 breaths per minute and oxygen saturation 98% on room air. Cardiovascular, neurological and respiratory examinations were normal. There was some abdominal tenderness.

What is the most likely cause?

A   Botulinum toxin
B   Ciguatera toxin
C   Pectenotoxin
D   Scombrotoxin
E   Tetrodotoxin

30. A 78-year-old white woman was referred to the cardiology clinic with worsening shortness of breath. She had a previous history of ischaemic heart disease and had had coronary artery bypass surgery 15 years ago. She also has type 2 diabetes mellitus, hypertension and depression.

    She was on gliclazide 40 mg twice daily, ramipril 10 mg once daily, simvastatin 40 mg once daily, aspirin 75 mg once daily, furosemide 80 mg twice daily, bisoprolol 7.5 mg once daily and citalopram 20 mg once daily. She had shortness of breath on walking 100 metres and used three pillows with occasional bouts of shortness of breath at night.

    On examination, her pulse was 50 beats per minute, blood pressure 130/68 mmHg, respiratory rate 18 breaths per minute, and oxygen saturation 96% on air. She had a 2/6 pansystolic murmur at the apex radiating to the axilla. Heart sounds were normal and there were no added sounds. Lung fields were clear.

    Investigations:

sodium 138 mmol/L (135–145)	creatinine 78 µmol/L (45–90)
potassium 3.9 mmol/L (3.5–5.0)	

    Echocardiogram:
    dilated left ventricle with lateral akinesia and ejection fraction of 30%
    mild mitral regurgitation
    mild tricuspid regurgitation and pulmonary artery systolic pressure 30 mmHg
    Myocardial perfusion scan did not show any reversible ischaemia

    What is the most appropriate next step in management?

    A Amiodarone
    B Amlodipine
    C Digoxin
    D Isosorbide mononitrate
    E Spironolactone

31. A 34-year-old woman presented with nausea and vomiting 4 hours after having taken an overdose of paracetamol. Her paracetamol level was above the treatment line and she was administered intravenous *n*-acetylcysteine (NAC) in 5% dextrose.

    Two hours after starting the infusion the patient complained of feeling hot. On examination, she had obvious facial flushing. Her temperature was 37.5°C, pulse 90 beats per minute, blood pressure 110/65 mmHg, respiratory rate 20 breaths per minute and oxygen saturation 95% on air. There was no angio-oedema and her chest was clear.

    What is the most appropriate next step in management?

    A Continue the NAC infusion at the same rate
    B Stop the NAC infusion and give oral methionine
    C Stop the NAC infusion but administer intravenous chlorpheniramine
    D Stop the NAC infusion but give oral NAC
    E Stop the NAC infusion but restart in 4 hours

32. A 19-year-old woman presented with fever, drowsiness and rash. She had no past medical history and was not taking any medication.

    On examination, her Glasgow Coma Scale score was 14/15. There was a non-blanching petechial rash over her trunk and limbs. There was neck stiffness and photophobia but no focal neurological signs.

    Investigations:

Cerebrospinal fluid microscopy: Gram-negative diplococci

What is most appropriate treatment?

A   Ceftriaxone
B   Cefuroxime
C   Chloramphenicol
D   Ciprofloxacin
E   Vancomycin and high-dose dexamethasone

33. A 21-year-old woman presented with left heel pain radiating into her left calf, particularly on walking, and progressing in severity over the last 48 hours. She had a past medical history of partial thyroidectomy for a nodule and had been recently treated with several courses of oral antimicrobials by her general practitioner for a urinary tract infection that had persisted.

On examination, the calf was soft and non-tender. There was focal tenderness over her heel with mild erythema but no oedema.

Over the past 2 months she had been treated with levothyroxine, cephalexin, nitrofurantoin, co-amoxiclav and ciprofloxacin.

What is the most likely diagnosis?

A   Cephalosporin myopathy
B   Nitrofurantoin tendinopathy
C   Penicillin myopathy
D   Pretibial myxoedema
E   Quinolone tendinopathy

34. A 24-year-old man presented with a painful, distorted neck 24 hours after commencing olanzapine for treatment of paranoid schizophrenia.

On examination, there was spasmodic torticollis.

Apart from stopping olanzapine, what is the most appropriate next step in management?

A   Intramuscular botulinum toxin
B   Intravenous dantrolene sodium
C   Intravenous procyclidine
D   Electroconvulsive therapy
E   Oral tizanidine

35. A 54-year-old woman presented to clinic with symptoms of tiredness, abdominal and back pain, and constipation. She had a past medical history of a major depressive illness and started medication for this 1 year ago.

Examination was unremarkable.

Investigations:

corrected calcium 2.9 mmol/L (2.2–2.6)	parathyroid hormone 8.5 pmol/L (0.9–5.4)
phosphate 0.3 mmol/L (0.8–1.4)	thyroid-stimulating hormone 0.1 mU/L (0.4–5.0)
alkaline phosphatase 577 U/L (45–105)	free thyroxine 4 pmol/L (10–25)

What is the most likely cause?

A   Amitriptyline
B   Fluoxetine
C   Lithium
D   Mirtazapine
E   Venlafaxine

36. A 54-year-old woman presented with a 3-day history of breathlessness, fever and a cough productive of rusty-coloured sputum. She was oriented and gave a clear history of paroxysmal

atrial fibrillation for which she was on beta blockers and warfarin. She had not recently travelled and had no pets.

On examination, her temperature was 38.1°C, pulse 125 beats per minute, blood pressure 125/85 mmHg, respiratory rate 16 breaths per minute and oxygen saturation 93% on air. Auscultation of the chest revealed focal bronchial breathing at the left base.

Investigations:

haemoglobin 12.8 g/dL (11.5–16.5)

white cell count 12.6 × 10⁹/L (4–11)

neutrophils 10.9 × 10⁹/L (1.5–7.0)

platelets 321 × 10⁹/L (150–400)

sodium 138 mmol/L (135–145)

potasssium 3.9 mmol/L (3.5–5.0)

urea 5.6 mmol/L (2.5–7.5)

creatinine 69 µmol/L (45–90)

C-reactive protein 127 mg/L (<5)

Chest X-ray (see **Figure 12.2**)

Figure 12.2

What is the most appropriate therapy?

A   Amoxicillin
B   Amoxicillin and clarithromycin
C   Co-amoxiclav and clarithromycin
D   Doxycycline
E   Levofloxacin

37. A 55-year-old non-diabetic man with a history of hypertension, atrial fibrillation and depression was admitted after taking an overdose of his medications. He was on amlodipine 10 mg and

digoxin 62.5-µg regularly and some empty packets of amlodipine were found beside him. It was not clear exactly what he had taken and when.

On arrival he was hypotensive with a blood pressure of 65/30 mmHg and bradycardic with a heart rate of 30 beats per minute. He was warm and vasodilated.

Which one of the following treatments should not be considered in this case?

A   Atropine
B   Calcium gluconate
C   Charcoal
D   Glucagon
E   Insulin/dextrose

38. A 28-year-old woman was admitted with a 36-hour history of flu-like illness during an epidemic of H1N1 influenza. She was 32 weeks' pregnant. She had been vaccinated against H1N1 influenza 6 weeks previously.

What is the most appropriate management?

A   Intravenous pooled human immunoglobulin
B   Intravenous zanamivir
C   Oral amoxicillin
D   Oral oseltamivir
E   Symptomatic treatment

39. A 45-year-old Lithuanian man was brought to the emergency department by his housemates in an acute confusional state. Earlier that evening he had been drinking home-made vodka. The patient did not speak English and was unable to give a history. His friends denied that he took drugs or other medication.

On examination, his Glasgow Coma Scale score was 12 (eyes 3, speech 4, motor 5). He was unkempt and smelt strongly of alcohol. His temperature was 37°C, pulse 104 beats per minute, blood pressure 90/58 mmHg, respiratory rate 28 breaths per minute and oxygen saturation 98% on air.

Cardiovascular, respiratory and abdominal examinations were normal. His pupils had normal and equal diameter but were slow to react to light. He could move all limbs. There was no neck stiffness, rash or marks on his skin.

Investigations:

sodium 131 mmol/L (135–145)	creatinine 102 µmol/L (60–110)
potassium 4.2 mmol/L (3.5–5.0)	chloride 104 mmol/L (95–107)
urea 8.6 mmol/L (2.5–7.5)	glucose 4.5 mmol/L (3.0–6.0)
Arterial blood gases (on air):	PO_2 12.3 kPa (11.3–12.6)
pH 7.29 (7.35–7.45)	bicarbonate 13 mmol/L (22–30)
PCO_2 3.0 kPa (4.7–6.0)	

The patient was initially treated with intravenous fluids, and an infusion of sodium bicarbonate to correct his acidosis.

What is the next most appropriate step in management?

A   Activated charcoal
B   Ethanol
C   Gastric lavage
D   Haemodialysis
E   Phenytoin

40. A 44-year-old man with a history of depression presented with nausea and vomiting, tinnitus and sweating after taking an overdose of an unknown substance a few hours earlier. He had no other past medical history.

     On examination, he was sweating and anxious. His temperature was 38°C, pulse 100 beats per minute, blood pressure 132/96 mmHg and respiratory rate 36 breaths per minute. Physical examination was unremarkable.

Investigations:

Arterial blood gases on air:	PO_2 13 kPa (11.3–12.6)
pH 7.51 (7.35–7.45)	base excess –6 mmol/L (± 2)
PCO_2 2.4 kPa (4.7–6.0)	bicarbonate 9 mmol/L (22–30)

What is the most likely diagnosis?

A   Ethylene glycol overdose
B   Methanol overdose
C   Organophosphate poisoning
D   Salicylate overdose
E   Tricyclic antidepressant overdose

41. A 59-year-old-man with newly diagnosed chronic myeloid leukaemia was referred for treatment.

Investigations:

haemoglobin 10.5 g/dL (13.0–18.0)	white blood cells 54 × 10⁹/L (4–11)
mean corpuscular volume 84 fL (80–96)	platelets 482 × 10⁹/L (150–400)

What is the most appropriate management?

A   Allogeneic stem cell transplantation
B   Daunorubicin combined with cytosine arabinoside
C   Hydroxyurea
D   Imatinib
E   Pegylated interferon-α

42. A 25-year-old man presented to his general practitioner with a 7-month history of diarrhoea associated with urgency and crampy abdominal pain. The pain was worse after eating and associated with abdominal bloating. He had not had any weight loss or rectal bleeding. He took no medications and there was no known family history of note.

     Physical examination was normal.

Investigations:

Full blood count: C-reactive protein and erythrocyte sedimentation rate normal
Tissue transglutaminase antibodies: negative

What is the most appropriate initial treatment?

A   Acupuncture
B   Amitriptyline
C   Hyoscine butylbromide (Buscopan)
D   Cognitive–behavioural therapy
E   Mesalazine

43. A 25-year-old woman was brought to the emergency department by a friend, 2 hours after allegedly taking an amitriptyline overdose. She had a history of depression and attempted suicide. She denied taking any other medications. The patient complained of blurred vision and palpitations.

On examination, she was tearful and agitated. Her Glasgow Coma Scale score was 14 (eyes 3, speech 5, motor 6), temperature 37.4°C, pulse 130 beats per minute, blood pressure 95/52 mmHg, respiratory rate 10 breaths per minute and oxygen saturation 98% on air. Cardiorespiratory examination was normal but neurological examination revealed dilated pupils.

Investigations:

sodium 136 mmol/L (135–145)	creatinine 98 µmol/L (45–90)
potassium 3.4 mmol/L (3.5–5.0)	chloride 107 mmol/L (95–107)
urea 7.3 mmol/L (2.5–7.5)	
Arterial blood gases (on air):	PO_2 11.9 kPa (11.3–12.6)
pH 7.31 (7.35–7.45)	bicarbonate 16 mmol/L (22–30)
PCO_2 4.9 kPa (4.7–6.0)	lactate 3.9 mmol/L (0.6–1.8)

ECG: sinus tachycardia with a widened QRS complex (140 ms) and prolonged QT interval

Apart from fluid resuscitation, what is the most appropriate next step in management?

A   Diazepam
B   Gastric lavage
C   Glucagon
D   Hyperventilation
E   Sodium bicarbonate

Answers

1. B Fomepizole

This patient has allegedly ingested a potentially fatal dose of antifreeze. She is exhibiting features consistent with acute ethylene glycol intoxication, and her blood tests show that she has a raised osmolar gap. Although her arterial blood gas is not presently greatly deranged this would be expected to deteriorate over the ensuing hours if no treatment is given. This is because ethylene glycol will be metabolised by alcohol dehydrogenase to glycoaldehyde, which in turn will be further metabolised to highly toxic entities including glycolic acid. The latter will cause a severe metabolic acidosis with high anion gap.

Therefore, the most appropriate step is to start treatment to prevent the metabolism of ethylene glycol (even though no serum ethylene glycol level has been recorded). This can be achieved by administering ethanol or fomepizole. Ethanol acts as a preferential substrate for alcohol dehydrogenase, therefore preventing the metabolism of ethylene glycol, whereas fomepizole is an inhibitor of alcohol dehydrogenase activity. Both prevent the formation of toxic ethylene glycol metabolites.

Fomepizole is licensed for treatment of ethylene glycol poisoning and, unlike ethanol, is not inebriating and does not require regular blood monitoring. Treatment should be continued until serum ethylene glycol falls below 50 mg/L.

Activated charcoal does not absorb ethylene glycol well. Gastric lavage is advised only if presentation is within 1 hour of ingestion. Intravenous lorazepam would be indicated if the patient were to develop frequent or prolonged seizures. Sodium bicarbonate may be indicated if severe metabolic acidosis develops. Haemodialysis is likely to be necessary in cases of severe poisoning.

Barceloux DG, et al. American Academy of Clinical Toxicology Practice Guidelines on the Treatment of Ethylene Glycol Poisoning. Ad Hoc Committee. J Toxicol Clin Toxicol 1999; 37(5):537.

2. E Methotrexate

Medical treatment for Crohn's disease, with the exception of methotrexate, should generally continue as the risks of stopping treatment usually outweigh the benefits. Methotrexate therapy has been shown to be teratogenic and embryotoxic in animal studies. It results in chromosomal damage and miscarriages and is contraindicated in pregnancy. Due to the long half-life of its metabolites it should be stopped at least 6 weeks before conception occurs. Thiopurines are generally considered safe in pregnancy. In the USA, they have a Food and Drug Administration (FDA) rating of D based on anecdotal reports of high abortion rates, but inflammatory bowel disease (IBD) follow-up studies of pregnancies during treatment with azathioprine and 6-mercaptopurine report normal deliveries and no excess rates of prematurity, low birthweight or chromosomal abnormalities. Studies of inhaled budesonide suggest that it is safe in pregnancy at the doses used, which are much higher than those used in IBD, so it is felt to be safe. There are no studies of oral budesonide in pregnancy. Infliximab use during pregnancy has been reported in 2 papers covering 92 pregnancies and no significantly increased risk of still births, ectopic pregnancies, spontaneous abortions and low birthweight was found. Congenital abnormalities occurred in two pregnancies but this may have been related to the underlying increased risk in women with IBD. Mesalazine has been shown to be safe in pregnancy in doses of up to 3 g per day.

van Assche G, et al. The second European evidence-based consensus on the diagnosis and management of Crohn's disease: Special situations. Journal of Crohn's and Colitis 2010; 4:63–101.

3. C Indometacin

Practically all patients with hemicrania continua respond to indometacin, which is typically administered at 75–150 mg/day in divided doses. Absolute resolution of symptoms usually occurs within 2 or 3 days of commencing treatment (and failure to respond should raise doubts about the diagnosis). Unfortunately, high relapse rates are observed on cessation of treatment.

Clarke C, et al (eds). Headache (Chapter 11). In: Neurology: A Queen Square Textbook. Oxford: Blackwell Publishing, 2009.

4. C Memantine

Alzheimer's disease is the most common form of dementia in the UK, affecting more than 350 000 people. Grading of severity is based on the Mini-Mental State Examination score: mild (21–26), moderate (10–20) or severe (<10). Disease progression is insidious, and median survival is approximately 7 years from symptom onset.

Any one of the acetylcholinesterase inhibitors (donepezil, galantamine or rivastigmine) can be used in the treatment of mild or moderate Alzheimer's disease. In contrast, the only pharmacological treatment licensed for the treatment of severe Alzheimer's disease in the UK is memantine, a voltage-dependent, moderate affinity, competitive n-methyl-D-aspartate receptor antagonist. This drug has been deemed cost-effective in the treatment of severe Alzheimer's disease at an incremental cost-effectiveness ratio of £26 500 per quality-adjusted life year (QALY) gained (when compared with best supportive treatment). Memantine does not prevent disease progression (although it does a have a small but significant effect in delaying the need for nursing home care), but improves symptoms and is particularly useful in agitated patients.

National Institute for Health and Clinical Excellence. NICE Guidelines. Donepezil, galantamine, rivastigmine and memantine for the treatment of Alzheimer's disease (TA217). London: NICE, 2011.

5. A Corticosteroids

Treatment of immune thrombocytopenia is not usually indicated unless the platelet count is <50. First-line treatments include corticosteroids and intravenous immunoglobulin. Anti-D may also be an appropriate first-line treatment in patients who are rhesus D positive, with no evidence of autoimmune haemolytic anaemia. Second-line agents include steroid-sparing immunosuppressants and rituximab. Romiplostim is a thrombopoietin receptor agonist that has been approved by the National Institute for Health and Clinical Excellence for use in patients with chronic immune thrombocytopenic purpura (lasting more than 12 months) which has failed to respond to standard active treatments and rescue therapies, or in those who have severe disease and a significant risk of haemorrhage that requires frequent rescue therapies. Splenectomy may be indicated if medical therapies prove unsuccessful; however, approximately 14% of patients will not respond to this treatment and, of those who do, 20% will relapse in the fullness of time. Platelet transfusion would be indicated only if the patient were actively bleeding. Plasma exchange has no role as a treatment in isolation.

Immune thrombocytopenic purpura is discussed in more detail elsewhere.

Hoffbrand V, Moss P, Pettit J. Bleeding disorders (Chapter 23). In: Essential Haematology, 5th edn. Oxford: Blackwell Publishing, 2006.
Provan D, et al. International consensus report on the investigation and management of primary immune thrombocytopenia. Blood 2010; 115:168–186.

6. C Increase dose of methadone

Four drugs – rifampicin, isoniazid, pyrazinamide and ethambutol – are used together in the initial phase of tuberculosis treatment to reduce the bacterial population and reduce the risk of drug resistance. Rifampicin is generally well tolerated but may cause mild gastrointestinal upset and/ or transient disturbance of liver function with elevated transaminases which does not require interruption of therapy. Occasionally more serious liver toxicity may occur requiring a change of treatment, particularly in those with pre-existing liver disease. Other major side effects include acute renal failure and thrombocytopenia. Patients should be warned that rifampicin will cause red discoloration of urine (useful for compliance monitoring) and other body fluids, and may discolour contact lenses.

Rifampicin induces hepatic enzymes which accelerate the metabolism of several drugs including oestrogens, corticosteroids, phenytoin, sulphonlyureas, opiates and anticoagulants. His symptoms are suggestive of opiate withdrawal. This is likely because of the increased metabolism of methadone, so the dose will need to be increased under close supervision. Similarly, in other patients taking concomitant medications specific advice and monitoring may be necessary, e.g. in women taking hormonal contraceptives alternative family planning advice should be offered.

Isoniazid is well tolerated. The major side effect is age-dependent hepatitis and there is increased toxicity with chronic alcohol abuse. Peripheral neuropathy is uncommon and the risk is reduced by administering pyridoxine. There is an increased risk of peripheral neuropathy in diabetes, chronic alcohol abuse, HIV, malnutrition, and pregnancy, and an increased dose of pyridoxine should be prescribed.

Pyrazinamide also causes gastrointestinal upset and drug-induced hepatitis. Ethambutol very rarely causes optic neuritis presenting with impairment of colour vision and/or loss of visual acuity.

Patients should receive appropriate counselling regarding the side effects associated with antituberculous therapy, and informed to seek advice if they develop symptoms including abdominal pain, nausea, vomiting, rash and/or jaundice, so that the appropriate action may be taken including checking liver function tests and full blood count.

National Institute for Health and Clinical Excellence. NICE Guideline No. 117: Tuberculosis. Clinical diagnosis and management of tuberculosis, and measures for its prevention and control. London: NICE, 2011.

7. B Coronary vasospasm

MDMA (3,4-methylenedioxy-N-methylamphetamine) ingestion can cause a variety of clinical manifestations. Minor side effects which are almost universal include tachycardia, hypertension, mydriasis, dry mouth, sweating, confusion, ataxia and bruxism (teeth gnashing and jaw clenching). More severe adverse effects include hyperpyrexia with rhabdomyolysis and multi-organ failure, serotonin syndrome, long QT syndrome, acute liver failure and hyponatraemia, and cerebral oedema. In rare cases cerebral venous sinus thrombosis, cerebral haemorrhage and aplastic anaemia have been reported. Coronary vasospasm is not associated with MDMA ingestion but is associated with cocaine ingestion.

Hall AP, Henry JA. Acute toxic effects of 'Ecstasy' (MDMA) and related compounds: overview of pathophysiology and clinical management. Br J Anaesth 2006; 96: 678–685.

8. E Reduction of oral hypotonic fluids to less than 500 mL/day

The patient has short bowel syndrome secondary to her previous mesenteric infarction and subsequent surgery. This has been complicated by a high-output stoma. Management of a high-output stoma in small bowel syndrome is challenging. The primary driver for stomal fluid loss is oral intake, and hypotonic fluids cause high stomal losses, so treatment begins with the patient restricting her total oral hypotonic intake to less than 500 mL/day. Fluid requirements can be maintained by the patient sipping a glucose/saline solution throughout the day, such as the modified WHO cholera rehydration solution. If there is marked sodium and water depletion then intravenous 0.9% saline may need to be given for 24–48 hours, while the patient is kept nil by mouth. Correcting electrolyte imbalances such as hypomagnesaemia is important, but correction of sodium and water depletion is an important first step in this process as it treats the secondary hyperaldosteronism caused by short bowel syndrome. Antimotility drugs will reduce stoma output by 20–30% by reducing small intestinal transit time, and so are important in the management of high-output stoma but reducing the high-output stoma drive is more important. Antisecretory medications can be used when there is a net secretory output (more than 3 L of stoma output is present in 24 hours) but absorption of energy, carbohydrate and lipids is not affected by proton pump inhibitors such as omeprazole and they do not reduce the severity of intestinal failure. Octreotide will reduce stomal output by 1–2 L in 24 hours but has no effect on energy, nitrogen or fat absorption, and should be used only in those with a net secretory output. Diet is important in the management of patients with short bowel and jejunostomy but the priority is correction of sodium and water imbalance.

Nightingale J, Woodward J M. Guidelines for management of patients with a short bowel. Gut 2006; 55(IV):iv1–iv12.

9. E Ropinirole

This patient has restless legs syndrome (RLS), a condition that can occur at any age. It tends to be more severe in older age, and affects women more frequently than men (2:1). It can occur as a primary disease, which has a familial tendency, or secondary to other factors (e.g. iron deficiency, renal failure, pregnancy, alcohol misuse). The diagnosis is clinical and requires the fulfilment of four criteria:

1. The presence of a compelling desire to move the lower limbs (often associated with an unpleasant dysaesthesia).
2. Motor restlessness (as movement tends to relieve, or improve, symptoms of dysaesthesia).
3. Worsening of symptoms at rest.
4. Circadian features, with symptoms being worse in the evening or at night.

Sleep disturbance and daytime fatigue are also common. Interestingly, patients diagnosed with RLS are often found to exhibit periodic limb movements of sleep (e.g. involuntary forceful dorsiflexion at the ankle) on polysomnography.

First-line treatments include ropinirole, pergolide and gabapentin. Clonazepam may be helpful as a hypnotic treatment, but is otherwise not thought to be useful. There is insufficient evidence for the use of dihydrocodeine in the treatment of RLS, but opiates may have a role. Perhaps, somewhat surprisingly, RLS may develop secondary to amitriptyline use. Baclofen is not indicated.

Vignatelli L, et al. EFNS guidelines on management of restless legs syndrome and periodic limb movement disorder in sleep. Eur J Neurol 2006;13:1049–1065.

10. C Inhibits mycobacterial RNA polymerase

Rifampicin is bactericidal and binds to the RNA polymerase deep within the RNA/DNA channel, preventing transcription to RNA and subsequent translation to proteins. It is lipophilic and is therefore a good agent in the treatment of tuberculous meningitis, which requires distribution to the central nervous system and penetration through the blood–brain barrier. Isoniazid is bacteriostatic and inhibits synthesis of mycolic acids in mycobacterial cell walls.

11. C Citalopram interaction with linezolid

This man is presenting with a serotonin syndrome caused by the interaction of the new antimicrobial linezolid with the patient's longstanding selective serotonin reuptake inhibitor (SSRI). Linezolid itself is a weak monoamine oxidase inhibitor and combination with all serotonin active agents should be avoided. Serotonin syndrome is characterised by somatic, autonomic and cognitive effects including hypo- and hypertension, tachycardia, sweating, excess bowel movements, hyperthermia, agitation, hallucinations, clonus and myotonia. There is no laboratory investigation to confirm the diagnosis but the clinical syndrome in the context of a relevant drug history is usually conclusive. Management is supportive – blood pressure can be modulated with a short-acting agent, hyperthermia and agitation with benzodiazepines (although on occasion intubation and sedation are required in severe cases), and the most crucial management step is withdrawal of the offending agent. The half-life of SSRIs is marked, but that of linezolid is relatively short and symptoms should resolve in less than 24 hours.

Tramadol itself does have some serotonin activity but would be unlikely to cause a serotonin syndrome; amitriptyline also has serotonin activity and has been documented to cause serotonin syndrome both in overdose situations and in conjunction with linezolid and citalopram, but at a dose of 25 mg is unlikely to be the cause in this case.

Bernard L, et al. Serotonin syndrome after concomitant treatment with linezolid and citalopram. *Clin Infect Dis* 2003; 36(9):1197.

12. D pH

The King's College criteria for transplantation in acute liver failure following paracetamol overdose after 24 hours of treatment are:
Arterial pH <7.25
OR
All of the following:
Creatinine >300 µmol/L, PT (prothrombin time) >100 s and grade 3/4 encephalopathy.

The King's College Criteria have a very good specificity (96%) but a limited sensitivity, meaning that the criteria do not accurately predict all those who will die without liver transplantation.

More recently the addition of a lactate of >3.5 on admission, or >3 after 24 hours of fluid resuscitation has been suggested to improve the sensitivity of the King's College criteria, but there has been discussion as to its utility. With the example given in the question, only pH <7.25 individually predicts the need for liver transplantation. The creatinine and prothrombin time (PT) are used in combination – on their own they are not sufficient for referral. The lactate value is not high enough to fulfil the predictive criteria, and bilirubin is not used as a factor to decide eligibility for liver transplantation.

O'Grady JG, et al. Early indicators of prognosis in fulminant hepatic failure. Gastroenterology 1989; 97:439.

13. D Modafinil

This patient has narcolepsy. Modafinil is the only medication in this list approved for treatment of narcolepsy in the UK. It is a novel wake-promoting agent, the precise mechanism of action of which remains unclear.

Ephedrine is most commonly used as a nasal decongestant. Mephedrone is an illegal stimulant drug, known as 'miaow miaow', which has no medical uses. Clomethiazole is a prescription drug used to treat insomnia. Promethazine is a sedating antihistamine.

Clarke C, et al (eds). Disorders of consciousness and sleep (Chapter 19). In: Neurology: A Queen Square Textbook. Oxford: Blackwell Publishing, 2009.

14. A Efavirenz-induced myositis

This man has a clinical and laboratory picture consistent with myositis and is on two agents likely to be the cause – simvastatin and efavirenz. The temporal drug history, with the statin having been introduced 3 years ago and the Atripla 3 months ago, makes it the efavirenz that is likely to be the cause of the myositis in this case. Simvastatin is metabolised via the cytochrome P450 3A4 (CYP3A4) isozymes and efavirenz is a mixed inducer and inhibitor of this pathway; however, co-administration of efavirenz and simvastatin actually decreases the plasma concentration of the statin and makes myositis from the statin less likely. Efavirenz itself does cause a myopathy and myositis in a small proportion of patients. Management is supportive, with removal of the offending agent, and fluids and renal support where necessary.

Metformin can cause a metabolic acidosis and this can manifest with systemic disturbance as exhibited in this case. The normal blood lactate precludes this as the cause in this case, however. Metformin-inducing myositis is not described. Similarly tenofovir can cause a lactic acidosis but, again, the normal blood lactate discounts this diagnosis in this case.

Klopstock T. Drug-induced myopathies. Curr Opin Neurol 2008; 21(5):590–595.

15. B Atropine

This patient is exhibiting signs of moderate-to-severe organophosphate poisoning, and needs to be treated aggressively. Organophosphates are frequently found in pesticides, and are a fairly common cause of intentional and unintentional poisoning worldwide, especially in poorer rural communities. Organophosphate poisoning can occur through ingestion, absorption through the skin, inhalation or injection. Organophosphates block the activity of acetylcholinesterase, preventing the degradation of acetylcholine within the nervous system. This, in turn, results in parasympathetic overactivity.

Atropine is usually considered the mainstay of treatment and should be started as early as possible. Many guidelines also advocate the combined early use of pralidoxime, a reactivator of phosphorylated acetylcholinesterase, but it should not be used without concomitant atropine because of possible worsening of symptoms through transient oxime-induced acetylcholinesterase inhibition.

Glycopyrrolate is an anticholinergic agent, but is not the first-line treatment. Intravenous diazepam would be appropriate should the patient develop seizures.

Eddleston M, et al. Management of acute organophosphorus pesticide poisoning. Lancet 2008; 371:597–607. Peter JV, et al. Oxime therapy and outcomes in human organophosphate poisoning: an evaluation using meta-analytic techniques. Crit Care Med 2006 34:502–510.

16. A Atenolol

Most phaeochromocytomas secrete adrenaline or noradrenaline or occasionally both. For control of hypertension and symptoms initially α-adrenoreceptor blockade is needed.

If initial β blockade is used, the unopposed α- action could lead to a hypertensive crisis. After adequate α blockade, β blockade determines the drug of choice. Hence a cardioselective β-blocker such as atenolol or metoprolol would be preferred. However, labetalol or carvedilol is not preferred as a single agent because its α:β ratio is poor.

Calcium channel blockers such as amlodipine could be used but are not among the list of options.

Bendrofluazide, furosemide and spironolactone may make the volume depletion in phaeochromocytoma worse.

Pacak K. Pre-operative management of the phaeochromocytoma patient. J Clin Endocrinol Metab 2007; 92(11):4069–4079.

17. A Allopurinol

There are many interactions involving immunosuppressive medications and it is important to be aware of these when prescribing any other drugs. Azathioprine is a thiopurine that is metabolised to 6-mercaptopurine, the active metabolite of the drug. This inhibits purine synthesis. It is used in transplant recipients as well as in the treatment of many autoimmune conditions, including rheumatoid arthritis, pemphigus and inflammatory bowel disease.

Allopurinol is a xanthine oxidase inhibitor often used in the treatment of gout. Xanthine oxidase is involved in the metabolism of 6-mercaptopurine and, by inhibiting it, metabolism is pushed preferentially along the pathway that results in 6-thioguanine nucleotide formation, which is responsible for the majority of the immunosuppressant activity, but also bone marrow suppression.

The interaction between allopurinol and azathioprine has been well documented, and deaths from bone marrow suppression have been recorded. In general, concomitant use should be avoided or, if deemed necessary, the dose of azathioprine should be dramatically reduced (to around 25% of the starting dose) and full blood count should be monitored weekly. Recovery of cell counts is typically seen within 4–8 weeks of withdrawal of either drug.

Amoxicillin is not particularly recognised as a cause of bone marrow suppression.

Clarithromycin should be used with caution, and preferably avoided, with calcineurin inhibitors (tacrolimus or ciclosporin) as it interferes with the CYP3A4 enzyme (one of the cytochrome P450 enzymes) and will result in much higher levels of these drugs, which can cause toxicity (but not bone marrow suppression). If a macrolide is deemed unavoidable then tacrolimus (or ciclosporin) doses should be pre-emptively cut and levels should be monitored regularly.

Prednisolone does not cause bone marrow suppression, and in fact a high white cell count is often seen on patients taking corticosteroids.

Gearry RB, et al. Allopurinol and azathioprine: A two-edged interaction. J Gastroenterol Hepatol 2010; 25(4):653–655.
Venkat RG. Azathioprine and allopurinol: a potentially dangerous combination. J Intern Med 1990; 228(1):69–71.

18. A Intravenous amphotericin B and flucytosine

This is a case of cryptococcal meningitis. The yeast, *Cryptococcus neoformans*, is commonly found in soil and the excreta of pigeons. Transmission is usually by inhalation, with pulmonary colonisation and subsequent haematogenous spread to the meninges. A granulomatous meningoencephalitis results. Immunosuppressed patients (HIV, immunosuppressant medications or reticuloendothelial malignancy) are at greatest risk of infection; further investigation for such causes is necessary in this patient. Typical presenting features of cryptococcal meningitis include headache and fever. Meningism and drowsiness may also be present. Less commonly, focal neurological signs occur. MRI of the brain may be normal, or otherwise it may show hydrocephalus, meningeal enhancement, cryptococcomas or enlarged perivascular spaces (Virchow–Robin spaces), surrounding blood vessels for a short distance as they enter the brain. Lumbar puncture often reveals raised opening pressure, indicative of raised intracranial pressure. Cerebrospinal fluid analysis may reveal a mononuclear pleocytosis, raised protein and reduced glucose. Serum cryptococcal antigen is a useful screening test. The detection of *Cryptococcus* species on an India ink stain of the cerebrospinal fluid is diagnostic of the condition.

First-line treatment is with intravenous amphotericin B and flucytosine. This induction regimen is usually continued for at least 4 weeks in HIV-negative, non-transplant patients who do not have neurological complications and whose cerebrospinal fluid yeast culture is negative after 2 weeks of treatment. In those with neurological complications, the induction regimen is continued for a total of 6 weeks. Consolidation therapy, in the form of oral fluconazole (400 mg once daily), is usually given for 8 weeks. Maintenance therapy, with oral fluconazole 200 mg once daily, may be given for a further 6–12 months. In HIV-positive patients, the induction and consolidation regimen differs and oral fluconazole is normally used as life-long prophylaxis. Other treatment may include serial lumbar punctures to reduce cerebrospinal fluid opening pressure to within normal limits; however, persistent raised intracranial pressure may necessitate a ventriculoperitoneal shunt.

Note: fluconazole is not licensed for intrathecal administration.

Caspofungin belongs to the echinocandin class of antifungal drugs. It is administered intravenously for the treatment of fungal infections, particularly in immunocompromised patients. It is most active against *Candida* and *Aspergillus* species.

Ketoconazole is inappropriate therapy as it does not readily cross the blood–brain barrier.

Oral pyrimethamine, sulfadiazine and folinic acid are used in the treatment of toxoplasmosis.

Perfect JR, et al. Clinical Practice Guidelines for the Management of Cryptococcal Disease: 2010 Update from the Infectious Diseases Society of America. Clin Infect Dis 2010; 50:291–322.

19. D Observation and follow-up

This patient is asymptomatic with chronic lymphocytic leukaemia (CLL). Her peripheral blood film clearly demonstrates numerous 'smudge cells' (fragile lymphocytes that have ruptured during slide preparation), which are typical of CLL. The patient has stage I disease according to the Rai staging system (see **Table 12.1**) and, as such, does not warrant medical intervention at present. Unfortunately, the condition is rarely cured with medical treatment; therefore, treatment tends to be instituted to achieve symptom control rather than normalisation of the blood profile. Many patients are managed conservatively throughout the course of their disease. However, the development of organomegaly, bone marrow suppression or haemolytic anaemia should prompt consideration of therapy.

Table 12.1 Rai staging system

Stage	Defining features	Median survival time from diagnosis
0	Lymphocytosis (>15 x 10^9/L)	150 months
I	Stage 0 and lymphadenopathy	101 months
II	Stage 0 and organomegaly ± lymphadenopathy	71 months
III	Stage 0 and anaemia (Hb <11 g/dL) ± organomegaly ± lymphadenopathy	19 months
IV	Stage 0 and thrombocytopenia (platelets <100 x 10^9/L) ± organomegaly ± lymphadenopathy	19 months

Note that the Binet system of staging is also often used for staging, either alone or in conjunction with the Rai system.

Rai KR, et al. Clinical staging of chronic lymphocytic leukemia. Blood 1975; 46(2):219.
Hoffbrand V, Moss P, Pettit J. Chronic lymphoid leukaemias (Chapter 15). In: Essential Haematology, 5th edn. Oxford: Blackwell Publishing, 2006.

20. E Varenicline

Varenicline avidly binds to the $\alpha_4\beta_2$ neuronal nicotinic acetylcholine receptor. Its partial agonist action helps to reduce symptoms of nicotine withdrawal and craving, and reduces the satisfaction of smoking. Varenicline is prescribed as a 12-week course and patients are twice as likely to quit smoking than using will-power or nicotine replacement therapy. Side effects of the treatment include gastrointestinal disturbance and it should be used with caution in patients with a history of psychiatric illness including depression. Patients should be counselled to stop treatment and seek advice if they notice a change in mood.

Bupropion has been used as an antidepressant and may be used to aid smoking cessation, but its mode of action is not clear and may involve an effect on noradrenaline and dopamine neurotransmission. Bupropion is contraindicated in patients with a history of seizures, central nervous system tumours, severe hepatic cirrhosis, and acute alcohol and benzodiazepine withdrawal. It should be used with caution in patients taking other drugs that may lower seizure threshold or with a history of alcohol abuse, head injury or diabetes.

Acamprosate and disulfiram may be helpful in maintaining abstinence in alcohol-dependent patients. Citalopram is a selective serotonin reuptake inhibitor and may be used for the treatment of depressive illness and panic disorder.

National Institute for Health and Clinical Excellence. NICE public health guidance. Smoking cessation services in primary care, pharmacies, local authorities and workplaces, particularly for manual working groups, pregnant women and hard to reach communities. London: NICE, 2010.

21. D Pyrazinamide-induced arthralgia

Adverse reactions to tuberculosis (TB) treatment are common and occur in around 10% of patients, often requiring a change in medication. Reactions are more common in patients receiving non-standard treatment and in HIV-positive individuals. TB therapy should be managed by physicians with a specialist interest in the disease.

Side effects of pyrazinamide include arthralgia, affecting about 1 in 100 patients. Other side effects of standard TB treatment (rifampicin, isoniazid, pyrazinamide and ethambutol) include: drug-induced hepatitis (most frequently caused by pyrazinamide); rash and pruritus; gastrointestinal disturbance; dysuria; interstitial nephritis; malaise; and rarely fever.

Ethambutol rarely causes optic toxicity. Baseline visual acuity using a Snellen chart should be documented, and patients and care-givers should be informed to stop the medication and seek immediate medical attention if they develop new visual symptoms. Mild arthralgia has been very rarely reported with the use of ethambutol.

Isoniazid side effects include rash, abnormal liver function tests, hepatitis, sideroblastic anaemia, peripheral neuropathy, mild central nervous system (CNS) effects and drug interactions. Peripheral neuropathy and CNS effects are due to pyridoxine (vitamin B_6) depletion, but are uncommon at doses of 5 mg/kg. Patients with conditions in which neuropathy is common (e.g. diabetes, uraemia, alcoholism, malnutrition, HIV infection), as well as pregnant women, should be given pyridoxine (vitamin B_6) supplementation (10–50 mg/day) with isoniazid. Isoniazid-induced systemic lupus erythematosus has been rarely reported; however, the antinuclear antibody is negative so this diagnosis is not supported.

Paradoxical reactions are seen after commencing antituberculous therapy. The reaction may consist of increased size of lymphadenopathy or increased volume of pleural effusion/ascites. The diagnosis including HIV status, culture results, drug sensitivities and compliance should be checked and treatment should be continued. Oral corticosteroids may be given to support selected patients.

The rheumatoid factor is mildly positive, but this may be raised because of the underlying inflammatory process. Anticyclic citrullinated protein (anti-CCP) antibodies are negative and therefore the diagnosis of rheumatoid arthritis in this setting is unlikely.

National Institute for Health and Clinical Excellence. NICE Guideline No. 117: Tuberculosis. Clinical diagnosis and management of tuberculosis, and measures for its prevention and control. London: NICE, 2011.

22. C Stop warfarin and prescribe 1 mg oral vitamin K

The British Society for Haematology guidelines recommend the cessation of warfarin and the prescription of 1–5 mg oral vitamin K in patients with an international normalised ratio (INR) >8.0 and no evidence of bleeding. The society recommends omitting one or two doses of warfarin in patients whose INR is 5.0–8.0, and in whom there is no evidence of bleeding. Fresh frozen plasma or factor IX complex is recommended in patients with elevated INR, in whom there is evidence of active bleeding.

Keeling, D et al. British Society for Haematology guidelines on oral anticoagulation with warfarin, 4th edition. Br J Haematol 2011; 154 (3):311–324.

23. D Skin rash

Lamotrigine is associated with the development of potentially life-threatening rashes. The patient should seek urgent medical attention if any rash appears. Typically, the rash will occur within the first 8 weeks of commencing the medication. In premarketing clinical trials for use of lamotrigine in epilepsy, serious rash with hospitalisation and discontinuation of lamotrigine occurred in 0.3% of adult patients. Rashes that have been reported include those associated with Stevens–Johnson syndrome, toxic epidermal necrolysis, angio-oedema and drug reaction with eosinophilia and systemic symptoms (DRESS). Other serious side effects include aseptic meningitis, blood dyscrasias and suicidal ideation.

Kanner, AM. Lamotrigine-induced rash: can we stop worrying? Epilepsy Curr 2005; 5(5):190–191.

24. D Use of dose-determining weight to dose gentamicin

This woman has streptococcal bacterial endocarditis. The UK guidelines for this outline a 6-week course of penicillin (although ceftriaxone can be similarly used particularly where outpatient antimicrobial therapy might be appropriate) with synergistic gentamicin for the first 2 weeks. The gentamicin should be dosed at 1 mg/kg three times daily. In those of a higher than ideal body weight the dose-determining weight should be used to arrive at the appropriate dose. Use of actual body weight will lead to overdosing of the gentamicin and high peak and trough levels, with the potential for renal toxicity. Use of ideal body weight will result in underdosing and a peak level that is below the target range, as in this case. This increases the likelihood of treatment failure and in case of bacterial endocarditis this can have serious sequelae. The dose-determining weight is used in the context of obesity to arrive at a dose likely to achieve the necessary therapeutic target range.

The dose-determining weight is calculated with:
IBW + 0.3 × [ABW – IBW]

[Where IBW = ideal body weight and ABW = actual body weight.]

Obesity leads to altered pharmacokinetics and pharmacodynamics for numerous reasons. The volume of distribution is obvious altered for lipid-soluble drugs, but in obesity glomerular filtration rate is increased (thus decreasing the half-life of many drugs) and hepatic metabolic pathways are also altered, again altering the half-life.

Wurtz R, et al. Antimicrobial dosing in obese patients. Clin Infect Dis 1997; 25(1):112–118.

25. E Stop pegylated interferon and ribavirin treatment

Current national and international guidelines for the treatment of chronic hepatitis C virus (HCV) recommend combination therapy with pegylated interferon and ribavirin. For patients with genotype 1, 4, 5 and 6 chronic hepatitis C virus, 12 weeks of therapy is initially recommended. If a 2 log drop in HCV RNA is NOT achieved by 12 weeks (termed an early viral response) there is a less than 3% chance of achieving a sustained viral response (defined as an undetectable HCV RNA 6 months after completion of treatment, and regarded as a cure), and therefore therapy should be stopped at this point. If there is a 2 log drop in HCV RNA at 12 weeks, combination therapy should be continued for 48 weeks to give the best chance of sustained viral response. If the patient is cirrhotic then continued therapy is less likely to be successful, but this is not a contraindication to treatment. Twenty-four weeks of pegylated interferon and ribavirin combination therapy is recommended for genotype 2 and 3 chronic HCV. Current practice is now to adopt response-guided therapy such that, if HCV RNA levels are undetectable after 4 weeks (a rapid viral response), then the duration of therapy can be shortened to 24 weeks' treatment instead of 48 weeks.

Ghany M, et al. Diagnosis, management and treatment of hepatitis C: an update. Hepatology 2009; 49(4):1335–1374.

26. E Quinine toxicity

Quinine is well documented to cause QT prolongation even at standard doses. Long QT intervals predispose the patient to an R-on-T phenomenon, which can initiate torsades de pointes. Sometimes pathological T-U waves may be seen in the ECG before the initiation of torsades. Torsades itself can initiate a syncopal episodes and can degenerate to ventricular tachycardia or ventricular fibrillation.

When quinine is given intravenously both UK and international guidelines suggest cardiac monitoring for precisely this reason. In this case the previously documented history of heart disease, itself a risk factor for further dysrhythmias, should have prompted a high index of clinical suspicion. In cases of malaria where there is a high risk of quinine-induced dysrhythmia alternative agents such as artesunate are available.

Digoxin produces a relative shortening of the QT interval, and although being relatively proarrhythmogenic in terms of atrial fibrillation it is unlikely to have been contributory to the development of torsades de pointes in this case. Hypomagnesaemia can contribute to dysrhythmias and specifically to torsades de pointes, and magnesium replacement, even in those found to be normomagnesaemic, can assist in terminating torsades. In this case the stable dose of furosemide is unlikely to have precipitously dropped the plasma magnesium levels although they should of course be checked. Both malaria and quinine can cause a hypoglycaemia and therefore when quinine is given intravenously capillary blood glucose should be regularly monitored. However, whilst hypoglycaemia can become a medical emergency it is unlikely to have contributed to the torsades de pointes in this case.

World Health Organization. Guidelines for the treatment of malaria, 2nd edn. Geneva: WHO, 2010.

27. A All-*trans*-retinoic acid

Acute promyelocytic leukaemia (AML-M3) is usually due to a t(15:17) translocation resulting in abnormal fusion of the promyelocytic (*PML*) gene on chromosome 15 with the retinoic acid receptor α gene, *RARα*, on chromosome 17. The abnormal PML–RARα fusion protein acts as a transcriptional repressor, via its interaction with the retinoid X receptor (RXR), and prevents differentiation of promyelocytes. In contrast, RARα normally acts as an activator through its interaction with RXR. Treatment with high-dose all-*trans*-retinoic acid (ATRA) enables the abnormal promyelocytes, which are in a state of arrested development, to proceed with their normal differentiation into mature myeloid cells through its competitive agonism of RXR. Treatment with high-dose ATRA alone, however, will not eradicate the abnormal clone – hence, the need for standard chemotherapy. However, this may be complicated by ATRA syndrome, which is characterised by fever, pulmonary infiltrates, hypoxia and neutrophilia; this is usually treated with intravenous dexamethasone in the first instance.

It is important to note that patients with AML–M3 are at risk of disseminated intravascular coagulation and potentially fatal haemorrhage. They may, therefore, require regular transfusions with platelets and fresh frozen plasma if there is any suggestion of abnormal coagulation.

Rituximab and thalidomide are not indicated in the treatment of AML–M3.

Hoffbrand V, Moss P, Pettit J. Management of haematological malignancy (Chapter 11). In: Essential Haematology, 5th edn. Oxford: Blackwell Publishing, 2006.

28. D High-flow oxygen therapy

Carbon monoxide poisoning presents with insidious clinical symptoms and can be difficult to diagnose as it mimic many other illnesses. The most common symptom is headache, but it may also present with dyspnoea on exertion, fatigability and irritability, difficulty concentrating, dizziness, syncope, confusion, respiratory failure, seizures, coma or death. It should always be borne in mind as a differential diagnosis in patients who present with any of these symptoms. Important details in the history are whether other family members or pets have been affected, as pets will often be affected earlier and more severely because of their small size. Enquiries should also be made as to whether the patient feels better at work, or home, and as to when their boiler or heating system was last serviced. Carbon monoxide poisoning can be rapidly fatal as carbon monoxide has an affinity for haemoglobin of 250–300 times that of oxygen. The clinical sequelae of CO poisoning all result from the subsequent tissue hypoxia. The management of CO poisoning is initially always high-flow oxygen. This reduces the half-life of CO from 240 minutes to 40–80 minutes. Hyperbaric oxygen is recommended in cases of severe CO poisoning, but there is debate as to what constitutes a severe case, and there is limited evidence to guide the use of hyperbaric oxygen. The recommendation is that hyperbaric oxygen should be given when there is a serum carboxyhaemoglobin concentration of over 40%.

Ilano AL, Raffin TA. Management of carbon monoxide poisoning. Chest 1990; 97:165–169.

29. D Scombrotoxin

Of the available answers scombrotoxin, ciguatera toxin and tetrodotoxin are most relevant to the ingestion of contaminated fish. Tetrodotoxin can be discounted since poisoning is usually associated with ingestion of the improperly prepared Japanese delicacy fugu (flesh of the Puffer fish); furthermore, it is a potent neurotoxin and its ingestion is often fatal. Scombrotoxin and ciguatera toxin poisoning can both be diagnosed clinically.

Scombrotoxin presents, as described above, with a self-limiting anaphylactoid response. Headache, flushing, tachycardia, palpitations, abdominal cramps and diarrhoea are common, as is blanching erythema, but weals are not typical. Wheezing can occur, but is said to occur more frequently in the context of existing asthma and histamine sensitivity. Management is supportive with intravenous fluids and antihistamines such as chlorpheniramine. Supplementary oxygen and bronchodilators may be necessary depending on respiratory involvement. Symptoms come on within 10 minutes to 2 hours of eating decaying fish, and usually resolve within 4–6 hours. The toxin forms when histidine is processed to histamine by bacterial decarboxylation; this occurs in the context of decay and is, obviously, associated with inappropriate storage of fish.

Ciguatera is the most common pathogenic marine toxin worldwide and is found principally in contaminated tropical reef fish. The affected individual typically presents within hours of ingestion of contaminated fish. There may be involvement of the gastrointestinal, neurological and cardiovascular systems. Abdominal pain, nausea, vomiting and diarrhoea are typical early features and may last for up to 2 days. Neurological involvement is variable, ranging from circumoral paraesthesia to reversal of temperature sensation, and from generalised weakness to respiratory paralysis and, rarely, coma. Cardiovascular involvement may include symptomatic bradycardia and hypotension. Management is supportive, and the prognosis is on the whole very good.

Botulism is, of course, principally associated with wound infection and ingestion of contaminated foodstuffs (typically canned foods). There are eight types of botulinum exotoxin which are produced by different strains of the anaerobe *Clostridium botulinum*. Types A and B are most common. Botulinum toxin is a neurotoxin that binds to the presynaptic membrane to prevent the release of acetylcholine at the neuromuscular junction. Ingestion of the heat-stable toxin or wound colonisation with *Clostridium botulinum* can be fatal.

Pectenotoxins are a group of toxins that have been implicated in diarrhoeal shellfish poisoning.

McLauchlin J, et al. Scombrotoxic fish poisoning. J Public Health 2006; 28:61–62.

30. E Spironolactone

This woman had New York Heart Association (NYHA) class III symptoms form heart failure.

The drugs which are known to reduce mortality in heart failure are angiotensin-converting enzyme (ACE inhibitors), beta-blockers and spironolactone. Angiotensin receptor blockers (ARBs) also confer a mortality advantage – but are not given as an option in this question.

Calcium channel blockers are helpful in symptom management as is furosemide, but they do not affect mortality. Similarly digoxin has symptomatic benefit especially in patients with concomitant atrial fibrillation, but no mortality benefits.

Isosorbide mononitrate and other vasodilators are useful in heart failure, but as an alternative if ACE inhibitors/ARBs or aldosterone antagonists are not tolerated. This is especially true in those of African origin.

Amiodarone has not been found to be beneficial in carotid–cavernous fistula (CCF); rather implantable cardioverter defibrillators are preferred to prevent sudden death in CCF. This person would, for example, qualify for implantable cardiac defibrillator implantation.

Spironolactone confers a mortality advantage in class 3/4 CCF and hence would be the next drug of choice in patients with preserved renal function and potassium <5 mmol/L.

Jessup WT, et al. Focused update: ACCF/AHA guidelines for the diagnosis and management of heart failure in adults: A report of the American College of Cardiology Foundation/American Heart Association Task Force on Practice Guidelines. J Am Coll Cardiol 2009; 53:1343–1382.

31. A Continue the NAC infusion at the same rate

Paracetamol overdose is a common cause of intentional and unintentional overdose, and causes a dose-dependent liver toxicity. A toxic metabolite of paracetamol, *N*-acetyl-*p*-benzoquinoneimine (NAPQI) is the cause of its hepatotoxicity. NAPQI is detoxified by interaction with glutathione, and so if sufficient glutathione is present the liver is protected. *N*-Acetylcysteine (NAC) prevents liver damage principally by restoring hepatic glutathione. Ten to twenty per cent of patients can experience adverse effects when given NAC which can vary from flushing to anaphylaxis.

Flushing itself is not an indication for stopping or slowing down the infusion. The development of angio-oedema or urticaria necessitates stopping the infusion and giving chlorpheniramine. Once the symptoms have abated then the NAC infusion can continue. Those patients who also experience hypotension or respiratory symptoms should be switched to oral NAC. There is no convincing evidence that slowing the rate of the infusion reduces the risk of developing anaphylactoid reactions. Methionine is an alternative to NAC but is used only if NAC is unavailable or if NAC cannot be tolerated.

Heard KJ. Acetylcysteine for acetaminophen poisoning. N Engl J Med 2008; 359:285–292.
Bailey B, McGuigan MA. Management of anaphylactoid reactions to intravenous N-acetylcysteine. Ann Emerg Med 1998; 31(6):710.

32. A Ceftriaxone

This patient has meningococcal meningitis (causative organism: *Neisseria meningitidis*). The European Federation of Neurological Societies currently lists benzylpenicillin, ceftriaxone and cefotaxime as first-line intravenous antibiotics. Alternatives include meropenem, chloramphenicol or moxifloxacin. Therefore, of the options given, the third-generation cephalosporin, ceftriaxone, would be most appropriate.

High-dose dexamethasone before or at initiation of antibiotic treatment for pneumococcal or *Haemophilus influenzae* type b meningitis is associated with a better prognosis; however, to date there is no evidence to suggest that high-dose dexamethasone improves outcome when given as an adjunct for the treatment of meningococcal meningitis. Regardless, some clinicians recommend the use of steroids in the treatment of all cases of community-acquired bacterial meningitis in which there is no evidence of septic shock (irrespective of the causative bacteria). It should be borne in mind, however, that it is thought that high-dose steroids may reduce central nervous system penetration of some antibiotics, such as vancomycin.

Chaudhuri A, et al. EFNS guideline on the management of community-acquired bacterial meningitis: report of an EFNS Task Force on acute bacterial meningitis in older children and adults. Eur J Neurol 2008; 15: 649–659.
Fitch MT, et al. Drug insight: steroids in CNS infectious diseases – new indications for an old therapy. Nat Clin Pract Neurol 2008; 4:97–104.

33. E Quinolone tendinopathy

This patient presents with an Achilles tendonitis and of the medications she has recently taken the ciprofloxacin is the most likely aetiological agent. Quinolone tendonitis is a well-described potential adverse event from quinolone use and is related to dose and to course length, and can be quite removed from when the course was taken: there are documented cases of it occurring up to 6 months after the drug was taken. The Achilles tendon is commonly involved and bilateral tendinitis is common, unlike with other causes. The exact mechanism of action is unclear but matrix-degrading, toxic and ischaemic processes have all been proposed. Treatment is with rest, splinting where necessary and, in sites other than the Achilles tendon, peritendinous steroid injection is advocated. This should be avoided in the Achilles itself as tendon rupture has been documented.

Penicillin and cephalosporins are a frequent cause of rash, with up to 4% of the population developing this side effect, but only 0.04% exhibiting true anaphylaxis. Myopathy is rare and tendonitis has not been described. Nitrofurantoin can cause a peripheral neuropathy if there is prolonged use in the context of renal impairment, but again myopathy and tendonitis have only rarely been described. The case is not consistent with pretibial myxoedema, although the dose of levothyroxine may be too low and thyroid function tests should be requested on this patient if not recently undertaken.

van der Linden PD, et al. Increased risk of Achilles tendon rupture with quinolone antibacterial use, especially in elderly patients taking oral corticosteroids. Arch Intern Med 2003; 163(15):1801–1807.

34. C Intravenous procyclidine

Acute dystonic reactions, such as the one described in the stem, are well-recognised complications of antipsychotic medications. After stopping the offending drug, the next most appropriate step is to promptly start treatment with a rapidly acting anticholinergic drug such as procyclidine or benztropine. These may be administered intravenously or intramuscularly. It is thought that the dopaminergic blockade caused by antipsychotic drugs (and, indeed, other agents such as metoclopramide) results in relative cholinergic overactivity in the basal ganglia, which may precipitate acute dystonic reactions. The rationale of treatment with an anticholinergic is that it should restore the normal balance of dopaminergic and cholinergic activity, and thus alleviate the acute dystonia.

Dantrolene sodium appears to act by disrupting the excitation–contraction coupling within skeletal muscle. It is thought that this is achieved through interference with the release of calcium from the sarcoplasmic reticulum of skeletal muscle cells. It may be used in the treatment of chronic spasticity resulting from upper motor neuron lesions. Additionally, it constitutes one of the pillars of management of malignant hyperthermia.

Electroconvulsive therapy has been approved by the National Institute for Health and Clinical Excellence for use in the treatment of severe depression, severe/prolonged mania, catatonia and some cases of schizophrenia. It is not used in the treatment of neuroleptic malignant syndrome itself.

Oral tizanidine is an α_2-adrenergic agonist that acts centrally to achieve muscle relaxation. It is commonly used for the treatment of spasticity resulting from multiple sclerosis or spinal cord injury.

Botox (OnabotulinumtoxinA, a form of botulinum toxin) is an injectable neurotoxin which acts at the neuromuscular junction by inhibiting the presynaptic release of acetylcholine. This, in turn, prevents muscular contraction. It has been approved in the UK for use in the treatment of a wide range of conditions including blepharospasm, hemifacial spasm, idiopathic cervical dystonia and focal limb spasticity. However, Botox would not be appropriate in this case, which almost certainly has a reversible cause.

Taylor D, Paton C, Kapur S. The Maudsley Prescribing Guidelines: 10th edn. The South London and Maudsley NHS Foundation Trust, Oxleas NHS Foundation Trust. London: Informa Healthcare, 2009.

35. C Lithium

The patient has biochemical and clinical evidence of hyperparathyroidism, and biochemical evidence of hypothyroidism. The incidence of both of these disorders is increased in patients who take lithium. Hypothyroidism and hyperparathyroidism are not associated with any of the other medications listed. Other side effects of lithium are a reduction in renal tubular function, and there are anecdotal reports that it may cause rashes or exacerbations of psoriasis.

McKnight RF, et al. Lithium toxicity profile: a systematic review and meta-analysis. Lancet 2012; 379:721–728.

36. A Amoxicillin

The patient in this vignette has community-acquired pneumonia and, given the rusty sputum and clinical and radiographic findings in keeping with lobar consolidation, this is most likely to be caused by *Streptococcus pneumoniae*. *Streptococcus pneumoniae* in the UK rarely exhibits penicillin resistance and hence β-lactam antimicrobials are the preferred choice. Although trusts have differing antimicrobial policies based upon local resistance patterns and other issues, the British Thoracic Society (BTS) has published guidelines specifically on community-acquired pneumonia and these are widely adhered to (see further reading). This patient has a CURB65 score of 0 and the BTS guidelines suggest amoxicillin 500 mg po three times daily for treatment of this. The CURB65 score is a prognostication tool utilised predominantly to delineate whether admission is indicated in cases of community-acquired pneumonia. The criteria are confusion, urea >7 mmol, respiratory rate >30 breaths per minute, systolic blood pressure <90 mmHg or diastolic <60 mmHg and age >65 years. A score of 2 or more warrants admission and those with a score of 1 should be considered for admission.

In penicillin-allergic patients doxycycline or clarithromycin is an appropriate alternative although empirical use of these must be with care as in some areas of the UK macrolide resistance approaches 15%. In this patient, there is additional need to avoid macrolides and quinolones as the anticipated international normalised ratio will be markedly deranged through interaction with the warfarin.

Lim WS, et al. BTS guidelines for the management of community acquired pneumonia in adults: update 2009. Thorax 2009; 64 (3):iii1–55.

37. B Calcium gluconate

This patient has presented with an overdose of medications which has resulted in him being bradycardic and hypotensive. Although it would seem that he has taken an overdose of amlodipine, it cannot be excluded that he has also taken an overdose of digoxin.

Amlodipine is a calcium channel blocker (CCB). Multiple cases of CCB overdose, many of which have been lethal, have been reported. The blockade of L-type calcium channels results in the clinical features of toxicity, including bradycardia, conduction delay, hypoinsulinaemia, hyperglycaemia, metabolic acidosis, peripheral vasodilatation and shock. Cardiac arrest may ensue.

Gastric lavage followed by activated charcoal may be useful in cases where there is early presentation post-overdose, and in particular with extended-release tablets.

Symptomatic bradycardia should be treated with atropine. Sympathomimetic agents may further be required to support heart rate and blood pressure.

Glucagon has an inotropic effect, probably related to an increase of adenosine cyclic monophosphate (cAMP) in the myocardium. It increases the heart rate, blood pressure and stroke volume. It should be given as a bolus followed by an infusion.

High-dose insulin is thought to enhance cardiac carbohydrate metabolism and has direct inotropic effects. It has been increasingly documented as being useful in CCB overdose and is thought to be possibly more efficacious than calcium, gluconate or catecholamines.

In an isolated CCB overdose calcium (the chloride salt is preferred to gluconate) is indicated for hypotension and conduction defects. It is, however, often ineffective and overtreatment can result in arrhythmias, central nervous system depression and death. In the context of CCB and digoxin overdose, as could well be the case here, calcium should be avoided as it may induce fatal cardiac arrhythmias.

Engebresten KM, et al. High-dose insulin therapy in beta-blocker and calcium channel-blocker poisoning. Clin Toxicol 2011; 49(4):277–283.

38. D Oral oseltamivir

Pregnant women are considered to be in a high-risk group during flu outbreaks and should be advised to seek early advice regarding treatment to reduce the chance of complications. Pregnant patients presenting with flu-like symptoms during a flu outbreak should be offered either oseltamivir or zanamivir (neuraminidase inhibitors active against influenza A and B viruses). This treatment should be started as soon as possible within the first 48 hours of symptoms. Oseltamivir is an oral preparation. Zanamivir is delivered by an inhaler (not intravenous).

There is no clear medical evidence that intravenous pooled human immunoglobulins improve outcome in H1N1 in pregnant women and it should not be given routinely. There is good evidence that a neuraminidase inhibitor should be offered to these patients early in the course of the illness and patients should be encouraged to present early. These patients are high risk and symptomatic treatment alone would not be the best advice in the scenario described. Amoxicillin would not be the agent of choice, unless there was evidence to suggest a superadded bacterial infection.

National Institute for Health and Clinical Excellence. NICE guidance: TA168. Amantadine, oseltamivir and zanamivir for the treatment of influenza. London: NICE, 2009.

39. B Ethanol

This patient has a metabolic acidosis with high anion gap and is most likely suffering from methanol poisoning. He has probably been consuming impure homemade vodka, and is exhibiting symptoms of toxicity. Some of these symptoms may mimic a 'hangover' from ethanol intoxication, but the abdominal pain and confusion are indicative of methanol toxicity. The sluggish pupillary responses, wide anion gap with metabolic acidosis, tachypnoea, tachycardia and hypotension add further weight to the clinical diagnosis. Blurred vision is also often associated with methanol toxicity.

Bicarbonate should be given to reverse the acidosis and reduce the amount of active formic acid. Methanol is first metabolised to formaldehyde by alcohol dehydrogenase, and this is subsequently metabolised by formaldehyde dehydrogenase to the toxic metabolite formic acid. Ethanol acts as a preferential substrate for alcohol dehydrogenase, therefore preventing the metabolism of methanol. Such treatment, thus, prevents the formation of toxic methanol metabolites and is continued until the unmetabolised methanol has been eliminated from the system.

There is no shortage of evidence to support the use of fomepizole, an alcohol dehydrogenase inhibitor, in the treatment of methanol poisoning.

Activated charcoal is not indicated as it is relatively ineffective against methanol. Gastric lavage would not be beneficial; ingestion was some hours earlier, and methanol is rapidly absorbed. Phenytoin would not be indicated unless the patient were to develop seizures.

Haemodialysis may be necessary in some cases if there is evidence of end-organ damage or if there are severe acid–base abnormalities not responding to medication.

Barceloux DG, et al. American Academy of Clinical Toxicology Practice Guidelines on the Treatment of Methanol Poisoning. Clin Tox 2002; 40(4):415–446.
Brent J, et al. Fomepizole for the treatment of methanol poisoning. N Engl J Med 2001; 344:424–429.

40. D Salicylate overdose

Salicylate overdose can present with vomiting, dehydration, vertigo, tinnitus, deafness, sweating and hyperventilation. It classically causes a mixed respiratory alkalosis and metabolic acidosis picture, as in this case. It should be managed with activated charcoal if the patient presents within 1 hour of ingestion of more than 250 mg/kg. Elimination of salicylate can be improved by urinary alkalinisation with 1.26% sodium bicarbonate. Haemodialysis is used in severe cases. Tricyclic antidepressant, ethylene glycol and methanol overdose all give a metabolic acidosis. Organophosphate poisoning can cause respiratory distress and sweating but it does not commonly cause a respiratory alkalosis.

Dargan PI, Wallace CI, Jones AL. An evidence based flowchart to guide the management of acute salicylate (aspirin) overdose. Emerg Med J 2002; 19:206–209.

41. D Imatinib

The current first-line agent in the treatment of chronic myeloid leukaemia is imatinib (Glivec), a specific inhibitor of bcr-abl kinase activity. This has largely supplanted the use of hydroxyurea, busulfan and pegylated interferon-α. It is a very effective medication, typically inducing a complete haematological remission (i.e. normalisation of the full blood count) within days to weeks, and is normally administered with allopurinol to protect against the development of hyperuricaemia.

Karyotypic and fluorescent *in situ* hybridisation (FISH) analyses are also used to measure cytogenetic response through detection of the Philadelphia chromosome in bone marrow. Reverse-transcriptase polymerase chain reaction (rtPCR) is used to measure the molecular response to treatment through the detection and quantification of the ratio of *bcr-abl* mRNA transcripts to normal *abl* mRNA transcripts in bone marrow or blood. Such blood and bone marrow tests are usually performed at 3- and 6-monthly intervals, respectively, in the first year of treatment.

Allogeneic stem cell transplantation is the only known cure for chronic myeloid leukaemia, but it is complicated by significant levels of morbidity and mortality, and is therefore primarily used for patients unresponsive to imatinib who are under the age of 65 years (and for whom a suitable sibling, or matched unrelated, donor is available).

Daunorubicin combined with cytosine arabinoside is a fairly standard chemotherapeutic regimen used in the treatment of acute myeloid leukaemia.

Hoffbrand V, Moss P, Pettit J. Chronic myeloid leukaemia (Chapter 13). In: Essential Haematology, 5th edn. Oxford: Blackwell Publishing, 2006.

42. C Hyoscine butylbromide (Buscopan)

This diagnosis is irritable bowel syndrome (IBS). This should be suspected in people who present with abdominal pain that is associated with altered bowel frequency or stool form, or relieved by defecation, and accompanied by at least two of the following symptoms: altered stool passage; abdominal bloating, distension, tension or hardness; symptoms made worse by eating; or passage of mucus. First-line management of IBS includes diet and lifestyle management and use of antispasmodics. Tricyclic antidepressants are second-line management if these measures do not work after 6 months. Acupuncture and mesalazine are not recommended in IBS, and cognitive–behavioural therapy is third-line management.

National Institute for Health and Clinical Excellence. NICE guidelines. Irritable bowel syndrome in adults: Diagnosis and management of irritable bowel syndrome in primary care. London: NICE, 2008.

43. E Sodium bicarbonate

This patient is symptomatic from an overdose of the tricyclic antidepressant amitriptyline. Furthermore, she is acidotic with widened QRS complexes on ECG. She, therefore, needs alkalinisation with intravenous sodium bicarbonate in the first instance. Hyperventilation is not appropriate therapy. Gastric lavage is appropriate only if performed within 1 hour of a life-threatening overdose. Intravenous diazepam would not be appropriate unless the patient were to develop seizures. Intravenous glucagon may have a role in treatment of myocardial depression and hypotension, but first the acidosis and ECG changes should be addressed.

Body R, et al. Guidelines in Emergency Medicine Network (GEMNet): guideline for the management of tricyclic antidepressant overdose. Emerg Med J 2011; 28:347–368.

Index